Nanomedicine, Nanotheranostics and Nanobiotechnology

Nanosized particles explored for therapeutics and diagnosis-related research areas need the latest updated information for budding researchers as well as academicians. Nanomedicine, nanotheranostics, and nanobiotechnology have been contemporary technological tools for diverse biomedical, pharmaceutical, and diagnostic solutions. The present book is divided into two sections.

The first section is dedicated to exclusive book chapters related to nanomedicine such as its history, regulatory aspects, scale-up, and regulatory toxicology. Additionally, this section includes chapters focusing on the application domain of nanomedicine for targeted cancer therapy, rheumatoid arthritis management, psoriasis treatment, ocular delivery, topical applications, oral bioavailability enhancement, and pulmonary delivery.

The second section is composed of chapters in the area of nanotheranostics and applications of nanobiotechnology. In brief, the latest topics such as gold nanoparticles in diagnostics and therapy, nanoparticles for siRNA delivery, carbon nanotubes for gene delivery, nanoparticles for vaccine delivery, nanobiotechnology in cell-based nanomedicines, nanotechnology in regenerative medicine, and nanocarriers in delivery of proteins and peptides are compiled.

KEY FEATURES

- A total of 26 emerging topics are covered in the book on cutting-edge research areas at the multi-disciplinary level.
- The chapters focus on fundamentals and applications, making the book attractive for beginners as well as experts.
- The chapters are written by well-known experts of the field in a simple scientific style with figures, schemes, and illustrations.

Dr. Rishi Paliwal and **Dr. Shivani Rai Paliwal**, editors of the book, are both domain experts who have been continuously exploring nanotechnological principles for diverse biomedical and pharmaceutical applications over the last two decades. As they are established nanomedicine scientists, the book has been edited using a profound knowledge base.

Nanomedicine, Nanotheranostics and Nanobiotechnology

Fundamentals and Applications

Edited by
Rishi Paliwal and Shivani Rai Paliwal

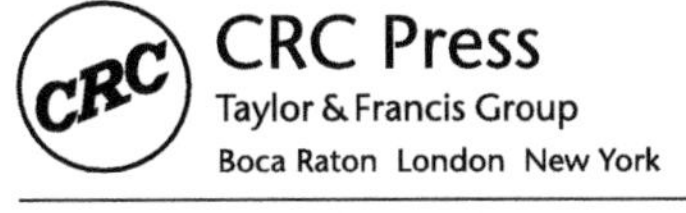

CRC Press
Taylor & Francis Group
Boca Raton London New York

CRC Press is an imprint of the
Taylor & Francis Group, an **informa** business

Designed cover image: © Shutterstock 2237785711

First edition published 2025
by CRC Press
2385 NW Executive Center Drive, Suite 320, Boca Raton FL 33431

and by CRC Press
4 Park Square, Milton Park, Abingdon, Oxon, OX14 4RN

CRC Press is an imprint of Taylor & Francis Group, LLC

ISBN: 978-0-367-65549-5 (hbk)
ISBN: 978-0-367-65550-1 (pbk)
ISBN: 978-1-003-13005-5 (ebk)

DOI: 10.1201/9781003130055

Typeset in Times LT Std
by Apex CoVantage, LLC

Contents

Chapter 4   Ocular Nanomedicine: Fundamentals and Recent Advances......................36

Abhishek K. Sah, Ishwari Choudhary, Nagendra Bhuwane, Shweta Ramkar,
Narayan Hemnani, and Preeti K. Suresh

Chapter 5   Skin as Attractive Target for Transdermal Nanomedicine..........................53

Neha Raina, Rakesh Pahwa, Bigul Yogeshver Bhardwaj, and Madhu Gupta

Chapter 6 Nanostructure-Based Pulmonary Drug Delivery Systems for
Respiratory Infections 66

*Vinay Kumar, Himani Singh, Sofiya Tarannum, Sanya Batheja,
Umesh Gupta, and Amit Kumar Goyal*

Chapter 7 Nanomedicines for Rheumatoid Arthritis 88

*Shradha Devi Dwivedi, Krishna Yadav, Deependra Singh,
and Manju Rawat Singh*

ix

Chapter 21 Nanoparticles for Controlled Delivery of Proteins and Peptides 267

Raghuraj Singh, Krishna Yadav, Eupa Ray, Kalpesh Vaghasiya, and Rahul Kumar Verma

Chapter 22 Nanotechnology and Regenerative Medicine..293

Taihaseen Momin, Anamika Sahu Gulbake, Shivaji Kashte, Rahul Tiwari, and Arvind Gulbake

Chapter 23 Nanomedicine for Cancer Immunotherapy 307

Renuka Khatik, Monika Dwivedi, Bhattarai Prapanna,
and Sushesh Srivatsa Palakurthi

Chapter 24 Carbon Nanotubes and Fullerenes in Nanotheranostics....................................320

Naveen Rajana, Padakanti Sandeep Chary, Valamla Bhavana,
and Neelesh Kumar Mehra

Chapter 25 Nanoparticles for Controlled Delivery of siRNA 332

Pramod Kumar

Chapter 26 Green Synthesis of Nanoparticles: From Protocols to Applications 352

Aanjaneya Mamgain, Nilosha Parveen, Rameshroo Kenwat,
Ravindra Shukla, Shivani Rai Paliwal, and Rishi Paliwal

Contributors

Alka
Department of Pharmaceutical Sciences
Babasaheb Bhimrao Ambedkar University
Vidya Vihar, Raebareli Road,
  Lucknow, India

Ashish Baldi
Maharaja Ranjit Singh Punjab Technical
  University
Bathinda, Punjab, India

Sanya Batheja
Department of Pharmacy, School of
  Chemical Sciences and Pharmacy
Central University of Rajasthan
Bandarsindri, Kishangarh, Ajmer,
  Rajasthan, India

Bigul Yogeshver Bhardwaj
Institute of Pharmaceutical
  Sciences
Kurukshetra University
Kurukshetra, Haryana, India

Samir Bhargava
Department of Pharmaceutics
Faculty of Pharmacy
School of Pharmaceutical and Population
  Health Informatics
DIT University
Dehradun, Uttarakhand, India

Kanchan Bharti
Department of Pharmaceutical Engineering
  and Technology
Indian Institute of Technology (Banaras Hindu
  University)
Varanasi, Uttar Pradesh, India

Valamla Bhavana
Pharmaceutical Nanotechnology
  Research Laboratory, Department
  of Pharmaceutics
National Institute of Pharmaceutical Education
  and Research (NIPER)
Hyderabad, Telangana, India

Nagendra Bhuwane
University Institute of Pharmacy, Faculty of
  Technology
Pt. Ravishankar Shukla University
Raipur, Chhattisgarh, India

Padakanti Sandeep Chary
Pharmaceutical Nanotechnology
  Research Laboratory, Department
  of Pharmaceutics
National Institute of Pharmaceutical Education
  and Research (NIPER)
Hyderabad, Telangana, India

Akash Chaurasiya
Department of Pharmacy
Birla Institute of Technology and Science, Pilani
Hyderabad, India

Ishwari Choudhary
University Institute of Pharmacy, Faculty of
  Technology
Pt. Ravishankar Shukla University
Raipur, Chhattisgarh, India

Monika Dwivedi
Department of Pharmaceutical Sciences and
  Technology
Birla Institute of Technology
Mesra, Ranchi, Jharkhand, India

Shradha Devi Dwivedi
University Institute of Pharmacy
Pt. Ravishankar Shukla University
Raipur, Chhattisgarh, India

Amit Kumar Goyal
Department of Pharmacy, School of Chemical
  Sciences and Pharmacy
Central University of Rajasthan
Bandarsindri, Kishangarh, Ajmer, Rajasthan, India

Anamika Sahu Gulbake
Faculty of Pharmacy
DIT University
Dehradun, Uttarakhand, India

Arvind Gulbake
Department of Pharmaceutics
National Institute of Pharmaceutical Education
    and Research
Guwahati, Assam, India

Madhu Gupta
Department of Pharmaceutics
Delhi Pharmaceutical Sciences & Research
    University
New Delhi, India

Umesh Gupta
Department of Pharmacy, School of Chemical
    Sciences and Pharmacy
Central University of Rajasthan
Bandarsindri, Kishangarh, Ajmer,
    Rajasthan, India

Ekta Gurnany
Department of Pharmaceutics
B. Pharmacy College
Rampura, Godhra, Gujrat, India

Narayan Hemnani
University Institute of Pharmacy, Faculty of
    Technology
Pt. Ravishankar Shukla University
Raipur, Chhattisgarh, India

Ankit Jain
Department of Materials Engineering
Indian Institute of Science
Bangalore, Karnataka, India

Keerti Jain
Department of Pharmaceutics
National Institute of Pharmaceutical Education
    and Research
Raebareli, Lucknow, Uttar Pradesh,
    India

Sanjay K. Jain
Pharmaceutics Research Projects Laboratory,
    Department of Pharmaceutical Sciences
Dr. Hari Singh Gour Central University
Sagar, Madhya Pradesh, India

Sushil K. Kashaw
Department of Pharmaceutical Sciences
Dr. Harisingh Gour Central University
Sagar, Madhya Pradesh, India

Varsha Kashaw
Sagar Institute of Pharmaceutical Sciences
Sagar, Madhya Pradesh, India

Shivaji Kashte
Centre for Interdisciplinary Research, D.Y.
    Patil Education Society
Institution Deemed to be University
Kolhapur, Maharashtra, India

Sumeet Katke
Department of Pharmacy
Birla Institute of Technology and Science
Pilani, Hyderabad, Telangana, India

Monika Kaurav
KIET Institute of Pharmacy
KIET Institute
Gaziabad, Uttar Pradesh, India

Rameshroo Kenwat
Nanomedicine and Bioengineering Research
    Laboratory, Department of Pharmacy
Indira Gandhi National Tribal University
Amarkantak, Madhya Pradesh, India

Disha Kesharwani
Department of Pharmaceutics
Columbia Institute of Pharmacy
Raipur, Chhattisgarh, India

Renuka Khatik
Department of Radiology
Washington University
St. Louis, Missouri

Pramod Kumar
Pulmonary Aerosol Delivery, Institute of Lung
    Health and Immunity
Helmholtz Zentrum
München, Neuherberg, Germany

Rajesh Kumar
School of Pharmaceutical Sciences
Lovely Professional University
Phagwara, Punjab, India

Vinay Kumar
Department of Pharmacy, School of Chemical
    Sciences and Pharmacy
Central University of Rajasthan
Bandarsindri, Kishangarh, Ajmer, Rajasthan, India

Rajkumari Lodhi
Bansal College of Pharmacy
Bhopal, Madhya Pradesh, India

Sabyasachi Maiti
Department of Pharmacy
Indira Gandhi National Tribal University
Amarkantak, Madhya Pradesh, India

Aanjaneya Mamgain
Nanomedicine and Bioengineering Research
  Laboratory, Department of Pharmacy
Indira Gandhi National Tribal University
Amarkantak, Madhya Pradesh, India

Priyanka Maurya
Department of Pharmaceutical
  Sciences
Babasaheb Bhimrao Ambedkar University
Vidya Vihar, Raebareli Road, Lucknow,
  Uttar Pradesh, India

Neelesh Kumar Mehra
Pharmaceutical Nanotechnology
  Research Laboratory, Department of
  Pharmaceutics
National Institute of Pharmaceutical Education
  and Research (NIPER)
Hyderabad, Telangana, India

Susmit Mhatre
Institute of Chemical Technology
Nathalal Parekh Road, Matunga, Mumbai,
  Maharashtra, India

Sunita Minz
Department of Pharmacy
Indira Gandhi National Tribal University
Amarkantak, Madhya Pradesh, India

Brahmeshwar Mishra
Department of Pharmaceutical Engineering
  and Technology
Indian Institute of Technology (Banaras Hindu
  University)
Varanasi, Uttar Pradesh, India

Nidhi Mishra
Department of Pharmaceutical Sciences
Babasaheb Bhimrao Ambedkar University
Vidya Vihar, Raebareli Road, Lucknow,
  Uttar Pradesh, India

Vijay Mishra
School of Pharmaceutical Sciences
Lovely Professional University
Phagwara, Punjab, India

Yachana Mishra
School of Bioengineering and Biosciences
Lovely Professional University
Phagwara, Punjab, India

Taihaseen Momin
Centre for Interdisciplinary Research, D.Y.
  Patil Education Society
Institution Deemed to be University
Kolhapur, Maharashtra, India

Shivraj Naik
Institute of Chemical Technology
Nathalal Parekh Road, Matunga, Mumbai,
  Maharashtra, India

Puja Nayak
Nanomedicine and Bioengineering
  Research Laboratory, Department
  of Pharmacy
Indira Gandhi National Tribal University
Amarkantak, Madhya Pradesh, India

Raquibun Nisha
Department of Pharmaceutical
  Sciences
Babasaheb Bhimrao Ambedkar University
Vidya Vihar, Raebareli Road, Lucknow,
  Uttar Pradesh, India

Rakesh Pahwa
Department of Pharmaceutics
Delhi Pharmaceutical Sciences &
  Research University
New Delhi, India

Ravi Raj Pal
Department of Pharmaceutical Sciences
Babasaheb Bhimrao Ambedkar University
Vidya Vihar, Raebareli Road, Lucknow,
  Uttar Pradesh, India

Sushesh Srivatsa Palakurthi
Department of Pharmaceutical Sciences, Irma
  Lerma Rangel College of Pharmacy
Texas A&M University College Station
Kingsville, TX

Shivani Rai Paliwal
Department of Pharmacy
Guru Ghasidas Vishwavidyalaya
    (A Central University)
Bilaspur, Chhattisgarh, India

Rishi Paliwal
Nanomedicine and Bioengineering Research
    Laboratory, Department of Pharmacy
Indira Gandhi National Tribal University
Amarkantak, Madhya Pradesh, India

Kanan Panchal
Department of Pharmacy
Birla Institute of Technology and Science
Pilani, Hyderabad, Telangana, India

Pritish Kumar Panda
Pharmaceutics Research Projects
    Laboratory, Department of
    Pharmaceutical Sciences
Dr. Hari Singh Gour Central University
Sagar, Madhya Pradesh, India

Nilosha Parveen
Nanomedicine and Bioengineering Research
    Laboratory
Department of Pharmacy, Indira Gandhi
    National Tribal University
Amarkantak, Madhya Pradesh, India

Shaik Rahana Parveen
School of Pharmaceutical Sciences
Lovely Professional University
Phagwara, Punjab, India

Parth Patel
Department of Pharmaceutics
National Institute of Pharmaceutical Education
    and Research (NIPER)
Raebareli, Lucknow, Uttar Pradesh, India

Vandana Patravale
Institute of Chemical Technology
Nathalal Parekh Road, Matunga,
    Mumbai, Maharashtra, India

Madhulika Pradhan
Rungta College of Pharmaceutical Sciences
    and Research
Kohka, Bhilai, Chhatisgarh, India

Bhattarai Prapanna
Department of Pharmaceutical Sciences
Irma Lerma Rangel College of
    Pharmacy, Texas A&M University
    College Station
Kingsville, TX

Neha Raina
Department of Pharmaceutics
Delhi Pharmaceutical Sciences & Research
    University
New Delhi, India

Sarjana Raikwar
Pharmaceutics Research Projects
    Laboratory, Department of
    Pharmaceutical Sciences
Dr. Hari Singh Gour Central University
Sagar, Madhya Pradesh, India

Naveen Rajana
Pharmaceutical Nanotechnology
    Research Laboratory, Department of
    Pharmaceutics
National Institute of Pharmaceutical Education
    and Research (NIPER)
Hyderabad, Telangana, India

Chetan Ram
Department of Pharmaceutics
Faculty of Pharmacy
School of Pharmaceutical and Population
    Health Informatics
DIT University
Dehradun, Uttarakhand, India

Shweta Ramkar
University Institute of Pharmacy, Faculty of
    Technology
Pt. Ravishankar Shukla University
Raipur, Chhattisgarh, India

Eupa Ray
Institute of Nano Science and Technology
Mohali, Punjab, India

Abhishek K. Sah
Department of Pharmacy
Shri Govindram Seksariya Institute of
    Technology & Science (SGSITS)
Indore, Madhya Pradesh, India

 xxi

Kantrol Kumar Sahu
Institute of Pharmaceutical Research
GLA University
Mathura, Uttar Pradesh, India

Prashant Sahu
Babulal Tarabai Institute of Pharmaceutical Science
Sagar, Madhya Pradesh, India

Priyanka Salunkhe
Institute of Chemical Technology
Nathalal Parekh Road, Matunga, Mumbai,
   Maharashtra, India

Shubhini A. Saraf
Department of Pharmaceutical Sciences
Babasaheb Bhimrao Ambedkar University
Vidya Vihar, Raebareli Road, Lucknow,
   Uttar Pradesh, India

Gaurav Saraogi
Sri Aurobindo Institute of Pharmacy
Indore, Madhya Pradesh, India

Satish Shilpi
School of Pharmaceuticals and Population
   Health Informatics
Faculty of Pharmacy
DIT University
Dehradun, Uttarakhand, India

Ravindra Shukla
Department of Botany
Indira Gandhi National Tribal University
Amarkantak, Madhya Pradesh, India

Shalini Shukla
Department of Pharmacy
Indira Gandhi National Tribal University
Amarkantak, Madhya Pradesh, India

Deependra Singh
University Institute of Pharmacy
Pt. Ravishankar Shukla University
Raipur, Chhattisgarh, India

Himani Singh
Department of Pharmacy, School of Chemical
   Sciences and Pharmacy
Central University of Rajasthan
Bandarsindri, Kishangarh, Ajmer, Rajasthan, India

Manju Rawat Singh
University Institute of Pharmacy
Pt. Ravishankar Shukla University
Raipur, Chhattisgarh, India

Neelu Singh
Department of Pharmaceutical Sciences
Babasaheb Bhimrao Ambedkar University
Vidya Vihar, Raebareli Road, Lucknow, India

Priya Singh
Department of Pharmaceutical Sciences
Babasaheb Bhimrao Ambedkar University
Vidya Vihar, Raebareli Road, Lucknow,
   Uttar Pradesh, India

Raghuraj Singh
Institute of Nano Science and Technology
Mohali, Punjab, India

Ramu Singh
Neuropharmacology Research
   Laboratory (NPRL), Department of Pharmacy
Indira Gandhi National Tribal University
Amarkantak, Madhya Pradesh, India

Sachin Kumar Singh
School of Pharmaceutical Sciences
Lovely Professional University
Phagwara, Punjab, India

Samipta Singh
Department of Pharmaceutical Sciences
Babasaheb Bhimrao Ambedkar University
Vidya Vihar, Raebareli Road, Lucknow,
   Uttar Pradesh, India

Veena Devi Singh
Shri Rawatpura Sarkar College of Pharmacy
Shri Rawatpura University
Raipur, Chhattisgarh, India

Vijay Kumar Singh
Shri Rawatpura Sarkar College of Pharmacy
Shri Rawatpura University
Raipur, Chhattisgarh, India

Tishya Srivastava
Institute of Chemical Technology
Nathalal Parekh Road, Matunga,
   Mumbai, Maharashtra, India

Kunjbihari Sulakhiya
Neuropharmacology Research
    Laboratory (NPRL), Department
    of Pharmacy
Indira Gandhi National Tribal University
Amarkantak, Madhya Pradesh, India

Preeti K. Suresh
University Institute of Pharmacy, Faculty of
    Technology
Pt. Ravishankar Shukla University
Raipur, Chhattisgarh, India

Sofiya Tarannum
Department of Pharmacy, School of Chemical
    Sciences and Pharmacy
Central University of Rajasthan
Bandarsindri, Kishangarh, Ajmer, Rajasthan,
    India

Rahul Tiwari
Faculty of Pharmacy
DIT University
Dehradun, Uttarakhand, India

Kalpesh Vaghasiya
Institute of Nano Science and Technology
Mohali, Punjab, India

Amit Verma
Pharmaceutics Research Projects Laboratory,
    Department of Pharmaceutical Sciences
Dr. Hari Singh Gour Central University
Sagar, Madhya Pradesh, India

Rahul Kumar Verma
Institute of Nano Science and Technology
Mohali, Punjab, India

Swati Verma
I.T.S. College of Pharmacy
Muradnagar, Ghaziabad, Uttar Pradesh, India

Sheetu Wadhwa
School of Pharmaceutical Sciences
Lovely Professional University
Phagwara, Punjab, India

Harsh Yadav
Department of Pharmacy
Indira Gandhi National Tribal University
Amarkantak, Madhya Pradesh, India

Krishna Yadav
University Institute of Pharmacy
Pt. Ravishankar Shukla University
Raipur, Chhattisgarh, India

Preface

The last three decades have witnessed a revolution in the customized and engineered drug delivery concept with the advances of nanotechnological and biotechnological innovations. Depending upon the functions and organizations, such applications in the biomedical domain have led to new terms such as "nanomedicine", "nanotheranostics", and "nanobiotechnology". Such research areas are rapidly growing and dynamic, with novel combinations of biomaterials, therapeutics, diagnostic, and sometimes site-specific driving ligands. A sufficient number of marketed products have been developed as new hopes contributing the better treatment regimen of the diseases using such novel drug delivery systems capable of manipulating cellular and sub-cellular machinery of dysfunction unhealthy cells.

We aimed to produce a single book covering the fundamentals and applications of emerging concepts related to nanomedicine, nanotheranostics, and nanobiotechnology. This book has 26 chapters. Each chapter is written by a leading expert and their team to describe core knowledge, with recent progress and outcomes of the topic covered.

Words are not enough to express thanks to our family members, our parents (Navin-Chanchala Paliwal and Laxmi Prasad-Anita Rai), and our sons Aaradhya and Swastik for their love, affection, and unconditional support during this project.

We are grateful to the chapter contributors, who dedicatedly put in hard effort in realization of our concept and shared their expertise with the readers of this book. We convey our humble regards to our mentor Prof. S. P. Vyas for sharing his knowledge and expertise with us as and when required. The encouragement, motivation, and support of our respective organizations are humbly acknowledged.

The timely help and support of the CRC publishing team, especially Ms. Renu and Ms. Jyotsna, from the beginning of the proposal to final book completion, is duly acknowledged.

We are confident that the book will be an asset for readers in many ways and expect that suggestions, comments, and remarks will be received in the near future from our beloved readers.

Editors,
Rishi Paliwal, PhD
Shivani Rai Paliwal, PhD

1 Nanomedicine
History, Progress, and Advances

*Rishi Paliwal, Shivani Rai Paliwal,
Shalini Shukla, and Puja Nayak*

1.1 INTRODUCTION

The concept of nanotechnology first arrived in the minds of physicists and other scientists for nanoscale assembly of various materials. The initial developments included scanning probe microscopes and determination of molecular structures called fullerenes, which later expanded to nanomaterials and nanomedicines. Nanomedicines currently being explored include liposomes, polymers (natural and synthetic), carbon nanotubes, grapheme and quantum dots [1]. A large number of nanomedicines have reached the market, and several of them are in clinical trials at the moment [2]. Nanomedicines have not only created a great revolution in the medical field, but it is also essential to carefully perform clinical trials in order to get safe and effective therapeutics. Some of the advantages of nanotechnology are:

- Better imaging and diagnostic tools are useful for earlier diagnosis and better treatment options.
- Nanotechnology is issued for controlled and sustained delivery of drugs.
- It helps to provide targeted drug delivery.
- It provides faster drug delivery and better medical care than conventional drug delivery systems.

1.2 PRE-NANOMEDICINE ERA

Up to the last century, the pharmaceutical industry had explored conventional pharmaceutical products, including tablets, capsules, suspensions and emulsions. Although such conventional dosage forms have been used commonly as they are convenient to use, manufacture, patient friendly and industry oriented including regulatory agencies. However, a large number of disadvantages of these systems restrict their successful use in achieving the desired pharmacokinetic and drug distribution due to either drug-related characteristics such as poor aqueous solubility, stability and a high first-pass metabolism leading to poor oral bioavailability and high dose administration. Apart from this, their inability to remove non-biodegradable residuals, leading to toxicity and high initial burst release after drug administration, is also one of the known issues. Scientists have been working continuously to combat these problems of conventional drug delivery systems. It takes longer for a conventional drug to pass all the clinical trials and enter the market. Further, it is an expensive and tedious process.

In order to minimize some of these issues, the concept of novel drug delivery systems came into practice, and it was suggested to modify existing drugs for prolonged and targeted delivery. This improved the safety-efficacy ratio of existing drugs, provided targeted delivery and lowered the research and development costs of new drugs [3–5]. The concept of nanomedicine was introduced in the year 1964, but it became a major idea in the pharmaceutical industry after1980s. Since then,

DOI: 10.1201/9781003130055-1

a lot of research work has been performed in this field, which has led to the development of many types of nanomedicines [6].

1.3 EVOLUTION OF NANOTECHNOLOGY

The term "nanotechnology" is derived from the Greek word "nano", which means "dwarf" or very small materials (one billionth of a meter). The National Nanotechnology Initiative (NNI) in the US defined nanotechnology as "a science, engineering, and technology conducted at the nanoscale (1 to 100 nm), where unique phenomena enable novel applications in a wide range of fields, from chemistry, physics and biology, to medicine, engineering and electronics".

Some of the remarkable milestones in developing nanomedicine are as follows:

- In 1959, the concept of nanotechnology was first introduced by American physicist and Nobel Prize winner Richard Feynman, who is also known as the father of modern nanotechnology.
- After 15 years, in 1974, Norio Taniguchi, a Japanese scientist, defined the term "nanotechnology" as: "nanotechnology mainly consists of the processing of separation, consolidation, and deformation of materials by one atom or one molecule".
- In the US, on January 21, 2000, the US president announced funding of research in the field of nanotechnology. After three years, the US signed into law the 21st-century Nanotechnology Research and Development Act. The legislation made nanotechnology research a national priority and created the National Nanotechnology Initiative.
- In 2006, the European Medicines Agency (EMA) published its first regulatory reflection paper related to nanotechnology-based medicinal products for human use.
- Some other counties and their regulatory bodies have launched respective guidelines for nanomedicine; for example, India launched guidelines for nanopharmaceuticals in 2019.
- In the past few decades, the application of nanotechnology in diagnostics, drug delivery and molecular imaging has been researched and has gotten good results.

Undoubtedly, nanomedicine has shown improved therapeutic interventions for the treatment of all almost all kinds of diseases. However, nanotechnology was first employed in the field of cancer, known as nano-oncology, by improving the efficacy of chemotherapeutic molecules against many types of cancers [7, 8]. Such nanotechnology-driven products remain helpful in targeting tumor sites, for example, by using nanoparticles anchored with antibodies and loaded with cytotoxic agents. Such nanosystems consequently specify drug delivery areas to modulate autophagy, metabolism or oxidative stress and hence exert better anticancer activity [9, 10]. In the past few decades, the United States Food and Drug Administration (USFDA) has approved about 100 nanotherapeutics, and many are under consideration. Along with chemotherapeutic drugs, various antifungal drugs in nanoformulation form are also available, such as liposomal amphotericin B. Other than liposomes, various other types of nanocarriers have been introduced and achieved great success in improved drug delivery, including but not limited to polymer-based nanoparticles (NPs), nanogels, protein-based NPs, inorganic nanoparticles and dendrimers [11, 12]. Figure 1.1 shows the progress in the area of nanomedicine and its major milestones.

1.4 FDA REGULATIONS FOR NANOMEDICINES

To date, there is no specific guidance document approved by the FDA exclusively for nanomedicines. This is because the FDA is not sure that nanomedicines work differently in comparison to other molecular drugs. However, in 2016, the FDA issued a document containing general regulations for all nanomaterials related to drugs, cosmetics and other devices. Scientists have a definite

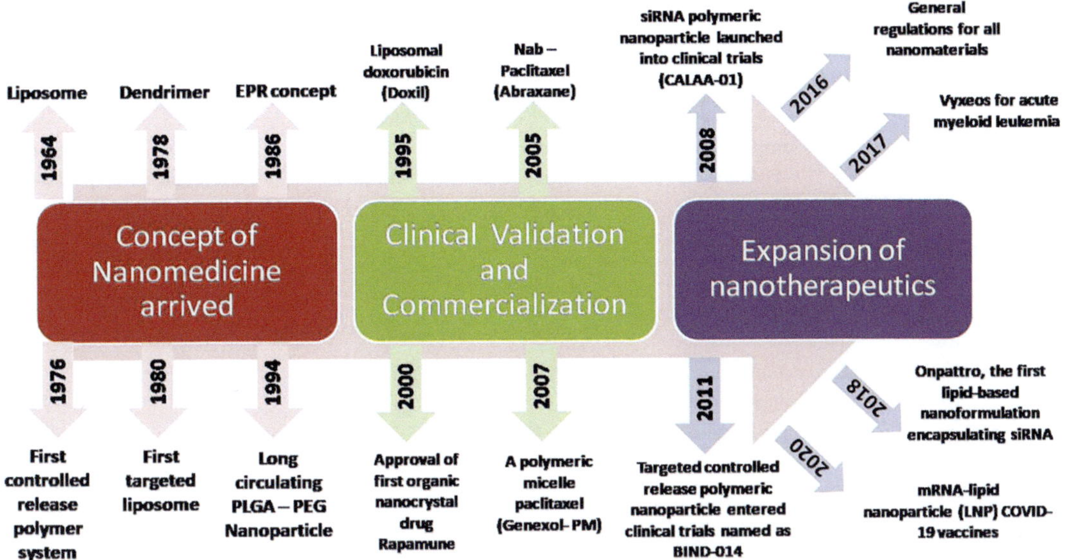

FIGURE 1.1 Progress in the field of nanomedicine, from concept to recent expansion.

idea that nanoparticles not only are beneficial due to their small size and surface area but also due to better therapeutics such as biodistribution, toxicity, pharmacokinetics and execution rates.

1.5 APPLICATIONS OF NANOTECHNOLOGY IN MEDICINE

The employment of nanotechnology in the pharmaceutical industries paved the way for the introduction of nanomedicine. Nanomedicine came up with potential benefits, overcoming the limitations of conventional drug delivery systems. One of them is the reduction in toxicity due to sustained, controlled or targeted release of drugs. Nanopharmaceuticals combine nanotechnology with biomedical and pharmaceutical sciences to improve drug delivery. Over the past three decades, significant growth in nanotherapeutic products has been observed. It is an established fact that nanotherapeutics often exhibit greater therapeutic efficacy than conventional small molecular drugs due to their size (10–100 nm). In this section, some well-known nano-drug carriers are discussed. Table 1.1 lists various types of nanocarriers and their related features.

1.5.1 LIPOSOMES

Liposomes were first discovered in the 1960s by Alec D Bangham at the Babraham Institute, University of Cambridge. Briefly, liposomes are special vesicles composed of a lipid bilayer membrane and an aqueous core. Hence, they are ampiphillic in nature and can incorporate both lipophillic as well as hydrophillic drugs. The first liposomal formulation was developed using natural lipids. However, today, we have large number of natural and synthetic phospholipids as well as surfactants for developing diverse types of liposomes such as pH-sensitive, magnetic, enzyme-sensitive and temperature-sensitive liposomes [3, 13].

Usually, the liposomes applied and developed for biomedical applications range between 50 and 450 nm. Liposomes are not to be confused with micelles, as micelles have only one lipid layer, with a polar head facing the outer environment and non-polar tail facing inward. On the other hand, liposomes are made of a phospholipid bilayer. In addition to this, liposomes have a more spacious core

TABLE 1.1

Nanocarriers Explored in the Development of Nanomedicine

Nanocarrier	Composition/ Feature	Proposed Year	Marketed Product Available	Representative Therapeutic Molecules Encapsulated
Inorganic NPs	Inorganic nanomaterials	1957	Yes	AuNPs, vaccine adjuvants
Liposomes	Phospholipid-based vesicular system	1961	Yes	Doxorubicin, Amphotericin B
Polymeric nanoparticles	PEGylated	1979	Yes	Estradiol, Leuprolide, Certolizumab
Dendrimers	Drugs conjugated with dendrimer structures	1982	Yes	Doxorubicin
Solid lipid nanoparticles	Solid lipid cored nanoparticles	Early 1990	Yes	Ciprofloxacin, Ambroxol
Drug nanocrystals	Drug crystals in nm size	2000	Yes	Immunosuppressants, antiemetics, Megestrol, Paclitaxel

than micelles. Liposomes are basically of two major types based on their structure: unilammellar vesicles (ULV) and multilamellar vesicles (MLV). ULVs have larger aqueous core and hence are employed for incorporation/encapsulation of hydrophilic drugs, whereas MLVs with many layers have been found useful for lipophilic drugs. When the rate kinetics is taken into consideration, it is found that ULVs with only one layer and a hydrodynamic diameter of 130 nm have a faster release than MLVs with many layers and a hydrodynamic diameter of 250 nm.

Second-generation liposomes led to modifications in composition of size and charge of the vesicle. Cholesterol was introduced in the lipid bilayer, which was helpful in reducing permeability and improving in vitro and in vivo stability issues [14]. Additionally, cholesterol helps in binding the layers and hence inhibits their transfer in high density lipoprotein (HDL) and low density lipoprotein (LDL). It also helps in stabilizing the core of the liposomes.

The first liposomal drug to get FDA approval was doxorubicin (Doxil) in 1995. The primary aim of liposomal therapeutics is to achieve targeted drug delivery along with protection from the surrounding environment, consequently improving drug stability and half life. The liposomal formulations currently available today include antifungal, anticancer and analgesic drugs. For the last 50 years, liposomes have been an interesting area of research and have been investigated extensively. Various types of liposomes with remote drug loading extruded for homogeneous size have been discovered so far, including long-circulating (PEGylated) liposomes, triggered release liposomes, liposomes containing nucleic acid polymers, ligand-targeted liposomes and liposomes containing combinations of drugs. Anticancer drug delivery systems based on liposomal formulations have been widely studied, and liposomal formulations of some drugs are in clinical trials, including cisplatin, irinotecan, paclitaxel and docetaxel. Similarly, some FDA-approved liposomal nanoformulations with the antifungal drug amphotericin B are Abelcet (Sigma Tau) in 1995, amphotec (Alkopharma) in 1996 and Ambisome (Astellas/Gilead) in 1997 [15].

Another similar type of nanostructure formed from surfactants is called niosomes. Although they are similar to liposomes, they have better properties and benefits than liposomes in a few areas, such as encapsulation of drugs at a higher capacity and more stability [16].

1.5.2 POLYMER-BASED NANOTHERAPEUTICS

Polymeric nanoparticles were first used in cancer therapy in 1979 when the adsorption of anti-cancer agents to polyalkylcyanoacrylate nanoparticles was studied [17]. Polymer-based nanomedicines possess many benefits and are used widely. The benefits include enhancing drug stability and half-life, targeting, improving biodegradability and enabling controlled release with the use of stimuli-responsive polymers. Polymer nanocarriers are made in a variety of structures, such as polymer drug conjugates, polymeric micelles, nanospheres and dendrimers. Stimuli-responsive polymer drug conjugates undergo structural transitions and release drugs in response to small changes in stimuli such as temperature or pH. Some polymers used in forming polymer drug conjugates include polyethylene glycol, polystyrene-maleic anhydride copolymer and N-(2-hydroxypropyl) methacrylamide. However, the clinical use of these polymer drug conjugates is narrow because non-biodegradable polymers cause insufficient circulation and less accumulation in target tissue. Hence, biodegradable polymers are still under investigation. Polymeric micelles are self-assembling amphiphilic nanocarriers that consist of a hydrophobic core and a hydrophilic surface. The hydrophobic core incorporates water-soluble drugs, and the hydrophilic exterior is used to provide solubility in aqueous solutions. Polymeric micelles also exhibit rapid uptake by reticuloendothelial system (RES); hence, they are PEGylated. Estrasorb is an FDA-approved micelle for treatment of the severe vasomotor symptoms of menopause.

1.5.3 DRUG NANOCRYSTALS

In the early 1990s, Elan Nanosystems came up with new structures called nanocrystals which took the place of microcrystals. Nanocrystals were introduced to overcome the problems of oral bioavailability enhancement as well as nanosuspensions for intravenous and pulmonary drug delivery. Drug nanocrystals are crystals of drugs at the nanometer scale and hence do not require drug carriers.

A large number of drug discovered so far are very promising in their pharmacological effect but possess low aqueous solubility; hence, suitable formulations are required for them. In order to tackle this problem, the nanocrystallization method was introduced. It involves two approaches: top down and bottom up. These methods successfully increase saturation solubility and dissolution velocity. Nanocrystal-based nanotherapeutics could be developed in diverse forms such as capsules, tablets, and pellets, and therefore can be administered by various routes. The first developed nanocrystal drug was Rapamune, which was developed in 2000 by Wyeth Pharmaceuticals (available as oral suspension and tablet), an immunosuppressant that prevents organ rejection in patients receiving kidney transplants. Subsequently, Emend was developed in 2001 (approved in 2003) by Merck. It was an antiemetic used in chemotherapy-induced vomiting. Some other drugs include Ticor (fenofibrate), Megace (megestrol) and Paxceed (paclitaxel) [18].

1.5.4 PROTEIN-BASED NANOTHERAPEUTICS

Protein-based nanomedicine is an ideal drug delivery system because it exhibits many advantages such as biocompatibility, low toxicity, renewable resources and immunogenicity. Some proteins frequently used for drug delivery purpose are albumin, collagen, ferritin or apoferitin protein cages, soy and whey protein, and gelatin. Protein-based nanotherapeutics is more beneficial than synthetic polymers, with little batch to batch variation. A suitable example of such a class is Abraxane (nab-paclitaxel), which is conjugated with albumin and put an end to toxic solvent used with paclitaxel.

1.5.5 METALLIC NANOPARTICLES

Metallic nanoparticles are versatile and have tunable size, shape and chemical properties. The inorganic materials employed are metals, metal oxides, semiconductors. In disease treatment, these were found useful in cancer therapy. Gold nanoparticles (AuNPs) began to be studied after Faraday's work in 1957. Various inorganic materials underwent clinical trials and were useful, for instance, Dexferrum, Feraheme, Infed and Feridex. Another example is recombinant human tumor necrosis factor (rhTNF) bound to colloidal gold (CYT-6091), which shows reduced toxicity and clearance rates in comparison to free rhTNF and has completed Phase I trials in patients with advanced cancer.

1.5.6 DENDRIMERS

Dendrimers are synthetic nanosized radially symmetrical molecules that have tree-like arms or branches. These small molecules were first discovered by Fritz Vögtle in 1978, Donald Tomalia in the 1980s and also independently by George R Newkome. Dendrimers have special features which make them useful in many applications. Dendrimers have applications in cancer treatment, as they are helpful in reducing enhanced permeation and retention effects (EPRs) caused by polymer drug conjugates due to increased permeability and accumulation in tumor tissues. In 1982, Maciejewski put forward the application of these branched structures as molecular containers. Dendrimers are also found to be useful in transdermal drug delivery systems (because of low water solubility and the presence of hydrophobic moieties) [19].

Dendrimers as nanocarriers have also been reported to be useful in gene therapy. For example, polyamidoamine (PAMAM) dendrimer–DNA complexes (called dendriplexes) maintain a positive net charge and bind to negatively charged surface molecules on cell membranes. Dendrimers are usually taken up into cells by nonspecific endocytosis and then degraded by lysosomes. Moreover, there is a new emerging field involving the combination of dendrimers and bioactive ligands dendrimer conjugates containing saccharides or peptides that can be exploited for therapeutic application in the delivery of antimicrobial and antiviral agents.

1.6 FUTURE SCOPE AND CHALLENGES

Although nanomedicine has existed for a while, not many nanomedicine-based formulations have been introduced on the market because the development of nanomedicines faces many obstacles (Table 1.2). Numerous issues need to be tackled in order to develop a successful nanoformulation.

TABLE 1.2
Nanomedicine under Clinical Trials

Drug Name	Delivery System	Disease	Phase	Company
ALN VSP02	LNP	Solid tumors	I Completed	Alnylam
SiRNA-EphA2-DOPAC	LNP	Advanced tumors	I completed	MD Anderson Cancer Center
ALN-PCS02	LNP	Hypercholesterolemia	I Completed	Alnylam
QPI-1007	Naked siRNA	Optic atrophy Ischemic optic neuropathy	I completed	Quark Pharmaceuticals
CALAA-01	Cyclodextrin NPs	Solid tumors	I active	Calando Pharmaceuticals
ARC-520	DPC	HBV	I Recruiting	Arrowhead Research
SGT-53	Liposome	Solid tumors	I	Synergene Therapeutics
MBP-Y003, MBP-Y004	Liposome	Lymphoma	Preclinical	Mebiopharm Co. Ltd
MCC-465	Liposome	Stomach cancer	I	Mitsubishi Tanabe Pharma Corp

Though the nanoparticle-based drug delivery system was introduced in the 1960s, it still has not gained the trust of the people and is not the first choice of patients and physicians. Hence, for the future market, it is necessary to create awareness among people regarding risk, benefits and safety concerns. Great advancement in nanomedicine, particularly for cancer therapeutics, has been seen and has shown satisfactory results clinically. One major challenge in the development of NPs is their ability to cause damage to healthy tissues [20]. They target not only lesions but also normal tissues. This is an important issue to tackle in the upcoming next-generation nanomedicines [21]. It is also important to regulate the circulation of NPs in the bloodstream. This can be done by proper selection of drug carriers. It has been seen that the abnormal vasculature and dense intestinal matrix in solid tumors can cause heterogenous drug distributions and hence poor penetration in tumors. The formation of ultrasmall nanoparticles can be a solution to this problem. They can penetrate deeply into tissues and also are easily eliminated by the renal route. Both these prospects could be united to form stimuli-sensitive NPs that have a better half life as well as good penetration in tissues, called stimuli-sensitive NPs (they change in size in response to the environment).

Researchers are working continuously to bring better and more efficacious nanomedicines into the market in newer domains, and some of the NPs produced so far have proved successful. For example, recently, extensive research has been performed in the field of Alzheimer's disease, which is a cause of dementia among the elderly.

In search of improved treatments for many diseases, scientists have investigated nutraceutical-based nanoparticles. Such nanoformulations improve the biological and chemical limits of nutraceuticals and hence prove more safe and effective. For example, quercetin-poly lactic-co-glycolic acid (PLGA) NPs, rutin-lipid polymers and curcumin nanogels are some representative reports.

Similarly, many new nano-immunotherapeutic agents have also been investigated, such as nanodiscs loaded with CpG, and pegylated doxorubicin is an immunogenic cell death (ICD)–inducing nanomedicine.

The respiratory system has a complicated defense mechanism, so in order to deliver drugs via this route, nanoparticles may play a role. They have been found to be effective in COVID-19 outbreaks. Various nanotechnology-based approaches have been used for disinfection purposes and for the development of COVID-19 diagnostic kits as well. Nanomedicines have provided many approaches to antiviral therapy, making it a good therapeutic option against COVID-19. Nanomedicine provides targeted and controlled delivery of drugs to the site of action, which in turn lowers the viral load and also lessens the risk of viral rebound. In this particular domain, dexamethasone nanomedicines have been hypothesized for COVID-19 management [22].

Despite their vast applications, some of the known challenges in the nanoformulation market are financial, ethical and regulatory challenges. For example, there is much financial assistance required for clinical trials, raw materials and equipment collection. A relatively low amount of funding has been raised in this area for research. Similarly, pharmaceutical industries are not willing to put their money into something that is not certain to be successful. A lot more nanomedicines are on the way, but each of them faces the problems of clinical translation, such as safety, efficacy, cost effectiveness and regulatory issues.

1.7 CONCLUSION

Nanotechnology has shown tremendous progress in every corner of science and technology, including the biomedical and pharmaceutical fields. It is one of the emerging fields in the pharmaceutical sciences that have been expanded for diverse applications. Nanoformulations are not new now, many developments have been seen since they were first introduced in the 1960s. However, they have not become as popular as conventional drugs, and there are still many challenges to tackle. However, ever-growing demands for better therapeutics have drawn the attention of the scientific community, which is evident from the increasing market revenues of nanomedicine-based products, which will further increase with advancements in knowledge and awareness in the coming years. To date, more than 100 nanomedicine products have been introduced, and many more are presently in clinical trials. The successful journey of nanomedicine products not only motivates but also creates a way forward for upcoming next-generation nanomedicine products.

REFERENCES

1. Paliwal R, Babu RJ, Palakurthi S. Nanomedicine scale-up technologies: feasibilities and challenges. *AAPS Pharmaceutical Science and Technology*. 2014 Dec;15(6):1527–34.
2. Min Y, Caster JM, Eblan MJ, Wang AZ. Clinical translation of nanomedicine. *Chemical Reviews*. 2015 Oct 14;115(19):11147–90.
3. Paliwal SR, Paliwal R, Agrawal GP, Vyas SP. Liposomal nanomedicine for breast cancer therapy. *Nanomedicine*. 2011 Aug;6(6):1085–100.
4. Etheridge ML, Campbell SA, Erdman AG, Haynes CL, Wolf SM, McCullough J. The big picture on small medicine: the state of nanomedicine products approved for use or in clinical trials. *Nanomedicine: Nanotechnology, Biology, and Medicine*. 2013 Jan;9(1):1.
5. Lombardo D, Kiselev MA, Caccamo MT. Smart nanoparticles for drug delivery application: development of versatile nanocarrier platforms in biotechnology and nanomedicine. *Journal of Nanomaterials*. 2019 Feb 27;2019:1–26.
6. Paliwal R, Kumar P, Chaurasiya A, Kenwat R, Katke S, Paliwal SR. Development of nanomedicines and nano-similars: recent advances in regulatory landscape. *Current Pharmaceutical Design*. 2022 Jan 1;28(2):165–77.
7. Paliwal SR, Kenwat R, Maiti S, Paliwal R. Nanotheranostics for cancer therapy and detection: state of the art. *Current Pharmaceutical Design*. 2020 Nov 1;26(42):5503–17.
8. Bayda S, Adeel M, Tuccinardi T, Cordani M, Rizzolio F. The history of nanoscience and nanotechnology: from chemical–physical applications to nanomedicine. *Molecules*. 2020 Jan;25(1):112.
9. Paliwal R, Paliwal SR, Vyas SP. Nanotherapeutics for cancer imaging and therapy. *Mini Reviews in Medicinal Chemistry*. 2017 Dec 1;17(18):1686–7.
10. Tekchandani P, Kurmi BD, Paliwal R, Paliwal SR. Galactosylated TPGS micelles for docetaxel targeting to hepatic carcinoma: development, characterization, and biodistribution study. *AAPS Pharmaceutical Science and Technology*. 2020 Jul;21(5):1–1.
11. Patra JK, Das G, Fraceto LF, Campos EV, del Pilar Rodriguez-Torres M, Acosta-Torres LS, Diaz-Torres LA, Grillo R, Swamy MK, Sharma S, Habtemariam S. Nano based drug delivery systems: recent developments and future prospects. *Journal of Nanobiotechnology*. 2018 Dec;16(1):1–33.
12. Kesharwani D, Mishra S, Paul SD, Paliwal R, Satapathy T. The functional nanogel: an exalted carrier system. *Journal of Drug Delivery and Therapeutics*. 2019 Apr 15;9(2-s):570–82.
13. Paliwal SR, Paliwal R, Vyas SP. A review of mechanistic insight and application of pH-sensitive liposomes in drug delivery. *Drug Delivery*. 2015 Apr 3;22(3):231–42.
14. Bozzuto G, Molinari A. Liposomes as nanomedical devices. *International Journal of Nanomedicine*. 2015;10:975.
15. Ventola CL. The nanomedicine revolution: part 2: current and future clinical applications. *Pharmacy and Therapeutics*. 2012 Oct;37(10):582.
16. Junyaprasert VB, Teeranachaideekul V, Supaperm T. Effect of charged and non-ionic membrane additives on physicochemical properties and stability of niosomes. *AAPS Pharmaceutical Science and Technology*. 2008 Sep;9(3):851–9.
17. Bolhassani A, Javanzad S, Saleh T, Hashemi M, Aghasadeghi MR, Sadat SM. Polymeric nanoparticles: potent vectors for vaccine delivery targeting cancer and infectious diseases. *Human Vaccines & Immunotherapeutics*. 2014 Feb 1;10(2):321–32.
18. Junghanns JU, Müller RH. Nanocrystal technology, drug delivery and clinical applications. *International Journal of Nanomedicine*. 2008 Sep;3(3):295.
19. Abbasi E, Aval SF, Akbarzadeh A, Milani M, Nasrabadi HT, Joo SW, Hanifehpour Y, Nejati-Koshki K, Pashaei-Asl R. Dendrimers: synthesis, applications, and properties. *Nanoscale Research Letters*. 2014 Dec;9(1).
20. Binda A, Murano C, Rivolta I. Innovative therapies and nanomedicine applications for the treatment of Alzheimer's disease: a state-of-the-art (2017–2020). *International Journal of Nanomedicine*. 2020;15:6113.

21. Shi Y, Lammers T. Combining nanomedicine and immunotherapy. *Accounts of Chemical Research.* 2019 May 23;52(6):1543–54.
22. Varahachalam SP, Lahooti B, Chamaneh M, Bagchi S, Chhibber T, Morris K, Bolanos JF, Kim NY, Kaushik A. Nanomedicine for the SARS-CoV-2: state-of-the-art and future prospects. *International Journal of Nanomedicine.* 2021;16:539.

2 Nanomedicine Development
Methods, Scale-up, and Challenges

Brahmeshwar Mishra and Kanchan Bharti

2.1 INTRODUCTION

The wide application of nanoparticles, ranging from the pharmaceutical industry to medicine, environmental science to agriculture and analytical chemistry, is the reason behind the huge amount of research going on in this field, along with different approaches for large-scale production of promising nanomaterials. When we look back in history, the term "nanotechnology" first came into the public consciousness in the book *Engines of Creation: The Coming Era of Nanotechnology*, written by K. Eric Drexler in 1986. From that era to the current scenario of research, it has reached a very advanced stage [1]. With the advent of more advanced research in nanomedicine, including but not limited to bacteria-mediated delivery of nanoparticles and drugs into cells, vaccination, gene therapy and cell therapy [2], these formulations have begun to play a major role in the field of healthcare. Nanomedicine is often described as a vehicle for drug delivery, contrast agents and diagnostic devices [3]. In 2006, the European Medicine Agency (EMA) defined nanomedicine as "the application of nanotechnology in view of making a medical diagnosis or treating or preventing diseases. It exploits the improved and often novel physical, chemical and biological properties of materials at nanometer scale". The nanometer scale is defined as 0.2–100 nm in the same document [4]. The advances made in nanomedicine research in terms of cellular, preclinical and clinical studies have mainly been used for cancer treatment, but problems like antibiotic resistance and artificial organs still need to be addressed. Although there is much evidence in the literature explaining many applications like magnetic nanoparticles for magnetic resonance imaging and targeting, gold nanoparticles for detection and analysis and polymeric and lipidic nanoparticles for drug delivery, very little of it sheds light on the challenges faced during the translation to successful commercial products. Due to this, products fail to reach the stage of even preclinical studies [5].

All the research going on in the field of nanomedicine aims to prove itself clinically superior to conventional dosage forms, along with its ability to become a commercially viable product. To fulfill this, products have to stand on the norms of regulatory bodies. This chapter gives an account on nanomedicine, widely used preparation methods, scale-up and challenges faced during formulation development.

2.2 METHODS OF NANOMEDICINE PRODUCTION

Broadly, the preparation method of nanomedicines can be categorized into top-down and bottom-up approaches. The method adopted for the preparation of nanomedicines decides their physical characteristics. The main objective of any method of production is to produce nanoparticles with properties like controlled particle size and polydispersity index, high drug loading, low batch-to-batch variation, feasibility for scale-up and compatibility with active pharmaceutical ingredient (API) irrespective of their properties. Top-down methods are simple and fast, show repeatability and are easy to scale up; at the same time, this approach is prone to contamination and is energy intensive. A bottom-up approach can be applied even for smaller batches and gives monodispersed particles, but it is not easy to scale up, it takes time to find suitable conditions, particle growth always need close monitoring and control and there is scope for solvent residues [6]. Some methods

DOI: 10.1201/9781003130055-2

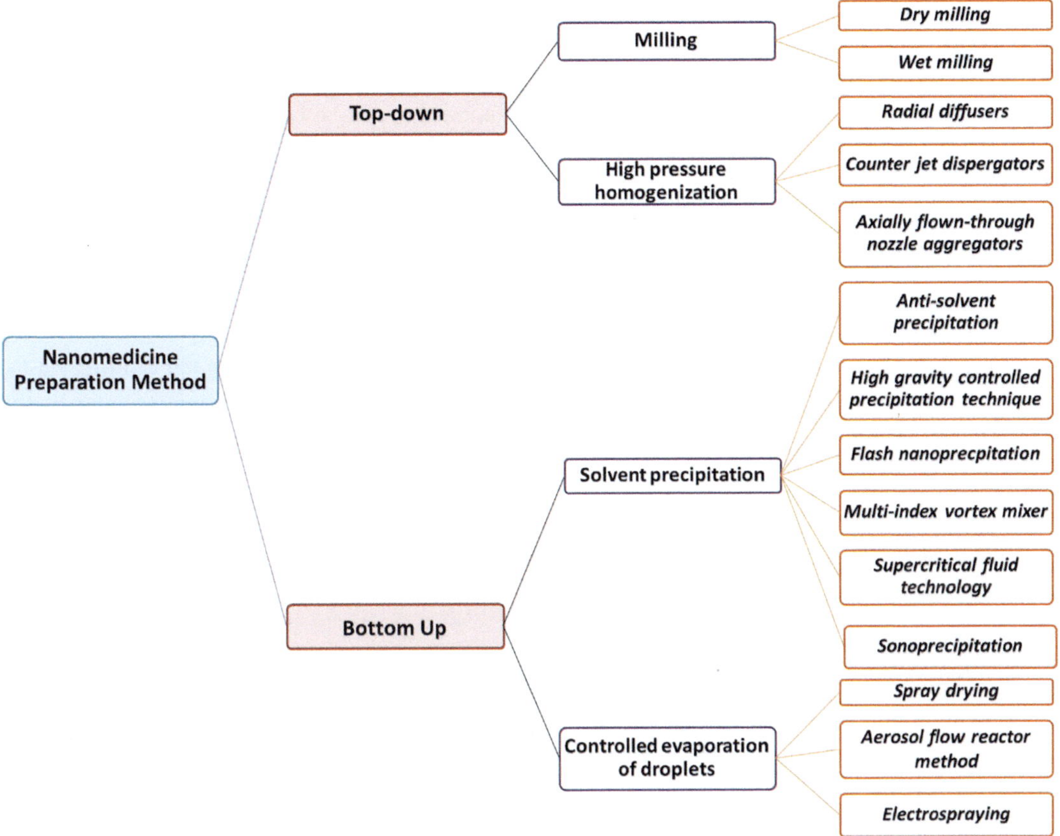

FIGURE 2.1   Various approaches for the preparation of nanomedicine.

of nanoparticle preparation have been discussed, showcasing their attributes for successful genera-tion of different types of nanoparticles. Figure 2.1 enumerates the methods differentiated on the basis of approach required for the production of nanomedicine.

2.2.1   TOP-DOWN METHODS

Milling and high-pressure homogenization are the most frequently employed methods for the top-down approach. However, this process struggles to produce smaller size particles, but particle size to 100 nm is achievable. The polydispersity index can be kept in check by increasing the number of milling and homogenization cycles. During milling, the particles tend to break and make agglomer-ates concurrently, but this can be resolved by using an appropriate stabilizer [6].

2.2.1.1   Milling

The milling technique consists of fluid-energy milling and dry ball milling. Large particles are crushed into smaller particles by applying forces like shear, attrition, impact or pressure. In cur-rent practice a liquid stabilizer system is required where the drug is dispersed and by the means of milling pearls. This method is mostly employed for the production of nanocrystals and has resulted in marketed products like aprepitant, fenofibrate, megesterol acetate, morphine sulfate, naproxen sodium and methylphenidate hydrochloride. Factors affecting the quality of products are milling speed and time, temperature of operation, properties of drugs and type of stabilizer used [7].

2.2.1.2 High-Pressure Homogenization

In the high-pressure homogenization (HPH) method, particle size reduction is achieved by shear and impact force, which happens due to media and particle collision. With respect to the milling method, HPH offers the advantage of less contamination that can be below the level of 1 ppm. In the literature, there are various subclassifications of the HPH method depending upon the type of nanoparticle preparation it is used for. For instance, there are designs like microfluidization and piston-gap design for nanocrystal preparation. For lipid-based nanoparticle preparation, the HPH method is classified into two approaches, hot homogenization and cold homogenization, depending upon the temperature at which they operate [8]. The units of HPH are a high-pressure pump and a high-pressure dispersion unit. This high-pressure dispersion unit is further subclassified into radial diffusers, counterjet dispergators and axially flown-through nozzle aggregates.

The most frequently used is the piston-gap design where the drug is dispersed in stabilizer solution and is passed at high speed and at high pressure of 1500–2000 bar through a narrow gap by the aid of piston. The cycle is repeated multiple times to obtain the desired characteristics. Dynamic pressure is generated at the narrow gap, and the static pressure is decreased due to increase in the kinetic energy, which causes the evaporation of the medium. This leads to the creation of many bubbles, which, when they leave the gap and enter the wide area, collapse to form nanosized particles of drug. This method solved many problems which were encountered in microfluidizer techniques [9].

2.2.2 Bottom-Up Approaches

The basic process of the bottom-up approach is precipitation of a drug in a supersaturated solution of the drug. Rapid evaporation (liquid atomization) or mixing with an antisolvent (antisolvent precipitation) is done to attain supersaturation. Control over particle size can be achieved by choosing a suitable stabilizer, which facilitates rapid mixing of drug to reach supersaturation, operating at appropriate temperature and pressure. However, this method has its own limitations; for example, it widely depends upon drug solubility, so poorly soluble drugs are difficult to process. The antisolvent precipitation technique further complicates it, as it demands drug solution miscibility in the antisolvent as well.

The solid state of the produced nanoparticles in the bottom-up approach depends upon the process conditions maintained. It can result in crystalline or amorphous nanoparticles, unlike top-down methods, where mainly crystalline particles are produced.

2.2.2.1 Solvent Precipitation

2.2.2.1.1 Anti-Solvent Precipitation

This method is simple and requires minimal equipment to produce amorphous nanoparticles. This precipitation technique results in the encapsulation of a wide range of material from synthetic drugs to natural compounds. Also this method employs protein-based polymers which give biocompatible drug nanoparticles like Ambraxane, which is albumin-based paclitaxel nanoparticles. This method includes three steps: i) solubilization of the drug in a suitable solvent, usually water; ii) addition of a suitable anti-solvent to precipitate the drug; and iii) addition of a crosslinking agent to fix the polymeric matrix. Water-miscible alcohols and multivalent ions present in the aqueous solution act as desolvating agent or antisolvents. The purpose of crosslinking is served by aldehydes, for example, glutaraldehyde for gelatin crosslinking [10]. During the scale-up of this process, the mixing of the aqueous and organic phases to induce polymer precipitation happens to be the most crucial step. Simplicity, ease of scaling and rapid and narrow size distribution of the particles are some of the advantages of this process [11]. The process has concerns like production of unstable nanosuspensions and the requirement of huge amounts of organic solvent to facilitate solubilization [12].

2.2.2.1.2 High-Gravity Controlled Precipitation Technique

In this method, the reactive precipitation occurs under high-gravity conditions and can be translated to commercial scale, which can be achieved by very few modifications in the experimental settings [13].

2.2.2.1.3 Flash Nanoprecipitation

This method can be done with the aid of a confined liquid impinging jet (CLIJ) where both drug solution and antisolvent come from different jets mounted in the same chamber, and when they mix, precipitation occurs under extreme turbulent conditions.

2.2.2.1.4 Multi-Index Vortex Mixer

This mixer was introduced to overcome the problem encountered during processing with confined liquid impinging jets. Here different flows of volumes can be mixed together to attain control over supersaturation and solvent composition [10].

2.2.2.1.5 Supercritical Fluid Technology

This method offers the advantage of rapid evaporation of the solvent and is considered a green method, as it uses supercritical CO_2 (SC CO_2), which is a safe non-toxic gas, for processing. SC CO_2 possesses high solubility with organic compounds which are insoluble in water [14]. Apart from SC CO_2, ethylene, tetrahydrofuran, ethane, nitrous oxide, sulfur hexafluoride, propane, ammonia, toluene and water are also used [15]. It can be elucidated that at critical temperature and pressure, SCF exists as liquid and vapor in a homogenous phase. This gives the dissolved solute high diffusivity because at critical points, the diffusivity and the viscosity of SCF are equal to the vapor phase. These properties and the high supersaturation of SCF help form nanosized particles. The SCF process for nanoparticle formation is divided into several categories, which are summarized in Figure 2.2. The process is suitable for thermolabile drugs and is a one-step rapid process with moderate operating temperature. However, the requirements of high pressure and auxiliary equipment and the high cost of processing limit its widespread use [16].

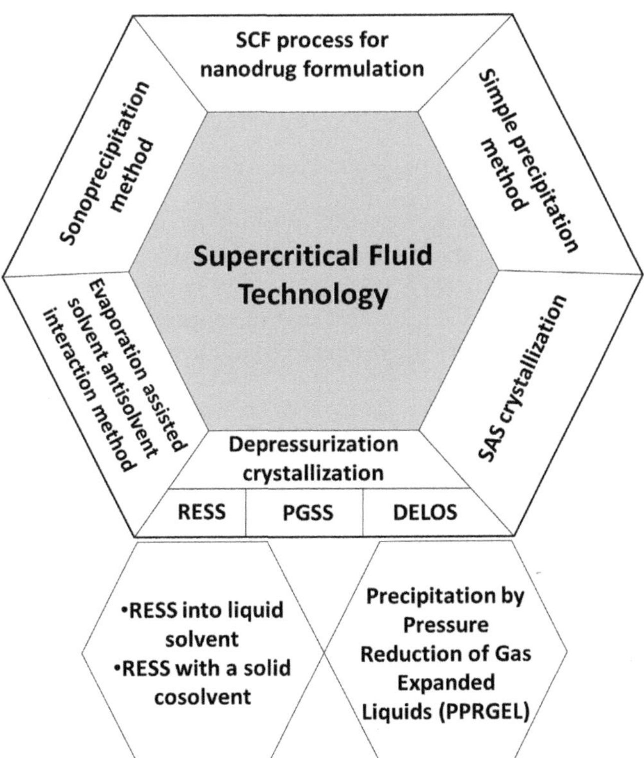

FIGURE 2.2 Types of supercritical fluid technology for nanomedicine formulation.

2.2.2.1.6   *Sonoprecipitation*

In this method, ultrasound is employed to make nanoparticles of controlled size by virtue of escalated mass transfer. This method is helpful in the case of those APIs where control over particle size is difficult because of particle growth and agglomeration [17]. Amplitude level and ultra-sonication time are some factors which affect the stability and dissolution profile of the API [18].

2.2.2.2   Controlled Evaporation of Droplets

2.2.2.2.1   *Spray Drying*

Spray drying is yet another commonly used method, which falls under the category of controlled evaporation of droplets for nanoparticle production. This method was not feasible earlier for the production of nanoparticles, since the cyclone was not able to collect such small particles until a modified version of a spray dryer was created with an electrostatic collector. Significant modification constitutes vibration less spray technology, which has the main role in particle generation in nano range. This method has been used to dry nanosuspensions to obtain dry powder for the reconstitution of lipid-based nanoparticles and sugar-based drug nanocrystals [19]. Apart from this, nanoparticles which need sophisticated processing parameters like protein and small interfering RNA nanoparticles have also been successfully prepared by this method [20]. Feed rate and the difference between inlet and outlet temperature are the driving force for particle drying. Residence time of the droplet and drying air temperature are the drying control parameters [10].

2.2.2.2.2   *Aerosol Flow Reactor Method*

This method is identical to spray drying in terms of atomization of drug solution. Droplets of drug solution pass through a heated laminar flow reactor in a carrier gas for drying. This is a single-step method intended to produce nanosized particles in more controlled manner to give unimodal size distribution. Temperature provided for the solvent to evaporate and the residence time of droplets are the factors affecting the final product quality [21].

2.2.2.2.3   *Electrospraying*

In this method, very fine submicron uniform-sized particles are produced by the impact of electrical forces. Solvent drying is facilitated by the coupling of drying gas to form nanoparticles [22].

2.3   SCALE-UP OF NANOMEDICINES

In a pharmaceutical company, the factors like type of nanoparticle, approach (top-down or bottom-up) and regulatory requirements majorly impact the scale-up of nanomedicines. Feasibility, robustness and cost-effectiveness are some key qualities a scale-up process must possess to produce nanomedicine with the desired physicochemical and therapeutic properties. Regulatory status of excipients and lack of nanotoxicity are the primary requirements for the large-scale production of nanomedicines [23].

At the lab scale, successful attempts have been made to scale up PLGA, lipid-based, chitosan and many other nanoparticles. Shegokar et al. reported the scaling up of stavudine-loaded solid lipid nanoparticles (SLNs) from lab scale of 40 g to medium scale of 10 Kg and large scale of 20/60 Kg. The use of piston-gap homogenizer for high-pressure homogenization of stavudine in the pre-emulsion made up of lipid melt dispersed in surfactant solution. Homogenizers with different features and capacity were used for different scales of production; for example, APV Micron LAB 40 and Micron LAB 60 piston gap homogenizers were used for lab scale and medium scale respectively. Gaulin 5.5 and Avestin C50 were used for large-scale production [24].

At the lab scale, chitosan nanoparticles are prepared by the lab-based ionotropic-gelation method. A study was done to compare the nanoparticles prepared by the spinning disc process with the lab scale method. Various advantages of SDP have been highlighted to support nanoparticle production by this method; adaptability for large-scale production is one of them. A major highlight of the work is that the nanoparticle characteristics seem to be more affected by the type and concentration of acid (acetic acid and tartaric acid) selected for the reaction rather than the processing parameters. There were no significant changes in the particle size of nanoparticles produced by conventional methods versus SDP. The process has been considered advantageous in terms of less waste production, safety during production, particle size growth and tunable feed rate [25].

Webb et al. investigated the capability of microfluidic manufacture for nanomedicine production where the GMP production requirement was fulfilled. They found that the type of mixer (herringbone mixer) used for lab-scale production was not fit to meet the GMP requirements, so they utilized another type (toroidal mixer) and a NanoAssemblr GMP system which had the capacity for a high flow rate ratio of aqueous:alcohol solution and total flow rate. The toroidal mixer offers the advantage of scale-independent production, as it uses the same parameter set points and normal operating range from lab scale to continuous production scale [26].

Table 2.1 lists some equipment along with its capacity to give insight into various scales on which this equipment can operate and its viability for industrial production of nanomedicines.

2.4 CHALLENGES OF NANOMEDICINE DEVELOPMENT

Research on nanomedicine from the workbench faces a lot of challenges for making it available at the bedside. As formulation development becomes more advanced, formulation scientists encounter new challenges. There are plenty of discussions highlighting the major hurdles of nanomedicine research; the most recent the discussion, the more diverse the challenges. The challenges are summarized in Table 2.2.

2.4.1 PHYSICOCHEMICAL CHARACTERIZATION

There are not any FDA guidelines for physicochemical characterization of nanomedicines, so there is an urgent need for standardized protocols and procedures. However, there are two product-specific draft guidance documents issued by the US FDA to deal with the emerging trend of nanotechnology used in the food and cosmetic industries. Physicochemical properties like size, surface

TABLE 2.1

Equipment Used in Various Methods of Nanoparticle Production, Capacity and Particle Size

Method	Equipment	Equipment Capacity	Particle Size Achieved by the Equipment	Ref.
High-pressure homogenization	Avestin EmulsiFlex-B3	0.5–3.5 ml	< 4000 nm	[27, 28]
	APV Micron Lab 40	40 ml	< 5000 nm	
	Panda homogenizer	10 L/hr	< 250 nm	
	NS 2006 homogenizer	35 L/hr	< 250 nm	
	NS3024 homogenizer	300 L/hr	< 250 nm	
Milling	Stirred pin mill (Labstar) milling system	555 ml	< 150 nm	[28]
	Stirred pin mill (LMZ2) milling system	1600 ml	< 150 nm	
	E_{max} high-energy ball mill	50 ml/125 ml	< 80 nm	
Flash nanoprecipitation	Confined impinging jet mixer	25 μL	< 45 nm	[29]
Sonoprecipitation	InsertMPC48	02L	< 1200 nm$^\$$	[30]
Spray Drying	Nano Spray Dryer B-90	5–20 ml	< 500 nm$^\&$	[29]

TABLE 2.2

Highlights of the Challenges Faced in Nanomedicine Development

S. No	Challenges	Possible Reasons	Outcomes
1	Physicochemical characterization	Shape and size, surface properties and composition Lack of standardized FDA guidelines for characterization Process involved in nanosizing	Aggregation, sedimentation, crystalline transformation, plasma and chemical instabilities Safety of nanomedicine Thermodynamic instability
2	Safety and toxicity of nanomedicines	Lack of chronic toxicity studies of nanoparticles Lack of study protocols for plasma concentration determination of nanomedicines	Cytotoxicity, immune response Hemolysis and inflammation, mitochondrial failure and bioenergetic crisis Under- or overtherapeutic effect
3	Bioavailability and targeting	Change in physiological properties Dynamic nature of cancer cells Tumor heterogeneity Small dose ratio w.r.t. administered dose reaching the targeted site	Changed pharmacokinetic properties Multiple organ interaction, side effects
4	Scale-up and manufacturing challenges	Scale-up under GMP Use of costly excipients Steps of manufacturing like homogenization, centrifugation, extrusion, lyophilization, sterilization	High cost of production Infrastructure requirement and scale-up challenges
5	Regulatory challenges	No specific guidelines in FDA, EMA, etc. Complicated and time consuming	Difficulty in making uniform guidelines for biological and non-biological products

properties, shape, composition, molecular weight, identity, purity, stability and solubility are critical parameters that are responsible for physiological interaction of nanomedicine related to their clinical benefits. Essential physicochemical properties have been characterized by techniques which are elementary for regulatory guidelines to ensure the safety of nanomedicine. The dynamic behavior of nanomedicine makes its characterization a tedious task [31]. The process of nanosizing creates new interfaces and positive Gibbs free energy that results in thermodynamically unstable systems. This can be seen in some of the very common stability issues like aggregation, sedimentation, crystalline transformation, plasma and chemical instabilities [32]. The size of nanomedicine, which is determined by the hydrodynamic diameter of the molecule, is responsible for circulation of nanomedicine in the bloodstream, accumulation around a localized area and even the generation of the cellular response. Smaller particle size is supposed to have more apoptosis than its bigger counterparts. This has been supported by many researches *viz.* bigger size of gold nanorods showed less penetration in brain and accumulated in other organs [33]. However, mitoxantrone loaded large particle size nanoparticles showed faster delivery to bladder cancer cells. These examples show how crucial particle size is, though the exact relation between efficacy and particle size cannot be defined. Similarly, it can be seen with particle size distribution that there has been evidence of similar average particle size but different PSD, which consequently can result in changes in targeting properties, drug release rate, biocompatibility, toxicity and in vivo behaviors. It can be elucidated by the research going on in the field of nanomedicines that physicochemical properties have a huge impact on toxicity. Even safe material which is considered biocompatible can be toxic due to its nano scale. Physicochemical properties can result in increased oxidative stress as a consequence of generation of free radicals. This problem can be assessed by the multifaceted characterization of nanomedicine to ensure batch-to-batch uniformity and fewer side effects.

2.4.2 SAFETY AND TOXICITY OF NANOMEDICINES

The study of the effect of nanomaterials on the environment and the population is inevitable in the case of development of products at the nano scale. Studies have been done to identify the potential risks at the molecular, cellular and tissue levels. Organ functions can be altered due to interaction of the nanoparticle–biological interface. The possibilities of genotoxicity have also been a matter of concern due to the generated oxidative stress. There are different studies which have emphasized the interaction of nanostructured material with cells and their cellular toxicology, cytotoxicity of nanoparticles, immune response on nanoparticles, nanotoxicology methodologies and methods to combat such toxic interactions [34]. Evidence of DNA damage and cell apoptosis due to high oxidative stress on a dose-dependent manner of nano-TiO$_2$ have been reported [35]. Semiconductor nanoparticles or quantum dots composed of toxic elements undoubtedly possess health risks [36].

Though there is plethora of research work published showing the toxicity profile of nanomaterials, nanotoxicity has itself become an entire domain to study. The generation of immune response due to nanoparticles needs to be studied, but there is lack of suitable animal models to do such studies. Also, when evaluating toxicity, one should take both acute and chronic toxicity studies into consideration. Acute toxicity studies have revealed mitochondrial failure and bioenergetic crisis on mitochondria, hemolysis and inflammation. The requirements of chronic toxicity studies will completely meet the safety requirements of nanomaterials, but they are time consuming and not incorporated in many promising studies on nanomedicines.

Another concern is the protocol of the determination of drug concentration in plasma to determine the pharmacokinetic profile of nanomedicine. Following the same methodology for nanomedicine as that of small-molecule drugs can result in erroneous data, leading to misinterpretation of the results and ultimately causing under- or overtherapeutic effects.

2.4.3 BIOAVAILABILITY AND TARGETING

In the oral route of administration, the major reasons for poor bioavailability are the drug having low aqueous solubility and poor permeability of drug across biological membranes. In the former case, efforts have been made to increase the aqueous solubility and intrinsic dissolution by decreasing the particle size and many other ways; however, in the latter case, a high dose is given to achieve the desired therapeutic concentration. Chemical and enzymatic barriers and P glycoprotein efflux present inside human gastrointestinal tract (GIT) also hinders oral bioavailability. To overcome such challenges, nanotechnology-based formulations facilitate oral bioavailability by mechanisms like increasing the surface area, providing protection against enzymatic and chemical degradation, higher drug permeation, reducing drug efflux, increasing aqueous solubility and dissolution rate, providing Peyer's patch-mediated transport and enhancing lymphatic transport. However, the limitations nanotechnology-based formulations suffer are maintenance of colloidal stability, particle size and use of appropriate stabilizers. For self-emulsifying nanoemulsions, incompatibility with capsule shells, drug precipitation and low-temperature storage conditions bar their extensive use. Due to stability concerns, despite being successful in providing sustained drug effects, lipid nanocarriers have still not made it to market [37].

The targeting of nanomedicines has provided a new avenue in the treatment of serious diseases where off-target effects, serious adverse effects and short circulation time can be avoided. Targeted drug delivery enables the higher accumulation of loaded drug to the diseased site irrespective of the method of administration. Targeting the tumor cells mainly happens by virtue of enhanced permeability and retention (EPR) effects. Many successful studies on ligand-modified PEGylated nanoparticles have been demonstrated, but in reality the total percentage accumulated at the targeted site is much less with respect to the total dose administered. The drug claimed to be targeted actually interacts with multiple organs and causes unwanted adverse effects. Factors like the dynamic nature of cancer cells and heterogeneity in tumors are likely to be focused to minimize the flaws of targeted drug delivery by nanoparticles. The ambiguity in the biodistribution and location of the targeted nanocarriers after administration limits the development and approval of more target-specific nanomedicines.

2.4.4 Scale-up and Manufacturing Challenges

Large-scale production of nanoformulations has to deal with the effects of scale-up and process limitations of preparative methods. Characteristics of nanomedicines such as particle size distribution, drug encapsulation, process residual materials, colloidal stability and surface morphology are majorly affected by the scale-up process. Keeping the industrial factorial design under consideration with controlled and reproducible manufacturing methods under good manufacturing practice is very important to achieve the desired properties [38]. Uniformity in properties ensures the desired clinical efficacy of the product. Steps of manufacturing like homogenization, centrifugation, extrusion, lyophilization and sterilization pose scale-up challenges. The processes need to be robust enough to produce products in the defined range. Production of nanomedicine requires the infrastructure to manage complex and higher-cost facilities like high-pressure homogenization, high energy milling equipment and lyophilizers [39]. An understanding of the interaction between the materials employed in preparation holds importance in successful scaling up of products. Also many times, the excipients are not cost effective, making the cost of the final product too high [29].

2.4.5 Regulatory Challenges

The regulatory pathway for a product based on nanotechnology faces several hurdles for its approval, as there is not any specific guidelines for such drug products either by the FDA, EMA or any other regulatory body. The complex nature of the product is the reason regulatory guidelines for preclinical development and characterization of nanomedicine products at biophysiological level are still lacking, making them inefficient to be used in clinical practice [39].

The development of a framework for the approval of any nanosimilar product in the case where the patent of the reference product expires is another major challenge. Still, this issue did not stop the USFDA abbreviated new drug application (ANDA) approval of doxorubicin hydrochloride liposome injection 2 mg/ml by Sun Pharma in 2013, according to the approved drug database. The approval was given after the evaluation of the safety, efficacy and bioequivalence of the reference product Doxil liposome injection, 2 mg/mL, of Janssen Research and Development, LLC. There is complete information on the label about the mechanism of action of the liposome-encapsulated drug. As we need more such nanosimilar products, more efficient guidelines are required.

The different categories of biological and nonbiological materials employed in nanoparticle preparation create another problem in the development of a uniform guideline. Though the regulatory approach for biological nanomedicines is under the framework of EMA, for non-biological complex drugs, the regulatory approach is still ongoing [31].

This all creates a complicated and time-consuming regulatory pathway with high-level expertise in innovative technology and a case-by-case basis evaluation in approval of nanomedicine. But the regulatory landscape is on the verge of improvement with definitions, guidelines and cooperation being established and improved. For example, it is a basic question whether a product is qualified to be called nanomedicine. The FDA criteria for a FDA-regulated product to come under the avenue of the application of nanotechnology is: Whether a material or end product is engineered to have at least one external dimension, or an internal or surface structure, in the nanoscale range (~1–100 nm) and whether a material or end product is engineered to exhibit properties or phenomena, including physical or chemical properties or biological effects, that are attributable to its dimension(s), even if these dimensions fall outside the nanoscale range, up to 1000 nm. There are developing collaborations of the FDA and European Technology Platform on Nanomedicine (ETPN) with the Nanotechnology Characterization Laboratory (NCL) and European Nano-Characterization Laboratory (EUNCL), respectively, in order to fuel the regulatory aspect and characterization of nanomedicines [40]. Hence, it can be seen that despite so many challenges, the regulatory landscape is continuously evolving to ensure more nanotechnology-based products reach the market.

REFERENCES

1. Eric, Drexler K. *Engines of Creation: The Coming Era of Nanotechnology.* Anchor Book (1986).
2. Jain, Kewal K. "Nanomedicine: application of nanobiotechnology in medical practice." *Medical Principles and Practice* 17, no. 2 (2008): 89–101.
3. Kim, Betty YS, James T. Rutka, and Warren CW Chan. "Nanomedicine." *New England Journal of Medicine* 363, no. 25 (2010): 2434–2443.
4. Satalkar, Priya, Bernice Simone Elger, and David M. Shaw. "Defining nano, nanotechnology and nanomedicine: why should it matter?" *Science and Engineering Ethics* 22, no. 5 (2016): 1255–1276.
5. Caruso, Frank, Taeghwan Hyeon, and Vincent M. Rotello. "Nanomedicine." *Chemical Society Reviews* 41, no. 7 (2012): 2537–2538.
6. Peltonen, Leena, Jouni Hirvonen, and Timo Laaksonen. "Drug nanocrystals and nanosuspensions in medicine." In *Handbook of Nanobiomedical Research: Fundamentals, Applications and Recent Developments: Volume 1. Materials for Nanomedicine*, pp. 169–197. World Scientific (2014).
7. Jarvis, Maria, Vinu Krishnan, and Samir Mitragotri. "Nanocrystals: a perspective on translational research and clinical studies." *Bioengineering & Translational Medicine* 4, no. 1 (2019): 5–16.
8. Paliwal, Rishi, R. Jayachandra Babu, and Srinath Palakurthi. "Nanomedicine scale-up technologies: feasibilities and challenges." *AAPS Pharmaceutical Science and Technology* 15, no. 6 (2014): 1527–1534.
9. Fateminia, SM Ali, Ziqiao Wang, and Bin Liu. "Nanocrystallization: an effective approach to enhance the performance of organic molecules." *Small Methods* 1, no. 3 (2017): 1600023.
10. Chan, Hak-Kim, and Philip Chi Lip Kwok. "Production methods for nanodrug particles using the bottom-up approach." *Advanced Drug Delivery Reviews* 63, no. 6 (2011): 406–416.
11. Rivas, Claudia Janeth Martínez, Mohamad Tarhini, Waisudin Badri, Karim Miladi, Hélène Greige-Gerges, Qand Agha Nazari, Sergio Arturo Galindo Rodríguez, Rocío Álvarez Román, Hatem Fessi, and Abdelhamid Elaissari. "Nanoprecipitation process: from encapsulation to drug delivery." *International Journal of Pharmaceutics* 532, no. 1 (2017): 66–81.
12. Truong-Dinh Tran, Thao, Phuong Ha-Lien Tran, Khanh Tu Nguyen, and Van-Thanh Tran. "Nanoprecipitation: preparation and application in the field of pharmacy." *Current Pharmaceutical Design* 22, no. 20 (2016): 2997–3006.
13. Chen, Jian-Feng, Yu-Hong Wang, Fen Guo, Xin-Ming Wang, and Chong Zheng. "Synthesis of nanoparticles with novel technology: high-gravity reactive precipitation." *Industrial & Engineering Chemistry Research* 39, no. 4 (2000): 948–954.
14. Elizondo, Elisa, Jaume Veciana, and Nora Ventosa. "Nanostructuring molecular materials as particles and vesicles for drug delivery, using compressed and supercritical fluids." *Nanomedicine* 7, no. 9 (2012): 1391–1408.
15. Kumar, Raj, Sameer Vishvanath Dalvi, and Prem Felix Siril. "Nanoparticle-based drugs and formulations: current status and emerging applications." *ACS Applied Nano Materials* 3, no. 6 (2020): 4944–4961.

16. Girotra, Priti, Shailendra Kumar Singh, and Kalpana Nagpal. "Supercritical fluid technology: a promising approach in pharmaceutical research." *Pharmaceutical Development and Technology* 18, no. 1 (2013): 22–38.

17. Jiang, Tongying, Ning Han, Buwen Zhao, Yuling Xie, and Siling Wang. "Enhanced dissolution rate and oral bioavailability of simvastatin nanocrystal prepared by sonoprecipitation." *Drug Development and Industrial Pharmacy* 38, no. 10 (2012): 1230–1239.

18. Tran, Thao Truong-Dinh, Phuong Ha-Lien Tran, Minh Ngoc Uyen Nguyen, Khanh Thi My Tran, Minh Nguyet Pham, Phuc Cao Tran, and Toi Van Vo. "Amorphous Isradipine nanosuspension by the sonoprecipitation method." *International journal of pharmaceutics* 474, no. 1–2 (2014): 146–150.

19. Chaubal, Mahesh V., and Carmen Popescu. "Conversion of nanosuspensions into dry powders by spray drying: a case study." *Pharmaceutical Research* 25, no. 10 (2008): 2302–2308.

20. Lee, Sie Huey, Desmond Heng, Wai Kiong Ng, Hak-Kim Chan, and Reginald BH Tan. "Nano spray drying: a novel method for preparing protein nanoparticles for protein therapy." *International Journal of Pharmaceutics* 403, no. 1–2 (2011): 192–200.

21. Eerikäinen, Hannele, Wiwik Watanabe, Esko I. Kauppinen, and P. Petri Ahonen. "Aerosol flow reactor method for synthesis of drug nanoparticles." *European Journal of Pharmaceutics and Biopharmaceutics* 55, no. 3 (2003): 357–360.

22. Yurteri, Caner U., Rob PA Hartman, and Jan CM Marijnissen. "Producing pharmaceutical particles via electrospraying with an emphasis on nano and nano structured particles-a review." *KONA Powder and Particle Journal* 28 (2010): 91–115.

23. Muller, Rainer H., Ranjita Shegokar, and Cornelia M. Keck. "20 years of lipid nanoparticles (SLN & NLC): present state of development & industrial applications." *Current Drug Discovery Technologies* 8, no. 3 (2011): 207–227.

24. Shegokar, R., K. K. Singh, and R. H. Muller. "Production & stability of stavudine solid lipid nanoparticles—from lab to industrial scale." *International Journal of Pharmaceutics* 416, no. 2 (2011): 461–470.

25. Loh, Jing Wen, Jessica Schneider, Michelle Carter, Martin Saunders, and Lee-Yong Lim. "Spinning disc processing technology: potential for large-scale manufacture of chitosan nanoparticles." *Journal of Pharmaceutical Sciences* 99, no. 10 (2010): 4326–4336.

26. Webb, Cameron, Neil Forbes, Carla B. Roces, Giulia Anderluzzi, Gustavo Lou, Suraj Abraham, Logan Ingalls et al. "Using microfluidics for scalable manufacturing of nanomedicines from bench to GMP: a case study using protein-loaded liposomes." *International Journal of Pharmaceutics* (2020): 119266.

27. Liedtke, S., S. Wissing, R. H. Muller, and K. Mäder. "Influence of high pressure homogenisation equipment on nanodispersions characteristics." *International Journal of Pharmaceutics* 196, no. 2 (2000): 183–185.

28. Nakach, Mostafa, Jean-René Authelin, Marc-Antoine Perrin, and Harivardhan Reddy Lakkireddy. "Comparison of high pressure homogenization and stirred bead milling for the production of nanocrystalline suspensions." *International Journal of Pharmaceutics* 547, no. 1–2 (2018): 61–71.

29. Hu, Jun, Wai Kiong Ng, Yuancai Dong, Shoucang Shen, and Reginald BH Tan. "Continuous and scalable process for water-redispersible nanoformulation of poorly aqueous soluble APIs by antisolvent precipitation and spray-drying." *International Journal of Pharmaceutics* 404, no. 1–2 (2011): 198–204.

30. Gajera, Bhavin Y., Dhaval A. Shah, and Rutesh H. Dave. "Development of an amorphous nanosuspension by sonoprecipitation-formulation and process optimization using design of experiment methodology." *International Journal of Pharmaceutics* 559 (2019): 348–359.

31. Soares, Sara, João Sousa, Alberto Pais, and Carla Vitorino. "Nanomedicine: principles, properties, and regulatory issues." *Frontiers in Chemistry* 6 (2018): 360.

32. Wang, Yancai, Ying Zheng, Ling Zhang, Qiwei Wang, and Dianrui Zhang. "Stability of nanosuspensions in drug delivery." *Journal of Controlled Release* 172, no. 3 (2013): 1126–1141.

33. Caster, Joseph M., K. Yu Stephanie, Artish N. Patel, Nicole J. Newman, Zachary J. Lee, Samuel B. Warner, Kyle T. Wagner et al. "Effect of particle size on the biodistribution, toxicity, and efficacy of drug-loaded polymeric nanoparticles in chemoradiotherapy." *Nanomedicine: Nanotechnology, Biology and Medicine* 13, no. 5 (2017): 1673–1683.

34. Singh, Surya. "Nanomedicine–nanoscale drugs and delivery systems." *Journal of Nanoscience and Nanotechnology* 10, no. 12 (2010): 7906–7918.

35. Meena, R., and R. Paulraj. "Oxidative stress mediated cytotoxicity of TiO2 nano anatase in liver and kidney of Wistar rat." *Toxicological & Environmental Chemistry* 94, no. 1 (2012): 146–163.

36. Lewinski, Nastassja, Vicki Colvin, and Rebekah Drezek. "Cytotoxicity of nanoparticles." *Small* 4, no. 1 (2008): 26–49.

37. Desai, Preshita P., Abhijit A. Date, and Vandana B. Patravale. "Overcoming poor oral bioavailability using nanoparticle formulations–opportunities and limitations." *Drug Discovery Today: Technologies* 9, no. 2 (2012): e87–e95.
38. Agrahari, Vibhuti, and Vivek Agrahari. "Facilitating the translation of nanomedicines to a clinical product: challenges and opportunities." *Drug Discovery Today* 23, no. 5 (2018): 974–991.
39. Agrahari, Vivek, and Praveen Hiremath. "Challenges associated and approaches for successful translation of nanomedicines into commercial products." *Nanomedicine* (2017): 819–823.
40. Hafner, Anita, Jasmina Lovrić, Gorana Perina Lakoš, and Ivan Pepić. "Nanotherapeutics in the EU: an overview on current state and future directions." *International Journal of Nanomedicine* 9 (2014): 1005.

3 Appraisal of Nanoformulations as a Tool for Oral Bioavailability Augmentation in Nanomedicine

*Alka, Priya Singh, Raquibun Nisha, Nidhi Mishra,
Neelu Singh, Samipta Singh, Ravi Raj Pal,
Priyanka Maurya, and Shubhini A. Saraf*

3.1 INTRODUCTION

Oral administration of drugs is most widely chosen owing to its immense benefits, such as painless administration, no aid, and patient compliance. Systemic absorption via the oral route primarily requires good solubility. Drugs with poor water solubility often have low and variable oral bioavailability. Stable and efficient means of solubilizing poorly water-soluble drugs are becoming an increasingly valuable part of pharmaceutical research. Poor oral bioavailability can lead to low efficacy and the requirement of higher dosages [1]. Examples include saquinavir (minimum effective concentration (MEC) is 100 ng/ml, but the oral dose required to achieve its MEC is 1200 mg/day, taken as 600 mg three times a day) [2], acetaminophen (paracetamol), and danazol (maximum therapeutic dose ranging from 600–800 mg twice a day; 6.2% bioavailability) [3]. Also, the high dosage of the drug eventually contributes to its wastage, which is not economical.

Bioavailability (BA) can be defined, according to the United States Food and Drug Administration (USFDA), as "the rate and extent to which a drug product absorbs the active ingredient or active moiety and is made accessible at the site of action" [4]. The bioavailability of a drug administered intravenously, by definition, is considered 100%. Delivery of drugs via other routes mostly decreases bioavailability because of inadequate absorption or first-pass metabolism.

In the vast area of nanomedicine, various nanoscale technologies have been applied to healthcare and nanoformulations or nanocarriers have gained considerable significance. They have established impressive performance over traditional dosage types in lipophilic or water-insoluble oral drug delivery [1, 5] by improving bioavailability, as shown in Figure 3.1. Also, the customized nanomedicine approach encompasses the right treatment strategy and associated theranostic approach. Therapy and diagnosis agents have merged for better output [6]. The purpose of theranostics is to establish the correct medication at the proper time and location. The knowledge of the condition and the genetic sequence makes it easier to treat individual patients. The reasons for poor bioavailability and approaches to enhancing oral bioavailability through different nanoformulations are the premise of this chapter. They are discussed in detail in the related sections.

3.2 REASONS FOR LOW BIOAVAILABILITY

Bioavailability is a complex phenomenon that depends on the attributes of a drug and the properties of biological membranes like the gut mucosa. Some crucial reasons for the low bioavailability of drugs are enumerated in the following.

DOI: 10.1201/9781003130055-3

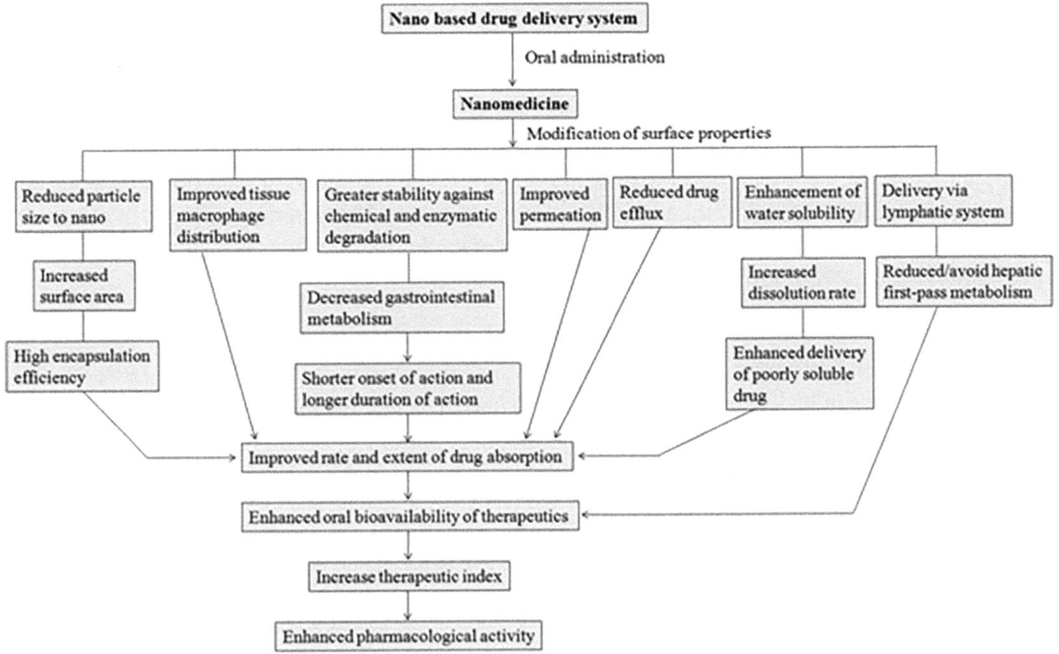

FIGURE 3.1 Schematic representation of the potential mechanism of enhancing oral BA.

3.2.1 Physiological Factors

3.2.1.1 Poor Aqueous Solubility

Solubility is important for drugs with low bioavailability. The gastrointestinal tract contents are aqueous. Thus, a substance with poor aqueous solubility has a low saturation solubility, generally associated with low dissolution rates of the dosage form, contributing to poor oral bioavailability [7].

3.2.1.2 Inappropriate Partition Coefficient

Exceedingly hydrophilic drugs cannot penetrate the gastrointestinal mucosa, since the gastrointestinal mucus membrane is lipophilic. A drug requires ample aqueous solubility to dissolve into the gastrointestinal content and permeate the water-filled capillaries called the tight junctions between adjoining cells. Log P and log D_x values help in defining the lipophilicity of a drug molecule. Adequate lipid solubility is required to make it easier to break into a lipid membrane by crossing through the cell and then into the systemic circulation to optimize its absorption. Drugs with a log P (log of partition coefficient at a pH where all molecules are neutral) value of 0 to 3 and Log D_x (log of distribution coefficient at particular pH where the molecules are in an ionic/neutral state) values of 1 to 3 often have better absorptivity than ones with log D_x above 3, where solubility could be lower and permeability could be greater. When log D_x is below 1, solubility could be high, but permeability could be low. Hence moderation of solubility and permeability is required for better bioavailability, which exists when the log D_x value is also moderate, that is, 1 to 3 [8].

3.2.1.3 First-Pass Metabolism

The intestinal wall and the liver are the common sites of metabolism, which must be passed through by oral drugs (metabolism of a drug before it reaches systemic circulation). A certain quantity of drug is lost in this transit. Consequently, many medications may be metabolized, and bioavailability decreases before sufficient plasma levels are reached [9].

3.2.1.4 High Gastric Emptying Rate

Typically, drugs are taken orally. They are not absorbed by the stomach, usually, but can be absorbed from the small intestines very easily. Factors that influence the gastric emptying rate can thus alter the absorption rate of most oral drugs. The rate of gastric drainage is affected by food; hormones; posture; peritoneal inflammation; extreme pain; stomach ulcers; diabetes; other metabolic diseases; drugs such as alcohol, anticholinergics, and opioids; and drugs blocking for ganglions, antacids, and metoclopramide. In most cases, the rise in gastric emptying and gastrointestinal motility improves the drug's absorption rate. In contrast, an absorption rate decline is correlated with an increase in gastrointestinal motility for digoxin and riboflavin [10].

3.2.1.5 High Molecular Weight of the Drug

The numbers of rotatable bonds decrease in larger molecules, while the polar surface increases, and so does the number of hydrogen bonds. All these relate to high molecular weight and low bioavailability [11].

3.2.1.6 Effect of Food

The concurrent administration of grapefruit juice is more likely to impact drugs with considerable first-pass metabolism, resulting in 5 to 30% less bioavailability. The absorption of tetracyclines can be decreased when chelates in the intestines are produced, with foodstuffs and dairy products with high calcium levels [12].

3.2.1.7 Restriction by Intestinal Barriers

The intestinal epithelium is the largest and most significant barrier to the outside world in a single-cell layer. It behaves as a selectively permeable barrier for the absorption and defense of intraluminal toxins, antigens, and enteric flora of nutrients, electrolytes, and water. The epithelium retains its selective barrier role by forming a complex network of proteins that bind adjacent cells mechanically to screen the intercellular region [13].

3.2.2 Physicochemical and Biopharmaceutical Factors

3.2.2.1 Lipinski's Rule of 5

The rule of 5 foresees weak absorption or permeation if there are more than five H-bond donors, ten H-bond receivers, a molecular weight higher than 500, and a measured log-P (cLog-P) higher than 5 in the drug discovery environment (Figure 3.2). However, Lipinski says that the rule of 5 only applies to compounds that are not active transporter substrates [14].

3.2.2.2 Polar Surface Area

Oral bioavailability depends upon molecular flexibility as well as the surface area of the polar portions. Increased rotational freedom can lead to a broader spread cross-section in the case of versatility, thereby affecting permeability adversely. On the other hand, such versatility may reduce the solution's crystallinity and thus improve aqueous solubility and absorption [15].

3.2.2.3 pH Partition Theory and pKa

Partition coefficients are useful for the calculation of the body's drug distribution. When a liquid or solid is put into a combination of two non-saturated liquids, it is split between the two phases to saturate each. Hydrophobic drugs are primarily absorbed by hydrophobic areas such as the cellular membrane and have a high partition coefficient. Conversely, hydrophilic medications are found mainly in water-rich parts, such as the cytoplasm, with low octanol/water partition coefficients [16]. Thus moderation is required to cross lipophilic membranes and solubilize in the cytoplasm. Hence the topic is not a simple, cut-and-dried solution but a complex phenomenon where extremes of hydrophilicity or lipophilicity do not work.

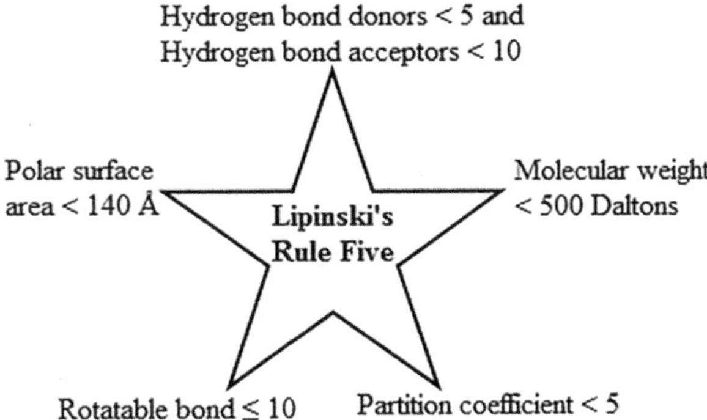

FIGURE 3.2 Diagrammatic representation of Lipinski's rule of five.

3.2.2.4 Particle Size

After reducing particle size, the dissolution velocity could significantly increase while at the same time improving bioavailability, improved saturation solubility, expanded surface area, and a thinner diffusion layer [17].

3.2.2.5 Polymorphism and Drug Amorphous Forms

The effect of medicines and their solubility, dissolution, and bioavailability are linked to drug polymorphism. The use of thermodynamically stable polymorphs is popular since no adjustments have to be made during storage. Better bioavailability can be provided by the most durable and less soluble form. A metastable way to achieve better clinical benefit can therefore be beneficial [18].

3.3 HUMAN INTESTINAL TRANSPORTERS AND THEIR ROLE IN BIOAVAILABILITY

Transporters play a vital role in medication disposal, pharmaceutical focusing, DDI interactions, and pharmaceutical toxicity. Transporters (SLCs) and effluxes (ABCs) contact medication pharmacokinetics and pharmacodynamics.

3.3.1 Primary Transporters Expressed on the Intestine

3.3.1.1 ATP-Binding Cassette Transporters

Transporters with a binding ATP cassette (ABC) form an entire family of integrative membrane proteins responsible for the multi-substrate membrane translocalization with the power of ATP. The nuclear-based motor, which drives transport, is supplied by highly preserved ABC domains of ABC carriers [19].

3.3.1.1.1 P-glycoprotein, MDR1, ABCB1

P-gp is the most common transport business of the ABC and was the first to be detected in humans where drug resistance in cancer therapies plays a critical function. The gene ABCB1/MDRI is present in various human tissues. P-glycoprotein utilizes these genes, and as a result, it is known to be a very significant transporter of the human transmembrane. It is found on the gut's apical surface, bile ducts, kidneys, placenta, luminous surface of the brain, and testes of the capillary endothelial cells [20].

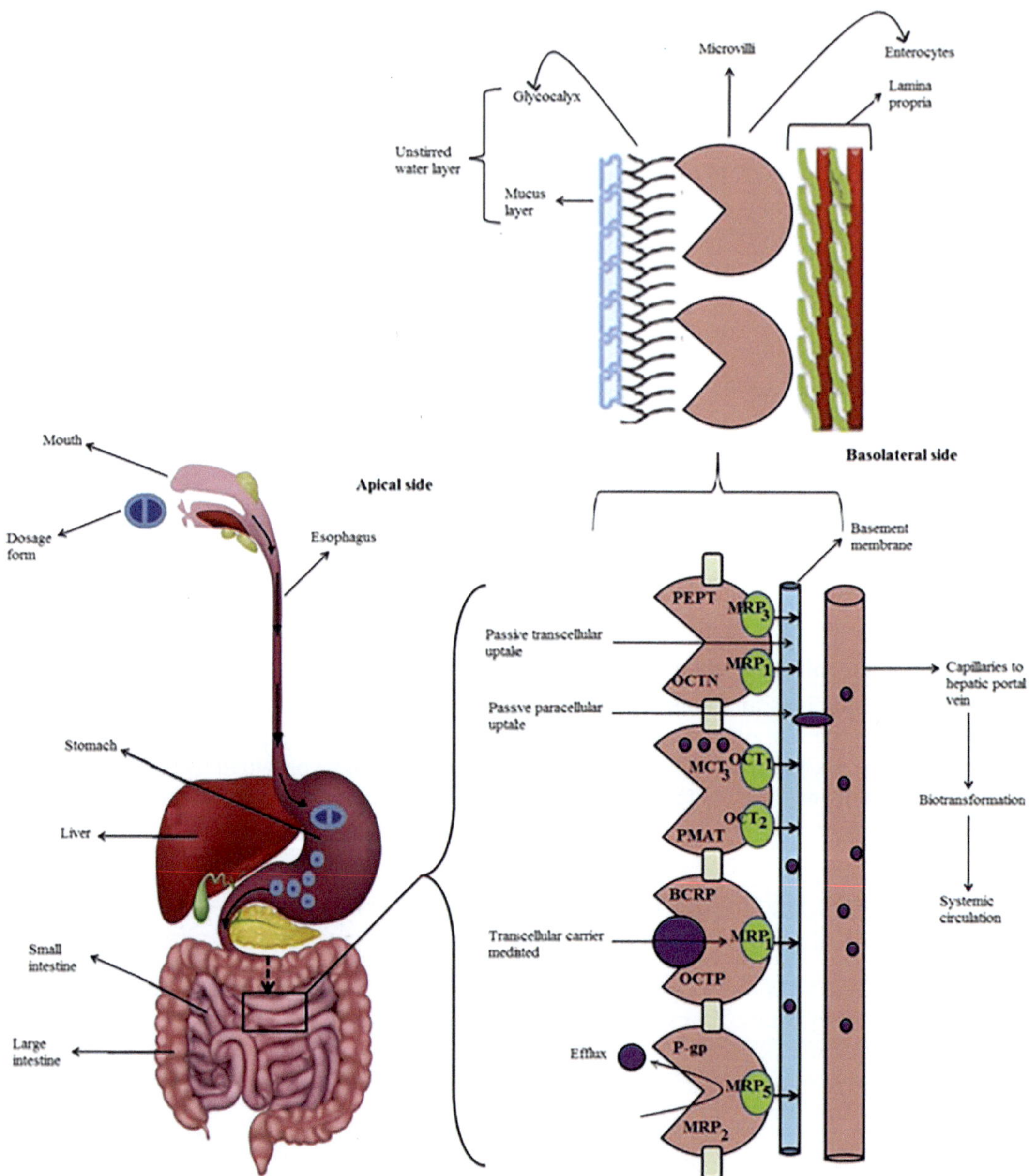

FIGURE 3.3 Targeted therapy via intestinal transporters for enhanced BA.

3.3.1.1.2 *Multidrug Resistance-Associated Protein 2, ABCC2*

MRP2 (ABCC2) carriers are another ATP-binding cassette present on the duodenum, jejunum, and renal proximal tubular epithelial cells, chain-like membrane as well on the apical membrane of enterocytes. It mediates glutathione, sulfate, and glucuronide conjugates of narcotically modified drugs, toxins, and bilious in the canaliculus. MRP2 can also hold some non-conjugated medicines, including ampicillin, ceftriaxone, methotrexate, irinotecan, and statins [21].

3.3.1.1.3 Breast Cancer Resistance Protein, ABCG2

The BCRP (gene symbol ABCG2) is an efflux transporter of the ABC. The name BCRP was given because of its origin. BCRP is known to throw out drugs from various locations such as the intestine and liver and may be responsible for the barrier function at the interface of the blood–brain, blood–placenta, and blood–testis barriers as part of the self-defense system for the organism. BCRP works physiologically. BCRP has recognized as target for many new anti-cancer drugs in clinical use, including traditional chemotherapy and targeted small therapeutic molecules [22].

3.3.1.2 Organic Ion Transporters

Numerous widely prescribed medications are critically affected by the organic anion transporters. These carriers have multiple conditions, including transcriptional control, sex-dependent regulation, and genetic change, which affect their expression and behavior. Besides, these transporters have been well reported. They have an essential role in managing the medications and the production of different conditions, such as nephrotoxicity and idiopathic hyperuricemia in the household [23].

3.3.1.2.1 Organic Cation Transporter, SLC22A

OCT is one of the heaviest liver transporters. OCTs are called poly-specific membrane carriers operating via the mediation of hepatic intakes, including dopamine, serotonin, and histamine, of hydrophilic compounds that are small and positive. In addition to OCTs' endogenous transportation, several different prescribed drugs such as antidiabetic agents and opioid analgesics have also been found as a drug transporter(s) [24].

3.3.1.2.2 Novel Organic Cation Transporter, SLC22A

SLC22-family transporters clades belong to members of major superfamily facilitators (MSFs) and are representative of a mechanistically different group of systems called organic anion transporters (OATs and URAT1). Although these are multi-selective, they play a key function in clearing endogenous as well as xenobiotic compounds in both renal and hepatic areas [25].

3.3.1.2.3 Organic Anion-Transporting Polypeptide, SLCO

Organic anion transporting polypeptides are part of the SLCO superfamily (OATPs). The 11 human OATPs consist of six families and ten subfamilies based on the identity of amino acids. These proteins are found throughout the body on the cellular plasma membrane. They have 12 TM domains and a multiplied putative glycosylation position intracellular terminal. A wide variety of amphiphilic substrates, including many drugs and toxins, mediate the sodium-independent use of OATPs since these proteins are multi-specific [26].

3.3.1.2.4 H+/peptide co-transporter, SLC15A1

H+-coupled oligopeptide symporters with predicted mucosal-topology are the H+-coupling transporters 1 and 2 (PEPT1, PEPT2, SLC15A1, SLC15A2, respectively). Recently, two new type 1 (PHT1, SLC15A4) and type 2 (PHT2, SLC15A3) peptide/histidine transporters have been identified in mammals. PEPT1 and PEPT2 are translocated to dipeptides and tripeptides that are made due to protein catabolism. They are pharmacologically essential because they may take a broad variety of mimetic medicines, like captopril, enalapril, and fosinopril, as well as antibiotics and penicillin classes [27].

3.4 NANOFORMULATION-BASED TECHNIQUES FOR ENHANCEMENT OF ORAL BIOAVAILABILITY

To overcome the shortcomings of poor oral bioavailability, nano-based systems are often utilized. The particle size reduction to nanometer scale improves the surface to volume ratio, thereby

TABLE 3.1

A Compilation of Research Reports on Nanoformulations for Oral Administration with Increased BA

Drug Delivery System	Drug	Core Constituent (Polymer/Lipid)	Method of Preparation	References
Solid lipid nanoparticles (SLNs)	Nimodipine	Palmitic acid	Hot homogenization and ultra-sonication method	[28]
Nano lipid carriers (NLCs)	Saquinavir	Dextran protamine, Precirol ATO15	High-pressure homogenization	[29]
Nanoparticles	Paclitaxel	Carbon (folate-polyethyleneimine functionalized)	Solvent evaporation	[30]
Solid self-emulsifying drug delivery system (SEDDS)	Dexibuprofen	Polyglycolyzed glycerides, oils	Pseudo-ternary phase diagram development followed by vortexing	[31]
Polymeric micelles	Paclitaxel	Pluronic F-127, Pluronic F-68	Dialysis	[32]
Nanoemulsion	Paclitaxel	Capryol 90, Labrasol, glycerol triacetate	Construction of the ternary phase diagram following the spontaneous method	[33]
Nanocrystals	Bicalutamide	Labrasol, Pluronic F-68	Antisolvent precipitation	[34]
Liposomes	Itraconazole	Lecithin and sodium deoxycholate	Thin-film hydration	[35]

increasing the drug's dissolution rate and achieving higher bioavailability. Different nanotechnology-based drug delivery systems are proposed (Table 3.1). Some common nanocarriers and their applications are outlined in the following.

3.4.1 Polymeric Nanoparticles

Drugs are encapsulated inside a matrix of various polymers depending upon the release characteristics desired from them, and suitable legands are attached to the surface for targeting. They can be prepared as nanospheres or nanocapsules using nano-precipitation, double emulsification, polymer coating, and emulsification diffusion. In the gastrointestinal (GI) tract, they have shown excellent stability, displaying required properties along with drug release and offering tremendous tissue targeting with enhanced cellular uptake. Polymeric nanoparticles prepared using zein have improved the oral bioavailability of insulin, per a study by Inchaurraga et al. [36].

3.4.2 Solid Lipid Nanoparticles

SLNs are composed of either one or a mixture of lipids with a high melting point. Since SLNs are made utilizing lipids, they also usually metabolized by the system in the way a lipid from food would be treated. Moreover, relative to liposomes and emulsions, these solid lipid carriers are known to be more robust and may thus offer superior protection for encapsulated drugs. SLNs enhanced the oral bioavailability of Felodipine (up to 3.17 times) [37], glibenclamide [38], and others.

3.4.3 Nanostructured Lipid Carriers

These are second-generation nanoparticles composed of a lipid blend. A film of surfactant is able to cover its surface, thereby minimizing the risk of coalescence. Since NLCs are composed of a blend of solid lipids and liquid lipids, they form lattice structures which enable higher drug loading. This is the reason NLCs are preferred over SLNs. NLCs have reported improving the bioavailability of many drugs such as candesartan cilexetil up to two-fold [39], nintedanib up to three-fold [40], and so on.

3.4.4 Lipid Drug Conjugates

Hydrophilic drugs are conjugated to lipids (e.g. with steroids, glycerides) to enhance their lipophilicity via LDCs and bioavailability. It also provides several other benefits, like delivering the drug with high loading capacity to improve targeting and reducing the drug's adverse effects. LDCs have been shown to enhance methotrexate bioavailability, and the lymphatic transport mechanism was demonstrated as the prevailing mechanism. Also, LDCs drastically augmented the intestinal lymphatics retention time [41].

3.4.5 Liposomes

A liposome is a phospholipidic drug delivery system derived from natural and synthetic sources. Phospholipids are the main ingredient along with cholesterol to maintain the uniformity and stability of the system. However, due to the aqueous and lipid organization structure, the phospholipid is more feasible for encapsulating both hydrophilic and hydrophobic drugs. Liposomes containing sodium deoxycholate improved the oral bioavailability of itraconazole up to nearly 1.67-fold compared to commercial capsules (SPORANOX) [35]. Per Bi et al. (2020), the AUC value of nifedipine was approximately 10 times improved via liposomes than free nifedipine [42].

3.4.6 Niosomes

Biocompatible, non-immunogenic niosomes produced by self-assembled nonionic surfactants can encapsulate both hydrophilic and lipophilic drugs. Niosomes have shown promising results in improving oral bioavailability, structurally similar to liposomes. The vesicles' small size could give a large interfacial area for intestinal absorption after oral administration. Nisha et al. (2020) developed β-sitosterol (BS)-loaded PEGylated niosomes (BSMF). The result showed that BSMF revealed significantly higher plasma t1/2, Cmax, and Tmax than pure BS [43].

3.4.7 Lipid-Polymer Hybrid Nanoparticles

LPHNPs have been widely developed to resolve the disadvantages of liposomes and polymeric nanoparticles. LPHNPs are polymeric nanoparticles protected by lipid bilayers and, as polymeric nanoparticles, have integrated properties of biocompatibility and integrity of lipids. The external lipid layer protects the release of hydrophilic drugs to maximize the performance of their encapsulation. Therefore, the inclusion of lipids in LPHNPs provides many advantages, such as lipophilic and hydrophilic drug encapsulation, precise targeting by surface modification, and enhancing the bioavailability of poorly soluble drugs. Tang et al. (2020) developed LPHNPs for improving oral absorption of enoxaparin. They concluded that the oral bioavailability of enoxaparin was distinctly augmented about 6.8-fold through LPHNs [44].

3.4.8 Self-Emulsifying Drug Delivery Systems

SEDDs consist of oil, surfactant, and cosolvent to emulsify in water under moderate gastrointestinal tract agitation conditions. SEDDS are isotropic mixtures that, upon GIT digestive motility, quickly generate o/w emulsions. The stability, water solubility, and bioavailability of lipophilic drugs are improved by SEDDS [45]. Zhang et al. (2019) prepared isoliquiritigenin (ISL)-loaded SMEDDS for the enhancement of oral bioavailability. It was revealed that the oral bioavailability of the ISL-SMEDDS improved 4.71-fold compared to free ISL solution [45].

3.4.9 POLYMERIC MICELLES

PMs are capable of self-aggregation similar to micelles. Because they are made of sections with hydrophilic as well as hydrophobic parts, they aggregate into micelle structures by aligning the hydrophilic ends together and conversely the hydrophobic portions towards the opposite ends. When drugs are enclosed in the hydrophilic or the hydrophobic channels thus formed, it results in bioavailability enhancement. Gu et al. (2020) prepared chrysophanol micelles (CLMs) for the enhancement of oral bioavailability. The outcome revealed that the bioavailability of CLM relative to free drugs was significantly improved (about 3.4 times) [46].

3.4.10 NANOCRYSTALS

NCs are characterized by surface stabilizers as nano-sized drug particles and have been extensively researched and discussed for their solubility saturation, dissolution rate improvement, and increased oral bioavailability. They can be developed through two primary methods, size reduction by mechanical attrition of nanoparticles of bulky crystals or aggregation of minute particles to form nanosized crystals [47]. Seto et al. (2019) developed a lutein nanocrystal (NC/LT) formulation with enhanced oral bioavailability. NC/LT administered orally showed 15.2 times greater oral absorption than crystalline LT [48]. Piet al. (2018) developed a baicalein nano-cocrystal (BE-NCT) to increase the dissolution rate and oral bioavailability. The result revealed that the bioavailability of BE-NCT was increased up to 6.02-fold as compared to BE coarse powder [47].

3.4.11 NANOEMULSIONS

NEs are thermodynamically stable, transparent water and oil dispersions. They are stabilized by an interfacial film of surfactant molecules at a droplet size of 100 nm. NE has a more significant solubilization potential and can be equipped with low energy inputs (heat or mixing) and long durability. Jha et al. (2020) prepared an etoposide nanoemulsion (ETP-NE) to enhance its oral bioavailability. The result showed that the ETP-NE oral bioavailability was enhanced up to 1752% and 224% compared to water-dispersed and commercial ETP emulsion [49].

3.5 IN-VITRO AND IN-VIVO PREDICTION MODELS

3.5.1 IN-VITRO PREDICTION MODELS

In-vitro high throughput–absorption distribution metabolism excretion (HT-ADME) tools may be utilized to assess and predict physiological properties such as permeability, metabolism, drug–drug interactions, and toxicities. *In-vitro* permeability prediction models depend on simulation with the intestinal epithelium. Various cell line models that simulate human epithelium like Caco-2 cells (human colon adenocarcinoma cells), Madin Darby Canine Kidney (MDCK) epithelial cells, LLCPK1 (pig kidney epithelial cells), 2/4/A1(rat fetal intestinal epithelial cells), HT-29 (human colon), TC-7(Caco-2 subclone), and IEC-18 (rat small intestine cell line) are utilized to estimate permeability [50]. Moreover, another model has been developed to estimate drugs in other parts of the body like the brain microvessel endothelial cells (BMEC) [51] and human-induced pluripotent stem cell (iPSC)–derived brain endothelial cells [52], which are utilized to predict unbound drugs in CNS.

IntrCaco2 is a tool developed by AstraZeneca to measure molecule permeability in the Caco-2 cell line. It is a concentration-independent permeability measurement that is not constrained by an active transport mechanism and is utilized to analyze the amount absorbed after oral administration [53]. Madin-Darby Canine Kidney is another cell line used for permeability appraisal [54]. MDCK cells are different from Caco-2 calls regarding their origin (dog kidney cells vs human colon carcinoma cells) and the cultivation period (3 weeks vs 3 days). They are also differentiated based upon the availability of active transporters and drug-metabolizing enzymes. Permeability and gut absorption relationship are less simulated in MDCK cells [55].

3.5.2 IN-VIVO PREDICTION MODELS/PRE-CLINICAL STRATEGIES

3.5.2.1 Invasive Methods

Despite several in-vitro models, the necessity of in-vivo experimentation cannot be overcome by in vitro efforts. Various animal species, such as rats and mice, are used to assess multiple parameters, such as Cmax, Tmax, AUC, MRT, and relative/absolute bioavailability in respective animals. Tmax and Cmax are directly obtained, which is the peak time and peak concentration obtained from each subject. After the dose is given, the drug's intravenous bolus concentrations are always declining [56]. The terminal half-life (t_2) is a half-life of mono-exponential functions. This parameter tells the decay of concentration of drug in the terminals [57]. The area under the curve is a parameter used in diverse ways that depend upon the experimental context. This is used as a catalogue for the drug's exposure in tissues compared to the drug levels in tissues [57].

3.5.2.2 Non-Invasive Methods

Some techniques may be used as non-invasive tools for assessing the pharmacokinetic profile, such as magnetic marker monitoring, gamma scintigraphy, and accelerator mass spectrometry [3].

3.6 PATENT REPORTS BASED ON NANOMEDICINE/NANOTECHNOLOGY

The present patent literature on nanomedicines for orally administered agents shows the potential of nanotechnology in drug delivery. The oral route can be explored to deliver therapeutics such as siRNA, chemotherapeutics, vaccines, and drugs that are degraded when administered in native forms. These inventions prove beneficial for drugs with low oral bioavailability as well as targeted drug delivery. There is now an ever-increasing trend in patenting the technology related to the oral administration of drugs. A few examples are listed in Table 3.2.

3.7 BASIC REGULATORY CONSIDERATIONS AND PROSPECTS IN BIOAVAILABILITY STUDIES

Under existing sanctuary authorities, the FDA regulates nano-products following the specific legal requirements for the specific type under its jurisdiction [3]. The Centre for Drug Evaluation and Research (CDER) of the FDA has been working for many years to ensure the properties of nanomaterials as a result of their application in drug products. Ongoing research projects of CDER include work related to identifying current test method limitations for assessing the safety and efficacy of nano-based therapeutics and nano-applications on product characteristics [63]. The FDA has issued several guidance documents on topics related to nanotechnology applications in FDA-regulated products [64]. The FDA Nanotechnology Task Force was established in August 2006 and is responsible for determining the regulatory approaches which encourage continued nano-based FDA regulated product development which is innovative, safe, and effective. It recognizes and proposes ways of solving any current expertise or policy discrepancies within the scientific community in nanotechnology [65]. In 2019, guidelines for nano-pharmaceuticals have also been issued by DBT, India, in coordination with CDSCO and ICMR, India [66].

TABLE 3.2
List of Patent Reports Based on Nanoformulations

S. No.	Title	Patent Number	API (Active Pharmaceutical Ingredient)	Inventors/References
1.	Self-micro/nanoemulsifying drug carrying system for oral use of rosuvastatin	WO2015142307	Rosuvastatin	[58]
2.	Lipophilic nanoparticles for drug delivery	US10568898B2	Doxorubicin	[59]
3.	Exosomal compositions and methods for the treatment of disease	US10799457B2	siRNA	[60]
4.	Pharmaceutical composition consisting of RNA with alkali metal as counter ion and formulated with dications	CA2821622C	RNA	[61]
5.	Dry powder composition comprising long-chain RNA	US10729654B2	Long-chain RNA	[62]

3.8　CONCLUSION AND FUTURE OUTLOOK

Nano-based formulations are vital to improving the oral absorption of poorly water-soluble drugs and their bioavailability profile. Significant advantages of nanoformulations include decreased dosage levels, bioavailability, drug effectiveness, reduced toxicity, and better patient acceptance. Oral bioavailability can be lowered because of the drug due to efflux carriers that transport drugs out of the cell. MDR1 and MRP2 were identified as necessary to improve oral bioavailability. However, nanomedicines do have certain application limitations, such as scale-up challenges, cost-effectiveness, and long-term stability problems. Obstacles such as these cannot deter the advancement and advantages of modern drug delivery technologies. Nanotechnology provides formulation scientists with the capability to broaden their technology base to suitably address existing medication problems and improve patient acceptance and therapeutic efficacy. Personalised nanotherapeutics, the design of a drug delivery device based on patient clinical phenotypes, is the future of drug delivery. All drugs will be administered at the appropriate time and correct dosing, for the precise duration, anywhere in the body with specificity, efficiency, and better outcomes, as the understanding of the human physiology advances.

REFERENCES

1. Sharma, M., R. Sharma, and D.K. Jain, Nanotechnology based approaches for enhancing oral bioavailability of poorly water soluble antihypertensive drugs. *Scientifica*, 2016. **2016**.
2. Hetal, T., P. Bindesh, and T. Sneha, A review on techniques for oral bioavailability enhancement of drugs. *Health*, 2010. **4**(3): p. 033.
3. Pathak, K. and S. Raghuvanshi, Oral bioavailability: issues and solutions via nanoformulations. *Clinical Pharmacokinetics*, 2015. **54**(4): p. 325–357.
4. Chow, S.C., Bioavailability and bioequivalence in drug development. *Wiley Interdisciplinary Reviews: Computational Statistics*, 2014. **6**(4): p. 304–312.
5. Ma, X. and R.O. Williams, Polymeric nanomedicines for poorly soluble drugs in oral delivery systems: an update. *Journal of Pharmaceutical Investigation*, 2018. **48**(1): p. 61–75.

6. Fornaguera, C. and M.J. García-Celma, Personalized nanomedicine: a revolution at the nanoscale. *Journal of Personalized Medicine*, 2017. **7**(4): p. 12.
7. Lennernas, H., Modeling gastrointestinal drug absorption requires more in vivo biopharmaceutical data: experience from in vivo dissolution and permeability studies in humans. *Current Drug Metabolism*, 2007. **8**(7): p. 645–657.
8. Vemulapalli, V., N. Ghilzai, and B.R. Jasti, Physicochemical characteristics that influence the transport of drugs across intestinal barrier. *AAPS Newsmagazine*, 2007. **18**: p. 18–21.
9. Derendorf, H., et al., Pharmacokinetics and oral bioavailability of hydrocortisone. *The Journal of Clinical Pharmacology*, 1991. **31**(5): p. 473–476.
10. Nimmo, W., Drugs, diseases and altered gastric emptying. *Clinical Pharmacokinetics*, 1976. **1**(3): p. 189–203.
11. Veber, D.F., et al., Molecular properties that influence the oral bioavailability of drug candidates. *Journal of Medicinal Chemistry*, 2002. **45**(12): p. 2615–2623.
12. Werle, M., A. Samhaber, and A. Bernkop-Schnürch, Degradation of teriparatide by gastro-intestinal proteolytic enzymes. *Journal of Drug Targeting*, 2006. **14**(3): p. 109–115.
13. Groschwitz, K.R. and S.P. Hogan, Intestinal barrier function: molecular regulation and disease pathogenesis. *Journal of Allergy and Clinical Immunology*, 2009. **124**(1): p. 3–20.
14. Benet, L.Z., et al., BDDCS, the rule of 5 and drugability. *Advanced Drug Delivery Reviews*, 2016. **101**: p. 89–98.
15. Lu, J.J., et al., Influence of molecular flexibility and polar surface area metrics on oral bioavailability in the rat. *Journal of Medicinal Chemistry*, 2004. **47**(24): p. 6104–6107.
16. Chaurasia, G., Effect of acidic, neutral and basic pH on solubility and partition-coefficient of benzoic acid between water-benzene system. *International Journal of Pharmaceutical Sciences and Research*, 2017. **8**(6): p. 2637–2640.
17. Sun, J., et al., Effect of particle size on solubility, dissolution rate, and oral bioavailability: evaluation using coenzyme Q10 as naked nanocrystals. *International Journal of Nanomedicine*, 2012. **7**: p. 5733.
18. Ainurofiq, A., et al., The effect of polymorphism on active pharmaceutical ingredients: a review. *International Journal of Research in Pharmaceutical Sciences*, 2020. **11**(2): p. 1621–1630.
19. Rees, D.C., E. Johnson, and O. Lewinson, ABC transporters: the power to change. *Nature Reviews Molecular Cell Biology*, 2009. **10**(3): p. 218–227.
20. Zhou, S.-F., Structure, function and regulation of P-glycoprotein and its clinical relevance in drug disposition. *Xenobiotica*, 2008. **38**(7–8): p. 802–832.
21. Hagenbuch, B., MRP2, multiple drug resistance protein 2, in *xPharm: The Comprehensive Pharmacology Reference*, S.J. Enna and D.B. Bylund, Editors. 2007, Elsevier: New York. p. 1–5.
22. Nakanishi, T. and D.D. Ross, Breast cancer resistance protein (BCRP/ABCG2): its role in multidrug resistance and regulation of its gene expression. *Chinese Journal of Cancer*, 2012. **31**(2): p. 73.
23. Riedmaier, A.E., et al., Organic anion transporters and their implications in pharmacotherapy. *Pharmacological Reviews*, 2012. **64**(3): p. 421–449.
24. Chandrasekaran, B., et al., Computer-aided prediction of pharmacokinetic (ADMET) properties, in *Dosage Form Design Parameters*. 2018, Academic Press. p. 731–755.
25. Pelis, R.M. and S.H. Wright, SLC22, SLC44, and SLC47 transporters—organic anion and cation transporters: molecular and cellular properties, in *Current Topics in Membranes*. 2014, Academic Press. p. 233–261.
26. Hagenbuch, B., SLC22 family of organic cation and anion transporters (version 2019.4) in the IUPHAR/BPS guide to pharmacology database. *IUPHAR/BPS Guide to Pharmacology CITE*, 2019. **2019**(4).
27. Scherrmann, J.M., 5.04—the biology and function of transporters, in *Comprehensive Medicinal Chemistry II*, J.B. Taylor and D.J. Triggle, Editors. 2007, Elsevier: Oxford. p. 51–85.
28. Chalikwar, S.S., et al., Formulation and evaluation of Nimodipine-loaded solid lipid nanoparticles delivered via lymphatic transport system. *Colloids and surfaces B: Biointerfaces*, 2012. **97**: p. 109–116.
29. Beloqui, A., et al., Dextran–protamine coated nanostructured lipid carriers as mucus-penetrating nanoparticles for lipophilic drugs. *International Journal of Pharmaceutics*, 2014. **468**(1–2): p. 105–111.
30. Wan, L., et al., Folate-polyethyleneimine functionalized mesoporous carbon nanoparticles for enhancing oral bioavailability of paclitaxel. *International Journal of Pharmaceutics*, 2015. **484**(1–2): p. 207–217.
31. Balakrishnan, P., et al., Enhanced oral bioavailability of dexibuprofen by a novel solid self-emulsifying drug delivery system (SEDDS). *European Journal of Pharmaceutics and Biopharmaceutics*, 2009. **72**(3): p. 539–545.

32. Dahmani, F.Z., et al., Enhanced oral bioavailability of paclitaxel in pluronic/LHR mixed polymeric micelles: preparation, in vitro and in vivo evaluation. *European Journal of Pharmaceutical Sciences*, 2012. **47**(1): p. 179–189.

33. Choudhury, H., et al., Improvement of cellular uptake, in vitro antitumor activity and sustained release profile with increased bioavailability from a nanoemulsion platform. *International Journal of Pharmaceutics*, 2014. **460**(1–2): p. 131–143.

34. Pokharkar, V.B., T. Malhi, and L. Mandpe, Bicalutamide nanocrystals with improved oral bioavailability: in vitro and in vivo evaluation. *Pharmaceutical Development and Technology*, 2013. **18**(3): p. 660–666.

35. Li, Z., et al., Development of Liposome containing sodium deoxycholate to enhance oral bioavailability of itraconazole. *Asian Journal of Pharmaceutical Sciences*, 2017. **12**(2): p. 157–164.

36. Inchaurraga, L., et al., Zein-based nanoparticles for the oral delivery of insulin. *Drug Delivery and Translational Research*, 2020. **10**: p. 1601–1611.

37. He, Y., et al., Enhanced oral bioavailability of felodipine from solid lipid nanoparticles prepared through effervescent dispersion technique. *AAPS Pharmaceutical Science and Technology*, 2020. **21**(5): p. 1–10.

38. Elbahwy, I.A., et al., Enhancing bioavailability and controlling the release of glibenclamide from optimized solid lipid nanoparticles. *Journal of Drug Delivery Science and Technology*, 2017. **38**: p. 78–89.

39. Anwar, W., et al., Enhancing the oral bioavailability of candesartan cilexetil loaded nanostructured lipid carriers: in vitro characterization and absorption in rats after oral administration. *Pharmaceutics*, 2020. **12**(11): p. 1047.

40. Zhu, Y., et al., Nanostructured lipid carriers as oral delivery systems for improving oral bioavailability of nintedanib by promoting intestinal absorption. *International Journal of Pharmaceutics*, 2020. **586**: p. 119569.

41. Agrawal, U., et al., Tailored polymer–lipid hybrid nanoparticles for the delivery of drug conjugate: dual strategy for brain targeting. *Colloids and Surfaces B: Biointerfaces*, 2015. **126**: p. 414–425.

42. Bi, Y., et al., A liposomal formulation for improving solubility and oral bioavailability of nifedipine. *Molecules*, 2020. **25**(2): p. 338.

43. Nisha, R., et al., Assessments of in vitro and in vivo antineoplastic potentials of β-sitosterol-loaded PEGylated niosomes against hepatocellular carcinoma. *Journal of Liposome Research*, 2020: p. 1–12.

44. Tang, B., Y. Qian, and G. Fang, Development of lipid–polymer hybrid nanoparticles for improving oral absorption of enoxaparin. *Pharmaceutics*, 2020. **12**(7): p. 607.

45. Zhang, K., et al., Enhancement of oral bioavailability and anti-hyperuricemic activity of isoliquiritigenin via self-microemulsifying drug delivery system. *AAPS Pharmaceutical Science and Technology*, 2019. **20**(5): p. 218.

46. Gu, M., et al., Improved oral bioavailability and anti-chronic renal failure activity of chrysophanol via mixed polymeric micelles. *Journal of Microencapsulation*, 2020. p. 1–19.

47. Pi, J., et al., A nano-cocrystal strategy to improve the dissolution rate and oral bioavailability of baicalein. *Asian Journal of Pharmaceutical Sciences*, 2019. **14**(2): p. 154–164.

48. Seto, Y., et al., Development of novel lutein nanocrystal formulation with improved oral bioavailability and ocular distribution. *Journal of Functional Foods*, 2019. **61**: p. 103499.

49. Jha, S.K., et al., Enhanced oral bioavailability of an etoposide multiple nanoemulsion incorporating a deoxycholic acid derivative–lipid complex. *Drug Delivery*, 2020. **27**(1): p. 1501–1513.

50. Yang, Y., et al., Chapter 12—oral drug absorption: evaluation and prediction, in *Developing Solid Oral Dosage Forms (Second Edition)*, Y. Qiu, et al., Editors. 2017, Academic Press: Boston. p. 331–354.

51. Liu, H., et al., Prediction of brain: blood unbound concentration ratios in CNS drug discovery employing in silico and in vitro model systems. *Drug Discovery Today*, 2018. **23**(7): p. 1357–1372.

52. Delsing, L., et al., Models of the blood-brain barrier using iPSC-derived cells. *Molecular and Cellular Neuroscience*, 2020. **107**: p. 103533.

53. Oprisiu, I. and S. Winiwarter, In silico ADME modeling, in *Systems Medicine*, O. Wolkenhauer, Editor. 2021, Academic Press: Oxford. p. 208–222.

54. Wang, M., et al., Permeability of exendin-4-loaded chitosan nanoparticles across MDCK cell monolayers and rat small intestine. *Biological and Pharmaceutical Bulletin*, 2014. **37**(5): p. 740–747.

55. Volpe, D.A., Variability in Caco-2 and MDCK cell-based intestinal permeability assays. *Journal of Pharmaceutical Sciences*, 2008. **97**(2): p. 712–725.

56. Urso, R. and L. Aarons, Bioavailability of drugs with long elimination half-lives. *European Journal of Clinical Pharmacology*, 1983. **25**(5): p. 689–693.

57. Urso, R., P. Blardi, and G. Giorgi, A short introduction to pharmacokinetics. *European Review for Medical and Pharmacological Sciences*, 2002. **6**: p. 33–44.

58. Karasulu, H., et al., Self-micro/nanoemulsifying drug carrying system for oral use of rosuvastatin, in *WO2015142307*. 2015.
59. Thaxton, C.S., et al., *Lipophilic nanoparticles for drug delivery*. 2020, Google Patents.
60. Zhang, H.-G., *Exosomal compositions and methods for the treatment of disease*. 2020, Google Patents.
61. Pascolo, S., *Pharmaceutical composition consisting of RNA having alkali metal as counter ion and formulated with dications*. 2017, Google Patents.
62. Eber, F.J., et al., *Dry powder composition comprising long-chain RNA*. 2020, Google Patents.
63. USFDA, *Center for Drug Evaluation and Research Nanotechnology Programs*. Nanotechnology Programs at FDA 2018 26/04/2018; Available from: www.fda.gov/science-research/nanotechnology-programs-fda/center-drug-evaluation-and-research-nanotechnology-programs.
64. USFDA, *Nanotechnology Guidance Documents*. Nanotechnology Programs at FDA 2018 23/03/2018; Available from: www.fda.gov/science-research/nanotechnology-programs-fda/nanotechnology-guidance-documents.
65. USFDA, *Nanotechnology Task Force*. Nanotechnology Programs at FDA 2020 15/10/2020; Available from: www.fda.gov/science-research/nanotechnology-programs-fda/nanotechnology-task-force.
66. Guidelines For Evaluation of Nanopharmaceuticals in India. Department of Biotechnology, Government of India, New Delhi. 2019, p. 1–14.

4 Ocular Nanomedicine
Fundamentals and Recent Advances

*Abhishek K. Sah, Ishwari Choudhary, Nagendra Bhuwane,
Shweta Ramkar, Narayan Hemnani, and Preeti K. Suresh*

4.1 INTRODUCTION OF OCULAR DELIVERY

The eye is an easily accessible site, but delivery of drugs to the eye remains a challenge for the ophthalmological researcher. The exceptional and complex anatomical and physiological features, along with various existing ocular barriers of the eyeball, render permeation of drugs into ocular tissue quite difficult. The eye is primarily spherical in shape; is approximately 24 mm in diameter; and consists of two main regions, the anterior and posterior segments. The front portion is small, and its appearance is one-sixth of the eyeball, while the posterior portion is the remaining part that is extremely delicate and highly vascularized but with limited accessibility for effective drug delivery. The posterior segment of the eye also contains the retina, a complex multicellular layer vital for visual acuity [1] (Figure 4.1). Various ocular diseases like conjunctivitis, ocular inflammation, cataract, uveitis, dry eye syndrome, glaucoma, age-related macular degeneration (AMD), diabetic retinopathy (DR), and diabetic macular edema (DME) require frequent dosing of drugs to maintain optimum ocular bioavailability; however, conventional formulations fail to achieve the requisite bioavailability (>1%) due to transient residence time on the precorneal surface, rapid tearing, and non-productive absorption of the drug from the cul-de-sac of the eyeball [2, 3].

The current drug therapeutic strategies fail to achieve the optimum therapeutic potential, and therefore development of novel ocular therapeutics has garnered considerable attention from researchers. In recent years, attention has shifted to nanodrug delivery platforms to explore new therapies for various ocular disorders. Nanotechnology and nanoscience are continuously emerging with the aim to improve the therapeutic potential of actives, and various techniques have been used to fabricate drug delivery systems in the nanoscale range [4–6]. Various nanotechnological approaches have been investigated to enhance the therapeutic potential for effective therapy by improving bioadhesive properties, controlled drug release patterns, specific targeted drug delivery, and stimuli-triggered systems, among others [7–9]. Although novel concept have been utilized for dosage forms like suspensions, emulsions, ocular inserts, eye ointments, and gel preparations, they offer scarce benefits in improving drug residence time on the precorneal segments. Additionally, they also have some shortcomings, like ocular irritation, blurring of vision, instability of the biomolecule in the ocular segment, and repeated administration of the dosage form, leading to poor patient compliance [10]. To overcome the limitations presented by the current therapy, there is an urgent need for fabrication of nano-based formulations which improve the therapeutic profile of drugs along with better patient compliance and open up new possibilities for pharmaco-ocular therapy. In this chapter, we review the recent advancements in nanomaterial-based formulations for ocular therapy, including nanoparticles, nanocapsules, nanospheres, solid lipid nanoparticles (SLNs), nanostructured lipid carriers (NLCs), liposomes, dendrimers, cubosomes, nanomicelles, hydrogels, contact lenses, and *in-situ* gels (Figure 4.2) and also report the clinical findings.

DOI: 10.1201/9781003130055-4

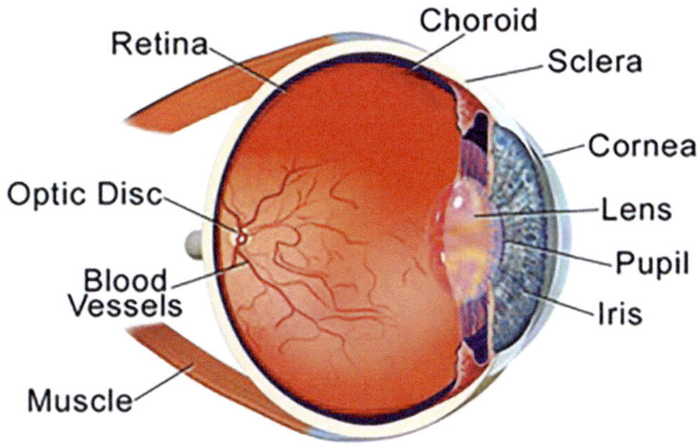

FIGURE 4.1 Structure of human eyeball.

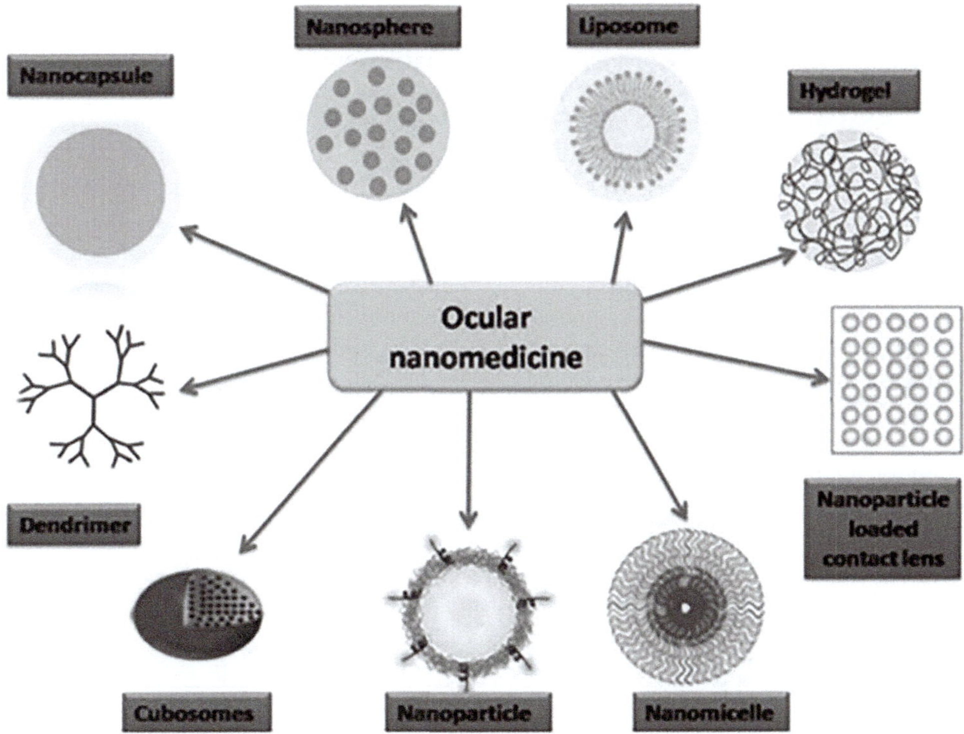

FIGURE 4.2 Different types of ocular nanomedicine.

4.2 APPROACHES FOR EFFICIENT DRUG DELIVERY

In recent years, various strategies have been explored to augment the therapeutic effect of drugs following ocular administration by achieving controlled drug release, improving the penetration profile, and/or enhancing retention time. Some of these approaches to address these objectives are discussed in the following section.

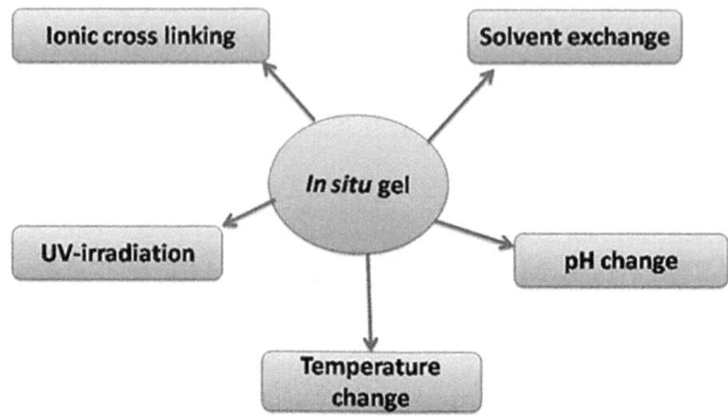

FIGURE 4.3 The trigger factors for *in situ* gel-based formulations.

4.2.1 *In Situ* Gel Formulation Systems

In situ gels are unique formulations based on phase transition which are in the liquid state at the time of instillation/administration and are converted into the gel state as and when they come into contact, even with minor alterations in terms of temperature, pH, or ionic strength within the physiological milieu of the eye. Thus, as compared to liquid formulations, better precorneal retention times are achieved with *in situ* gels. The prime advantage of *in situ* gelling systems over already-gelled formulations is the prospect of administering accurate and reproducible quantities [11, 12]. The various factors that trigger *in situ* gel formation are depicted in Figure 4.3 [13, 14].

Various *in situ* gel formulations have been investigated to improve the therapeutic potential of actives and enhance ocular bioavailability. Gupta et al. (2007) investigated a timolol maleate–loaded *in situ* gel formulation based on thermo- and pH-responsive polymers for the effective management of glaucoma. Pluronic F-127 and chitosan were used in combination as a thermo-responsive and pH-responsive polymer, respectively. The prepared formulation was characterized *in vitro* for various parameters including clarity, gelation temperature, pH, isotonicity, sterility, rheological behavior, drug release profile, transcorneal permeation profile, and ocular irritation. The prepared formulations were found to be transparent and isotonic and changed their physical sol state to gel state above 35°C at pH 6.9 to 7.0. A better drug penetration profile across the corneal tissue along with improved retention time was also observed. The results suggested that this formulation would be a better alternative than conventional formulations for the effective management of glaucoma and various other ocular disorders. An acetazolamide-loaded nanoemulsion (NE) based on electrolyte-triggered *in situ* gel for ocular delivery in the effective management of glaucoma has been reported. These novel NE formulations were prepared by using peanut oil, Tween 80, and Cremophor EL as a surfactant and Transcutol P and propylene glycol as cosurfactant. Gellan gum was used separately and with xanthan gum, HPMC, and Carbopol for inducing *in situ* gelling. The prepared formulation was found to have an improved drug release profile over a longer duration of time, along with uniform spherical size distribution (Figure 4.4). Additionally, these formulations had better stability at different temperature levels excluding gellan/Carbopol. Gellan/xanthan and gellan/HPMC revealed improved therapeutic property along with prolonged intraocular pressure (IOP), lowering efficacy as compared to eye drops and oral tablets. These results showed that prepared *in situ* gel formulations would be promising agents for electrolyte-triggered *in situ* gels for ocular delivery of acetazolamide [15, 16]. Other *in situ* gel formulations are listed in Table 4.1.

4.2.2 Mucoadhesive Systems

Mucoadhesive systems are also one of the approaches that has been continuously investigated with an aim to provide sustained drug release, improve drug retention on precorneal segments, and provide

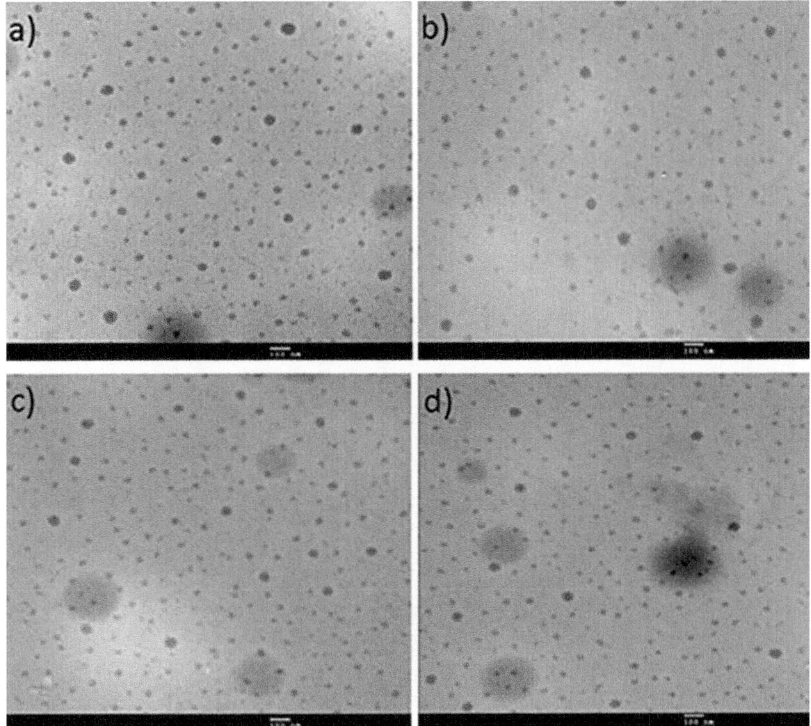

FIGURE 4.4 TEM images of a) nanoemulsion, b) nanoemulsion *in situ* gel gellan/xanthan, c) nanoemulsion *in situ* gel gellan/HPMC, d) nanoemulsion *in situ* gel gellan/Carbopol [16].

better patient compliance, along with circumventing other limitations of conventional formulation. In this context, Bhatta et al. (2012) reported the natamycin-loaded lecithin/chitosan mucoadhesive nanoparticle for effective treatment of ocular bacterial infection. The prepared formulations were characterized for various parameters like particle size, encapsulation efficiency, drug loading, zeta potential, *in vitro* drug release profile, and *in vitro* antifungal activity. The drug release pattern had an initial burst release followed by a biphasic release. Similar *in vitro* antifungal activity against *Candida albicans* and *Aspergillus fumigates* was evident as compared with a marketed suspension and free drug solution. The formulation also showed better mucin adhesion properties. These results strongly argued that lecithin/chitosan may be a better alternative for improving drug residence time and achieving prolonged drug release with reduced frequency of ocular administration [47]. Some other mucoadhesive ocular formulations are listed in Table 4.1.

4.2.3 CONTACT LENSES

Therapeutic or drug-eluting contact lenses have been explored to address the limitations of conventional ocular formulation by enhancing the drug residence time on the precorneal surface to increase bioavailability and maximize drug efficacy with minimal systemic toxicity [48, 49]. Although prolonged drug release can be achieved with therapeutic contact lenses, the problem remains ocular discomfort in long-term use, especially for patients who are not using contact lenses for vision correction. Another issue with contact lenses is that the drug in the pre-lens tear film (between the cornea and the lens), also possess a similar clearance pathway as with topical application [46]. Nanomaterials may provide controlled drug release, but alternatively the drug may get trapped up

TABLE 4.1

Various Drug-Loaded Ocular Formulations for the Improvement of the Therapeutic Profile in the Treatment of Various Ocular Diseases

Polymer/Lipid	Drug	Novel Formulations	Disease	Major Outcomes	Reference
Methylcellulose	Tranilast nanoparticles	*In situ* gel	Ocular inflammation	Prolonged drug release profile, along with enhanced drug residence time on the precorneal surface, better anti-inflammatory efficacy with longer duration	[17]
Triacetin, Transcutol P, Poloxamer 407, Poloxamer188	Acyclovir (ACV)	*In situ* gel	Ocular viral infection	Sustained drug pharmacokinetic profile as compared with control solution, drug permeation profile about 2.8-fold higher than control solution, along with established safety profile	[18]
Compritol 888 ATO, Miglyol 812	N-palmitoylethanolamide	NLCs	Retinal disease, diabetic retinopathy	Improved delivery of the drug to the retinal tissue, better therapeutic profile, significantly inhibits the TNF-α level in streptozocine induced diabetic rats	[19]
Precirol ATO5, Tween 80, Poloxamer 188	Ciprofloxacin	NLCs	Bacterial endophthalmitis	Sustained *invitro* drug release profile of the drug up to 24 h, increased permeation of the drug as compared with commercial eye drops, enhanced drug bioavailability along with prolonged antimicrobial features	[20]
Carboxymethyl chitosan and poloxamer 407, cross-linker genipin	Quercetin	NLCs with hydrogel	–	Quercetin-loaded NLC hydrogel crosslinked with genipin showed improved cytocompatibility with less ocular irritation as compared with NLC crosslinked with glutaraldehyde. Cellular uptake better in NLC and NLC-hydrogel. Improved penetration profile confirmed by *ex vivo* fluorescence imaging technique along with prolonged drug precorneal residence time and high drug bioavailability	[21]
–	Polymyxin B, Dexamethasone acetate	NLCs	Ocular infections	Improved physicochemical properties, higher stability profile, improved antimicrobial activity against *Pseudomonas aeruginosa* and anti-inflammatory activity	[22]
Chitosan oligosaccharide	Valylvaline-stearic acid	Nanomicelles	Ocular inflammation	Established safety profile confirmed by *in vitro* cell line studies in human corneal epithelial cells (HCEpiC) and human conjunctival epithelial cells (HConEpiC). Better *ex vivo* penetration efficacy of fluorescence-loaded nanomicelles	[23]

D-α-tocopheryl polyethylene glycol succinate (TPGS), Pluronic F127/ Pluronic F68	Posaconazole	Micelles	Ocular fungal infections	Better encapsulation efficiency, ultra nano size of 20 nm, prolonged *in vitro* drug release profile of drug-loaded micellar formulation as compared with conventional suspension	[24]
–	Resveratrol	Micelles	Corneal wound healing	Drug-loaded micellar formulation exhibited high drug chemical stability profile as compared with plain drug solution. Improved permeation *in vitro* and *in vivo* profile, high cellular uptake as compared with plain drug suspension	[25]
–	–	Liposomes	Ocular cancer	Prolonged corneal transient time along with improved corneal permeability by iRGD tailored liposomal formulations	[26]
Leucaena leucocephala galactomannan (LLG)	Dorzolamide hydrochloride	Polymeric nanoparticles	Intraocular pressure	Better transcorneal permeation profile of 87, 88, and 65% as compared with conventional formulations. Prolonged IOP-lowering efficacy	[27]
–	Isoniazid	SLNs	Ocular bacterial infection	Drug-loaded SLNs exhibited sustained drug release profile up to 48 h along with better penetration profile against excised rat cornea. Established safety profile confirmed by *in vitro* cell line studies. Significantly improved uptake of fluorescein-labeled SLNs *in vitro* and *in vivo*, along with high ocular bioavailability	[28]
Sodium deoxycholate and chitosan, PVA	Prednisolone acetate	Nanoparticle	Ocular inflammation	Prolonged drug release up to 24 h along with better pharmacokinetic profile. Improved therapeutic efficacy	[29]
PEG-PLGA	Antioxidant	Nanoparticles	Diabetic retinopathy and diabetic cataracts	Prepared antioxidant loaded PEG-PLGA nanoparticles reduced the efficacy of diabetic cataract in an experimental animal by preventing epithelial tissue form oxidative stress, and restrict α-crystallin glycation also maintained the transparency of ocular lens	[30]
Poloxamer 188	Lutein ester	Nanoparticles	AMD	Improved bioavailability along with better antioxidant and scavenging properties in the ocular tissue	[31]

(Continued)

TABLE 4.1 (Continued)

Various Drug-Loaded Ocular Formulations for the Improvement of the Therapeutic Profile in the Treatment of Various Ocular Diseases

Polymer/Lipid	Drug	Novel Formulations	Disease	Major Outcomes	Reference
Compritol ATO 888 and Transcutol P	Propranolol hydrochloride	NLCs	Glaucoma	Better *in vitro* drug permeation profile across excised rabbit cornea	[32]
Eudragit L100–55	Econazole nitrate (EN)	Mucoadhesive SEDDS	Ocular fungal infection	Prolonged ocular residence time on to the precorneal surface by mucoadhesive SEDDS along with nano-size dimension with 2.5-fold high mucoadhesive profile as compared with blank SEDDS. Also sustained the drug release profile up to 8 h with no corneal toxicity	[33]
Stearic acid, Tween 80, sodium deoxycholate	Levofloxacin	SLN	Conjunctivitis	Optimized formulation in nano-size range of 237.82 nm along with higher EE of 78.71%. Prolonged *in vitro* drug release profile followed by Korsmeyer–Peppas model release pattern. Similar antibacterial efficacy against *Staphylococcus aureus* and *Escherichia coli* as compared with commercial eye drops. Formulation showed safety profile and non-irritant confirmed by HET-CAM model	[34]
HPMC, PLGA	Dexamethasone	*In situ* gel	Intraocular inflammation	Sustained the drug release up to 7–10 days	[35]
Chitosan oligosaccharide lactate, glycerin or PEG 400	Ofloxacin	NLC-based insert	Bacterial keratitis	Improved pharmacokinetic profile by mechanism of diffusion and swelling, prolonged precorneal drug retention up to 24 h along with sixfold high bioavailability as compared with commercial formulation, better antimicrobial activity against *Staphylococcus aureus* and keratitis within 7 days without toxicity	[36]
PVA, stearic acid, palmitic acid	Itraconazole	SLNs	Ocular infection	Nano-size range with better permeation profile by drug-loaded stearic acid SLNs as compared with palmitic acid SLNs. Efficient *in vitro* antibacterial efficacy against *Aspergillus flavus* confirmed by zone of inhibition	[37]

Medium-chain triglycerides, lanolin or petrolatum, polyvinyl pyrrolidone	–	Nanoscale-dispersed eye ointments (NDEO), nanoemulsion	Dry eye disease	Improved drug therapeutic efficacy, better drug retention on precorneal segment, along with enhanced formulation stability profile at freezing temperature of 4°C and safe ocular application	[38]
Poloxamer 188 and Tween 80, Compritol 888 ATO	Indomethacin	SLN	Ocular inflammation	Significantly improved drug ocular bioavailability, along with chemical stability. Better penetration profile showed by drug loaded SLN as compared with plain drug solution- (0.1% w/v) and indomethacin hydroxypropyl-beta-cyclodextrin–based formulations (0.1% w/v)	[39]
PVA/EVA	Ganciclovir	Implant	Cytomegalovirus retinitis cased by AIDS	Sustained drug release up to 8 months duration without any systemic toxicity	[40]
–	Cyclosporine A	SLN	Ocular inflammation	Sustained the drug release profile up to 48 h, improved drug transient time on precorneal surface, better penetration profile due to nanodimension of formulation, along with better stability parameters	[41]
Silicone with PVA	Fluocinolone acetonide	Insert, implant	DME, chronic uveitis	Controlled the drug release up to 3 years, improved visual acuity	[42–45]
PLGA, pHEMA	Ciprofloxacin	Contact lens	Ocular infection	Controlled drug release profile up to 4 weeks, better therapeutic efficacy	[46]

NPs: Nanoparticles, SEDDS: Self-emulsifying drug delivery systems, PLGA: Poly(lactic-co-glycolic) acid, pHEMA: Poly(hydroxyethyl methacrylate), DME: Diabetic macular edema, PVA: Polyvinyl alcohol, PEG: Poly ethylene glycol, EVA: Ethylene vinyl alcohol, AIDS: Acquired immunodeficiency syndrome, HPMC: Hydroxypropyl methyl cellulose, IOP: Intra-ocular pressure, AMD: Age-related macular degeneration, NLCs: Nano-structured lipid carrier, EE: Entrapment efficiency, SLNs: Solid lipid nanoparticles, SLN: Solid lipid nanoparticle

permanently within the hydrogel matrix. This was exhibited in PLGA–pHEMA layers with only approximately 10% of the total drug releasing from the contact lens. The addition of nanomaterials to the contact lens must not compromise the intrinsic features of the latter, including wettability, user comfort, optical transparency, biocompatibility, oxygen permeability, mechanical properties, and non-irritant profile. Apart from the promises of these therapeutic contact lenses, they have certain limitations that need to be addressed. First and foremost, the nanoscale surface roughness is a significant aspect for transfer of bacteria from contact lenses and deposit formation composed of tear proteins on the surface and may influence bacterial adhesion to surface [50]. This may be responsible for undesirable effects on eye irritation and infection. Also, since these nanoconstructs may not be covalently bound to the polymeric matrices of contact lenses, the free nanocarriers can be a source of irritation to the eye [51]. Another major issue that necessitates due attention is the possibility of drug loss and/or leaching from therapeutic contact lenses.

4.2.4 OPHTHALMIC IMPLANTS

Ocular implants offer exclusive features for site-specific drug delivery for both anterior as well as posterior segment diseases, including uveitis, macular edema, diabetic macular edema, Irvine–Gass syndrome, ocular inflammation of posterior segment, cytomegalovirus retinitis, and proliferative vitreoretinopathy (PVR) [52–56]. In the past decades, ocular implants were formulated using non-biodegradable polymers, which led to patient compliance problems since it required twin surgeries, one at the time of installation of the implant and a second for the removal of the drug-exhausted device. From the patient's perspective, these types of medications were not user friendly, were more painful, and carried the risk of other ocular complications like cataracts, retinal detachment, and hemorrhage [57–59]. Therefore, lately the focus has shifted to biodegradable implants, which have received considerable attention due to their superior features of biodegradability, biocompatibility, and sustained drug release profile [59]. Various biodegradable polymers that have been employed include polylactic acid (PLA), polylactide co-glycolic acid (PLGA), polycaprolactones, and polyglycolic acid (PGA) [60]. The various implants for the ocular diseases are reported in Table 4.1 and marketed products in Table 4.2.

4.3 NANOMEDICINE IN OCULAR DRUG DELIVERY

Nanomedicine for ocular delivery has its own benefits in terms of controlled drug delivery, avoidance of systemic toxicity, and better patient compliance, along with improved therapeutic outcomes. Owing to the special features of nano-based formulations, researchers have focused on various nanocarriers for ocular delivery. These include polymeric nanoparticles, nanostructured lipid carriers, solid lipid nanoparticles, micelles, liposomes, niosomes, and dendrimers [3]. These nanocarriers improved the therapeutic potential while overcoming the limitations associated with current conventional ocular medications with confirmed, controlled, and targeted delivery of biomolecules [61–63].

4.3.1 POLYMERIC NANOPARTICLES

Polymeric nanoparticles are generally solid colloidal particles consisting of biodegradable and biocompatible polymers. These have been extensively investigated as nano-vehicles for ocular application due to their unique features and propensity to improve residence time on the precorneal surface [64, 65]. The nanodimensions with size ranging from 10 to 1000 nm assist in avoiding irritation within the eye cavity and facilitate prolonged drug release as compared with conventional eye drop formulations. Various polymers like polyethylene glycol, chitosan, and hyaluronic acid (HA) are mixed in the nanoparticulate formulation to improve drug retention on the precorneal surface, with the additional feature of mucoadhesiveness [66, 67]. Recently scholars investigated

TABLE 4.2

Some Marketed Products of Ocular Implants Available for Ocular Disease

Brand Name	Formulations	Compositions	Disease	Manufacturer
Retisert	Ocular implants	Fluocinolone acetonide	Posterior uveitis	Bausch + Lomb, NY
Vitrasert		Ganciclovir	CMV	Control Delivery System, Inc (pSivida)
Iluvien	Ocular implants	Fluocinolone acetonide	DME	Alimera Sciences, Alpharetta, GA
Yutiq	Ocular implants	Fluocinolone acetonide	Chronic noninfectious uveitis	Eye-Point Pharmaceuticals, Watertown, MA
Retisert	Ocular vitreal implants	Fluocinolone acetonide	Chronic noninfectious uveitis	Bausch + Lomb, Rochester, NY
Surodex	Ocular implants	Dexamethasone	Macular edema	Allergan, Inc., Irvine, CA, USA
Ozurdex, Novadur	Ocular implants	Dexamethasone	Intraocular inflammation	Allergan, Irvine, CA
Lucentis	Ocular implants	Ranibizumab	nAMD	Genentech, South San Francisco, CA
XIPERE, CLS-TA	Suprachoroidal drug delivery	Triamcinolone acetonide	Macular edema associated with noninfectious uveitis	Clearside Biomedical, Alpharetta, GA
Eylea	Suprachoroidal drug delivery	Aflibercept	DME	Regeneron, Tarrytown, NY

DME: Diabetic macular edema, nAMD: Neovascular age-related macular degeneration, CMV: Cytomegalovirus.

antioxidant-loaded polymeric nanoparticles for ocular delivery in the effective treatment of age-related eye disorders like senile cataracts [68]. In this research, topically applied lutein-loaded poly (lactic-co-glycolic acid) nanoparticles were prepared, and their antioxidant potential was investigated in selenite-induced cataracts in rats. The Cy5-labeled PLGA nanoparticles and lutein-loaded PLGA nanoparticles were characterized for zeta potential, particle size distribution, stability, and bio-distribution. The formulation had a good stability profile at a freezing temperature of 4°C devoid of alteration in morphology and size as compared to the higher temperatures of 25°C, 26°C, and 37°C. Lutein-loaded nanoparticles exhibited more protective action to photo degradation as compared to pure lutein solution upon 6 hours UV exposure. The ocular retention of a Cy5-labled nanoparticle formulation was also investigated in experimental animals for 15, 30, or 60 min. The intensity of fluorescence Cy5-labled nanoparticles on different anterior ocular tissues like the cornea, episcleral tissue, sclera, and posterior tissue of the choroid were assessed and found to have improved fluorescence intensity in treatment of experimental animals as compared to the control group. Furthermore, lowering of fluorescence intensity was found in anterior as well as posterior ocular tissue after 30 and 60 min, indicating easy elimination. The results advocated for its potential application in ocular delivery, along with an improved penetration profile. Additionally, drug-loaded nanoparticles incorporated within thermo-responsive hydrogel to improve the precorneal residence time were tested on experimental animals. Lutein-loaded PLGA nanoparticles showed better drug concentration of 1,278 μg/mL, with the highest lowering capacity in selenite-induce cataracts as compared with other treated and untreated groups of animals [68]. Other investigated nanoparticles are listed in Table 4.1.

4.3.2 Nanostructured Lipid Carriers

Nanostructured lipid carriers are biocompatible carriers consisting of solid lipid(s), liquid lipid(s), surfactant, and water and have a size range of 50 to 1000 nm. They form a complex with the mucus layer of the cornea, and due to its mucoadhesiveness, it can prolong the transcorneal residence time and subsequently enhance drug bioavailability [69, 70]. Recently Baig et al. (2020) investigated a besifloxacin-loaded cationic nanostructured lipid carrier (CNLC) for ocular delivery in the treatment of bacterial infection. These novel formulations were prepared by using Gelucire 50/13, Compritol 888 ATO, and Labrafac PG as a stabilizer, solid lipid, and liquid lipid, respectively. The CNLCs were characterized for various parameters, including particle size, polydispersity index (PDI), morphology by TEM, entrapment efficiency, cytotoxicity, and cellular infiltration by 2- and 3-dimentional conjunctival tissue model. The results for particle size, PDI, and zeta potential indicated that they retained their stability for up to 2 weeks with 80% entrapment efficiency. In the compatibility studies, the FTIR spectra showed no significant dissimilarity between dummy CNCLs, besifloxacin-loaded CNLC nanoformulation, and pure drug samples, confirming that the drug was completely immersed in the CNLC devoid of any interaction (Figure 4.5). A better penetration profile was found by the 3D model, and MTT cytotoxicity exhibited 60% cell viability on a conjunctival fibroblast model upon addition of 0.6 mg/ml of besifloxacin (Figure 4.6) [71]. Other NLCs investigated for ocular applications are listed in Table 4.1.

4.3.3 Solid Lipid Nanoparticles

SLNs are a colloidal carrier system with a lipid matrix consisting of a solid lipid or mixture of solid lipids (0.1% to 30% w/w) mixed in an aqueous media and have been investigated as a potential nanocarrier for the delivery of various therapeutic agents [72]. They offer several benefits, including better drug stability, non-toxicity, self-degradable profile, and biocompatibility, along with lipid composition analogous to biological lipids, targeted delivery, improved drug loading efficacy, loading of both lipophilic as well as hydrophilic drugs, and ease of commercial manufacturing [73–75]. Recently Wadetwar et al. investigated bimatoprost nanoparticle-laden pH-responsive *in-situ* gel for

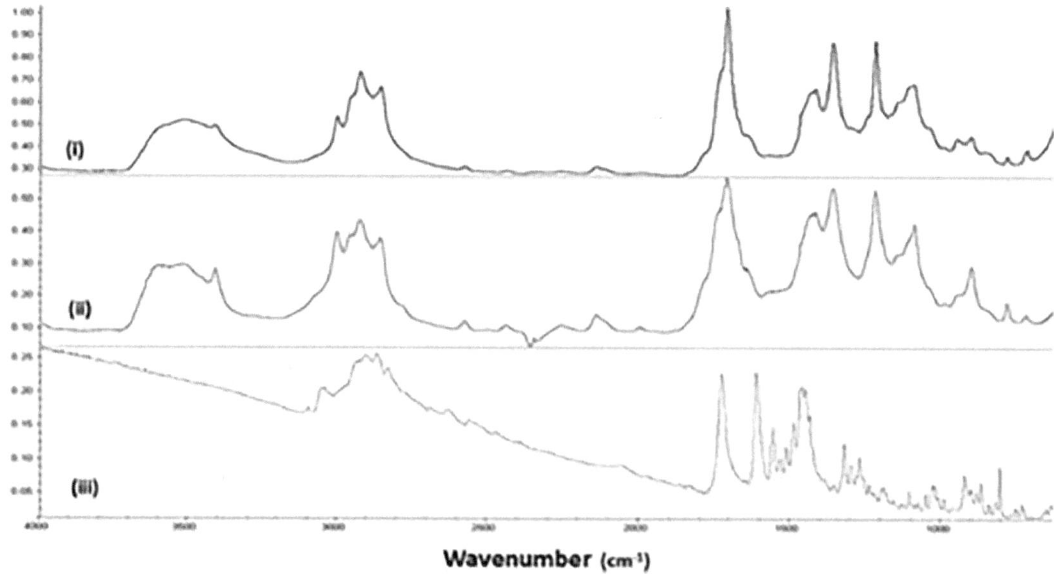

FIGURE 4.5 FTIR image for compatibility study between (i) dummy CNLC formulations, (ii) besifloxacin-loaded CNLC nanoformulation, and (iii) pure besifloxacin hydrochloride drug [71].

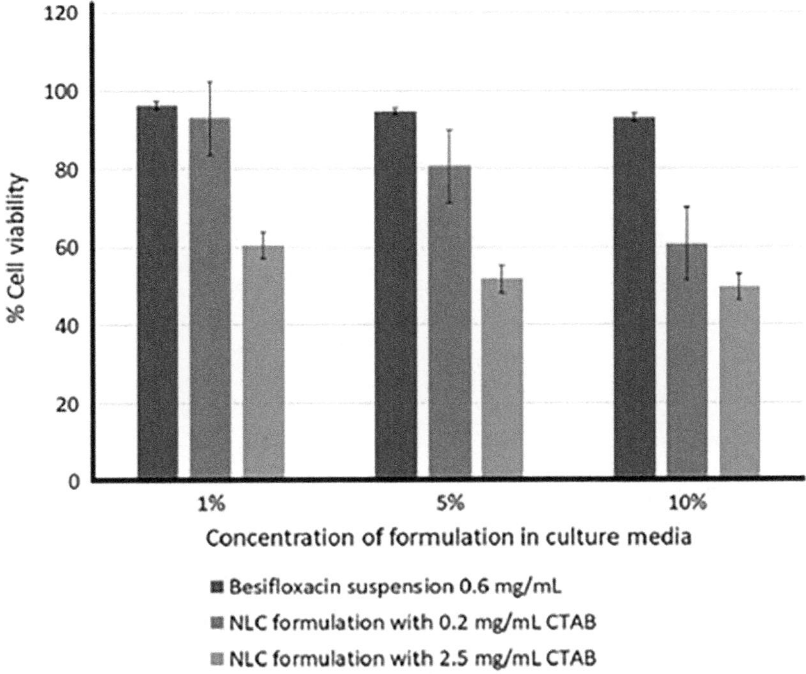

FIGURE 4.6 MTT assay graph indicating % cell viability when incubating with 1% besifloxacin suspension (0.6 mg/mL) or 1% NLC formulation with 0.2 mg/mL CTAB or 1% NLC formulation with 2.5 mg/mL CTAB (n = 3) [71].

ocular application for the effective treatment of glaucoma. In this formulation, glyceryl monostearate and Tween 80 were used as solid lipid and surfactant and fabricated by using high-pressure homogenization followed by sonication. The optimized formulations were further characterized for *in vitro* and *ex vivo* drug release profiles, irritation potential by HET-CAM model, and alteration of cellular structure by histopathological studies. The results showed a prolonged drug release pattern for a longer duration of time, along with non-irritant behavior. Additionally, no ultrastructural changes were found in the cellular tissues (Figure 4.7). Bimatoprost nanoparticle-laden pH-responsive *in situ* gel may be explored for the effective treatment of glaucoma [76]. Various other investigated SLNs are summarized in Table 4.1.

4.3.4 MICELLES

Grimaudo et al. investigated corneal wound healing efficacy of ferulic acid (antioxidant) nanocomposite-loaded nanogels and micelles. Solubility of the drug was also assessed and was found to be similar to 1.9 ± 0.3 and 3.4 ± 0.3 for 50 and 100 mg/ml Pluronic F68 micellar solutions. Hyaluronans were also included in the dummy and ferullic acid–loaded micelles thereafter cross-linked with ε-polylysine. Nanodimensions and positive zeta potential were exhibited by hyaluronan nanogel. The micellar formulation was also characterized for various parameters, including rheological profile, biocompatibility, wound healing efficacy, *in vitro* drug release, and penetration profile across excised bovine corneas. The sustained release parameter was found for up to 48 h followed by rapid release as compared with Pluronic micelles. In addition, fibroblast growing efficacy followed by *in vitro* wound healing were observed by micelles nanogel formulation along with accumulation of ferulic acid within normal and injured corneas (>100 μg/cm^2) [77]. Various other micellar formulations are listed in Table 4.1.

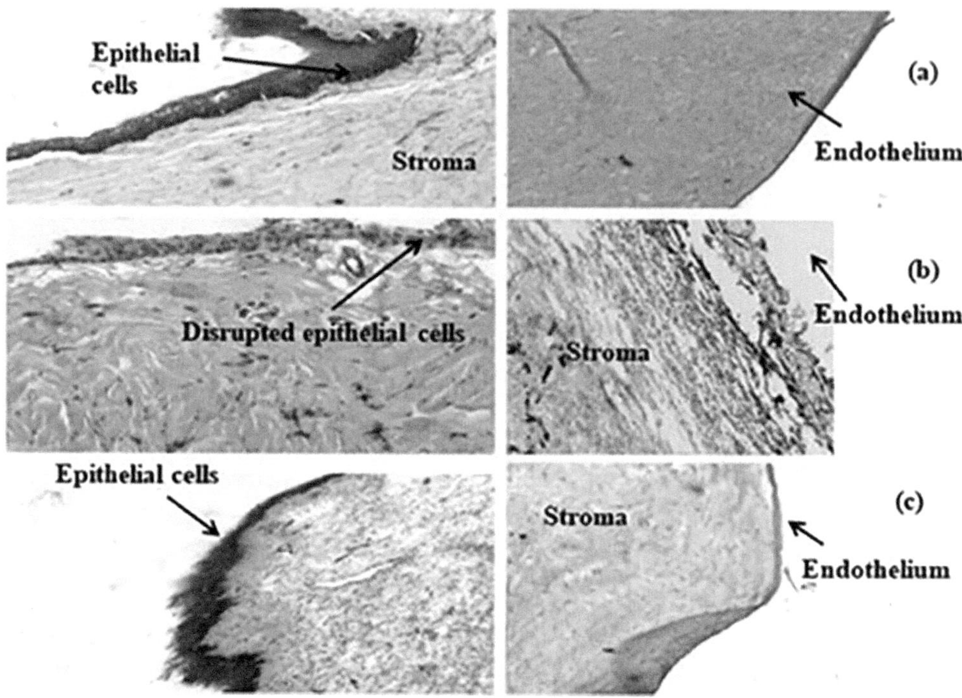

FIGURE 4.7　Histopathological slides of the excised goat cornea: (a) normal saline (control), (b) isopropyl alcohol (positive control), and (c) SLN-ISG3 [76].

4.3.5　LIPOSOMES

Liposomes are spherical colloidal nanocarriers consisting of one or more phospholipid bilayer(s) surrounding an aqueous core. They have shown new possibilities for ocular application due to their multiple beneficial features of size, biocompatibility, biodegradability, low toxicity, and capacity to encapsulate drugs irrespective of their hydrophilic, lipophilic, or amphiphilic nature. Additionally, they offer better residence time on precorneal segments and prolonged drug half lives in vitreous fluids, along with less toxicity. However, due to lack of bioadhesive features, penetration into the deeper layer of ocular tissues is inadequate; therefore various polymers and ligand-based formulations have been investigated to improve the therapeutic profile of the liposomes [78–82]. Lai et al. investigated berberine hydrochloride and chrysophanol-loaded liposomes for the treatment of age-related macular degeneration. These drug-loaded liposomes coated with polyamidoamine dendrimer (PAMAM G3.0) showed higher permeability across human corneal epithelial cells, along with high bioadhesive properties in experimental animal models. These liposomes exhibited higher berberine hydrochloride bioavailability, along with protective efficacy in human retinal pigment epithelial cells and in rat retina on photo-oxidative–induced retinal injury. No ultrastructural changes were found on the ocular surface in a rabbit model. These results suggest their promise for ocular application in various disorders [78]. Other liposomal formulations are listed in Table 4.1.

4.4　CURRENT AND FUTURE RESEARCH

Delivery of drugs to ocular tissue for both the anterior as well as the posterior segment is crucial and challenging for the effective treatment of different ocular disorders. In recent years, various nanocarriers have been investigated for ocular delivery. However, the main challenges for the better development of nanoparticulate formulations are the desired nano-size range, better entrapment efficacy, and established safety profiles. Various nanocarriers showed prolonged drug release features, high drug bioavailability, and high penetration efficacy, along with better patient compliance over conventional formulations. Further investigation is needed *in vitro* and *in vivo*, which will provide practical utility and correlate the *in vivo* performance of these nanomedicines.

4.5 ACKNOWLEDGMENTS

The authors are thankful to the director, University Institute of Pharmacy and Pt. Sunderlal Sharma Central library, Pt. Ravishankar Shukla University, Raipur, India, for providing necessary infrastructure facilities and Inflibnet e-resources. One of the authors (AKS) is also thankful to the director, SGSITS, Indore and Central Library, for providing necessary facilities and e-resources.

REFERENCES

1. Suresh PK, Barsa G, Sah AK, Daharwal SJ. Ocular implants as drug delivery device in ophthalmic therapeutics: An overview. *Research Journal of Pharmacy and Technology.* 2014 Jun 1; 7 (6):665.
2. Sah AK, Suresh PK. Medical management of glaucoma: Focus on ophthalmologic drug delivery systems of timolol maleate. *Artificial Cells, Nanomedicine, and Biotechnology.* 2017 Apr 3; 45 (3):448–59.
3. Sah AK, Bhuwane N, Choudhary I, Ramkar S, Suresh PK. Application of biocompatible nanocarriers in glaucoma: Challenges and advances. *Nanoformulations in Human Health: Challenges and Approaches.* 2020:207–26.
4. Raghava S, Goel G, Kompella UB. Ophthalmic applications of nanotechnology. In: Tombran-Tink J, Colin JB, eds. *Ocular Transporters in Ophthalmic Diseases and Drug Delivery.* Totowa: Humana Press. 2008: 415–35.
5. Bell AT. The impact of nanoscience on heterogeneous catalysis. *Science.* 2003 Mar 14; 299 (5613):1688–91.
6. Meyer E, Gyalog T, Overney RM, Dransfeld K. *Nanoscience: Friction and Rheology on the Nanometer Scale.* Singapore: World Scientific. 1998: 392.
7. Zarbin MA, Montemagno C, Leary JF, Ritch R. Nanotechnology in ophthalmology. *Canadian Journal of Ophthalmology.* 2010; 45:457–76.
8. Bucolo C, Maltese A, Drago F. When nanotechnology meets the ocular surface. *Expert Review of Ophthalmology.* 2008 Jun 1; 3 (3):325–32.
9. Ideta R, Tasaka F, Jang WD, Nishiyama N, Zhang GD, Harada A, Yanagi Y, Tamaki Y, Aida T, Kataoka K. Nanotechnology-based photodynamic therapy for neovascular disease using a supramolecular nanocarrier loaded with a dendritic photosensitizer. *Nano Letters.* 2005 Dec 14; 5 (12):2426–31.
10. Sah AK, Suresh PK. Recent advances in ocular drug delivery, with special emphasis on lipid based nanocarriers. *Recent Patents on Nanotechnology.* 2015 Aug 1; 9 (2):94–105.
11. Gurny R., Ibrahim H., Buri P. The development and use of in situ formed gels triggered by pH. In: Edman, Y., ed. *Biopharmaceutics of Ocular Drug Delivery.* Boca Raton, FL: CRC Press. 1993: 81–90.
12. Cohen S, Lobel E, Trevgoda A, Peled Y. A novel in situ-forming ophthalmic drug delivery system from alginates undergoing gelation in the eye. *Journal of Controlled Release.* 1997 Feb 17; 44 (2–3):201–8.
13. Ruel-Gariepy E, Leroux JC. In situ-forming hydrogels—review of temperature-sensitive systems. *European Journal of Pharmaceutics and Biopharmaceutics.* 2004 Sep 1; 58 (2):409–26.
14. Varshosaz J, Tabbakhian M, Salmani Z. Designing of a thermosensitive chitosan/poloxamer in situ gel for ocular delivery of ciprofloxacin. *The Open Drug Delivery Journal.* 2008 Aug 21; 2 (1).
15. Gupta H, Jain S, Mathur R, Mishra P, Mishra AK, Velpandian T. Sustained ocular drug delivery from a temperature and pH triggered novel in situ gel system. *Drug Delivery.* 2007 Jan 1; 14 (8):507–15.
16. Morsi N, Ibrahim M, Refai H, El Sorogy H. Nanoemulsion-based electrolyte triggered in situ gel for ocular delivery of acetazolamide. *European Journal of Pharmaceutical Sciences.* 2017 Jun 15; 104:302–14.
17. Nagai N, Minami M, Deguchi S, Otake H, Sasaki H, Yamamoto N. An in situ gelling system based on methylcellulose and tranilast solid nanoparticles enhances ocular residence time and drug absorption into the cornea and conjunctiva. *Frontiers in Bioengineering and Biotechnology.* 2020 Jul 7; 8:764.
18. Mahboobian MM, Mohammadi M, Mansouri Z. Development of thermosensitive in situ gel nanoemulsions for ocular delivery of acyclovir. *Journal of Drug Delivery Science and Technology.* 2020 Feb 1; 55:101400.

19. Puglia C, Santonocito D, Ostacolo C, Maria Sommella E, Campiglia P, Carbone C, Drago F, Pignatello R, Bucolo C. Ocular formulation based on palmitoylethanolamide-loaded nanostructured lipid carriers: Technological and pharmacological profile. *Nanomaterials.* 2020 Feb 8; 10 (2):287.

20. Youssef A, Dudhipala N, Majumdar S. Ciprofloxacin loaded nanostructured lipid carriers incorporated into in-situ gels to improve management of bacterial endophthalmitis. *Pharmaceutics.* 2020 Jun; 12 (6):572.

21. Yu Y, Xu S, Yu S, Li J, Tan G, Li S, Pan W. A hybrid genipin-cross-linked hydrogel/nanostructured lipid carrier for ocular drug delivery: Cellular, ex vivo, and in vivo evaluation. *ACS Biomaterials Science & Engineering.* 2020 Feb 5; 6 (3):1543–52.

22. Rocha ED, Ferreira MR, dos Santos Neto E, Barbosa EJ, Löbenberg R, Lourenço FR, Bou-Chacra N. Enhanced in vitro antimicrobial activity of polymyxin B–coated nanostructured lipid carrier containing dexamethasone acetate. *Journal of Pharmaceutical Innovation.* 2021 Mar; 16:125–35.

23. Xu X, Sun L, Zhou L, Cheng Y, Cao F. Functional chitosan oligosaccharide nanomicelles for topical ocular drug delivery of dexamethasone. *Carbohydrate Polymers.* 2020 Jan 1; 227:115356.

24. Durgun ME, Kahraman E, Güngör S, Özsoy Y. Optimization and characterization of aqueous micellar formulations for ocular delivery of an antifungal drug, posaconazole. *Current Pharmaceutical Design.* 2020 Apr 1; 26 (14):1543–55.

25. Li M, Zhang L, Li R, Yan M. New resveratrol micelle formulation for ocular delivery: Characterization and in vitro/in vivo evaluation. *Drug Development and Industrial Pharmacy.* 2020 Dec 1; 46 (12):1960–70.

26. Huang H, Yang X, Li H, Lu H, Oswald J, Liu Y, Zeng J, Jin C, Peng X, Liu J, Song X. iRGD decorated liposomes: A novel actively penetrating topical ocular drug delivery strategy. *Nano Research.* 2020 Nov; 13:3105–9.

27. Mittal N, Kaur G. Leucaena leucocephala (Lam.) galactomannan nanoparticles: Optimization and characterization for ocular delivery in glaucoma treatment. *International Journal of Biological Macromolecules.* 2019 Oct 15; 139:1252–62.

28. Singh M, Guzman-Aranguez A, Hussain A, Srinivas CS, Kaur IP. Solid lipid nanoparticles for ocular delivery of isoniazid: Evaluation, proof of concept and in vivo safety & kinetics. *Nanomedicine.* 2019 Feb; 14 (4):465–91.

29. Hanafy AF, Abdalla AM, Guda TK, Gabr KE, Royall PG, Alqurshi A. Ocular anti-inflammatory activity of prednisolone acetate loaded chitosan-deoxycholate self-assembled nanoparticles. *International Journal of Nanomedicine.* 2019 May 29:3679–89.

30. Zhou Y, Li L, Li S, Li S, Zhao M, Zhou Q, Gong X, Yang J, Chang J. Autoregenerative redox nanoparticles as an antioxidant and glycation inhibitor for palliation of diabetic cataracts. *Nanoscale.* 2019; 11 (27):13126–38.

31. Wu M, Feng Z, Deng Y, Zhong C, Liu Y, Liu J, Zhao X, Fu Y. Liquid antisolvent precipitation: An effective method for ocular targeting of lutein esters. *International Journal of Nanomedicine.* 2019 Apr 15:2667–81.

32. Sharif Makhmal Zadeh B, Niro H, Rahim F, Esfahani G. Ocular delivery system for propranolol hydrochloride based on nanostructured lipid carrier. *Scientia Pharmaceutica.* 2018; 86 (2):16.

33. Elbahwy IA, Lupo N, Ibrahim HM, Ismael HR, Kasem AA, Caliskan C, Matuszczak B, Bernkop-Schnürch A. Mucoadhesive self-emulsifying delivery systems for ocular administration of econazole. *International Journal of Pharmaceutics.* 2018 Apr 25; 541 (1–2):72–80.

34. Baig MS, Ahad A, Aslam M, Imam SS, Aqil M, Ali A. Application of box–Behnken design for preparation of levofloxacin-loaded stearic acid solid lipid nanoparticles for ocular delivery: Optimization, in vitro release, ocular tolerance, and antibacterial activity. *International Journal of Biological Macromolecules.* 2016 Apr 1; 85:258–70.

35. Lee DJ. Intraocular implants for the treatment of autoimmune uveitis. *Journal of Functional Biomaterials.* 2015 Jul 31; 6 (3):650–66.

36. Üstündağ-Okur N, Gökçe EH, Bozbıyık Dİ, Eğrilmez S, Ertan G, Özer Ö. Novel nanostructured lipid carrier-based inserts for controlled ocular drug delivery: Evaluation of corneal bioavailability and treatment efficacy in bacterial keratitis. *Expert Opinion on Drug Delivery.* 2015 Nov 2; 12 (11):1791–807.

37. Mohanty B, Majumdar DK, Mishra SK, Panda AK, Patnaik S. Development and characterization of itraconazole-loaded solid lipid nanoparticles for ocular delivery. *Pharmaceutical Development and Technology.* 2015 May 19; 20 (4):458–64.

38. Zhang W, Wang Y, Lee BT, Liu C, Wei G, Lu W. A novel nanoscale-dispersed eye ointment for the treatment of dry eye disease. *Nanotechnology.* 2014 Feb 26; 25 (12):125101.

39. Hippalgaonkar K, Adelli GR, Hippalgaonkar K, Repka MA, Majumdar S. Indomethacin-loaded solid lipid nanoparticles for ocular delivery: Development, characterization, and in vitro evaluation. *Journal of Ocular Pharmacology and Therapeutics*. 2013 Mar 1; 29 (2):216–28.

40. Kuno N, Fujii S. Biodegradable intraocular therapies for retinal disorders: Progress to date. *Drugs Aging*. 2010; 27:117–34.

41. Başaran E, Demirel M, Sırmagül B, Yazan Y. Cyclosporine-A incorporated cationic solid lipid nanoparticles for ocular delivery. *Journal of Microencapsulation*. 2010 Jan 1; 27 (1):37–47.

42. Campochiaro PA, Brown DM, Pearson A, Chen S, Boyer D, Ruiz-Moreno J, Garretson B, Gupta A, Hariprasad SM, Bailey C, Reichel E. Sustained delivery fluocinolone acetonide vitreous inserts provide benefit for at least 3 years in patients with diabetic macular edema. *Ophthalmology*. 2012 Oct 1; 119 (10):2125–32.

43. Hebson CB, Srivastava SK. A functional, nonfunctioning Retisert implant. *Ocular Immunology and Inflammation*. 2011 Jun 1; 19 (3):210–1.

44. Jaffe GJ, Martin D, Callanan D, Pearson PA, Levy B, Comstock T. Fluocinolone acetonide uveitis study group. Fluocinolone acetonide implant (Retisert) for noninfectious posterior uveitis: Thirty-four-week results of a multicenter randomized clinical study. *Ophthalmology*. 2006 Jun; 113 (6):1020–7.

45. Jancevski M, Foster CS. The Retisert experience. *Investigative Ophthalmology & Visual Science*. 2010 Apr 17; 51 (13):5852.

46. Ciolino JB, Hoare TR, Iwata NG, Behlau I, Dohlman CH, Langer R, Kohane DS. A drug-eluting contact lens. *Investigative Ophthalmology & Visual Science*. 2009 Jul 1; 50 (7):3346–52.

47. Bhatta RS, Chandasana H, Chhonker YS, Rathi C, Kumar D, Mitra K, Shukla PK. Mucoadhesive nanoparticles for prolonged ocular delivery of natamycin: In vitro and pharmacokinetics studies. *International Journal of Pharmaceutics*. 2012 Aug 1; 432 (1–2):105–12.

48. Bengani L, Chauhan A. Are contact lenses the solution for effective ophthalmic drug delivery? *Future Medicinal Chemistry*. 2012 Nov; 4 (17):2141–3.

49. Li CC, Chauhan A. Modeling ophthalmic drug delivery by soaked contact lenses. *Industrial & Engineering Chemistry Research*. 2006 May 10; 45 (10):3718–34.

50. Mitik-Dineva N, Wang J, Mocanasu RC, Stoddart PR, Crawford RJ, Ivanova EP. Impact of nano-topography on bacterial attachment. *Biotechnology Journal: Healthcare Nutrition Technology*. 2008 Apr; 3 (4):536–44.

51. Whitesides GM. Nanoscience, nanotechnology, and chemistry. *Small*. 2005 Feb; 1 (2):172–9.

52. Dong X, Chen NA, Xie L, Wang S. Prevention of experimental proliferative vitreoretinopathy with a biodegradable intravitreal drug delivery system of all-trans retinoic acid. *Retina*. 2006 Feb 1; 26 (2):210–3.

53. Del Amo EM, Urtti A. Current and future ophthalmic drug delivery systems: A shift to the posterior segment. *Drug Discovery Today*. 2008 Feb 1; 13 (3–4):135–43.

54. Fialho SL, Silva Cunha AD. Manufacturing techniques of biodegradable implants intended for intra-ocular application. *Drug Delivery*. 2005 Jan 1; 12 (2):109–16.

55. Fialho SL, Rêgo MB, Siqueira RC, Jorge R, Haddad A, Rodrigues Jr AL, Maia-Filho A, Silva-Cunha A. Safety and pharmacokinetics of an intravitreal biodegradable implant of dexamethasone acetate in rabbit eyes. *Current Eye Research*. 2006 Jan 1; s31 (6):525–34.

56. Kunou N, Ogura Y, Hashizoe M, Honda Y, Hyon SH, Ikada Y. Controlled intraocular delivery of ganciclovir with use of biodegradable scleral implant in rabbits. *Journal of Controlled Release*. 1995 Nov 1; 37 (1–2):143–50.

57. Souto EB, Dias-Ferreira J, López-Machado A, Ettcheto M, Cano A, Camins Espuny A, Espina M, Garcia ML, Sánchez-López E. Advanced formulation approaches for ocular drug delivery: State-of-the-art and recent patents. *Pharmaceutics*. 2019 Sep 6; 11 (9):460.

58. Mittal S, Miranda O. Recent advancements in biodegradable ocular implants. *Current Drug Delivery*. 2018 Feb 1; 15 (2):144–54.

59. Sánchez-López E, Egea MA, Davis BM, Guo L, Espina M, Silva AM, Calpena AC, Souto EM, Ravindran N, Ettcheto M, Camins A. Memantine-loaded PEGylated biodegradable nanoparticles for the treatment of glaucoma. *Small*. 2018 Jan; 14 (2):1701808.

60. Ng XW, Liu KL, Veluchamy AB, Lwin NC, Wong TT, Venkatraman SS. A biodegradable ocular implant for long-term suppression of intraocular pressure. *Drug Delivery and Translational Research*. 2015 Oct; 5:469–79.

61. Girdhar V, Patil S, Banerjee S, Singhvi G. Nanocarriers for drug delivery: Mini review. *Current Nanomedicine (Formerly: Recent Patents on Nanomedicine)*. 2018 Aug 1; 8 (2):88–99.

62. Singhvi G, Patil S, Girdhar V, Dubey SK. Nanocarriers for topical drug delivery: Approaches and advancements. *Nanoscience & Nanotechnology-Asia.* 2019 Sep 1; 9 (3):329–36.

63. Gorantla S, Rapalli VK, Waghule T, Singh PP, Dubey SK, Saha RN, Singhvi G. Nanocarriers for ocular drug delivery: Current status and translational opportunity. *RSC Advances.* 2020; 10 (46):27835–55.

64. Kaur H, Ahuja M, Kumar S, Dilbaghi N. Carboxymethyl tamarind kernel polysaccharide nanoparticles for ophthalmic drug delivery. *International Journal of Biological Macromolecules.* 2012 Apr 1; 50 (3):833–9.

65. Sah AK, Suresh PK, Verma VK. PLGA nanoparticles for ocular delivery of loteprednol etabonate: A corneal penetration study. *Artificial Cells, Nanomedicine, and Biotechnology.* 2017 Aug 18; 45 (6):1156–64.

66. Omerović N, Vranić E. Application of nanoparticles in ocular drug delivery systems. *Health and Technology.* 2020 Jan; 10: 61–78.

67. Bu HZ, Gukasyan HJ, Goulet L, Lou XJ, Xiang C, Koudriakova T. Ocular disposition, pharmacokinetics, efficacy and safety of nanoparticle-formulated ophthalmic drugs. *Current Drug Metabolism.* 2007 Feb 1; 8 (2):91–107.

68. Swetledge SM. *Polymeric Nanoparticles as an Antioxidant Delivery System for Age-Related Eye Disease.* Baton Rouge, LA: Louisiana State University and Agricultural & Mechanical College. 2020.

69. Balguri SP, Adelli GR, Majumdar S. Topical ophthalmic lipid nanoparticle formulations (SLN, NLC) of indomethacin for delivery to the posterior segment ocular tissues. *European Journal of Pharmaceutics and Biopharmaceutics.* 2016 Dec 1; 109:224–35.

70. Üner M, Yener G. Importance of solid lipid nanoparticles (SLN) in various administration routes and future perspectives. *International Journal of Nanomedicine.* 2007 Dec 1; 2 (3):289–300.

71. Baig MS, Owida H, Njoroge W, Yang Y. Development and evaluation of cationic nanostructured lipid carriers for ophthalmic drug delivery of besifloxacin. *Journal of Drug Delivery Science and Technology.* 2020 Feb 1; 55:101496.

72. Ramkar S, Sah AK, Bhuwane N, Choudhary I, Hemnani N, Suresh PK. Nano-lipidic carriers as a tool for drug targeting to the pilosebaceous units. *Current Pharmaceutical Design.* 2020 Aug 1; 26 (27):3251–68.

73. Wadetwar RN, Agrawal AR, Kanojiya PS. In situ gel containing Bimatoprost solid lipid nanoparticles for ocular delivery: In-vitro and ex-vivo evaluation. *Journal of Drug Delivery Science and Technology.* 2020 Apr 1; 56:101575.

74. Seyfoddin A, Al-Kassas R. Development of solid lipid nanoparticles and nanostructured lipid carriers for improving ocular delivery of acyclovir. *Drug Development and Industrial Pharmacy.* 2013 Apr 1; 39 (4):508–19.

75. Pal Kaur I, Kanwar M. Ocular preparations: The formulation approach. *Drug Development and Industrial Pharmacy.* 2002 Jan 1; 28 (5):473–93.

76. Wadetwar RN, Agrawal AR, Kanojiya PS. In situ gel containing Bimatoprost solid lipid nanoparticles for ocular delivery: In-vitro and ex-vivo evaluation. *Journal of Drug Delivery Science and Technology.* 2020 Apr 1; 56: 101575.

77. Grimaudo MA, Amato G, Carbone C, Diaz-Rodriguez P, Musumeci T, Concheiro A, Alvarez-Lorenzo C, Puglisi G. Micelle-nanogel platform for ferulic acid ocular delivery. *International Journal of Pharmaceutics.* 2020 Feb 25; 576:118986.

78. Lai S, Wei Y, Wu Q, Zhou K, Liu T, Zhang Y, Jiang N, Xiao W, Chen J, Liu Q, Yu Y. Liposomes for effective drug delivery to the ocular posterior chamber. *Journal of Nanobiotechnology.* 2019 Dec; 17: 1–2.

79. Diebold Y, Jarrín M, Sáez V, Carvalho EL, Orea M, Calonge M, Seijo B, Alonso MJ. Ocular drug delivery by liposome–chitosan nanoparticle complexes (LCS-NP). *Biomaterials.* 2007 Mar 1; 28 (8):1553–64.

80. Bochot A, Fattal E, Boutet V, Deverre JR, Jeanny JC, Chacun H, Couvreur P. Intravitreal delivery of oligonucleotides by sterically stabilized liposomes. *Investigative Ophthalmology & Visual Science.* 2002 Jan 1; 43 (1):253–9.

81. Ravar F, Saadat E, Gholami M, Dehghankelishadi P, Mahdavi M, Azami S, Dorkoosh FA. Hyaluronic acid-coated liposomes for targeted delivery of paclitaxel, in-vitro characterization and in-vivo evaluation. *Journal of Controlled Release.* 2016 May 10; 229:10–22.

82. Wang JL, Liu YL, Li Y, Dai WB, Guo ZM, Wang ZH, Zhang Q. EphA2 targeted doxorubicin stealth liposomes as a therapy system for choroidal neovascularization in rats. *Investigative Ophthalmology & Visual Science.* 2012 Oct 1; 53 (11):7348–57.

5 Skin as Attractive Target for Transdermal Nanomedicine

Neha Raina, Rakesh Pahwa, Bigul Yogeshver Bhardwaj, and Madhu Gupta

5.1 INTRODUCTION

An effective route for the delivery of drugs is the skin, the largest organ in humans, as it circumvents many drawbacks of the oral route. Because of skin's benefits, it has intrigued investigators in recent years. This vital body organ acts as an ultimate interface between the external environment and body and constitutes about 16% of the total adult body weight (1). Homeostasis in the body is maintained by the skin through regulating the clearance and entrance of various substances, thus averting loss of water and maintaining the temperature of the body (2, 3). The skin is a complex barrier with three layers: the epidermis (outermost layer); the middle layer, the dermis (contains various connective fibers, sensory receptors and sweat glands); and the hypodermis, a subcutaneous layer (which has adipose tissue and anchors the other two skin layers for support). This route has been explored to a great extent for delivery of drugs because of its user friendliness and larger surface area. The skin is primarily employed as a drug administration route for topical (dermal) delivery, where a drug is located in skin layers, or transdermal delivery, where a drug passes via the dermis and finally enters the blood (4). Nowadays scientists have shown great interest in the delivery of drugs through the skin in a controlled manner. In addition, transdermal devices have been fabricated for several therapeutic agents such as fentanyl, clonidine, testosterone, fentanyl, scopolamine, nitroglycerin and estradiol (5). But a few inadequacies of transdermal route make difficult to pass drugs through the stratum corneum, the topmost layer of the skin. The outstanding skin barrier property is a main hindrance to the efficient transport of drugs via this path (6, 7). Skin permeation resistance in this layer is due to its unique arrangement, which further reduces the passage of large molecules, especially those larger than 500 daltons. But nanoparticles can solve this problem to a large extent because nanoparticles have size range of 1–100 nm (8, 9). However, nanoparticles in the range of 50–500 nm are also suitable depending on the route of administration for the purpose of drug delivery. Due to their smaller particle size, nanoformulations or nanocarriers show better targeting, drug retention and specificity (10). These features make them perfect transdermal drug delivery systems (TDDS). In the late 1970s, TDDSs were introduced into the US market, and this route is employed for enhancement of bioavailability of lipophilic poorly soluble and low-permeable drugs (BCS II & IV). Patient compliance is another advantage of TDDS, as self administration is possible and easy. It prevents gastrointestinal degradation of some therapeutic agents as well as avoiding hepatic first-pass metabolism, which causes degradation of the majority of the drugs (11). The numerous benefits of TDDS include being trouble-free, causing negligible skin injury (as it does not affect the structure of SC of the skin and does not abolish the skin barrier function), and encouraging macromolecular drug permeation, which is currently a very popular research area in TDDSs (12).

5.2 SKIN DISORDER TREATMENT BY TRANSDERMAL DELIVERY

Skin, the largest organ in humans, is an efficient route for the delivery of drugs as it circumvents several disadvantages of the oral route (Figure 5.1). Skin is primarily employed as a drug administration

DOI: 10.1201/9781003130055-5

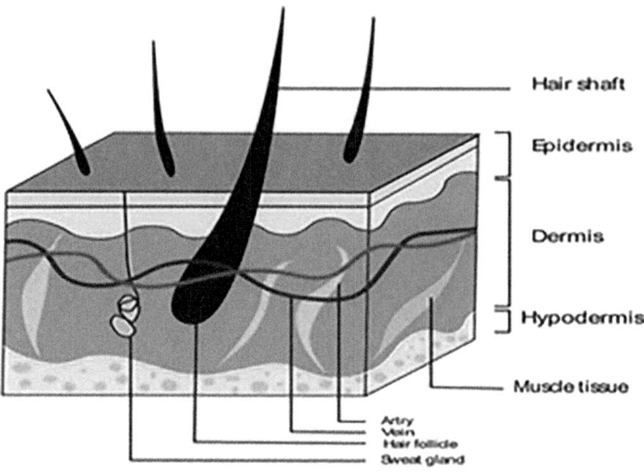

FIGURE 5.1 Skin structure with layers.

route for topical (dermal) delivery, where a drug is located in skin layers, or transdermal delivery, where a drug passes via the dermis and finally enters the blood (1, 2). Various skin disorders treated by the nanotechnology approach are mentioned in the following (Figure 5.2).

5.3 PSORIASIS

Psoriasis is a long-term inflammatory multifactorial skin disorder condition, driven by hyperproliferative epidermis responses due to development and hyperactivation of immature keratinocytes (13–16). Recent investigations on patients for psoriasis include ethosomal and liposomal formulations loaded with anthralin for improving efficacy and safety. These formulations have been integrated into different gel bases to ease administration. Ex vivo permeability tests found that in comparison with liposomal gel, anthralin ethosomal gel had substantially greater permeation via rat abdominal tissue. The clinical evaluation results of these formulations demonstrated minimized side effects of the drug. Results have shown that anthralin ethosomal gel in psoriatic patients is an efficient and secure treatment that justifies its ability to improve the effectiveness and safety of the drug (17).

5.4 ATOPIC DERMATITIS

Atopic dermatitis (AD) or eczema is a skin condition with chronic inflammation that exhibits signs of extreme swelling, oozing, itching and redness (18–20). The current investigation for this disorder involves the use of Cephalosprorin A (CsA) nanocapsules (NCs) topically. Drug penetration was enhanced in several layers of porcine ear skin with the CsA-NCs. In terms of better protection of the integrity of the skin barrier, a decline in systemic pro-inflammation markers and decreased skin inflammation were seen with the use of the topical formulation of CsA-NCs. In comparison with the current topical therapeutic drugs in AD, the overall experimental findings indicate that this novel topical platform is capable of providing better efficacy in AD treatment (21).

5.5 ACNE

Acne is a skin condition that affects appearance, is accompanied by chronic inflammation and occurs in the sebaceous glands, usually in the back and face area (22, 23). The factors responsible for acne development are colonization of propionibacterium acnes, excessive androgen level,

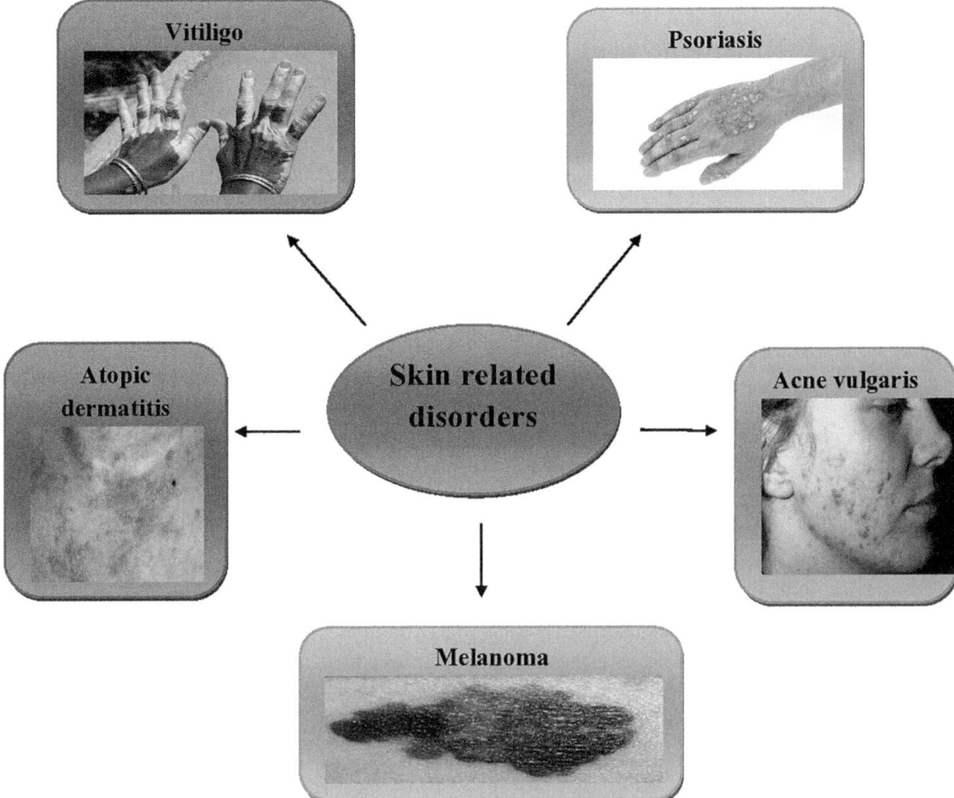

FIGURE 5.2 Common skin disorders.

pro-inflammatory cytokine release and abnormal keratinization of the sebaceous glands (24–26). One research study focused on 3D-printed niosomal hydrogel (3DP-NH) containing cryptotanshinone (CPT) as a topical acne therapy using the reverse phase evaporation technique. Three-dimensional (3D) printing technologies have the ability to facilitate the personalized treatment of acne (27).

5.6 MELANOMA

The deadliest type of skin cancer is melanoma. Its successful treatment is possible in the initial stage with the help of surgery alone, and it has a higher rate of survival; however, the survival rates decrease considerably after metastasis (28, 29). Therefore, the topical application of chemotherapy is an effective route for successful skin cancer treatment (30, 31). A 5-Flurouracil (FU) chitosan-based loaded pH-responsive biodegradable nanogel (FCNGL) was fabricated through the ion gelation technique for melanoma treatment. The formulation was effective against melanoma at even the lowest concentration (0.2% w/v) and showed selective accumulation of the drug at the melanoma site. Hemolysis and study of coagulation demonstrated high protection, while FCNGL was successful in MTT and apoptosis experiments. Evaluation such as immunohistochemistry (IHC) analysis of the tumor displayed enhancement of subcutaneous layer alignment and epithelial skin layer renewal. The results clearly show that for topical chemotherapy, FCNGL has potential for effective delivery of 5-FU in a sustained manner (32).

5.7 VITILIGO

Vitiligo is a depigmentation skin disease accompanied by macules of white color without melanocytes (33, 34). It has severe impacts psychologically and can even cause suicidal thoughts (35, 36). To treat this particular condition, a topical formulation of an ethosome-based hydrogel loaded with methoxsalen was fabricated. Accumulation of ethosomal formulation in dermal and epidermal layers resulted in increased skin permeation. Thus, formulation improved percutaneous penetration of methoxsalen and therefore can be employed for vitiligo treatment (37).

5.8 NANOCARRIERS FOR TRANSDERMAL DRUG DELIVERY

Nanocarriers are structures with a particle size below 500 nm. Because of their size, new properties arise that ultimately help in better therapeutic action. Currently the focus is on topically applied nanocarriers, as the skin offers a huge area for the application of such systems. For dermal treatment, it is important to distinguish between the desired effects of the formulation: the local effect on the top or inside of the skin (penetration only) or the systemic effect followed by skin permeation (38). It is also possible to differentiate between the goals of the production of nanocarriers, which could be safety of the active ingredients; the targeted delivery to the desired organ; and/or the controlled release of the active ingredient (39). As the most promising revolutionary research field of drug delivery, the transdermal route is now competing with oral therapy, with about 40% of drug delivery candidate products under clinical evaluation linked to transdermal or dermal systems (40). Obviously, the drug must be able to penetrate the skin (Figure 5.3) barrier and meet its delivery target in order for transdermal drug delivery systems to be successful. The barrier layer of the dermis exists in its outermost layer, the stratum corneum (41). This layer is a thick matrix (10–15μm) comprising dead and dehydrated keratinocytes (corneocytes) surrounded by a lipid matrix (42). In general, the penetration of topically applied solutes is considered to occur through the lipid portion of the matrix, historically modeled as organized among corneocytes into multiple bilayer structures that are in turn adhered to each other to stabilize the matrix through protein rivets called desmosomes (43, 44). The transdermal route has the ability to be an extremely successful delivery site for protein and peptide drugs. The permeation of the entire nanosystem or the drug itself is a prerequisite for the efficacy of a nanocarrier in the case of transdermal drug delivery (45–48). Innovative systems of drug delivery for this purpose are developed with massive efforts that include nanoparticular systems and vesicular transport systems (Table 5.1) (49).

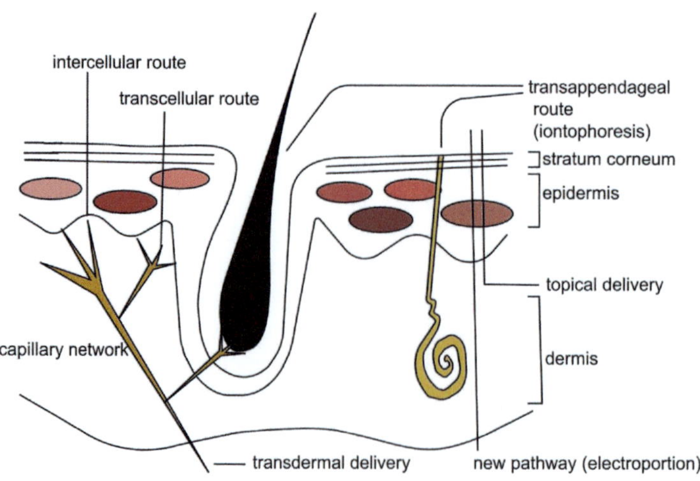

FIGURE 5.3 Transport of drugs through skin.

TABLE 5.1

Nanocarriers for Transdermal Drug Delivery

Drug	Nanoformulation	Treatment	Description	References
Ammonium glycyrrhizate	Ultradeformable liposomes	Skin inflammation	Study reveals that ultradeformable liposomes loaded with ammonium glycyrrhizate reduced inflammation of skin. So, this formulation shows potential as a topical drug delivery system used for anti-inflammatory therapy.	(50)
Tacrolimus and curcumin	Liposphere gel	Psoriasis	The results validate that liposphere gel comprising tacrolimus and curcumin can be an effectual strategy for psoriasis treatment.	(51)
Azelaic acid	Nanostructured lipid carriers	Acne vulgaris	Study highlighted a nanostructured lipid carrier gel was an efficient vehicle for enhancing the tissue targetability and efficacy of azelaic acid.	(52)
Nano-CUR and sulphoraphane	Ethosomal nanogel	Cancer therapy	Optimized ethosome NGs exhibited significant anticancer effect in B16-F10 murine tumor cell line.	(53)
Tetracycline HCl and tretinoin	Liposome formulations	Acne vulgaris	Results presented a dual active ingredient with comedolytic and bacteriostatic effects in a single, safe and stable liposome formulation.	(54)
Mangifera indica L.	Nanoemulsions	Acne	Such results might provide promising anti-acne nanoemulsions with the notable capacities of extract stabilization and permeation enhancing which will be further clinically evaluated.	(55)
Mulberry leaves, quercetin	Transfersomal gel	Acne vulgaris	It is evident from this study that mulberry leaves extract transfersomes gel is a promising prolonged delivery system for quercetin and has reasonably good stability characteristics and can potentially be used in the treatment of acne vulgaris through a transdermal drug delivery system.	(56)
Psoralen and resveratrol	Ultradeformableliposomes (UDLs)	Vitiligo	Psoralen and resveratrol co-loaded UDLs act in vitiligo through dual mechanisms of action: stimulation of melanin and tyrosinase activity and antioxidant activity, and they have promising therapeutic potential for the treatment of vitiligo.	(57)

(Continued)

TABLE 5.1   (Continued)

Nanocarriers for Transdermal Drug Delivery

Drug	Nanoformulation	Treatment	Description	References
Thymoquinone	Ethosomes	Acne	The developed thymoquinone-loaded ethosome formulation was a safe, less irritating and well-tolerated formulation for topical delivery and effective treatment option for acne vulgaris and various skin disorders.	(58)
Berberine chloride and evodiamine	Ethosomes	Melanoma	Studies like cell viability tests proved the optimized ethosomes increased the inhibitory effect on B16 melanoma cells, so ethosomes containing a combination of BBR and EVO are a promising delivery system for potential use in melanoma therapy.	(59)
Tazarotene	Transfersomes	Acne vulgaris	The developed tazarotene transfersomal gel has the ability to overcome the barrier properties of the skin and increase drug release.	(60)
Cyclosporine (CYC)	Cationic liposomes	Psoriasis	Topical application of CYC liposomal gels reduced the symptoms of psoriasis and levels of key psoriatic cytokines such as tumor necrosis factor-α, IL-17 and IL-22. This developed liposomal carrier of CYC was found to be effective and can find application in treatment of psoriasis.	(61)

Some new technologies for transdermal transport of drug are explained in the following (Figure 5.4).

Microemulsions: They are thermodynamically stable colloidal dispersions formed spontaneously without any energy input. Spontaneously, microemulsions emerge, mixing a suitable amount of a surfactant framework, a lipophilic component and a hydrophilic component (62, 63). They can occur over a broad range or only exist in narrow ranges depending on the components involved in the device (64). The process of formation includes a highly fluid interfacial film and low interfacial tension between the oil and the aqueous phase (65).

5.9   SOLID LIPID NANOPARTICLES

Solid lipid nanoparticles (SLNs) are usually called emulsion-based carriers of lipophilic bioactive compounds, have biocompatibility and are considered efficient carriers for antimicrobial agents (66). A recent study is based on transdermal delivery, which includes testosterone enanthate-loaded solid lipid nanoparticles (TESLNs), and its permeation through excised rat skin was explored. Through the results of evaluation of the nanoparticles, no cellular toxicity was seen, so fabricated TE-SLNs can be useful as potential carriers for testosterone-enanthate delivery via the transdermal route (67).

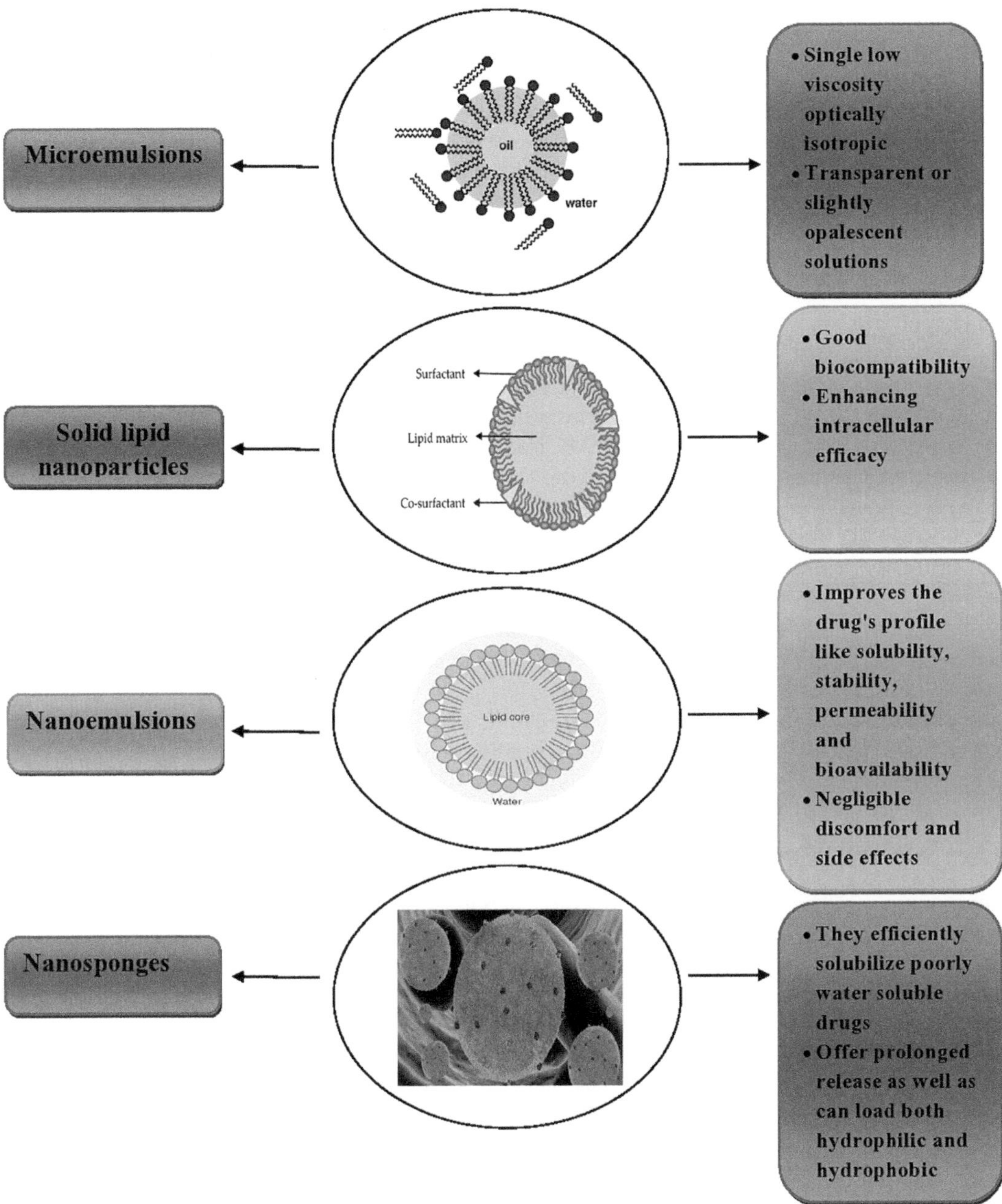

FIGURE 5.4 Nanocarriers for transdermal delivery.

5.10 MICROSPONGES

Microsponges are considered advanced systems for delivery of drugs that have the ability to encapsulate various agents, like anti-acne agents, essential oils, anti-inflammatory agents and fragrances (68, 69). Their diameter ranges from 5 to 300 μm; microcarriers are therefore chosen as a medium for the topical delivery of medicines, as they can prolong drug duration (70). Microsponges are efficient carriers that are capable of decreasing local unwanted effects of dermatological agents.

A naringenin-loaded microsponge gel using polymer ethyl cellulose was produced for dermatitis. Carbopol added in the optimized microsponge batch was incorporated to prepare a 1% naringenin-loaded microsponge gel (NGMSG 1%). In vivo studies were conducted on albino Wistar rats. In animals studies, no skin irritation was observed with NGMSG formulations, and NGMSG 1% demonstrated healing at a faster rate, and a considerable decrease in swollen earflap thickness, WBC count and elevated drug deposition were also observed. Therefore, this microsponge gel can be used for atopic dermatitis treatment (71).

5.11 NANOEMULSIONS

Nanoemulsions are isotropic scattered solutions of two non-miscible liquids, typically consisting of an oily system dispersed in an aqueous system or an aqueous system dispersed in an oily system but comprising nanometer-sized droplets or other oily phases (72, 73). This strengthens the functionality of the drug, such as solubility, durability, permeability and bioavailability, by encapsulating it into a droplet core oil and water (74). Nanoemulsion has been effective in supplying active drugs at therapeutically relevant levels to the target organ, with minimal pain and adverse effects (75). Nanoemulsions have stronger propagating properties in the skin than conventional emulsions, which is why they are used in dermatology to enhance the distribution of medications to and from the stratum corneum (76, 77). Nanoemulsions have been well used for numerous drugs, including pharmaceuticals, phytopharmaceuticals, cosmeceuticals, nutritional and nutraceuticals, to improve human health (78). Research was conducted on nanoemulsions (NEs) produced using alginate and chitosan for topical delivery of the cytotoxic agent piplartine (piperlongumine) against skin cancer. The formulation increased drug penetration, and its effects on 3D melanoma tissues were concentration-related; at 1%, piplartine caused destruction of the epidermis. These findings encourage the possible applicability of piplartin-containing chitosan-modified nanoemulsions as a new approach for local skin cancer treatment (79).

5.12 NANOSPONGES

Nanosponges are hyper-cross-linked cyclodextrin polymers that are nanostructured to form 3D networks and are acquired with a cross-linker like carbonyldiimidazole by complexing cyclodextrin (80, 81). There are typically numerous polymer chains in their crystal architecture that can construct unique microdomains appropriate for the co-encapsulation of two drugs of a distinct chemical composition (82). Nanosponges used widely because they effectively solubilize poorly water-soluble drugs and have extended release simultaneously, and because of their inner hydrophobic cavities and external hydrophilic branching, they can load both hydrophilic and hydrophobic drug molecules (83). These small sponges will circulate within the body to accomplish precise targeted delivery before they encounter their target location to activate the drug in a controlled and configured manner (84). To enhance the efficacy, durability, permeation and bioavailability of pharmacotherapeutic drugs, there are many implementations of nanosponges in transdermal drug delivery. Cyclodextrin nanosponges (CDNSs) were prepared for topical delivery of clobetasol propionate (CP) for psoriasis. An in vivo study was also carried out using a mouse tail model. Evaluation results clearly show the potential of fabricated CP nanogels in topical psoriasis treatment, with enhanced patient compliance (85).

5.13 TOXICITY ASPECTS

The main challenges faced by drug delivery systems include toxicological and safety issues. Cellular responses are greatly influenced by the form and charge of nanocarriers. The topographical surface characteristics and surface roughness of nanocarriers regulate biological responses either by exerting a direct impact on the cytoskeleton or through protein alignment indirectly (86). The reduced size of nanocarriers allows proteins to adsorb onto their surface, creating epitopes on the surface of the protein (87). The scale of nanocarriers has been given more attention; as the size decreases to the nanometric range, the ratio of surface to volume increases exponentially. Consequently, toxicity and reactivity escalate in the cells. Particle size below 50 nm has significantly increased necrotic cell death, although less toxicity was seen above 100 nm (88, 89).

5.14 CONCLUSION

The recent technical advancements in delivery via the transdermal route have come about as a result of a deeper understanding of the molecular-level structure of the stratum corneum and the permeation pathways through the skin. The transdermal route is becoming a widely accepted drug administration route because of its better ability to apply drugs to the site of action without cracking the skin membrane. Nanotechnology is newly developed as a favorable technique to resolve the skin's barrier function. This chapter covered widely employed nanoparticulate carriers for improving the transport of drugs through the dermis. The previously discussed findings showed a superior relationship between nanoparticulate carriers and skin structures to facilitate drug delivery. Research has focused on the development of newer nanoparticulate carriers with desirable properties for skin applications in the near future, with developments in material engineering, manufacturing and characterization techniques. Future studies, however, should guarantee the benefits and determine the risk ratio for several therapeutic agents loaded in nanocarriers.

REFERENCES

1. Kamble P, Sadarani B, Majumdar A, Bhullar S. Nanofiber based drug delivery systems for skin: A promising therapeutic approach. *Journal of Drug Delivery Science and Technology.* 2017;41:124–33.
2. Tobin DJ. Introduction to skin aging. *Journal of Tissue Viability.* 2017;26(1):37–46.
3. Schäfer-Korting M, Mehnert W, Korting HC. Lipid nanoparticles for improved topical application of drugs for skin diseases. *Advanced Drug Delivery Reviews.* 2007;59(6):427–43.
4. Neubert RH. Potentials of new nanocarriers for dermal and transdermal drug delivery. *European Journal of Pharmaceutics and Biopharmaceutics.* 2011;77(1):1–2.
5. Barry BW. Mode of action of penetration enhancers in human skin. *Journal of Controlled Release.* 1987;6(1):85–97.
6. Barry BW. *Dermatological Formulations: Percutaneous Absorption.* Marcel Dekker, New York, NY & Basel, 1983.
7. El Maghraby GM, Williams AC, Barry BW. Skin hydration and possible shunt route penetration in controlled estradiol delivery from ultradeformable and standard liposomes. *Journal of Pharmacy and Pharmacology.* 2001;53(10):1311–22.
8. Prausnitz MR, Mitragotri S, Langer R. Current status and future potential of transdermal drug delivery. *Nature Reviews Drug Discovery.* 2004;3(2):115–24.
9. Escobar-Chávez JJ, Díaz-Torres R, Rodríguez-Cruz IM, Domínguez-Delgado CL, Morales RS, Ángeles-Anguiano E, Melgoza-Contreras LM. Nanocarriers for transdermal drug delivery. *Research and Reports in Transdermal Drug Delivery.* 2012;1:3–17.
10. Barry BW. Novel mechanisms and devices to enable successful transdermal drug delivery. *European Journal of Pharmaceutical Sciences.* 2001;14(2):101–14.
11. Rizwan M, Aqil M, Talegaonkar S, Azeem A, Sultana Y, Ali A. Enhanced transdermal drug delivery techniques: An extensive review of patents. *Recent Patents on Drug Delivery & Formulation.* 2009;3(2):105–24.
12. Paudel KS, Milewski M, Swadley CL, Brogden NK, Ghosh P, Stinchcomb AL. Challenges and opportunities in dermal/transdermal delivery. *Therapeutic Delivery.* 2010;1(1):109–31.
13. Gudjonsson JE, Johnston A, Sigmundsdottir H, Valdimarsson H. Immunopathogenic mechanisms in psoriasis. *Clinical & Experimental Immunology.* 2004;135(1):1–8.
14. Marepally S, Boakye CH, Patel AR, Godugu C, Doddapaneni R, Desai PR, Singh M. Topical administration of dual siRNAs using Fusogenic lipid nanoparticles for treating psoriatic-like plaques. *Nanomedicine.* 2014;9(14):2157–74.

15. Lowes MA, Bowcock AM, Krueger JG. Pathogenesis and therapy of psoriasis. *Nature.* 2007;445(7130):866–73.

16. Cornell RC. Clinical trials of topical corticosteroids in psoriasis: Correlations with the vasoconstrictor assay. *International Journal of Dermatology.* 1992;31:38–40.

17. Fathalla D, Youssef EM, Soliman GM. Liposomal and ethosomal gels for the topical delivery of anthralin: Preparation, comparative evaluation and clinical assessment in psoriatic patients. *Pharmaceutics.* 2020;12(5):446.

18. Boneberger S, Rupec RA, Ruzicka T. Complementary therapy for atopic dermatitis and other allergic skin diseases: Facts and controversies. *Clinics in Dermatology.* 2010;28(1):57–61.

19. Oranje AP, Devillers AC, Kunz B, Jones SL, DeRaeve L, Gysel DV, De Waard-van der Spek FB, Grimalt R, Torrelo A, Stevens J, Harper J. Treatment of patients with atopic dermatitis using wet-wrap dressings with diluted steroids and/or emollients. An expert panel's opinion and review of the literature. *Journal of the European Academy of Dermatology and Venereology.* 2006;20(10):1277–86.

20. Devillers AC, Oranje AP. Efficacy and safety of 'wet-wrap' dressings as an intervention treatment in children with severe and/or refractory atopic dermatitis: A critical review of the literature. *British Journal of Dermatology.* 2006;154(4):579–85.

21. Badihi A, Frušić-Zlotkin M, Soroka Y, Benhamron S, Tzur T, Nassar T, Benita S. Topical nano-encapsulated cyclosporine formulation for atopic dermatitis treatment. *Nanomedicine.* 2020;24:102140.

22. Tan JK, Bhate K. A global perspective on the epidemiology of acne. *British Journal of Dermatology.* 2015;172:3–12.

23. Dessinioti C, Katsambas AD. The role of Propionibacterium acnes in acne pathogenesis: Facts and controversies. *Clinics in Dermatology.* 2010;28(1):2–7.

24. Poomanee W, Chaiyana W, Mueller M, Viernstein H, Khunkitti W, Leelapornpisid P. In-vitro investigation of anti-acne properties of Mangifera indica L. kernel extract and its mechanism of action against Propionibacterium acnes. *Anaerobe.* 2018;52:64–74.

25. Krautheim A, Gollnick HP. Acne: Topical treatment. *Clinics in Dermatology.* 2004;22(5):398–407.

26. Eady EA, Gloor M, Leyden JJ. Propionibacterium acnes resistance: A worldwide problem. *Dermatology.* 2003;206(1):54–6.

27. Wang Z, Liu L, Xiang S, Jiang C, Wu W, Ruan S, Du Q, Chen T, Xue Y, Chen H, Weng L. Formulation and characterization of a 3d-printed cryptotanshinone-loaded niosomal hydrogel for topical therapy of acne. *AAPS Pharmaceutical Science and Technology.* 2020;21:1–3.

28. Singh S, Zafar A, Khan S, Naseem I. Towards therapeutic advances in melanoma management: An overview. *Life Sciences.* 2017;174:50–8.

29. Tracey EH, Vij A. Updates in melanoma. *Dermatologic Clinics.* 2019;37(1):73–82.

30. Luo C, Shen J. Research progress in advanced melanoma. *Cancer Letters.* 2017;397:120–6.

31. Brys AK, Gowda R, Loriaux DB, Robertson GP, Mosca PJ. Nanotechnology-based strategies for combating toxicity and resistance in melanoma therapy. *Biotechnology Advances.* 2016;34(5):565–77.

32. Sahu P, Kashaw SK, Sau S, Kushwah V, Jain S, Agrawal RK, Iyer AK. pH responsive 5-fluorouracil loaded biocompatible nanogels for topical chemotherapy of aggressive melanoma. *Colloids and Surfaces B: Biointerfaces.* 2019;174:232–45.

33. Garg BJ, Garg NK, Beg S, Singh B, Katare OP. Nanosized ethosomes-based hydrogel formulations of methoxsalen for enhanced topical delivery against vitiligo: Formulation optimization, in vitro evaluation and preclinical assessment. *Journal of Drug Targeting.* 2016;24(3):233–46.

34. Doppalapudi S, Mahira S, Khan W. Development and in vitro assessment of psoralen and resveratrol co-loaded ultradeformable liposomes for the treatment of vitiligo. *Journal of Photochemistry and Photobiology B: Biology.* 2017;174:44–57.

35. Hann SK, Cho MY, Im S, Park YK. Treatment of vitiligo with oral 5-methoxypsoralen. *The Journal of Dermatology.* 1991;18(6):324–9.

36. George WM, Burks JW. Treatment of vitiligo with psoralen derivatives. *AMA Archives of Dermatology.* 1955;71(1):14–8.

37. Garg BJ, Garg NK, Beg S, Singh B, Katare OP. Nanosized ethosomes-based hydrogel formulations of methoxsalen for enhanced topical delivery against vitiligo: Formulation optimization, in vitro evaluation and preclinical assessment. *Journal of Drug Targeting.* 2016;24(3):233–46.

38. Schroeter A, Engelbrecht T, Neubert RH, Goebel AS. New nanosized technologies for dermal and transdermal drug delivery. A review. *Journal of Biomedical Nanotechnology.* 2010;6(5):511–28.

39. Godin B, Touitou E. Transdermal skin delivery: Predictions for humans from in vivo, ex vivo and animal models. *Advanced Drug Delivery Reviews.* 2007;59(11):1152–61.

40. Neubert RH. Potentials of new nanocarriers for dermal and transdermal drug delivery. *European Journal of Pharmaceutics and Biopharmaceutics.* 2011;77(1):1–2.
41. Cross SE, Roberts MS. Physical enhancement of transdermal drug application: Is delivery technology keeping up with pharmaceutical development? *Current Drug Delivery.* 2004;1(1):81–92.
42. Barry BW. Novel mechanisms and devices to enable successful transdermal drug delivery. *European Journal of Pharmaceutical Sciences.* 2001;14(2):101–14.
43. Potts RO, Guy RH. Predicting skin permeability. *Pharmaceutical Research.* 1992;9(5):663–9.
44. Bala P, Jathar S, Kale S, Pal K. Transdermal drug delivery system (TDDS)-a multifaceted approach for drug delivery. *Journal of Pharmacy Research.* 2014;8(12):1805–35.
45. Bos JD, Meinardi MM. The 500 Dalton rule for the skin penetration of chemical compounds and drugs. *Experimental Dermatology: Viewpoint.* 2000;9(3):165–9.
46. Beignon AS, Briand JP, Muller S, Partidos CD. Immunization onto bare skin with synthetic peptides: Immunomodulation with a CpG-containing oligodeoxynucleotide and effective priming of influenza virus-specific CD4+ T cells. *Immunology.* 2002;105(2):204–12.
47. Pannatier A, Jenner P, Testa B, Etter JC. The skin as a drug-metabolizing organ. *Drug Metabolism Reviews.* 1978;8(2):319–43.
48. Lampe MA, Williams ML, Elias PM. Human epidermal lipids: Characterization and modulations during differentiation. *Journal of Lipid Research.* 1983;24(2):131–40.
49. Jijie R, Barras A, Boukherroub R, Szunerits S. Nanomaterials for transdermal drug delivery: Beyond the state of the art of liposomal structures. *Journal of Materials Chemistry B.* 2017;5(44):8653–75.
50. Barone A, Cristiano MC, Cilurzo F, Locatelli M, Iannotta D, Di Marzio L, Celia C, Paolino D. Ammonium glycyrrhizate skin delivery from ultradeformable liposomes: A novel use as an anti-inflammatory agent in topical drug delivery. *Colloids and Surfaces B: Biointerfaces.* 2020;193:111152.
51. Jain A, Doppalapudi S, Domb AJ, Khan W. Tacrolimus and curcumin co-loaded liposphere gel: Synergistic combination towards management of psoriasis. *Journal of Controlled Release.* 2016;243:132–45.
52. Malik DS, Kaur G. Exploring therapeutic potential of azelaic acid loaded NLCs for the treatment of acne vulgaris. *Journal of Drug Delivery Science and Technology.* 2020;55:101418.
53. Soni K, Mujtaba A, Akhter MH, Zafar A, Kohli K. Optimisation of ethosomal nanogel for topical nano-CUR and sulphoraphane delivery in effective skin cancer therapy. *Journal of Microencapsulation.* 2020;37(2):91–108.
54. Eroğlu İ, Aslan M, Yaman Ü, Gultekinoglu M, Çalamak S, Kart D, Ulubayram K. Liposome-based combination therapy for acne treatment. *Journal of Liposome Research.* 2020;30(3):263–73.
55. Poomanee W, Khunkitti W, Chaiyana W, Leelapornpisid P. Optimization of Mangifera indica l. kernel extract-loaded nanoemulsions via response surface methodology, characterization, stability, and skin permeation for anti-acne cosmeceutical application. *Pharmaceutics.* 2020;12(5):454.
56. Nangare S, Dhananjay B, Mali R, Shitole M. Development of novel freeze-dried mulberry leaves extract-based transfersomal gel. *Turkish Journal of Pharmaceutical Sciences.* 2021;18(1):44–55.
57. Doppalapudi S, Mahira S, Khan W. Development and in vitro assessment of psoralen and resveratrol co-loaded ultradeformable liposomes for the treatment of vitiligo. *Journal of Photochemistry and Photobiology B: Biology.* 2017;174:44–57.
58. Kausar H, Mujeeb M, Ahad A, Moolakkadath T, Aqil M, Ahmad A. Optimization of ethosomes for topical thymoquinone delivery for the treatment of skin acne. *Journal of Drug Delivery Science and Technology.* 2019;49:177–87.
59. Lin H, Lin L, Choi Y, Michniak-Kohn B. Development and in-vitro evaluation of co-loaded berberine chloride and evodiamine ethosomes for treatment of melanoma. *International Journal of Pharmaceutics.* 2020:119278.
60. Sahu JP, Khan AI, Maurya R, Shukla AK. Formulation development and evaluation of Transferosomal drug delivery for effective treatment of acne. *Advance Pharmaceutical Journal.* 2019;4(1):26–34.
61. Walunj M, Doppalapudi S, Bulbake U, Khan W. Preparation, characterization, and in vivo evaluation of cyclosporine cationic liposomes for the treatment of psoriasis. *Journal of Liposome Research.* 2020;30(1):68–79.
62. Aliberti AL, de Queiroz AC, Praça FS, Eloy JO, Bentley MV, Medina WS. Ketoprofen microemulsion for improved skin delivery and in vivo anti-inflammatory effect. *AAPS Pharmaceutical Science and Technology.* 2017;18(7):2783–91.
63. Nastiti CM, Ponto T, Abd E, Grice JE, Benson HA, Roberts MS. Topical nano and microemulsions for skin delivery. *Pharmaceutics.* 2017;9(4):37.

64. Cichewicz A, Pacleb C, Connors A, Hass MA, Lopes LB. Cutaneous delivery of α-tocopherol and lipoic acid using microemulsions: Influence of composition and charge. *Journal of Pharmacy and Pharmacology.* 2013;65(6):817–26.

65. Praça FG, Viegas JS, Peh HY, Garbin TN, Medina WS, Bentley MV. Microemulsion co-delivering vitamin A and vitamin E as a new platform for topical treatment of acute skin inflammation. *Materials Science and Engineering: C.* 2020;110:110639.

66. Meng K, Chen D, Yang F, Zhang A, Tao Y, Qu W, Pan Y, Hao H, Xie S. Intracellular delivery, accumulation, and discrepancy in antibacterial activity of four enrofloxacin-loaded fatty acid solid lipid nanoparticles. *Colloids and Surfaces B: Biointerfaces.* 2020;194:111196.

67. Tajbakhsh M, Saeedi M, Akbari J, Morteza-Semnani K, Nokhodchi A, Hedayatizadeh-Omran A. An investigation on parameters affecting the optimization of testosterone enanthate loaded solid nanoparticles for enhanced transdermal delivery. *Colloids and Surfaces A: Physicochemical and Engineering Aspects.* 2020;589:124437.

68. Junqueira MV, Bruschi ML. A review about the drug delivery from microsponges. *AAPS Pharmaceutical Science and Technology.* 2018;19(4):1501–11.

69. Bhuptani RS, Patravale VB. Starch microsponges for enhanced retention and efficacy of topical sunscreen. *Materials Science and Engineering: C.* 2019;104:109882.

70. Devi N, Kumar S, Prasad M, Rao R. Eudragit RS100 based microsponges for dermal delivery of clobetasol propionate in psoriasis management. *Journal of Drug Delivery Science and Technology.* 2020;55:101347.

71. Nagula RL, Wairkar S. Cellulose microsponges based gel of naringenin for atopic dermatitis: Design, optimization, in vitro and in vivo investigation. *International Journal of Biological Macromolecules.* 2020;164:717–25.

72. Gheorghe I, Saviuc C, Ciubuca B, Lazar V, Chifiriuc MC. Nanodrug delivery systems for transdermal drug delivery. In *Nanomaterials for Drug Delivery and Therapy* (pp. 225–244). William Andrew Publishing, Elsevier, 2019 Jan 1.

73. Zhengguang L, Jie H, Yong Z, Jiaojiao C, Xingqi W, Xiaoqin C. Study on the transdermal penetration mechanism of ibuprofen nanoemulsions. *Drug Development and Industrial Pharmacy.* 2019;45(3):465–73.

74. Abdulbaqi MR, Rajab NA. Apixaban ultrafine o/w nano emulsion transdermal drug delivery system: Formulation, in vitro and ex vivo characterization. *Systematic Reviews in Pharmacy.* 2020;11(2):82–94.

75. Sarheed O, Shouqair D, Ramesh KV, Khaleel T, Amin M, Boateng J, Drechsler M. Formation of stable nanoemulsions by ultrasound-assisted two-step emulsification process for topical drug delivery: Effect of oil phase composition and surfactant concentration and loratadine as ripening inhibitor. *International Journal of Pharmaceutics.* 2020;576:118952.

76. Harwansh RK, Deshmukh R, Rahman MA. Nanoemulsion: Promising nanocarrier system for delivery of herbal bioactives. *Journal of Drug Delivery Science and Technology.* 2019;51:224–33.

77. Sutradhar KB, Amin ML. Nanoemulsions: Increasing possibilities in drug delivery. *European Journal of Nanomedicine.* 2014;6(1):53.

78. Sun Y, Xia Z, Zheng J, Qiu P, Zhang L, McClements DJ, Xiao H. Nanoemulsion-based delivery systems for nutraceuticals: Influence of carrier oil type on bioavailability of pterostilbene. *Journal of Functional Foods.* 2015;13:61–70.

79. Giacone DV, Dartora VF, de Matos JK, Passos JS, Miranda DA, de Oliveira EA, Silveira ER, Costa-Lotufo LV, Maria-Engler SS, Lopes LB. Effect of nanoemulsion modification with chitosan and sodium alginate on the topical delivery and efficacy of the cytotoxic agent piplartine in 2D and 3D skin cancer models. *International Journal of Biological Macromolecules.* 2020;165:1055–65.

80. Gangadharappa HV, Prasad SM, Singh RP. Formulation, in vitro and in vivo evaluation of celecoxib nanosponge hydrogels for topical application. *Journal of Drug Delivery Science and Technology.* 2017;41:488–501.

81. Tannous M, Trotta F, Cavalli R. Nanosponges for combination drug therapy: State-of-the-art and future directions. *Future Medicine.* 2020;15(7):643–46.

82. Jain A, Prajapati SK, Kumari A, Mody N, Bajpai M. Engineered nanosponges as versatile biodegradable carriers: An insight. *Journal of Drug Delivery Science and Technology.* 2020:101643.

83. Iriventi P, Gupta NV, Osmani RA, Balamuralidhara V. Design & development of nanosponge loaded topical gel of curcumin and caffeine mixture for augmented treatment of psoriasis. *Daru: Journal of Faculty of Pharmacy, Tehran University of Medical Sciences.* 2020;28(2):489–506.

84. Pushpalatha R, Selvamuthukumar S, Kilimozhi D. Cyclodextrin nanosponge based hydrogel for the transdermal co-delivery of curcumin and resveratrol: Development, optimization, in vitro and ex vivo evaluation. *Journal of Drug Delivery Science and Technology.* 2019;52:55–64.

85. Kumar S, Prasad M, Rao R. Topical delivery of clobetasol propionate loaded nanosponge hydrogel for effective treatment of psoriasis: Formulation, physicochemical characterization, antipsoriatic potential and biochemical estimation. *Materials Science and Engineering: C.* 1920;119:111605.
86. Rahmati M, Mozafari M. Nano-immunoengineering: Opportunities and challenges. *Current Opinion in Biomedical Engineering.* 2019;10:51–9.
87. Albanese A, Tang PS, Chan WC. The effect of nanoparticle size, shape, and surface chemistry on biological systems. *Annual Review of Biomedical Engineering.* 2012;14:1–6.
88. Abdel-Mottaleb MM, Try C, Pellequer Y, Lamprecht A. Nanomedicine strategies for targeting skin inflammation. *Nanomedicine.* 2014;9(11):1727–43.
89. Nel A, Xia T, Mädler L, Li N. Toxic potential of materials at the nanolevel. *Science.* 2006;311(5761):622–7.

6 Nanostructure-Based Pulmonary Drug Delivery Systems for Respiratory Infections

Vinay Kumar, Himani Singh, Sofiya Tarannum, Sanya Batheja, Umesh Gupta, and Amit Kumar Goyal

6.1 INTRODUCTION

In the United States, the prevalence of obstructive lung diseases entails approximately 25 million cases, and the majority of these are treated with inhalation medications. Respiratory disease encompasses a group of diseases which mainly affect the lungs locally, such as asthma and chronic obstructive pulmonary disease (COPD). Mucus hypersecretion, severe inflammation, and airway defense are the major hurdles in drug delivery and therapeutic efficiency in respiratory disease. Chronic airway inflammation and mucus hypersecretion are the hallmark manifestations of COPD and cystic fibrosis (C.F.). In asthma, inflammation appears to be aggravated by allergen-specific Th2 cells, resulting in eosinophilia, while in COPD and C.F., inflammatory response facilitates the hypersecretion of mucus in the disease. The chronic stage of the disease is also associated with widespread damage to the bronchial epithelium. However, all these diseases also deteriorate other body functions. Depending on the individual size, different deposition patterns can be observed in the inhalable range. At the same time, smaller particles reach the peripheral lung areas, and larger ones preferentially deposit in the central part.

During breathing, the lungs are more prone to exposure to foreign airborne particles, including bacteria and pollens. The foreign particles quickly get fixed in the upper conducting airway region of the respiratory tract. The less available surface area of the pulmonary epithelium in the trachea region restricts the particles in its absorption process. Particle deposition occurs under the influence of dynamics in the respiratory tract (1). Pulmonary delivery depends upon various parameters: flow properties, mucus interaction, non-compressibility, aerodynamics surface area, and temperature. Particles with a greater diameter can also accumulate under the inertial impaction process. Even particles with a lower diameter (less than 1 nm) may deposit through the alveoli diffusion process. In general, particles with a diameter of 1–3 μm offer a significant deposition. Moreover, there are no statistical equations available to justify a relationship between particle velocity and its deposition behavior. Thus, determining particle trajectories, inertia, and diffusion influenced by the synchronized conditions is essential to envisage inhaled particles' distribution patterns.

The earliest techniques involving burning and inhaling aromatic leaves, especially tobacco, to achieve the desired pharmacological effect. Understanding the characteristics and features of medicinal plants, the preparation of a nasal snuff from the powder form of aromatic plants and oils was used in earlier days (2). In the respiratory system, lungs permit a greater surface area for absorption and lead to escalated blood circulation, making a way to transport therapeutics via a non-invasive approach. Localized delivery approaches are utilized in the most promising way to treat respiratory diseases, especially tuberculosis, asthma, influenza, and chronic obstructive pulmonary disease; additionally, they reduce systemic toxicity. Alternatively, systemic drug delivery could be

DOI: 10.1201/9781003130055-6

achieved by targeting the alveolar region. The appropriate bioavailability can be achieved by targeting the alveolar area, where drugs can be easily absorbed into the systemic circulation through a thin layer of epithelial cells. This approach also leads to modulated permeability, a quicker onset of action, and restriction to the first-pass metabolism. Moreover, frequent medical scientific advances exhibit immense potential for efficient pulmonary delivery of bioactive or proteins that cannot be taken orally and require parenteral delivery (3).

Drug inhalation enables rapid drug deposition in the lungs and has fewer side effects as compared to administration by other routes. The plausible benefits of aerosolized delivery drive innovation and development in the medical field, especially in pulmonary disorders. There are limitless advantages of aerosols, including non-invasive targeted approaches, a greater surface area, potentially fewer systemic side effects, decreased drug metabolism, and patient compliance (4). An aerosolized device could be utilized to deliver therapeutics sustainably and in a controlled way. A number of drugs have been successfully delivered via pressurized metered-dose inhalers (pMDI) (5), dry powder inhalers (DPIs) (6), or nebulizers (7). In addition, other drugs have been delivered through aerosol techniques. Nanocarrier-based approaches have been exploited extensively to treat pulmonary diseases using aerosolized lung delivery. In general, nanocarrier-mediated transportation to the lungs could be a fascinating concept due to the prolonged release of particle retention in the lungs. Alternatively, nanoparticles with a size range below 250 nm are less taken up by the macrophages in the alveolar regions. The combined effects might improve local respiratory drug therapy. Pulmonary drug delivery systems require nanoformulations for inhaling therapeutics in the lower respiratory region. Moreover, it is the most convenient route to deposit an adequate amount of drug at disease-specific sites, with lower dosage, localized pharmacological effect, and circumventing the first-pass metabolism effect, which reduces the drug's metabolism. Thus, targeted approaches are being substantially geared toward the pulmonary delivery of therapeutics by reducing the systemic complications related to long-term medicament administration.

Recent medical advances have established that small-airway passage significantly leads to obstructive airway passage (8). Many researchers have contributed to the delivery of suitable medications by targeting small airways, thus modulating their bioavailability within the nanocomposite (9). Aerosolized drug delivery is a crucial component in managing respiratory diseases, especially asthma and COPD. Therefore, opting for the most suitable device to meet a personalized patient's needs is crucial in clinical applications. Asthma and COPD disease patients could be treated with an integral inhalable formulation system. Different varieties of inhalers with distinctive features are available on the market. Therefore, individual choice depends upon the most appropriate device, which is important per clinical consideration.

6.1.1 Pulmonary Drug Delivery—An Overview

For delivering drugs directly to the lungs, the preferred routes are:

a) **Intranasal delivery**: It generally consists of the delivery of drugs in aerosolized form via the nasal route through the nasal passage (10).
   - **Advantages**: Intranasal delivery is recommended when frequent dosing is needed. It is non-invasive and thus a good option for pulmonary delivery with techniques like nasal high-flow and low-flow therapy.
   - **Disadvantages**: Conventional aerosol delivery with size 3–7 μm is restricted in the nose region, as these get filtered. This prevents the bioavailability of the drug (85%) reaching systemic circulation when delivered as small particles through this route (11).

b) **Oral inhalation delivery:** It is further categorized into
   i) **Intra-tracheal instillation**: In this technique, drugs are administered in the trachea regions with the help of a syringe. Its applicability is restricted only to preclinical trials (1).

ii) **Intra-tracheal inhalation:** Drug-containing particles are delivered to the lungs through aerosol technology. This technique favors both higher penetration and uniform distribution. It could effectively deliver small-sized particles with a minimum drug loss (20%) (12).

6.1.1.1 Mechanism of Pulmonary Drug Deposition

a) **Inertial impaction:** This occurs as the inertia of the particles restricts their movement with respect to the flow of air, where the collision of particles along the walls makes them settle. Particles with greater aerodynamic diameters (>3 μm) generally get easily deposited at the bronchial region due to inertial impaction, as shown in Figure 6.1. Particle mass, hyperventilation, respiration frequency, and air velocity affect impaction (13). Dry powder inhalations and metered-dose inhalers (MDIs) work via this mechanism.

b) **Sedimentation** indicates the deposition of small particles (of diameter 1–8 μm) on the walls of the small airways and alveoli due to gravity. Breath-holding mainly affects this mechanism, as it gives particles sufficient time to deposit in the lungs under the influence of gravity, outweighing the air resistance (14).

c) **Brownian diffusion:** Small particles (diameter < 5 μm) undergo deposition through diffusion from high to low concentration, which is mainly dependent on Brownian motion. The particle's shape is accountable for this mechanism. Particles settle in a low-airflow region (nasopharynx) like small airways of alveolar regions and bronchioles (14).

Some other mechanisms are interception (particle deposition due to their shape and size, e.g., fibers), turbulent mixing (non-uniform fluctuations in particles containing fluid due to turbulent motion) (15), and electrostatic precipitation (electrostatic attraction between charged particles).

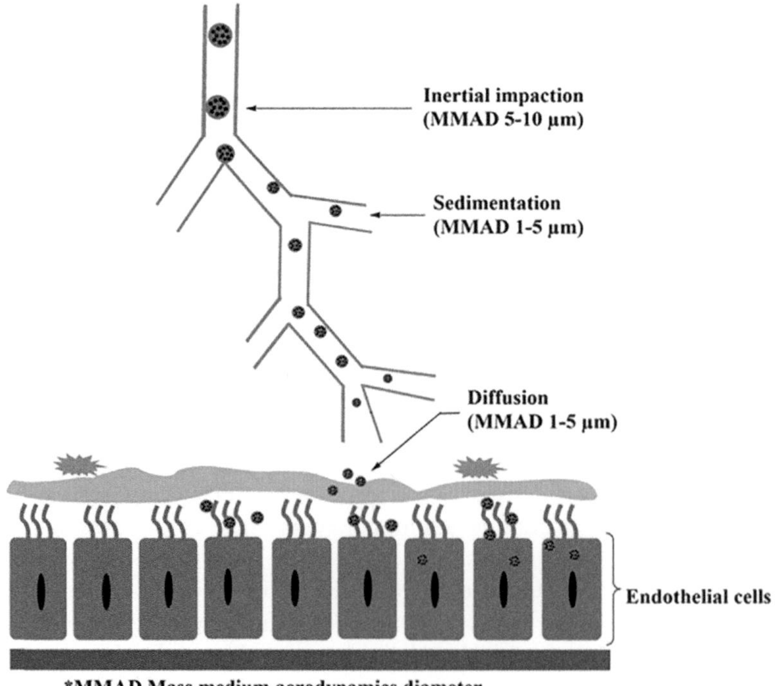

FIGURE 6.1   Mechanism of deposition of particulate systems in lungs.

6.1.2 Particle-Based Pulmonary Delivery

Inhalation could be an efficient approach to deliver following aerosolization (10). The aerosolization technique efficiently expels the compressed or liquefied drug from the container as gas/mist with or without propellant (16). The physicochemical characteristics of the particles are immensely important in aerosolized delivery approaches. The determination of the deposited particles and their flow behavior depends on the aerosolized device's structural framework and the lung's anatomical structure. The drug absorbance and its clearance rate from the systemic circulation depend upon the efficient delivery approaches as well as the physiological framework of the organ.

Some of the critical parameters that need to be considered in these approaches are as follows:

a) Particle size in aerosolized delivery
b) Physical stability
c) Particle density and shape
d) pH and osmolarity
e) Viscosity

a) **Particle size in aerosolized delivery**—Homogenous aerosol formulations are widely considered a delivery tool by the pharmaceutical industry. Per the requirements of measuring particle size, the nominal diameter range of particles is usually considered a reference for the standard spherical geometries. Particle size and size distribution play a key role in developing homogenous aerosolized formulations. In addition to the geometric particle size, factors influencing particle deposition are physical state, shape, density, and velocity (17). Geometric particle size can be measured via two techniques:

i. Direct measurement—using a microscope
ii. Indirect measurement—using inertial impactors and laser light scattering

The aerodynamics diameters of drug particles are considered when the optimum range (0.4–7 μm) is used to treat pulmonary disease. The greater surface area of the lung (i.e., 100 m^2) and thickness of the thin epithelial membrane (0.2 to 0.7 μm) allows the advantages of improved efficiency with minimal side effects (18). Thus, the ideal particle size in designing aerosolized formulation should be between 2 and 6 μm. However, the spatial distribution of larger particles (> 6 μm) intervenes in the upper airway region of the lung, whereas deposition of small particles (< 2 μm) takes place in the alveolar region of the lung (15). Moreover, the cohesive and adhesive interactions between particle and cell surface are significant parameters for designing an inhalable formulation. A series of dynamic forces, especially Van der Waal's forces, hydrostatic interaction, mechanical interlocking, and electrostatic interaction, are basic contributors to the interactions observed in the lungs (19).

b) **Physical stability**—Physical stability is one of the most crucial factors for delivering medications through aerosolized devices, as the aerosol consists of dense particles in less solvent, leading to inter-particle interactions such as aggregation or repulsion. Inter-particle interaction could cause instability in the formulation during storage conditions, thereby reducing the efficacy and potency of the formulations (19). Thus, stabilizers such as mannitol and trehalose could be incorporated into the formulations to avoid physical instability. It could improve the physical stability of formulations and the performance of aerosolized dosage forms (20). The spray-dried formulation is the best example of an amorphous drug when stored in high humidity conditions, as gain in moisture tends to modulate aerodynamic diameter, leading to instability of the formulation (21).

c) **Particle density and shape**—Another essential factor is particle density, and shape plays a vital role in modulating the pulmonary drug delivery system (22). As stated earlier, the aerodynamic diameter of the particles is the critical parameter in the deposition process. Also, density and shape are essential factors for determining the particle's aerodynamic diameter. Parameters affecting the aerodynamic diameter are the drag forces generated during the formation of different shapes of the particles (such as oblate ellipsoids, elliptical disks, rectangular disks, spheres, and worm-like shapes) (22) and the terminal settling velocities observed when particles settle under the influence of gravitational force. The change in the shape of particles with a decrease in aerodynamic diameter tends to increase the surface roughness. Hence, deeper lung penetration can be observed compared to spherical particles (23). The particle shape also depends on inter-particle interactions, and utilizing van der Waals force helps to prevent particle aggregation and improve the performance of the aerosolization technique (24). Interception-based particle deposition will be experienced by highly elongated particles unsuitable for the aerosolization technique due to higher attraction forces (25).

d) **pH and osmolarity**—The optimum pH and osmolarity achieved in aerosolized formulations has always been a challenge. Mucus secretion in the respiratory tract requires a neutral pH (26). An acidic pH, along with the non-isotonic nature of the formulation, induces bronchoconstriction, which is quite risky to asthmatic patients. Thus, optimum pH and tonicity of the aerosol formulation are required for its stability. It can be maintained and achieved using several salts like NaCl and NaOH. Sodium chloride helps maintain the formulation's tonicity, whereas sodium hydroxide and hydrochloric acid help keep the formulation's optimum pH.

e) **Viscosity**—Inhaled particles, using the aerosolization technique, generally adhere to the respiratory mucosal membrane before reaching the alveolar region. The primary mechanism involved in mucosal adhesion is the formation of polyvalent adhesive interactions (26). At low shear rates, the bulk viscosity of respiratory mucus is typically 1000–10,000 times higher than the water. Hence, the viscosity of a formulation plays an essential role in its fabrication. An increase in viscosity can be achieved by increasing the droplet size or by simply decreasing the temperature. Thus, a change in viscosity affects particle size shape and modifies the deposition mechanism (10).

Other than the characteristics mentioned previously, particle surface charge, lipophilicity, pKa, protein binding of the drug, and permeability across epithelial barriers are also important parameters to be considered while formulating the pulmonary delivery system (27).

6.1.3 PULMONARY DELIVERY DEVICES

Pulmonary drug delivery systems are delivery devices used for administering medications in the form of various formulations to the pulmonary organs of the human body (10). Several factors that assist the selection of a delivery device are as follows:

- Nature and formulation of the drug
- Administration site
- Pathophysiology of the lungs (27)

This selection of delivery devices directly affects the aerosolization of particles and the pattern of deposition that ultimately ensures the efficacy of the delivered drug. Inhaler devices should possess characteristics such as being portable, small in size, easy to handle, and compatible to use, and they should be able to deliver particles to the specified site with a specific aerodynamic diameter (4). Three types of delivery devices are used to administer drugs to the lungs: pressurized metered dose inhalers, dry powder inhalers, and nebulizers.

a) **Pressurized—metered dose inhalers (pMDIs):** pMDIs are a commonly used delivery device for treating respiratory illness. All drugs are inhalable and can be administered via pMDIs as single or in combination. pMDIs are composed of the following components:

- Metal canister
- Mouthpiece
- Actuator
- Metered valve

Solution and suspension formulations are available for pMDIs and suitable excipients like cosolvents, surfactants, and propellants. The mechanism and functioning of pMDIs start when the particles of the drug come in contact with air. Due to the difference in the boiling temperature of the formulation and the room temperature, the aerosolization of the drug particles takes place due to evaporation. The size of the particles may vary from medication to medication (10). Several advantages of the pMDIs are as follows:

- It is a compact and portable device.
- It provides multiple as well as consistent dosing.
- It possesses resistance to bacterial contamination and humidity.
- It is a cost-effective device.

Along with advantages, it has some disadvantages, as it is difficult to activate this device because of poor grip strength. This causes less coordination between hands and breathing, leading to less lung bioavailability of drugs. Conventional devices contain chlorofluorocarbons (CFCs) as the propellant that causes the drugs' cold-freon effect and high throat deposition. This all ultimately delivers uneven or no drug to the lungs. Hence, CFCs were replaced with hydrofluoroalkane (HFA). These propellants provide warmer and softer sprays of fine particles, overcoming the limitations of CFCs, which is a cold-freon effect (28). These are mainly used in asthma and COPD (28). Three techniques are applicable for pMDIs, as follows:

- Modulite technology
- Breath-actuated technology
- Co-suspension delivery technology

b) **Dry powder inhalers:** DPIs constitute the second class of pulmonary drug delivery devices. These are employed for the delivery of powdered forms of drugs requiring less coordination between the breathing process and the actuation process (10). They are mainly designed to deliver proteins, therapeutics, and drugs to the lungs (27). The devices involve complex structural frameworks to have therapeutics accurately and precisely due to dried powder particles. The components of DPIs are:

- Mesh
- Cyclone
- Manifold
- Spiral chamber (10)

Traditionally, DPIs administer dry, powdered micronized drug particles and use excipients of large sizes, such as lactose, sucrose, and glucose, for increment in the flow and reduction in the aggregation. DPIs utilize fluidization techniques, meaning sweeping particles by air on inhalation. When the device is activated, the fluidized formulation enters the airway, and the drug separates from the

TABLE 6.1

List of Available Marketed Nebulizers Used in the Treatment of Pulmonary Disease

Type of Marketed Formulation	Drug	Device	Manufacturer
AeroEclipse II BAN	Methacholine	Breath-actuated nebulizer	Monaghan Medical Corp.
AKITAJET	Tobramycin	Vibrating mesh nebulizer	Activaero GmbH
UltibroBreezhaler	Glycopyrronium bromide and indacaterol maleate	Dry powder inhaler	Novartis Pharmaceuticals Ltd.
CompAIRCompressor	Iloprost	Jet nebulizer	Omron Dalian Co., Ltd.
FloventDiskus	Fluticasone propionate	Metered dose inhalers	GlaxoSmithKline LLC
I-neb AAD	α-1 antitrypsin	Vibrating mesh nebulizer	Philips-Respironics Ltd.
MicroAir NE-U22	Budesonide	Vibrating mesh nebulizer	Omron Healthcare
PARI LC Plus	Tobramycin	Breath-enhanced nebulizer	PARI GmbH
Sidestream Plus	Salbutamol	Breath-enhanced nebulizer	Philips-Respironics Ltd.

carrier and moves into the lungs (27). DPIs have proven their utility, delivering formulations without propellant use. Second, they ensure the patient's compliance and auto-functioning without the aid of inhalation and actuation processes. Due to the usage of dry formulations, they possess good chemical stability (27). The only drawback of the DPIs is that there are chances of drug clumping, which leads to inconsistent dosing of drugs (27). DPIs are available as single-dose, multiple-unit dose, and multiple-dose reservoirs (10). They require an inspiratory force of 30–60 L/min. DPIs main use two main systems. A system that requires energy for aerosolizing particles from inhalation is called a passive system. The systems need some kind of mechanical device like an impeller attached to it, named active systems (27). Marketed formulations are listed in Table 6.1.

c) **Nebulizers:** Nebulizers are the third category of pulmonary drug delivery devices. They can efficiently deliver therapeutics via the nasal route. They can produce aerosol droplets in the size range of 1–5 μm in a developed solution or suspension formulation, as shown in Figure 6.1. These delivery devices are utilized for unresponsive patients who are unable to use DPIs and pMDIs (27). Various factors can affect optimized medication delivery, such as air pressure, drug solution volume, viscosity of the drug solution, and type of mouthpiece selected. This class of devices possesses various advantages; no coordination is required between actuation and inspiration processes, and aerosolized particles of smaller size are produced efficiently. Hence, they are good at delivering large doses. Along with the advantages, some disadvantages are also associated, like the complex setup of devices, high cost, lack of portability, need for daily cleaning, inconvenient loading of each dose, and a longer period being needed to inhale a higher dose of the medications. Three main types of nebulizers can be seen on the market with different mechanisms, which are as follows:

- **Jet nebulizers**: These types require a compressed gas source, which generates high pressure near the nozzle, producing smaller aerosolized particles in response. These nebulizers should be able to return droplets in the reservoir, as it defines their output and efficiency.
- **Mesh nebulizers**: A perforated membrane, aperture, or plate is utilized to produce aerosolized particles with a piezo-element for vibration purposes. These types of nebulizers can deliver suspensions, aqueous solutions, and aerosols.
- **Ultrasonic nebulizers**: Nebulizers of this type utilize high-frequency ultrasonic waves converted from electrical energy to produce smaller particles in aerosolized form from the liquid formulation (27).

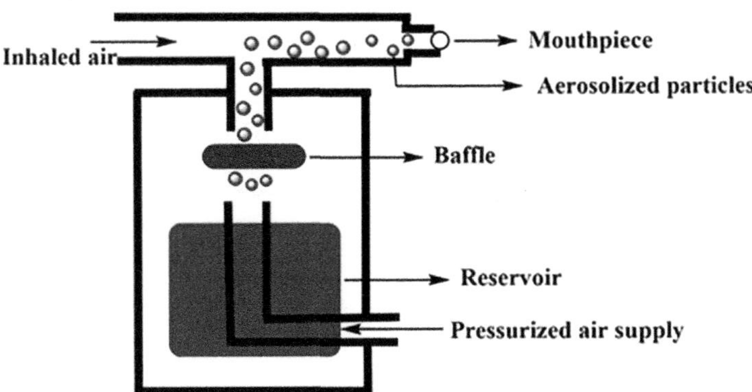

FIGURE 6.2 Schematic representation of jet nebulizer exhibiting the functional structural framework of nebulizers.

6.2 NOVEL DRUG DELIVERY SYSTEMS

6.2.1 LIPOSOMAL FORMULATIONS

Liposomes have been one of the most extensively studied nanocomposites in nanomedicine since the 1960s (27, 29). Liposomes are small vesicles comprising lipid bilayer membranes (usually phospholipids) and cholesterol, which tend to self-enclose the hydrophilic core between the bilayer membranes, as shown in Figure 6.3. The lipid component consists of surfactant, lecithin, soya-lecithin, and neutral phospholipids utilized in the preparation of liposomes. Liposomes tend to self-assemble drugs or bioactives in their spherical vesicular structure (10). Liposomes can be distinguished based on the particle size, ranging from 20 nm to 1 μm based on their distinctive lamellarity and composition (30). Among these nanostructures, a small unilamellar vesicle (SUV) is the most-studied nanocarrier to deliver drugs, enzymes, DNA, and siRNA due to bypassing of the reticuloendothelial system (RES) (31). So far, it is the biocompatible multifunctional nano-vehicle approved by the USFDA for delivering inhalable therapeutics. The distinctive inherited features include its biocompatibility, biodegradability, thermodynamic stability, and easy surface modifications to make it a versatile nanocarrier to transport drugs in systemic circulation. The ligand/antibody-anchored nanostructures encased with drug molecules could achieve efficacious outcomes via drug-targeting mechanisms for pulmonary drug delivery.

Liposomes can minimize localized lung irritation with prolonged duration of drug release and sustained action with less toxicity. Moreover, the outer lipidic membranes, composed of phospholipids, facilitate the intake of therapeutics to the alveolar macrophages via intracellular targeting (10). Multifunctional liposomal nanoformulations are used in numerous clinical advancements through inhalation for the treatment of various diseases such as cystic fibrosis, tuberculosis, pulmonary infections, pneumonia, bronchitis, asthma, and lung cancer. The treatment of respiratory diseases has been challenging since the 1900s due to the hydrophobic nature of therapeutic moieties. This leads to an issue in the development of nano-formulations due to a few drawbacks, such as stability, solubility, and undefined toxicity problems (32).

The first approved inhalable liposome was Alveofact (natural surfactant), obtained from a phospholipid fraction from bovine lung for the treatment of immature lungs developed in premature babies in 1980.

Caimmi and colleagues highlighted the difficulty in eradicating *Mycobacterium abscessus,* which is responsible for exacerbating lung diseases (like cystic fibrosis). USFDA-approved liposome-based nanoformulations like Arikayce (amikacin-loaded liposomal inhalable suspension) have been proven to treat non-tuberculous mycobacterial infections such as those caused

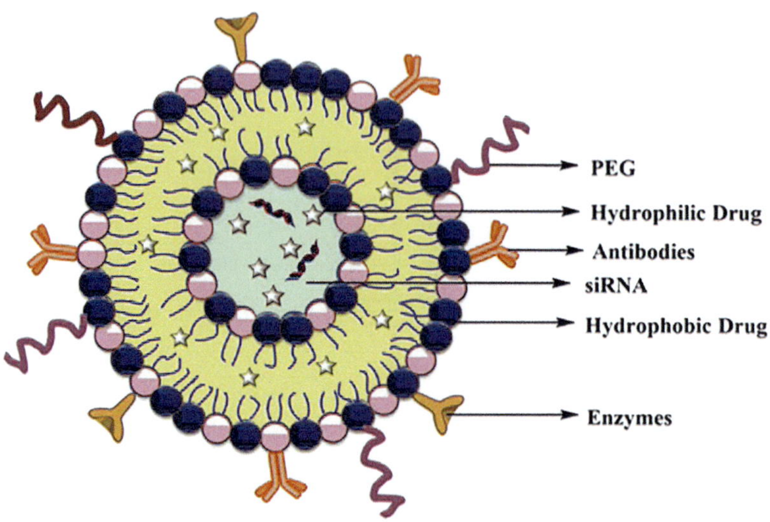

FIGURE 6.3 Multifunctional liposomes are made of phospholipids and cholesterol and may contain distinctive targeting ligands to the specific site, a prominent approach utilized in the treatment of lung cancer.

by *Mycobacterium abscessus* (33). Another research group has developed folic-acid conjugated docetaxel liposomes (LP-DTX-FA) for the treatment of lung cancer. Liposomes consisting of phosphatidylcholine and cholesterol (6:1 proportion) were prepared using a thin lipid film hydration method (34). Furthermore, many other liposomal formulations, such as lipoplatin and L-NDDP, are in different phases of clinical trials. The approval for these formulations depends upon factors like better therapeutic efficacy, rapid onset of action, prolonged and sustained effects at the targeted sites, minimal side effects, targeting potency, patient compliance, and cost-effectiveness.

6.2.2 Micellar Formulations

Polymeric micelles are a type of colloidal system that possess a core-shell type in their nanostructure. Amphiphilic polymers (e.g., PLGA, PLA-PEG) are the micellar nanoformulations' main constituent, as shown in Figure 6.4. When dispersed in aqueous systems above critical micelle concentration (CMC), these polymers tend to undergo self-emulsification under the influence of free energy reduction. The self-assembly leads to a reduction in contact with the aqueous molecules, forming a core-shell type of nanostructures. The micellar system consists of an interior hydrophobic core and a hydrophilic exterior shell. This sequence of steps leads to the formation of hydrogen bonds with water molecules and the water-loving constituent of the polymer, thereby reducing the contact between hydrophilic and lipophilic constituents for micelles formation. The lipophilic molecules get entrapped in hydrophobic regions. The common type of amphiphilic polymers used for this purpose can have the composition of bi- or tri-block polymers, phospholipids, and conjugates of polymers and lipids. The advantages of micellar-type formulations are as follows:

- Encapsulation of hydrophilic as well as hydrophobic drugs is possible in the shell and core of the micelles, respectively.
- Ease of surface engineering to design tailor-made multifunctional nanostructures.
- Escalated bioavailability of therapeutics in systemic circulation.
- Prolonged duration of drug release at infected organs.
- The favorable physiochemical nature of the drug leads to better encapsulation efficiency.
- They exhibit excellent pharmacokinetics behavior.

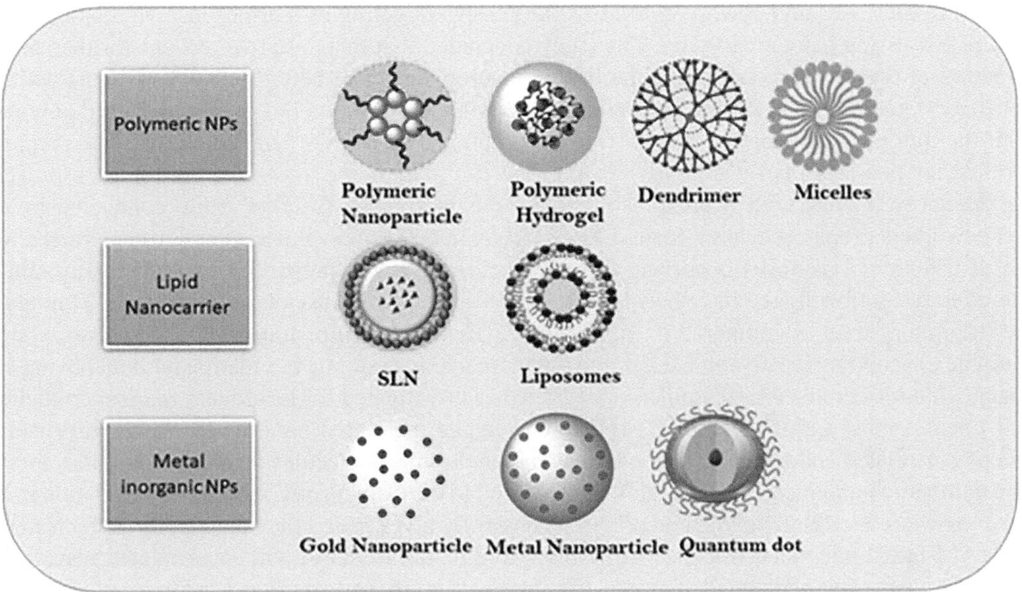

FIGURE 6.4 Schematic representation of micellar formulations showing hydrophilic shell and hydrophobic core representing (A) unloaded micelles, (B) loaded micelles.

The disadvantages of micellar-type formulations are as follows:

- The stability of micelles depends on the CMC, increasing the chances of bursting in unfavorable conditions.
- The lower number of amphiphilic polymers for the micellar systems restricts its applicability. Scale-up of a micellar system for large scaling is difficult, needing improvisation (35).

The evaluation of micellar systems is a critical consideration in the delivery of drugs. Blanco and coworkers studied the preclinical aspects of a new therapeutic agent named β-lapachone encased in micellar formulation. The developed nanoformulations sufficiently expedited the treatment of orthotropic lung tumors, with minimum adverse effects and reduced hemolytic anemic reaction (36).

Gill and coworkers conducted a study evidencing the delivery of paclitaxel-loaded PEG_{5000}–DSPE-based micelles via the pulmonary route. Unlike the intravenously administered formulation, the intrathecal-administered drug was proven to be less cytotoxic to the normal cells that did not need to be targeted. The hemocompatibility study also showed the prepared formulation's safety profile (37).

In another study, Gilani and coworkers developed a chitosan and stearic acid-based nanofiller formulation that entrapped amphotericin B as the model drug. This formulation was able to provide greater encapsulation along with an increment in the solubility of amphotericin B. A jet nebulizer showed better delivery when a comparative study was done against a twin-impinger apparatus (38). Banginski and colleagues prepared a nano-formulation of salmon calcitonin encased in the DSPE-PEG_{2000} micellar system. This nanostructure effectively delivered against pulmonary infections, showing the protection of bioactives against enzymatic degradation, thus providing better bioavailability of therapeutics to reach systemic circulation (39).

In one study, Lee and coworkers studied the passive targeting of thermosensitive diblock copolymers possessing biocompatibility. The study concluded that there are two reasons for the passive targeting of drugs: reduction of uptake by the macrophages and better delivery to lungs with no *in-vitro* cytotoxicity (40). Rosere and colleagues developed nanomicelles of folate-grafted polymers with the aim of increasing the solubility of hydrophobic drugs like temozolomide. The prepared formulation possessed perfect aerodynamic properties to be in the lower respiratory tract for treating adenocarcinomas with overexpressed folate receptors (35). Another study conducted by Hu and coworkers prepared nylered-loaded PEG-PLGA micelles to evaluate the pharmacokinetic and bio-distribution of naturally occurring compound curcumin. The prepared formulation was administered to rats following the intrathecal route, with a sustained release of medication for 24 hours in the respiratory tract as compared to intraventory parenteral administration. This nanoformulation was able to penetrate the alveoli barrier and blood, reaching systemic circulation without having any change in its structure. This formulation was further investigated for its efficacy against epithelium cell lines, namely Calu-3 and NCCI-H441. The ligand-fabricated nanostructure was involved in receptor-mediated endocytosis, with clathrin and cholesterol molecules, leading to cellular uptake. The number of nanomicelles was highly internalized to the Calu-3 cells, which had deposition in the upper airways (41, 42). Kim and coworkers successfully investigated the conjugation of cholesterol-PAMAM-based polymeric micelles with complexed luciferase DNA and encapsulated resveratrol. The *in-vivo* studies concluded that the formulation significantly reduced inflammation in lung infections (43). A study conducted by Wang and coworkers successfully conjugated pluronic with succinylated-gelatin loaded with paclitaxel. The developed formulation was administered via inhalation to treat lung carcinoma (44). Bio-distribution studies indicated that the desired concentration was achieved in the lungs similar to IV administration. Additionally, the intrathecal route provided less drug deposition in rat lungs when compared with clinical trials. However, this formulation leads to increased sensitivity to tumor cells and reduction of toxicity in normal cells.

6.2.3 Nanoparticles

a) **Polymeric nanoparticles:** Polymers encapsulate drugs and offer targeting in a controlled and sustained manner in this colloidal nanocarrier system, as shown in Figure 6.5. Polymeric nanoparticles also protect drugs from enzymatic degradation and increase their lung residence time. Both natural and synthetic origin polymers could be employed in designing polymeric nanoparticles. These are further divided into two types:
   Polymeric nanocapsules: Polymers facilitate the encapsulation of drugs.
   Polymeric nanospheres: Drugs dispersed in the polymer matrix.

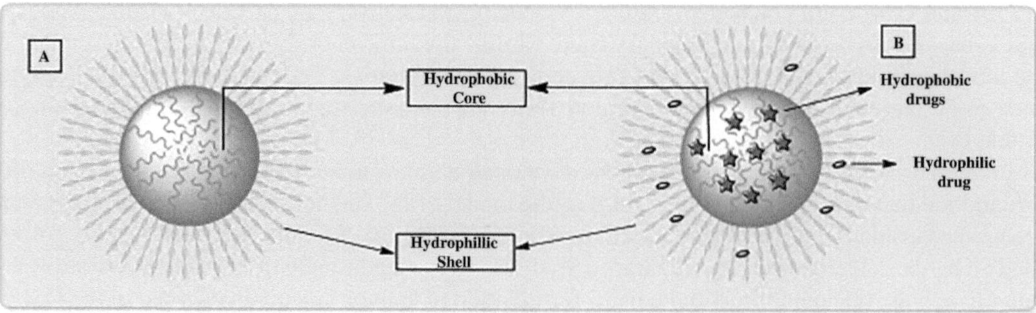

FIGURE 6.5 Various types of nanocomposites utilized in the effective delivery of therapeutics in the treatment of pulmonary diseases.

Deacon and colleagues prepared tobramycin-loaded alginate/chitosan-based nanoparticles for the treatment of cystic fibrosis targeting *P. aeruginosa*, and dornasealfa increased nanoparticle penetration (45). Costa-Gouveia and coworkers loaded ethionamide into β-cyclodextrin nanoparticles and reported a log reduction in mycobacterial load when studies were done *in vivo* on mice lungs (46). Yoo and coworkers reported PLGA nanoparticles incorporating hydroxyl benzyl alcohol (HBA) and poly oxalate (HPOX), treating airway inflammation and asthma in ovalbumin-induced mice when given intratracheally. Adi and coworkers reported ciprofloxacin and doxycycline-loaded PVA nanoparticles showed a sustained effect (47). Russo and coworkers reported that the foscarnet chitosan nanoparticles crosslinked with glutaraldehyde prolonged its residence time in the blood and *in vivo* exposure to infected lung cells (48). Choi and coworkers reported albumin nanoparticles, which were able to deliver DOX and TRAIL simultaneously against the cell lines of lung cancer (49).

b) **Solid-lipid nanoparticles:** Solid lipid nanoparticles (SLNs) are efficient nanocomposites made up of lipids. These consist of a solid lipophilic core, a surface coated with phospholipids, and a high melting point with the material to be encapsulated, as shown in Figure 6.5. SLNs are potential nanocarriers of pharmacologically active substances for localized or systemic delivery. SLNs protect the encapsulated drugs from degradation and can deliver drugs to targeted sites at a controlled rate. These carriers can target drugs passively due to their small size, and ligand-anchored delivery is also one possibility that ensures active targeting. Rosiere and coworkers studied paclitaxel-encapsulated SLNs to target lung tumors efficiently (35). Ji et al. formulated SLNs encapsulating naringenin, which resulted in a remarkable increase in the bioavailability of the hydrophobic drug (50). Makled et al. prepared inhalable SLNs incorporating sildenafil-citrate for pulmonary hypertension therapy (51). Gaspar et al. evaluated the potential of SLNs encapsulating antibiotics, as these were able to reduce *Mycobacterium tuberculosis* growth in mouse lungs when given through DPI (52). Liu et al. reported that insulin-loaded SLNs using sodium cholate and soybean phosphatidylcholine could reduce hyperglycemia. Patil-Gadhe and colleagues formulated a nanostructured lipidic carrier using Precirol AT05 and Capriol-90 incorporating water-soluble montelukast sodium and showed efficient targeting towards the lungs and biocompatibility (27, 53).

c) **Inorganic nanoparticles:** Nanoparticles comprising inorganic metals like platinum, iron, zinc, and gold lie in the nanometric size range, as shown in Figure 6.3. Inorganic nanoparticles have been widely exploited for treating and detecting various diseases like HIV-AIDS, influenza, and hepatitis. Inorganic nanoparticles are capable of treating viral and other diseases/disorders, as the metals themselves have the property of attacking viruses from numerous sites. Metal nanoparticles may interact with the host cells either intracellularly or extracellularly. They communicate with gp120 proteins and competitively inhibit the binding of the virus to the host cell's site, restricting the attachment of the virus with the cells and thereby showing their intrinsic antiviral properties. Ramalingam and coworkers successfully conjugated doxorubicin with polyvinylpyrrolidone-gold nanoparticles (PVP-Au NPs) and evaluated its enhanced cytotoxicity against A549 cells (54). Halwani and colleagues designed antibodies (IL4Rα) fabricated with superparamagnetic iron oxide nanoparticles (SPION-anti-IL4Rα NPs) that could suppress inflammation in asthmatic OVA-sensitized mice (55). Wu and coworkers fabricated hollow calcium phosphate nanoparticles coated with phospholipids and successfully co-delivered paclitaxel and doxorubicin, utilized in lung cancer treatment. The nano-formulation induced apoptosis and lowered viable cell counts on the A549 cells via *in-vitro* cytotoxicity assays (56). Morris et al. prepared silver nanoparticles (AgNPs), which were able to slow down the replication of respiratory syncytial virus (RSV) and the synthesis of cytokines (57). Verma and coworkers formulated quercetin-loaded Fe_3O_4 magnetic nanoparticle aerosolized delivery systems wrapped with PLGA, which could reduce the viable cell count against

A549 pulmonary cells (58). Tarantula and colleagues fabricated mesoporous silica NPs (MSNs) and loaded them with anti-cancer drugs (DOX and CIS) and MRP1and BCL2 mRNA-targeted siRNA, which induced apoptosis and suppressed pump/non-pump resistance in cells. Jeremiah and colleagues prepared a variety of Ag NPs of divergent sizes and concentrations. The prepared nanoparticles, with a size of 10 nm, efficiently inhibited extracellular SARS-CoV-2 at 1–10 ppm, whereas they displayed cytotoxic properties at 20 ppm and above concentration.

6.3 APPLICATIONS

6.3.1 Inhalable Antiviral Formulations

Various viruses account for respiratory infections, such as influenza virus, coxsackie virus, adenovirus, respiratory syncytial virus, rhinovirus, corona virus, human bocavirus, avian influenza H5N1, and tenovirus. Among these, the influenza virus is primarily responsible for serious airway infections across the globe. Meanwhile, the respiratory syncytial virus and parainfluenza virus are also responsible for lower respiratory tract infections among infants.

Hedrick and colleagues established the potential of Relenza, whose every blister dose carries combination drugs (5 mg zanamivir + 20 mg lactose). Influenza patients (5–12 years old) who inhaled two blisters two times daily for 5 days observed that the median time to relieve the symptoms was reduced. Ison and coworkers evaluated the potential of zanamivir in combination with rimantadine administered in nebulized form and well tolerated by influenza-infected patients (59). Kubo and coworkers also proved that Inavir [laninamiviroctanoate (LANI)] could be retained in the lungs for more than 5 days, and a single inhalation was sufficient for showing efficacy towards the various viruses (H1N1/H275Y, H1N1, H3N2, and influenza Betc) (60). Verreault and coworkers formulated micronized dry powder of Cidofovir (NanoFOVIRTM; Nf), treated rabbitpox virus (RPXV) in the rabbit model, and observed lessening of RPX-induced symptoms. The authors concluded that Cidofovir can be seen as a practicable antiviral for treating poxviruses such as smallpox (61). Stankova and coworkers reported that ribavirin was delivered through the inhalation route and was utilized in treating parainfluenza 3-virus in immune-compromised newborn infants (62). Douglas and coworkers reported that interferon was administered effectively through the nasal route, thus preventing rhinovirus-induced colds for a short duration in family contacts who got viral exposure (63). Turner and colleagues investigated nano-formulation in preclinical studies to deliver interferon through a nasal route that expedites protection against both coronavirus and influenza A virus (64). Giudice and coworkers developed a carboxymethylatedglucan-based nano-vehicle to deliver therapeutics like resveratrol in infected sites and preserve its biological activity against enzymatic degradation. These nanoformulations lower the severity and reappearance of respiratory infections among children (65).

6.3.2 Inhalable Antifungal Formulations

Pulmonary fungal infections are subject to increase because of patients whose immune systems are compromised. Fungal infections can be due to any species, like *Histoplasma capsulatum*, *Sporothrix schenkii*, *Coccidioides* species, *Blastomyces dermatiditis*, *Aspergillus*, *Candida*, and *Pneumocystis*. Orally and intravenously administrable antifungal drugs are available on the market, including amphotericin B, caspofungin, voriconazole, and itraconazole.

a) **Amphotericin B**: Standard therapy for fungal infections utilizes amphotericin B but also leads to cardiotoxicity and nephrotoxicity. Some marketed preparations based on novel carriers available for Amphotericin B are AmBisome, Fungizone, and Abelcet. The inhalable drugs are covered here one by one. AmB belongs to the class of polyene macrolides applied in pulmonary aspergillosis infection in patients of AIDS and those who have gone through any organ transplantation. A liposomal preparation of AmB, which DPIs can administer, was intended to be used in life-threatening critical conditions of pulmonary infections (66).

b) Further studies focused on the detrimental part of the preparation formula, which was found to be deoxycholate, as studied by Kuiper et al. They found that the pulmonary surfactant did not cause any toxicity, as it did with deoxycholate. This study focused on encapsulated and liposomal preparations (67). A study showed that chitosan oligosaccharide micelles grafted with a stearic acid preparation that was prepared for pulmonary administration using an air-jet nebulizer showed results equal to those of fungizone but were less toxic. Recently, the reported data passed on the information that liposomal preparation of AmB is far better among all the available formulation types, with a prolonged half-life and good safety profile leading to better tolerability.

c) **Itraconazole:** Itraconazole is an azole antifungal used against pulmonary aspergillosis. As it has low aqueous solubility and a low absorption profile, preparing a formulation that can be inhaled was important. Yang and their group conducted a comparative study between inhalable itraconazole formulation and a marketed preparation named Sporanox. This study stated that the nebulized formulation delivered the drug better to the site, thereby improving the bioavailability of the drug compared to the marketed formulation administered orally. Continuing this study further, Yang and coworkers compared the bioavailability of nanoamorphous and crystalline formulations of the drug, concluding that increased bioavailability of amorphous version tended to increase the dissolution of the drug from the carrier (68).

d) **Voriconazole** is an antifungal agent with a broad spectrum of activity marketed as Captisol and Vfend and administered via intravenous and oral routes. The inhalable formulation came into the limelight when systemic preparations showed deadly effects and were withdrawn from the market. This drug also has low aqueous solubility but 700 times more than itraconazole. Using the thin film freezing technique, Beinborn et al. prepared a DPI formulation of this drug. The pharmacokinetics of the microcrystalline type of preparation was better than that of the nano-aggregates. Voriconazole remains in amorphous nano-aggregates form in the lungs for a shorter time period, leading to better pharmacokinetics (69).

e) **Pentamidine:** Pentamidine is an antifungal drug used by AIDS and lung transplant patients in *Pneumocystis* pneumonia (PCP) infection. It is used as a prophylaxis for the treatment of PCP. Studies were conducted that resulted in effective inhalation therapy but only for those who do not respond to the first-line drugs. The rise of any secondary infection because of *Candida, Herpes zoster,* or influenza is the only limitation of this drug, along with some side effects (15).

6.3.3 Inhalable Anti-Asthmatic Formulations

Asthma is the most common respiratory disease, infecting many humans worldwide. It is a chronic disorder characterized by constriction and inflammation in airway passage caused by fungal species, especially *Aspergillus* and *Alternaria*, and other inhalable allergens (like pollen, dust mites, pet dander, etc.). It causes a variant degree of airflow obstruction and hyper-responsiveness of the airway (28). A scientific committee, the Global Initiative for Asthma (GINA), was established in 1993 by the World Health Organization (WHO) in association with the National Heart, Lung, and Blood Institute to gain interest in the public domain for the awareness, diagnosis, management, and prevention of asthma (70). According to GINA guidelines (2019), short-acting beta-agonists (SABA) such as salbutamol should not be administered alone to treat asthma in adults or adolescents. SABA is recommended to be administered in emergencies, along with the optimum dose of inhalable corticosteroids for acute asthma. Several researchers have reported and contributed research related to dry powder inhalation therapy since the 1950s (71). The frequent advancement and improvement in aerosolized delivery devices such as pressurized metered dose inhalers has the key advantage of breath-actuators and transports measured doses of marketed formulations such as Easibreathe and Azmacort.

Furthermore, both multi-dose liquid inhalers, DPIs, and nebulizers (Respimat), which possess systematically designed unique, distinctive features, were utilized in the delivery of medications. Examples of dry-powder inhaler spacers, holding chambers, and other new-generation devices are shown in Figure 6.6. MDI is specially designed for the expulsion of drugs in the form of soft mist,

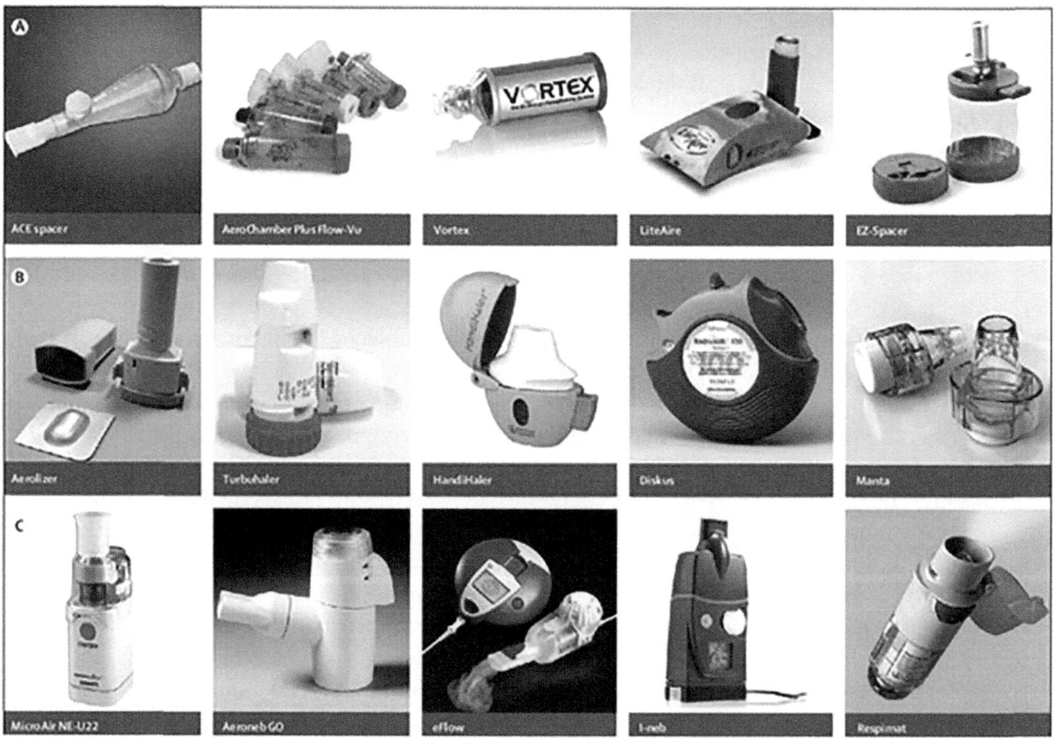

FIGURE 6.6 Examples of marketed spacers and holding chambers, dry-powder inhalers available by prescription or in development, and nebulizers that incorporate new-generation technology. The ACE spacer (Smiths Medical, Rockland, MA, USA), the EZ-Spacer (FSC Laboratories, Charlotte, NC, USA), and the Inspirease spacer (not shown) are examples of reverse-flow designs; AeroChamber Plus Flow-Vu (Trudell Medical International, London, ON, Canada), Vortex (PARI Respiratory Equipment, Midlothian, VA, USA), and Nebuchamber (AstraZeneca, Lund, Sweden; not shown) are examples of metal or non-conducting valved holding chambers. The LiteAire (Thayer Medical, Tucson, AZ, USA) is a collapsible, disposable, valved paper spacer. The Aerolizer (Schering Plough, Kenilworth, NJ, USA) and Handihaler (Boehringer-Ingelhein, Ingelheim, Germany) dry-powder inhalers are capsule devices; the Turbuhaler (AstraZeneca, Lund, Sweden) is a reservoir dry-powder inhaler; the Diskus (GlaxoSmithKline, Ware, UK) is a multi-unit dose dry-powder inhaler with single doses of drug encapsulated in foil blisters; the Manta single-dose dry-powder inhaler (Manta Devices, Boston, MA, USA) is a disposable, low-cost inhaler that uses a foil blister for drug storage with a unique internal opening technology. The MicroAir NE-U22 (Omron, Vernon Hills, IL, USA), Aeroneb GO (Aerogen, Galway, Ireland), eFlow (PARI, Midlothian, VA, USA), and I-neb (Respironics, Murrysville, PA, USA) incorporate vibrating mesh or vibrating plate aerosol generators. I-neb and Prodose (Profi le Therapeutics, Bognor Regis, UK; not shown) use adaptive aerosol delivery technology for drug delivery. The Respimat inhaler (Boehringer-Ingelheim, Ingelheim, Germany) is the first of a new class of hand-held inhalers called soft mist inhalers. Both the Respimat and the AERx (Aradigm, Hayward, CA, USA; not shown) are high efficiency devices that use precise dosimetric systems. The Respimat inhaler has a multi-dose capability. Reprinted with permission from Elsevier publication (Dolovich et al., 2011).

which is similar to the case of nebulizers. Nevertheless, the preferred inhalers utilized for rehabilitation therapy for asthmatic disorders are MDIs. Leukotriene receptor antagonists such as montelukast, zafirlukast, and zafirlukast can be taken into consideration as an alternative option, delivered in combination with SABA. Since 2007, long-acting beta-agonists (LABA)–low-dose ICS combinations have also shown promising results in treating mild asthma. For example, a budesonide–formoterol combination was used in a single inhaler for Symbicort maintenance and reliever therapy (SMART, AstraZeneca). Tulbah et al. designed nano-formulations to enhance the efficacy of simvastatin on airway inflammation and developed an inhalable solution showing a reduction in inflammation of chronic lung disease (72). The only drawback observed in a few patients is non-compliance during inhalable therapy. The majority of patients cannot use these devices precisely due to various factors such as a mismatch of breathing pattern with actuation of the device, improper breath-hold after inhalation, manual dexterity, and strength in hands. Thus, proper demonstration should be given to asthmatic patients during inhalation therapy (73).

6.3.4 Inhalable Anti-Tuberculosis Formulations

Today, 10 million people are infected with dangerous tuberculosis worldwide every year, and 2 million deaths result from this disease. In 2016, the World Health Organization stated a higher mortality rate of 10.40 million. The WHO also demonstrated that the most effective first-line drug, rifampicin, is associated with resistance to approximately 0.60 million people and 0.49 million related to multidrug-resistant TB (MDR-TB). The WHO has set a goal to reduce TB incidence by up to 90% by 2035. In general, MTB infections provoke a weak immune response and result in higher death tolls among HIV patients. In animals and humans, the lung is considered the most complex organ. Approximately 300 million alveoli are present in the human lungs, with a 70–160 m^2 surface area. The rapid emergence of drug-resistant TB has aggravated the epidemic situation globally. In most instances, the bacillus is transmitted through inhalation, leads to pulmonary diseases, and affects most other organs. Sometimes those cases are untreatable by available anti-TB drugs (Global TB report). Both multiple drug-resistant and extensively drug-resistant TB (MDR and XDR-TB) influence the development of an integrated delivery system for the treatment of tuberculosis. The elimination rate of target TB is still lower than its incidences (28 times). Resistant TB (XDR-TB) is a critical form of TB that could be cured with fewer marketed anti-tubercular medications. Developing newer drugs could be an attractive approach to improving the current TB situation. Several benefits of inhalable anti-tubercular formulations include greater specific site targeting, greater bioavailability of the drug, increased retention time, and minimum dosing frequency. The first-line drug treatment regimen for TB involves rifampicin (RIF), streptomycin, isoniazid (INH), and pyrazinamide (PZA) (74, 75). The advent of ongoing clinical trials of newer regimens, including pretomanid, bedaquiline, and linezolid, has been utilized to treat tuberculosis (76).

Aerosol-based inhaled therapy is a distinctive and progressive approach that may reduce the use of conventional drug delivery systems. Tuberculosis is the second most infectious disease after AIDS, causing deaths worldwide. In the conventional approach, inhalation permits the quick absorption of drugs with short-duration localized effects. It also necessitates a nanocomposite design for the controlled release of formulations to localized action in the respiratory system (77). Aerosolized delivery also provides patient compliance compared to other administration routes, such as intravenous (78). The fine particle fraction or aerodynamic size of less than 5 µm in the aerosolized delivery has excellent therapeutic potential. In nebulizers, dry powders for inhalation are considered more stable, and higher dose formulations are suitable in metered-dose inhalers. Nanocarrier-based DPIs are more reliable in achieving localized higher concentrations of anti-TB drugs by either passive or active targeting. Nanocarriers can overcome the drawbacks related to the conventional route of administration (oral and parenteral). Rifampicin and clofazimine have specific issues, mostly lower water solubility due to hydrophobicity. DPIs seem to be an excellent option for delivering these drugs. Nasiruddin and coworkers demonstrated nano carrier-based approaches for the treatment of TB. Costa and coworkers used polymeric and lipid-based nanoparticles to have anti-tubercular drugs in the form of DPIs. Hoppentocht and colleagues focused on the severe challenges of disease consideration with practical and technical tasks for antibiotic formulations to treat TB. The Nahar group studied and reviewed *in-vitro*, *ex-vivo*, and *in-vivo* models for particle deposition and absorption for anti-tubercular therapy.

Current delivery approaches do not efficiently do intracellular targeting; a severe lack of therapeutics for a disease like tuberculosis leads to macrophage cell infection (79). Therefore, the current approach would be focused more on intracellular targeting achieved to treat tuberculosis (80, 81). It is desirable to choose alternative methods; distinctive formulations have been developed to achieve optimum drug concentration in the infected cellular tropics rather than the plasma blood pool. However, inhalation delivery devices offer advantages over other delivery routes like the parenteral and oral routes. Aerosolized delivery is superior to the alternative route for treating localized lung diseases such as asthma, pulmonary infections, and cystic fibrosis. Moreover, pulmonary delivery might be appropriate for treating systemic diseases due to the thinness of lung epithelium tissue, greater surface area in the alveolar region, and escape of first-pass hepatic effect, resulting in enhanced drug absorption to the systematic circulation.

6.4 FUTURE PERSPECTIVES

The pulmonary route has the potential to deliver pharmacologically active agents in treating respiratory diseases. Pulmonary absorption of drugs across the pulmonary membrane depends on the release kinetics. Recent technological advances encourage the development of new delivery devices intended to deliver therapeutics in the lungs via envisaging the use of pulmonary administration for systemic drug delivery. It also executes nanotechnology's latest concepts and innovations to design versatile nanosystems (nanoparticles, liposomes, dendrimers, and micelles) to deliver therapeutic agents to sites specific organs or tissues. It is highly recommended to use newer strategies to target specific tissues and restrict distribution throughout the lungs. Developing newer propellants made aerosol delivery promising using inhalers by restricting chlorofluorocarbons' toxic effects on the stratospheric ozone. Developing hydrofluoroalkanes (HFA 134a and HFA 227) that have no ozone-damaging potential and are safe have improved aerosol technology. Nanoparticulate systems exhibit great potential to transport therapeutic agents. The core of these nanostructures encapsulates a variety of drugs, therapeutics, and siRNAs. Lipoprotein- and polysaccharide-based nanoparticles can efficiently deliver pharmacological active agents for pulmonary infections. Advanced refined techniques can overcome a few drawbacks and ensure the reproducibility of dose and precise delivery to the lungs. The newer inhalation systems are potentially superior to classical nebulizers or MDIs. Novel technologies provide significant clinical advantages to increase delivery efficiency and targeting of specific regions. Drug delivery to the lungs by aerosolized inhalation could be achieved in optimum dosage by repetitive inhalation (82, 83).

REFERENCES

1. Lizio R, Marx D, Nolte T, Lehr CM, Sarlikiotis AW, Borchard G, et al. Development of a new aerosol delivery system for systemic pulmonary delivery in anaesthetized and orotracheal intubated rats. *Lab Anim [Internet]*. 2001 Jun 23 [cited 2022 Jul 6];35(3):261–70. Available from: https://journals.sagepub.com/doi/abs/10.1258/0023677011911589
2. Stein SW, Thiel CG. The history of therapeutic aerosols: A chronological review. *J Aerosol Med Pulm Drug Deliv [Internet]*. 2017 Feb 1 [cited 2023 Dec 6];30(1):20–41. Available from: www.liebertpub.com/doi/10.1089/jamp.2016.1297
3. Sung JC, Pulliam BL, Edwards DA. Nanoparticles for drug delivery to the lungs. *Trends Biotechnol*. 2007 Dec 1;25(12):563–70.
4. Andrade F, Rafael D, Videira M, Ferreira D, Sosnik A, Sarmento B. Nanotechnology and pulmonary delivery to overcome resistance in infectious diseases. *Adv Drug Deliv Rev*. 2013 Nov 30;65(13–14):1816–27.

5. Newman SP. Drug delivery to the lungs: Challenges and opportunities. *Ther Deliv [Internet]*. 2017 Jul 1 [cited 2022 Jul 6];8(8):647–61. Available from: www.future-science.com/doi/10.4155/tde-2017-0037

6. Ziffels S, Bemelmans NL, Durham PG, Hickey AJ. In vitro dry powder inhaler formulation performance considerations. *J Control Release*. 2015 Feb 10;199:45–52.

7. Ari A, De Andrade AD, Sheard M, Alhamad B, Fink JB. Performance comparisons of jet and mesh nebulizers using different interfaces in simulated spontaneously breathing adults and children. *J Aerosol Med Pulm Drug Deliv [Internet]*. 2015 Aug 1 [cited 2023 Dec 6];28(4):281–9. Available from: www. liebertpub.com/doi/10.1089/jamp.2014.1149

8. Thompson PJ. Drug delivery to the small airways. *Am J Respir Crit Care Med [Internet]*. 1998 [cited 2023 Dec 6];157(5 Pt 2). Available from: https://pubmed.ncbi.nlm.nih.gov/9606321/

9. Ariyananda PL, Agnew JE, Clarke SW. Aerosol delivery systems for bronchial asthma. *Postgrad Med J [Internet]*. 1996 [cited 2023 Dec 6];72(845):151. Available from: www.ncbi.nlm.nih.gov/pmc/articles/ PMC2398392/?report=abstract

10. Mishra B, Singh J. Novel drug delivery systems and significance in respiratory diseases. *Target Chronic Inflamm Lung Dis Using Adv Drug Deliv Syst*. 2020 Jan 1;57–95.

11. Ghadiri M, Young PM, Traini D. Strategies to enhance drug absorption via nasal and pulmonary routes. *Pharmaceutics [Internet]*. 2019 Mar 1 [cited 2023 Dec 6];11(3). Available from: www.ncbi.nlm.nih.gov/ pmc/articles/PMC6470976/

12. Lippmann M, Yeates DB, Albert RE. Deposition, retention, and clearance of inhaled particles. *Br J Ind Med [Internet]*. 1980 [cited 2023 Dec 6];37(4):337. Available from: www.ncbi.nlm.nih.gov/pmc/articles/ PMC1008751/?report=abstract

13. Caimmi D, Martocq N, Trioleyre D, Guinet C, Godreuil S, Daniel T, et al. Positive effect of liposomal amikacin for inhalation on mycobacterium abcessus in cystic fibrosis patients. *Open Forum Infect Dis [Internet]*. 2018 Mar 1 [cited 2023 Dec 6];5(3). Available from: www.ncbi.nlm.nih.gov/pmc/articles/ PMC5846290/

14. Martonen TB, Katz IM. Deposition patterns of aerosolized drugs within human lungs: Effects of ventilatory parameters. *Pharm Res [Internet]*. 1993 [cited 2023 Dec 6];10(6):871–8. Available from: https:// pubmed.ncbi.nlm.nih.gov/8321856/

15. Darquenne C. Aerosol deposition in health and disease. *J Aerosol Med Pulm Drug Deliv [Internet]*. 2012 Jun 1 [cited 2023 Dec 6];25(3):140–7. Available from: https://pubmed.ncbi.nlm.nih.gov/22686623/

16. Lachman L, Lieberman HA, Kanig JL. Theory and practice of industrial pharmacy. 1994 [cited 2023 Dec 6];902. Available from: https://archive.org/details/TheTheoryAndPracticeOfIndustrialPharmacy ByLachmanAndLieberman3rdEditnsameep104

17. Carvalho TC, McConville JT. The function and performance of aqueous aerosol devices for inhalation therapy. *J Pharm Pharmacol [Internet]*. 2016 May 1 [cited 2023 Dec 6];68(5):556–78. Available from: https://pubmed.ncbi.nlm.nih.gov/27061412/

18. Kleinstreuer C, Feng Y, Childress E. Drug-targeting methodologies with applications: A review. *World J Clin Cases WJCC [Internet]*. 2014 Dec 12 [cited 2023 Dec 6];2(12):742. Available from: www.ncbi. nlm.nih.gov/pmc/articles/PMC4266823/

19. Mortensen NP, Durham P, Hickey AJ. The role of particle physico-chemical properties in pulmonary drug delivery for tuberculosis therapy. *J Microencapsul [Internet]*. 2014 Dec 1 [cited 2023 Dec 6];31(8):785–95. Available from: https://pubmed.ncbi.nlm.nih.gov/25090595/

20. Shetty N, Park H, Zemlyanov D, Mangal S, Bhujbal S, Zhou Q (Tony). Influence of excipients on physical and aerosolization stability of spray dried high-dose powder formulations for inhalation. *Int J Pharm*. 2018 Jun 10;544(1):222–34.

21. Chen L, Okuda T, Lu XY, Chan HK. Amorphous powders for inhalation drug delivery. *Adv Drug Deliv Rev*. 2016 May 1;100:102–15.

22. Dabbagh A, Abu Kasim NH, Yeong CH, Wong TW, Abdul Rahman N. Critical parameters for particle-based pulmonary delivery of chemotherapeutics. *J Aerosol Med Pulm Drug Deliv [Internet]*. 2018 Jun 1 [cited 2023 Dec 6];31(3):139–54. Available from: www.liebertpub.com/doi/10.1089/jamp.2017.1382

23. Tang P, Chan HK, Raper JA. Prediction of aerodynamic diameter of particles with rough surfaces. *Fac Eng—Pap [Internet]*. 2004 Jan 1 [cited 2023 Dec 6];147(1–3):64. Available from: https://ro.uow.edu.au/ engpapers/1464

24. Zeng XM, Martin GP, Marriott C, Pritchard J. The influence of carrier morphology on drug delivery by dry powder inhalers. *Int J Pharm*. 2000 Apr 25;200(1):93–106.

25. Larhrib H, Martin GP, Prime D, Marriott C. Characterisation and deposition studies of engineered lactose crystals with potential for use as a carrier for aerosolised salbutamol sulfate from dry powder inhalers. *Eur J Pharm Sci*. 2003 Jul 1;19(4):211–21.

26. Lai SK, Wang YY, Hanes J. Mucus-penetrating nanoparticles for drug and gene delivery to mucosal tissues. *Adv Drug Deliv Rev [Internet]*. 2009 Feb 2 [cited 2023 Dec 6];61(2):158. Available from: www.ncbi.nlm.nih.gov/pmc/articles/PMC2667119/

27. Patil JS, Sarasija S. Pulmonary drug delivery strategies: A concise, systematic review. *Lung India [Internet]*. 2012 Jan [cited 2022 Jul 6];29(1):44–9. Available from: https://pubmed.ncbi.nlm.nih.gov/22345913/

28. Onoue S, Misaka S, Kawabata Y, Yamada S. New treatments for chronic obstructive pulmonary disease and viable formulation/device options for inhalation therapy. *Expert Opin Drug Deliv [Internet]*. 2009 Aug [cited 2022 Jul 6];6(8):793–811. Available from: www.tandfonline.com/doi/abs/10.1517/17425240903089310; http://dx.doi.org/101517/17425240903089310

29. Pattni BS, Chupin VV, Torchilin VP. New developments in liposomal drug delivery. *Chem Rev [Internet]*. 2015 Oct 14 [cited 2022 Jul 6];115(19):10938–66. Available from: https://pubs.acs.org/doi/full/10.1021/acs.chemrev.5b00046

30. Kumar V, Khan I, Gupta U. Lipid-dendrimer nanohybrid system or dendrosomes: Evidences of enhanced encapsulation, solubilization, cellular uptake and cytotoxicity of bortezomib. *Appl Nanosci [Internet]*. 2020 Nov 1 [cited 2023 Dec 6];10(11):4049–62. Available from: https://link.springer.com/article/10.1007/s13204-020-01515-7

31. Bassetti M, Vena A, Russo A, Peghin M. Inhaled liposomal antimicrobial delivery in lung infections. *Drugs [Internet]*. 2020 Sep 1 [cited 2023 Dec 6];80(13):1309–18. Available from: https://link.springer.com/article/10.1007/s40265-020-01359-z

32. Adler-Moore J, Proffitt RT. AmBisome: Liposomal formulation, structure, mechanism of action and preclinical experience. *J Antimicrob Chemother [Internet]*. 2002 Jan 1 [cited 2023 Dec 6];49(suppl_1):21–30. Available from: https://dx.doi.org/10.1093/jac/49.suppl_1.21

33. Caimmi D, Martocq N, Trioleyre D, Guinet C, Godreuil S, Daniel T, et al. Positive effect of liposomal Amikacin for inhalation on mycobacterium abcessus in cystic fibrosis patients. *Open Forum Infect Dis [Internet]*. 2018 Mar 1 [cited 2023 Dec 7];5(3). Available from: https://dx.doi.org/10.1093/ofid/ofy034

34. Zhu X, Kong Y, Liu Q, Lu Y, Xing H, Lu X, et al. Inhalable dry powder prepared from folic acid-conjugated docetaxel liposomes alters pharmacodynamic and pharmacokinetic properties relevant to lung cancer chemotherapy. *Pulm Pharmacol Ther*. 2019 Apr 1;55:50–61.

35. Rosière R, Gelbcke M, Mathieu V, Van Antwerpen P, Amighi K, Wauthoz N. New dry powders for inhalation containing temozolomide-based nanomicelles for improved lung cancer therapy. *Int J Oncol [Internet]*. 2015 Sep 1 [cited 2023 Dec 6];47(3):1131–42. Available from: www.spandidos-publications.com/10.3892/ijo.2015.3092/abstract

36. Blanco E, Bey EA, Khemtong C, Yang SG, Setti-Guthi J, Chen H, et al. β-lapachone micellar nanotherapeutics for non-small cell lung cancer therapy. *Cancer Res [Internet]*. 2010 May 15 [cited 2022 Jul 6];70(10):3896–904. Available from: https://aacrjournals.org/cancerres/article/70/10/3896/559516/Lapachone-Micellar-Nanotherapeutics-for-Non-Small

37. Gill KK, Nazzal S, Kaddoumi A. Paclitaxel loaded PEG5000–DSPE micelles as pulmonary delivery platform: Formulation characterization, tissue distribution, plasma pharmacokinetics, and toxicological evaluation. *Eur J Pharm Biopharm*. 2011 Oct 1;79(2):276–84.

38. Gilani K, Moazeni E, Ramezanli T, Amini M, Fazeli MR, Jamalifar H. Development of respirable nanomicelle carriers for delivery of amphotericin B by jet nebulization. *J Pharm Sci [Internet]*. 2011 Jan 1 [cited 2023 Dec 6];100(1):252–9. Available from: https://onlinelibrary.wiley.com/doi/full/10.1002/jps.22274

39. Baginski L, Gobbo OL, Tewes F, Salomon JJ, Healy AM, Bakowsky U, et al. In vitro and in vivo characterisation of PEG-lipid-based micellar complexes of salmon calcitonin for pulmonary delivery. *Pharm Res [Internet]*. 2012 Jun 10 [cited 2023 Dec 6];29(6):1425–34. Available from: https://link.springer.com/article/10.1007/s11095-012-0688-6

40. Lee RS, Lin CH, Aljuffali IA, Hu KY, Fang JY. Passive targeting of thermosensitive diblock copolymer micelles to the lungs: Synthesis and characterization of poly(N-isopropylacrylamide)-block-poly(ε-caprolactone). *J Nanobiotechnology [Internet]*. 2015 Jun 18 [cited 2023 Dec 6];13(1):1–12. Available from: https://jnanobiotechnology.biomedcentral.com/articles/10.1186/s12951-015-0103-7

41. Hu X, Yang FF, Quan LH, Liu CY, Liu XM, Ehrhardt C, et al. Pulmonary delivered polymeric micelles—pharmacokinetic evaluation and biodistribution studies. *Eur J Pharm Biopharm*. 2014 Nov 1;88(3):1064–75.

42. Hu X, Yang FF, Liu CY, Ehrhardt C, Liao YH. In vitro uptake and transport studies of PEG-PLGA polymeric micelles in respiratory epithelial cells. *Eur J Pharm Biopharm*. 2017 May 1;114:29–37.

43. Kim G, Piao C, Oh J, Lee M. Self-assembled polymeric micelles for combined delivery of anti-inflammatory gene and drug to the lungs by inhalation. *Nanoscale [Internet]*. 2018 May 14 [cited 2022 Jul 6];10(18):8503–14. Available from: https://pubmed.ncbi.nlm.nih.gov/29693671/

44. Wang X, Chen Q, Zhang X, Ren X, Zhang X, Meng L, et al. Matrix metalloproteinase 2/9-triggered-release micelles for inhaled drug delivery to treat lung cancer: Preparation and in vitro/in vivo studies. *Int J Nanomedicine [Internet]*. 2018 [cited 2023 Dec 7];13:4641–59. Available from: www.tandfonline.com/action/journalInformation?journalCode=dijn20

45. Deacon J, Abdelghany SM, Quinn DJ, Schmid D, Megaw J, Donnelly RF, et al. Antimicrobial efficacy of tobramycin polymeric nanoparticles for Pseudomonas aeruginosa infections in cystic fibrosis: Formulation, characterisation and functionalisation with dornase alfa (DNase). *J Control Release*. 2015 Jan 28;198:55–61.

46. Costa-Gouveia J, Pancani E, Jouny S, Machelart A, Delorme V, Salzano G, et al. Combination therapy for tuberculosis treatment: pulmonary administration of ethionamide and booster co-loaded nanoparticles. *Sci Rep [Internet]*. 2017 Dec 1 [cited 2022 Jul 6];7(1). Available from: https://pubmed.ncbi.nlm.nih.gov/28710351/

47. Adi H, Young PM, Chan HK, Salama R, Traini D. Controlled release antibiotics for dry powder lung delivery. *Drug Dev Ind Pharm [Internet]*. 2010 Jan [cited 2023 Dec 6];36(1):119–26. Available from: www.tandfonline.com/doi/abs/10.3109/03639040903099769

48. Russo E, Gaglianone N, Baldassari S, Parodi B, Cafaggi S, Zibana C, et al. Preparation, characterization and in vitro antiviral activity evaluation of foscarnet-chitosan nanoparticles. *Colloids Surf B Biointerfaces*. 2014 Jun 1;118:117–25.

49. Choi SH, Byeon HJ, Choi JS, Thao L, Kim I, Lee ES, et al. Inhalable self-assembled albumin nanoparticles for treating drug-resistant lung cancer. *J Control Release*. 2015 Jan 10;197:199–207.

50. Ji P, Yu T, Liu Y, Jiang J, Xu J, Zhao Y, et al. Naringenin-loaded solid lipid nanoparticles: Preparation, controlled delivery, cellular uptake, and pulmonary pharmacokinetics. *Drug Des Devel Ther [Internet]*. 2016 Mar 1 [cited 2022 Jul 6];10:911–25. Available from: www.dovepress.com/naringenin-loaded-solid-lipid-nanoparticles-preparation-controlled-del-peer-reviewed-fulltext-article-DDDT

51. Makled S, Nafee N, Boraie N. Nebulized solid lipid nanoparticles for the potential treatment of pulmonary hypertension via targeted delivery of phosphodiesterase-5-inhibitor. *Int J Pharm*. 2017 Jan 30;517(1–2):312–21.

52. Gaspar DP, Gaspar MM, Eleutério CV, Grenha A, Blanco M, Gonçalves LMD, et al. Microencapsulated solid lipid nanoparticles as a hybrid platform for pulmonary antibiotic delivery. *Mol Pharm [Internet]*. 2017 Sep 5 [cited 2022 Jul 6];14(9):2977–90. Available from: https://pubs.acs.org/doi/full/10.1021/acs.molpharmaceut.7b00169

53. Patil-Gadhe A, Kyadarkunte A, Patole M, Pokharkar V. Montelukast-loaded nanostructured lipid carriers: Part II pulmonary drug delivery and in vitro-in vivo aerosol performance. *Eur J Pharm Biopharm [Internet]*. 2014 [cited 2022 Jul 6];88(1):169–77. Available from: https://pubmed.ncbi.nlm.nih.gov/25078860/

54. Ramalingam V, Varunkumar K, Ravikumar V, Rajaram R. Target delivery of doxorubicin tethered with PVP stabilized gold nanoparticles for effective treatment of lung cancer. *Sci Reports [Internet]*. 2018 Feb 28 [cited 2023 Dec 7];8(1):1–12. Available from: www.nature.com/articles/s41598-018-22172-5

55. Halwani R, Sultana Shaik A, Ratemi E, Afzal S, Kenana R, Al-Muhsen S, et al. A novel anti-IL4Rα nanoparticle efficiently controls lung inflammation during asthma. *Exp Mol Med [Internet]*. 2016 Oct 7 [cited 2023 Dec 6];48(10):e262–e262. Available from: www.nature.com/articles/emm201689

56. Wu C, Xu J, Hao Y, Zhao Y, Qiu Y, Jiang J, et al. Application of a lipid-coated hollow calcium phosphate nanoparticle in synergistic co-delivery of doxorubicin and paclitaxel for the treatment of human lung cancer A549 cells. *Int J Nanomedicine [Internet]*. 2017 Oct 31 [cited 2023 Dec 6];12:7979–92. Available from: www.tandfonline.com/action/journalInformation?journalCode=dijn20

57. Morris D, Ansar M, Speshock J, Ivanciuc T, Qu Y, Casola A, et al. Antiviral and immunomodulatory activity of silver nanoparticles in experimental RSV infection. *Viruses [Internet]*. 2019 Aug 1 [cited 2022 Jul 6];11(8). Available from: https://pubmed.ncbi.nlm.nih.gov/31398832/

58. Verma NK, Crosbie-Staunton K, Satti A, Gallagher S, Ryan KB, Doody T, et al. Magnetic core-shell nanoparticles for drug delivery by nebulization. *J Nanobiotechnology [Internet]*. 2013 Jan 23 [cited 2022 Jul 6];11(1):1–12. Available from: https://jnanobiotechnology.biomedcentral.com/articles/10.1186/1477-3155-11-1

59. Ison MG, Gnann JW, Nagy-Agren S, Treanor J, Paya C, Steigbigel R, et al. Safety and efficacy of nebulized zanamivir in hospitalized patients with serious influenza. *Antivir Ther [Internet]*. 2003 Apr 1 [cited 2023 Dec 6];8(3):183–90. Available from: https://journals.sagepub.com/doi/abs/10.1177/135965350300800301; https://doi.org/101177/135965350300800301

60. Kubo S, Kakuta M, Yamashita M. In vitro and in vivo effects of a long-acting anti-influenza agent CS-8958 (laninamivir octanoate, Inavir) against pandemic (H1N1) 2009 influenza viruses. *Jpn J Antibiot [Internet]*. 2010 Oct 1 [cited 2023 Dec 6];63(5):337–46. Available from: https://europepmc.org/article/med/21268406

61. Verreault D, Sivasubramani SK, Talton JD, Doyle LA, Reddy JD, Killeen SZ, et al. Evaluation of inhaled Cidofovir as postexposure prophylactic in an aerosol rabbitpox model. *Antivir Res*. 2012 Jan 1;93(1):204–8.

62. Stankova J, Carret AS, Moore D, McCusker C, Mitchell D, Davis M, et al. Long-term therapy with aerosolized ribavirin for parainfluenza 3 virus respiratory tract infection in an infant with severe combined immunodeficiency. *Pediatr Transplant [Internet]*. 2007 Mar 1 [cited 2023 Dec 6];11(2):209–13. Available from: https://onlinelibrary.wiley.com/doi/full/10.1111/j.1399-3046.2006.00607.x

63. Douglas RM, Moore B, Miles HB, Pinnock CB. Could preventive intranasal interferon lower the morbidity in children prone to respiratory illness? *Med J Aust [Internet]*. 1990 May 1 [cited 2023 Dec 6];152(10):524–8. Available from: https://onlinelibrary.wiley.com/doi/full/10.5694/j.1326-5377.1990.tb125353.x

64. Turner RB, Felton A, Kosak K, Kelsey DK, Meschievitz CK. Prevention of experimental coronavirus colds with intranasal α-2b interferon. *J Infect Dis [Internet]*. 1986 Sep 1 [cited 2023 Dec 6];154(3):443–7. Available from: https://dx.doi.org/10.1093/infdis/154.3.443

65. Miraglia Del Giudice M, Maiello N, Capristo C, Alterio E, Capasso M, Perrone L, et al. Resveratrol plus carboxymethyl-β-glucan reduces nasal symptoms in children with pollen-induced allergic rhinitis. *Curr Med Res Opin [Internet]*. 2014 Oct 1 [cited 2023 Dec 6];30(10):1931–5. Available from: www.tandfonline.com/doi/abs/10.1185/03007995.2014.938731

66. Shah SP, Misra A. Development of liposomal amphotericin B dry powder inhaler formulation. *Drug Deliv [Internet]*. 2004 Jul [cited 2023 Dec 6];11(4):247–53. Available from: www.tandfonline.com/doi/abs/10.1080/10717540490467375

67. Kuiper L, Ruijgrok EJ. A review on the clinical use of inhaled amphotericin B. *J Aerosol Med Pulm Drug Deliv [Internet]*. 2009 Sep 14 [cited 2023 Dec 6];22(3):213–27. Available from: www.liebertpub.com/doi/10.1089/jamp.2008.0715; https://home.liebertpub.com/jamp

68. Yang W, Peters JI, Williams RO. Inhaled nanoparticles—a current review. *Int J Pharm [Internet]*. 2008 May 22 [cited 2022 Jul 6];356(1–2):239–47. Available from: https://pubmed.ncbi.nlm.nih.gov/18358652/

69. Zhou QT, Leung SSY, Tang P, Parumasivam T, Loh ZH, Chan HK. Inhaled formulations and pulmonary drug delivery systems for respiratory infections. *Adv Drug Deliv Rev*. 2015 May 1;85:83–99.

70. Grandbastien M, Piotin A, Godet J, Abessolo-Amougou I, Ederlé C, Enache I, et al. SARS-CoV-2 pneumonia in hospitalized asthmatic patients did not induce severe exacerbation. *J Allergy Clin Immunol Pract*. 2020 Sep 1;8(8):2600–7.

71. Chandel A, Goyal AK, Ghosh G, Rath G. Recent advances in aerosolised drug delivery. *Biomed Pharmacother*. 2019 Apr 1;112:108601.

72. Tulbah AS, Ong HX, Colombo P, Young PM, Traini D. Novel simvastatin inhalation formulation and characterisation. *AAPS Pharm Sci Tech [Internet]*. 2014 May 8 [cited 2022 Jul 6];15(4):956–62. Available from: https://link.springer.com/article/10.1208/s12249-014-0127-6

73. Purucker ME, Rosebraugh CJ, Zhou F, Meyer RJ. Inhaled fluticasone propionate by diskus in the treatment of asthma: A comparison of the efficacy of the same nominal dose given either once or twice a day. *Chest*. 2003 Oct 1;124(4):1584–93.

74. Sloan DJ, Davies GR, Khoo SH. Recent advances in tuberculosis: New drugs and treatment regimens. *Curr Respir Med Rev [Internet]*. 2013 Jun 6 [cited 2022 Jul 6];9(3):200. Available from: www.ncbi.nlm.nih.gov/pmc/articles/PMC3968807/

75. Sloan D, Davies G, Khoo S. New drugs and treatment regimens. *Curr Respir Med Rev*. 2013 Aug 15;9(3):200–10.

76. Murray S, Mendel C, Spigelman M. TB alliance regimen development for multidrug-resistant tuberculosis. *Int J Tuberc Lung Dis*. 2016 Dec 1;20(12):S38–41.

77. Taylor KMG, Taylor G, Kellaway IW, Stevens J. The influence of liposomal encapsulation on sodium cromoglycate pharmacokinetics in man. *Pharm Res [Internet]*. 1989 [cited 2022 Jul 6];6(7):633–6. Available from: https://pubmed.ncbi.nlm.nih.gov/2508078/

78. Carter KC, Puig-Sellart M. Nanocarriers made from non-ionic surfactants or natural polymers for pulmonary drug delivery. *Curr Pharm Des*. 2016 Apr 20;22(22):3324–31.

79. Bhardwaj A, Kumar L, Narang RK, Murthy RS. Development and characterization of ligand-appended liposomes for multiple drug therapy for pulmonary tuberculosis. *Artif Cells, Nanomedicine, Biotechnol [Internet]*. 2013 [cited 2023 Dec 6];41(1):52–9. Available from: www.tandfonline.com/doi/abs/10.3109/10731199.2012.702316

80. Pandey R, Ahmad Z. Nanomedicine and experimental tuberculosis: Facts, flaws, and future. *Nanomedicine Nanotechnology, Biol Med*. 2011 Jun 1;7(3):259–72.

81. Pandey P, Nandkeoliar T, Tikku AP, Singh D, Singh MK. Prevalence of dental caries in the Indian population: A systematic review and meta-analysis. *J Int Soc Prev Community Dent [Internet]*. 2021 May 1 [cited 2023 Mar 14];11(3):256. Available from: www.ncbi.nlm.nih.gov/pmc/articles/PMC8257015/

82. Adi H, Young PM, Chan HK, Salama R, Traini D. Controlled release antibiotics for dry powder lung delivery. *Drug Dev Ind Pharm [Internet]*. 2010 Jan [cited 2021 Jan 27];36(1):119–26. Available from: www.tandfonline.com/doi/abs/10.3109/03639040903099769

83. Paranjpe M, Müller-Goymann CC. Nanoparticle-mediated pulmonary drug delivery: A review. *Int J Mol Sci [Internet]*. 2014 Apr 8 [cited 2022 Jul 6];15(4):5852. Available from: www.ncbi.nlm.nih.gov/pmc/articles/PMC4013600/

7 Nanomedicines for Rheumatoid Arthritis

*Shradha Devi Dwivedi, Krishna Yadav,
Deependra Singh, and Manju Rawat Singh*

7.1 INTRODUCTION

Rheumatoid arthritis (RA) is an inflammatory autoimmune disorder. It causes chronic systemic disorder that is characterized by bone erosion, joint destruction, and synovial dysplasia (1). According to ongoing measurements of the WHO (2019) and Global RA organizations, around the world, 23 million individuals are influenced by RA. Globally, the prevalence of RA varies from 0.5% to 1% (2). However, the ongoing advances in science have investigated the particular etiology of RA, yet at the same time, it requires all the more understanding and examination. RA is a kind of heterogeneous disease caused due to genetic and environmental factors. Environmental factors cause anti-citrulline antibodies and epigenetic regulation at the gene expression level. Genetic and environmental associations demonstrate the effect of autoantibodies on citrulline antigen subtlety in RA. These anti-citrulline antibodies may also be detected in patients with RA before the initiation of signs of joint damage. According to the accessible details, 67% of patients with RA showed the existence or absence of anti-citrulline antibodies. In this manner, these can be utilized as an asymptomatic tool for the early distinguishing proof of RA (3).

These discoveries recommend that for autoimmunity, the joint may not be the only main site. Other agents that trigger and enhance the risk of RA are exposed lung to harmful agents such as liquor, smoke, tobacco, and microbes like *Aggregatibacter actinomycetemcomitans* and *Porphyromonas gingivalis* (4). Generally, tobacco smoking is viewed as a danger factor since it affects cell demise and triggers mucosal toll-like receptors. These further invigorate antigen-introducing cells, for example, dendritic cells and B cells. Besides, tobacco smoking causes an exceptionally high convergence of free extremists, which associate with DNA and lead to transformation. The genetic and environmental factors initiate and recruit the macrophages, mast cells, natural killer cells, and dendritic cells that affect the joint sites. Activated synoviocytes, synovial macrophages, CD 8+ T and CD 4+ cell plays an essential role in inflammatory activity by the constant release of pro-inflammatory cytokines such as interleukins (IL) IL-1 and IL-6, TNF α and nuclear factor κ β activator. Abnormal proliferation and differentiation of osteoclast have been provoked by TNF α. Further, TNF α along with IL-6 encourages the synovial cell to produce matrix metalloproteinase and tissue degrading enzyme leads to bone erosion (5). Still, intracellular signaling pathways and autoantigens act in RA is remaining unclear due to which its cure is not possible. An ongoing examination uncovered that the signal transduction pathway, the Janus kinase signaling pathway responsible for the progression of RA (Figure 7.1) (6). Consequently, Intracellular signaling pathways repressing therapeutics have been formulated and are right known accessible in the market for successful RA treatment (6). Even though new biological and conventional dosage form demonstrates the therapeutical impact, somewhat they possess a harmful impact due to improper and higher dosing (6, 7). Hence, the patient needs novel potential therapeutics that diminished the side effect of the conventional dosage form. Nanomedicine act as a novel delivery system having numerous advantages in RA treatment like enhanced efficacy, the pharmacological profile of active agents, and target specification of the therapeutical agent in inflammable joints (7). This book chapter focus on nanomedicine used in RA treatment includes liposome, nanoparticles, etc.

DOI: 10.1201/9781003130055-7

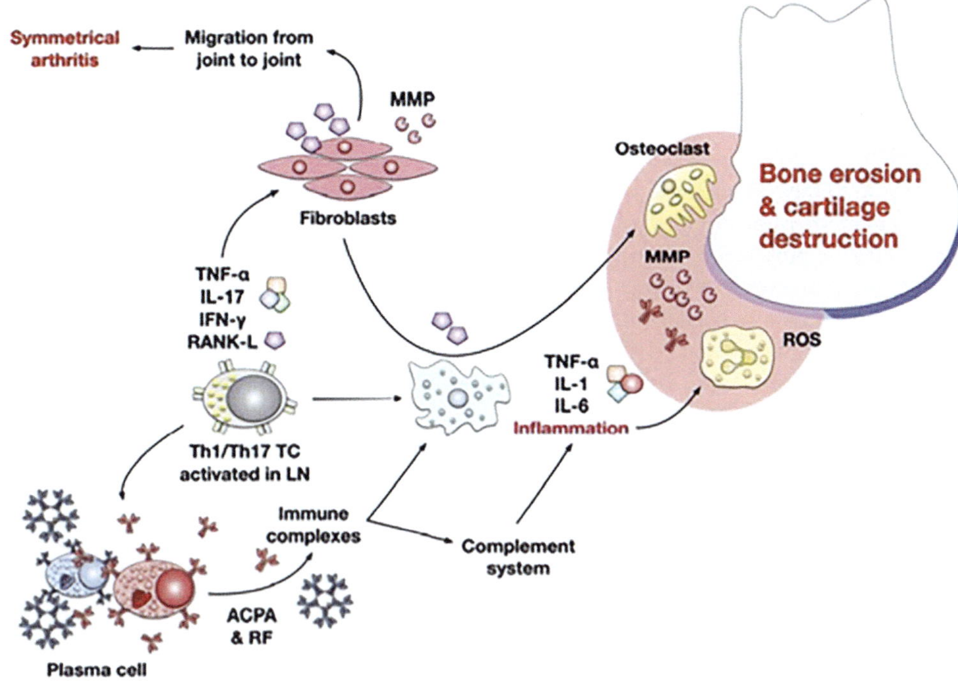

FIGURE 7.1 Pathophysiology of rheumatoid arthritis (8).

7.2 CURRENT TREATMENT OF RA

The primary aim for RA treatment consists of joint pain suppression, reduction of joint inflammation and swelling, prevent erosion of bone, and restore mobility and function of joint. To accomplish this goal various medicament were prescribe to patients. Generally, there are three categories of RA medicament are available like disease-modifying agents (DMARD), corticosteroid, nonsteroidal anti-inflammatory drug (NSAID). They are administered to the patient by various routes includes oral route, intra-articular and subcutaneous injections. Among them, NSAID has mostly prescribed medicament for symptomatic relief in RA patients (9). NSAID act by blocking the cyclooxygenase enzyme that inhibits prostaglandin (PG) biosynthesis. In this manner, it provides an excellent anti-inflammatory and analgesic action (10). NSAID shows dose-dependent action i.e. in lower concentration it shows analgesic action while in higher concentration it shows anti-inflammatory action. Mainly prescribed NSAIDs include diclofenac, ibuprofen, Celecoxib, flurbiprofen, meloxicam, naproxen, and piroxicam. Extensive administration of NSAID may cause severe side effects such as duodenal or peptic ulcer, gastrointestinal distress, erosion of small bowel, hypertension, heart failure, stroke, delay in wound healing, and seizure.

Another commonly administered anti-rheumatoid agent is a corticosteroid that may prescribe alone or along with other active agents like DMARDs or NSAID. Corticosteroids slow down the RA progression and prevent cartilage and bone damage (11). Corticosteroid act by suppressing the release of inflammatory cytokines and inhibit the migration of leukocytes but it has certain limitations including lipid abnormalities, loss of bone from lumbar spines, adrenal suppression, and osteoporosis. Several shreds of evidence demonstrate that a combination of another agent like DMARD with corticosteroids provides remission of swift, delay in the disease progression, and prevents bone and cartilage erosion (1).

DMARDs are well known to improve RA symptoms, reduce the damage of cartilage and joints, downregulate disease progression, and enhance function and mobility of joints. DMARD should prescribe at the earlier stage of RA that results in the rescission of disease and improve the overall function of joints. There are two DMARDs a) conventional DMARDs and b) biological DMARDs. Conventional DMARDs include Methotrexate, Hydroxychloroquine, Sulfasalazine, and Leflunomide. Methotrexate is a first-line drug for moderate to chronic RA. Biological DMARD includes Tocilizumab, etanercept, abatacept, and rituximab. Depending upon the disability and chronicity, tolerability, position of joint injury, comorbidities, and economical status of the patient, DMARDs may be prescribed alone or in combination with other active agents such as DMARDs, corticosteroids. Numerous evidences show that a combination regimen of DMARDs with other therapeutical agents shows higher suppression of disease progression and its symptoms as compared to DMARDs alone. However, DMARDs play a significant role in remission of the disease, but the long-term treatment of DMARDs often results in mild (stomatitis, vomiting, nausea, and rashes) severe side effect.

Even though, conventional therapeutic agents show their pharmacological action up to a limited extend. Along with these, its long-term treatment or escalation of dose may result in life-threatening side effects. This side effect may occur due to their uneven distribution and accretion in unspecified sites such as cells, sub-cellular domains, tissue, and organ. Hence, it is essential to develop new strategies for drug delivery having specific targeting, negligible systemic and local toxicity, and enhance therapeutical outcomes.

7.3 NANOTECHNOLOGY AND ADVANCEMENT

Despite a wide range of effective therapeutics, available for RA treatment, still, RA therapy remains a crucial challenge as commonly prescribed medicament hardly leads to complete recovery and frequently involves adverse effects and drug resistance. This can be overcome by using Nanomedicine. Nanomedicine appears as novel therapeutical strategies that involve the application of nanotechnology to achieve effective and targeted delivery. Nano-medicine helps to overcome the disadvantages of conventional medicine that include poor bioavailability, unspecified drug accumulation, high drug plasma protein binding, low pharmacological response, and internalization into the target tissue. Because of the remarkable physiological characteristic of nanomedicine like surface charge, nanoscopic size, loading efficacy, high entrapment; nanomedicine shows therapeutical and pharmacological feasibility. In addition to this nanomedicine, act as a shielding agent for active agent against premature degradation on exposure to physiochemical and chemical environment, enhanced circulation time, controlled/sustained release behavior and improve therapeutic efficacy (12). There is a certain barrier that must be overcome to achieve the desired effects of RA treatment; the first barrier that occurs just after intravenous or intra-articular administration of nanomedicine is opsonization and reorganization of nanomedicine by the reticuloendothelial system (RES), which leads to rapid clearances from plasma and decrease the efficacy of nanomedicine deliver to the inflammatory site. The second challenge was inflammable vascular endothelium. Any inflammatory stimulation endothelial cell promotes the release of matrix degradation enzymes. Matrix degrading enzymes digest the basal membrane then migrate and disassociate to develop primitive angiotubes that further develop into angiogenesis (13). Administered nanomedicine either has to enter the joint cavity through the endothelium and activate other RA symptoms like inflammation or to eliminate angiogenesis by targeting this abnormal vasculature. Thirdly, the conjugated ligand with nanomedicine must be specific to corresponding receptors and molecules that were only revel in the targeted site, for minimum side effects.

To treat RA, the nanomedicine must have to meet the following requirement a) nanomedicine have desired size (range from 10nm to 100nm) and surface charge (anion and neutral charge) b) propagation of circular time through PEGylation c) conjugation with a specific ligand. The desired size of nanomedicine enhances its circulation time by avoiding its reorganization by the liver (smaller than 100nm) and filtration through the kidney (greater than 10nm) (14). In the last two decades, nanotechnology plays a significant role in the treatment of disease, especially via its active targeting ability. Hence, this review is based on the pharmaceutical significance of nanomedicine in RA treatment. Different kind of nanomedicine used in the treatment of rheumatoid arthritis is mention in table 7.1.

TABLE 7.1

Different kind of nanomedicine used in the RA treatment

Therapeutic/ imagining agents	Type of nanocarriers	Remark	Reference
Morin	Liposome	1. surface modification with mannose 2. Enhances macrophage uptake 3. Suppress the mRNA expression of pro-inflammatory cytokines	(15)
Prednisolone (PD)	Liposome	1. PEGylated surface 2. Enhanced circulation time. 3. Minimum clearance mediated by RES. 4. Higher homing of PD in inflamed joints in animals. 5. Suppression of osteoclast and of RANKL	(16, 17)
Morin	Liposome	1. Surface modification with mannose 2. Improve macrophages uptake. 3. Diminish mRNA expression and downregulate inflammatory cytokines, angiogenic factors, transcription factor and inflammatory enzyme. 4. abate protein expression of STAT-3, TNF-α, p-STAT-3, interleukins, RANKL, with higher expression of osteoprotegerin (OPG)	(15)
DEX	Liposome	1. Conjugation of the surface with anti-VCAM-1 2. Specific targeting to VCAM-1 and suppress its expression	(18, 19)
indomethacin	Liposome	1. Encapsulation of indomethacin in liposomes reduces the toxic effects	(20)
superoxide dismutase	Liposome	1. enhanced accumulation of superoxide dismutase at inflammable site 2. long-lasting circulation time	(21)
fullerene	Liposome	1. suppress ROS level 2. Inhibit signaling pathway of NF-κB	(22)
clodronate	Liposome	1. Systemic elimination of macrophages	(23)
Dexamethasone palmitate	Liposome	1. larger accumulation in the inflammatory joints 2. the higher anti-inflammatory outcome in terms of RA control	(24)
Cyclosporin A	Micelles	1. Polysialic acid (PSA) as an ingredient to synthesis polymeric micelles 2. Non-receptor mediated endocytosis 3. Elevated uptake by synovial fibroblasts.	(25)
Dexamethasone	Micelles	1. To encapsulate dexamethasone in micelles [poly (ethylene glycol)–poly (ε caprolactone)] has been used.	(26)

(*Continued*)

TABLE 7.1 (Continued)

Different kind of nanomedicine used in the RA treatment

Therapeutic/ imagining agents	Type of nanocarriers	Remark	Reference
Camptothecin (CPT)	Micelles	1. Surface PEGylation with vasoactive intestinal peptide (VIP) provide active targeting to VIP receptors. 2. Higher uptake by monocytes, synovial macrophages, fibroblasts 3. dwindle joint inflammation	(27)
Laenoxicam	Micelles	1. It shows the anti-inflammatory and anti-arthritic effect	(28)
Methotrexate and Nimesulide	Micelles	1. reduces bone erosion 2. Decrease the serum levels of inflammatory cytokines. 3. In arthritic rats it help in the recovering of bone microstructure	(29)
Tocilizumab	Metallic nanoparticles	1. Tocilizumab is loaded within gold nanoparticles 2. It shows dual targeting towards IL-6R and VEGF and suppress its expression	(30)
Methotrexate	Metallic nanoparticles	1. Methotrexate encapsulated in gold half-shell nanoparticles 2. It shows photo-thermal treatments	(31)
Mesenchymal stem cells	Metallic nanoparticles	1. Mesenchymal stem loaded within Iron oxide nanoparticles 2. Iron oxide nanoparticles generate a magnetic field in synovial fibroblasts 3. It is used to repair and restore the function of damaged tissue	(32)
betamethasone phosphate (BP)	Polymeric nanoparticles	1. PEGylation is done by adsorption or grafting of polyethylene glycol on the surfaces of NPs 2. It prolongs plasma half-life and drug release 3. In comparision to non-PEGylated polymeric NPs, PEGylated polymeric NPs shows higher anti-RA efficacy.	(33)
Prednisolone	Polymeric nanoparticles	1. Prednisolone loaded pH-sensitive liposomes conjugated with hyaluronic acid allow the targeted delivery to the inflamed synovial cells. 2. It enhances potentially diminish off-target toxicity	(34)
Methotrexate	Polymeric nanoparticles	1. Dextran–methotrexate NPs modified with Folate considerably suppress inflammation, and selectively accumulation in inflamed synovium, 2. reduces proinflammatory cytokine	(35)
Dexamethasone	Polymeric nanoparticles	1. Dexamethasone loaded nanoparticles coated with Hyaluronic acid with reduced damage of cartilage and bone	(36)
Dexamethasone and Methotrexate	Chitosan nanoparticle	1. Chitosan nanoparticles loaded with Dexamethasone and Methotrexate demonstrate superior therapeutic efficacy along with lower toxicity	(37)
Actarit	Solid Lipid Nanoparticles (SLNs)	1. The injectable actarit loaded Solid Lipid Nanoparticles exhibit enhanced therapeutic efficacy 2. It reduces adverse-effects allied with oral administration of actarit	(38)
Celecoxib	Solid lipid nanoparticle (Tristearin)	1. Celecoxib loaded within SLNs shows higher anti-inflammatory and anti-rheumatic arthritic effect	(39)
Etoricoxib	Albumin Nanoparticles	1. Folic acid modified nanoparticles exhibited potential targeting towards activated macrophages cells, amplified bioavailability and spatial delivery	(40)
Tacrolimus	Human serum albumin	1. Tacrolimus encapsulated within human serum albumin enhances the anti-rheumatic arthritic effect	(41)

7.3.1 LIPOSOME

Liposomes are spherical vesicles with single or multiple bilayers. It is mainly composed of cholesterol and phospholipids that form a bilayer of lipid having an aqueous center. It can encapsulate both hydrophobic compounds and hydrophilic submerge in different lamellae with the help of van der walls force (42, 43). Phospholipids are a crucial component of liposomes that provides a specific feature to liposomes like encapsulating tendency and activity in the organism (44). Property of liposome not only affected by its composition, but also by its surface charge, size, and lamellae layer, bilayer rigidity, preparation method, and modification of surface (45) for example, higher accumulation of amphipathic drug (Doxirubin) is observed on using ammonium sulfate method (42). Traditional liposomes rapidly cleared from circulation via the reticuloendothelial system (RES). The incorporation of liposome by PEG polymer yields a stealth liposome that enhances circulation time by remaining unrecognized by RES. Stealth liposomes can be formulated by encapsulating liposomes with a polymer like poly-(amino acid)(PAA) and poly-(vinyl alcohol) (PVA) (46). Moreover, the lipid shell was further modified with specific ligands and stimuli-response agents to achieve higher distribution at targeted sites.

Metselaar et al. report that intravenous administration of GCS loaded PEGylated liposome, temporarily reduces arthritis. In addition to these, the lower sized PEG-liposome (100 nm) have higher accumulation in targeted sites and lower accumulation in the spleen and liver; as compared to larger size liposome (450 nm) (16, 47). PEGylated liposome is also used to enhance the efficacy of DMARDs (like MTX), NSAIDs (like indomethacin), and biologics (like superoxides dismutase). Cationic liposomes are used to deliver nucleic acid. CD40 is a characteristic marker of RA that is overexpressed in the surface synoviocytes, synovial monocytes, and dendritic cells (DCs). Overexpression of CD40L and CD40 leads to activate DCs, synovial monocytes in the inflammatory synovium, and release TNF α and IL-1β. This enhances joint inflammation, swelling, and severalty of RA. An antisense oligonucleotide (ASO) based approach is used for gene splicing and specific delivery to inflammable synovium (48). Andreakos et al. (49) develop a novel liposome having amphoteric characteristics for CD40-ASO targeting delivery. It is incorporated with CD40—CD154 for targeted delivery and interaction in inflammable synovium with good tolerability, devoid of severe toxicity, and superior anti-arthritis activity as compared to the naked liposome. Moreover, it reduces the expression of CD40 monocytes, inflammatory cells, DCs, and cytokines (IL-6, IL-17, and TNF-α) (48). This evidence support that the incorporation of liposome with a targeted ligand on its surface enhances its targetability efficacy and permeability for RA treatment (50). Recently, a surface modification of liposome with mannose—mediating agent act as a novel strategy that optimized liposome site-specification towards activated macrophage and efficacy (51). Mannose modified liposome was formulated for targeted delivery of dietary products, phenol, and morin. Treatment of AIA rat model with mannose-modified liposome significantly improve macrophage uptake, reduce expression of mRNA of crucial pro-inflammatory cytokines (IL-17, IL-1β, IL-6, TNF α), inflammatory enzymes (iNOS), transcriptional factor (NF-$\kappa\beta$-p65), and angiogenic factors. Morin-loaded liposomes not only decrease inflammation of the joint but also diminish osteoclastogenesis and downregulate osteoporosis (15).

Despite the targeted delivery of therapeutical payload, the desired biocompatibility, and clinical applicability of liposome, may still have some limitations. Liposomes were quickly opsonized by the RES due to which it rapidly undergoes metabolic degradation and systemic clearance results in lower plasma half-life. This can be overcome by alternating its composition (such as type of phospholipids and side-chain) and physicochemical property (zeta potential, size). Modification of surface with PEG only results in partial enhancement of the pharmacodynamic and pharmacokinetic profile of nanomedicine. For instance, PEGylated nanomedicine only results in a reduction of plasma half-life but it hinders the interaction of nanomedicine to the targeted site while conjugation of nanomedicine with targeted ligand enhances its efficacy and penetration through receptor-mediated endocytosis that overcomes the RES opsonization. Interestingly, the application of all these strategies together has emerged to formulate a superior nanomedicine and these kinds of strategies are called multifunctionalization. In multifunctional strategies, the surface of nanomedicine was conjugated with multiple targeted ligands. Inspired by these strategies, Vannieainghe et al. (52) formulate a multi-functionalized nanomedicine that consists of HA1; RGD tagged PEGylated PD-encapsulated nanomedicine for its targeted delivery to specific sites. RGD peptides recognize $\alpha v\beta 3$ integrin, $\alpha 1\beta 3$ integrin antagonist act as promising therapeutical strategies for mitigation of angiogenesis in the synovial site, cartilage erosion, and inflammation (53).

7.3.2 Micelles

Micelles are shell or core-like structures formed from a block of amphiphilic molecules i.e. di-block and Tri-blocks. Amphillic blocks aggregate into a nanosized colloidal structure having a hydrophobic core with a hydrophilic exterior in the aqueous phase (54). Formation of self assembles structure micelles generally occur when each unimers are dissolved in an aqueous solution that is above a specific critical micelles concentration (CMC) and a critical micelles temperature (CMT) (55). Payloads that have low aqueous solubility were encapsulated in a hydrophobic core. Due to well-defined structure, colloidal stability, physiochemical property, nanoscopic size, higher solubility, enhanced loading capacity, higher plasma life, and sustained release profile micelles have earned a remembrance reorganization as the versatile nanocarrier. Owning a sophisticated feature and intrinsic versatility, polymeric micelles have a great ability for target delivery with a wide range of pharmacological and diagnostics molecules to inflammable synovium for RA treatment (55). To achieve targeted delivery of therapeutical and diagnostic payload must be optimized through specific targeting of higher expressed molecules or receptors at the targeted site. This can be achieved by identifying the upregulated receptor or molecules and deliver a payload in targeted sites without its distribution to other sites. In RA, NF-$\kappa\beta$ a transcription factor plays a crucial role in the regulation of inflammatory cascades. Activated NF-$\kappa\beta$ enhanced expression of several genes that respond to T helper cell, activation, differentiation, and proliferation of FLS, proinflammatory cytokines secretion, osteoclast leads to cartilage damage and progression of the disease (56, 57). This inflammatory cascade cans downregulate by using SiRNA (58). Wang et al. (59) used a similar kind of amphiphilic copolymer i.e. polycaprolactone polyethylene glycol (PCL-PEG) and polycaprolactone poly-ethylenimine (PCL-PEI) to formulate hybrid polymeric micelles to deliver dexamethasone (DEX) and SiRNA together. Co-loaded hybrid polymer micelles inhibit NF-κ β signaling and decrease the release of pro-inflammatory cytokines i.e. TNF-α, IL-1β, decrease activation and recruitment of macrophage, T cell response, and decrease cartilage and bone erosion, the severity of arthritis and thickness of paw (59).

Multifunctional micelles boost site—selection targetability like conjugation of folic acid (FA) and polysialic acid (PSA). Polysialic is a natural polymer with hydrophobic nature. PSA enhances plasma half-life, receptor targeting, and enhance therapeutical outcome. Zhang et al. (60) engineered multifunctional micelles of FA and PSA to deliver DEX to inflammatory synovium. These micelles improve cellular uptake, suppress activation of macrophages, decrease the release of pro-inflammatory cytokines, and RA progression. From the various study, it has been found that multifunctional micelles show greater plasma half-life for RA treatment (60). The targeted delivery of MTX has been achieved by polymeric hybrid micelles by conjugating its surface with sialic acid (SA) (61). It enhances aggregation of MTX in the inflammable synovium and activates macrophages via SA conjugated MTX-loaded micelles. It not only inhibits activated and recruitment of macrophage but also prevent side effects associated with commercial administration of MTX like creatine, urea nitrogen, aspirate aminotransferase, and alanine aminotransferase level. Another innovative strategy for the controlled release of payload in an acidic environment is pH-sensitive polymeric micelles. Local inflammation at inflammable synovium enhances metabolic action, insufficient oxygen level, and sifting towards lactate formation and anaerobic glycolysis that leads to pH alteration at inflammable joints. By utilizing this concept sensitive micelles Li-et al. formulate pH-sensitive micelles (62).

In pH, sensitive micelles payloads were conjugated with APN through hydrazone bond which provides sensitivity towards acidic pH.

7.3.3 Metallic Nanoparticles

Metallic nanoparticles have been emerged as latest the development due to their promising biodegradability, biocompatible, versatile modification, magnetic property, unique size, and higher optical absorption (63). Metallic nanoparticles consist of silica-gold nanoshells, iron oxides nanoparticles, quantum dots, and gold nanoparticles. The implementation of metallic nanoparticles can give multifunctional nanoparticles that show desired therapeutical efficacy. Among all these metallic nanoparticles, gold nanoparticles (AU-NPS) have been extensively exploited for their biocompatibility, optical absorption, and RA treatment. AU-NPS act as a natural anti-angiogenesis agent via actively binding with vascular endothelial growth factor (VEGF) in inflammable synovium. Moreover, AU-NPS is known to have anti-oxidant action by scavenging reactive oxygen species (ROS), which leads to the formation of RANKL-induced osteoclast and results in cartilage and bone erosion (64) and act as potential therapeutical agents for RA. A study conducted by Leet et al. (65) engineered a dual-targeting multifunctional AU-NP, loaded with TCZ and functionalized with hyaluronic acid (HA). HA-AU-NPS/TCZ promising diminish the release of pro-inflammatory cytokines by inhabiting IL-6 receptor and VEGF-induced proliferation that ultimately diminish the rate of inflammation and joint destruction (65). In another study, a novel nanomedicine was formulated by encapsulating MTX and functionalized with RGD peptide to target $\alpha V\beta3$ in the highly vascularized area in combination with near-infrared florescence's (NIRF) irradiation, it shows a lower concentration of MTX with enhanced therapeutical Index compared with conventional MTX-treatment (66). Another metallic nanoparticle that is widely used in RA treatment is Iron oxide nanoparticles. Iron oxide nanoparticles were used for both passive and active targeting delivery. Iron oxide nanoparticles are also known as super magnetic iron oxide nanoparticles (SPION). SPION serves as a target carrier for specific distribution of payloads in the response of the external magnetic field (67). SPION has unique benefits like excellent magnetic property, biocompatibility, and easy surface modification for further targetability. SIPON consists of an iron oxide core with a hydrophilic coat of biocompatible compound. SPION is mainly implicated as magnetic (Fe3O4) or magnetite core (γ Fe3O4) (68). Butoescu et al. (69) develop a PLGA microparticle that is encapsulated with both DEX and SPION to alleviate arthritis. Due to SPION magnetic property it shows prolongs retention in joints. From the current study, SPION was functionalized with PEI and loaded with siRNA. PEI-SPION/SiRNA significantly enhances cellular uptake and aggregation of SiRNA in the inflammatory site which is achieved with help of external magnetic agents. PEI-SPION/SiRNA NP has an anti-inflammatory action (70).

7.3.4 Polymeric Nanoparticles

Polymeric nanoparticles (NP) act as a promising carrier for the effective delivery of various agents such as vaccines, biological macromolecules, imaging agents, and active agents (71). A common polymer that is employed for the formulation of Nanomedicines in RA treatments is poly(lactic-co-glycolic acid) (PLGA). PLGA NP is significantly used to deliver betamethasone phosphate (BP) for a sustained period. BP-loaded PLGA NPs reduce inflammation and enhance its efficacy. Zincs play a crucial role in the development of PLGA NPS as it alters its physiological characteristic such as practical size, poly-dispersibility index, and surface charge, and encapsulation efficacy, release ability. An intra-articular administration of BP-loaded PLGA NPs demonstrates higher inflammatory response, reduces joint swelling, sustain release of BP in synovial fluid, and prevent articular damage and remission of RA progression.

PH sensitive polymeric NPs play a pivotal role in the delivery of payload agents at lower pH microenvironment of inflammable sites. Alam et al. (72) formulate a pH-sensitive polymeric nanoparticle that consists of PEGylated hyaluronic acid (P-HA) which acts as a hydrophilic shell, 5-β-Cholanic phosphate (cap) as a pH-sensitive agent, for targeted delivery of MTX. MTX-HA-NPs-MP is multifunctional nanomedicine that demonstrates sustain release and enhances drug release with higher circulation time and reduces opsonization of RES and decreases renal clearance, as compared with MTX-HA-NPs (72). Folic acid receptors (FR) are highly upregulated on the surface of macrophages that act as a molecular target for specific targeting. Moural et al. (73) engineered a multifunctional nanocarrier by encapsulating SPIONS (contrast agent) and MTX (as anti-RA agent) into PLGA NPS. SPIONS/MTX-PLGA NPS was further modified with the anti-CD64 monoclonal antibody. CD64 receptors are upregulated in the surface of macrophages in RA patients (74). Endocytosis of anti-CD64 conjugated SPIONS/MTX/PLGA NPS demonstrates a significant enhancement of cellular uptake and greater cytotoxicity against LPS-activated RAW 264.7 cell as compared to non-conjugated MTX-PLGA NP and SPIONS/MTX PLGA NP (73).

7.3.5 NATURAL POLYSACCHARIDES BASED NANOPARTICLES

Natural polymers like HA, alginates, and chitosan are applicable in RA treatment. HA is a kind of natural polysaccharides that occurs in the extracellular matrix in humans, which is applicable for both targeting ligand and drug carriers. It has been reported that the inhibition of γ-secretase effectively reduces inflammatory arthritic by inhibiting the Notch signaling pathway. Park et al. engineered a halurinated nanoparticles (HA-NP) loaded with γ-secretase inhibitor (DAPT). DAPT-HA-NP demonstrate a potential therapeutical action in collagen-induced arthritis (CIA) mouse model, that significantly reduce arthritic level, tissue damage and infiltration of neutrophil (75). Chitosan is a naturally occurring poly-Saccharides; it is a biodegradable mucoadhesive agent with and non-toxic nature. Chitosan have positive charge which act as an effective carrier for negative charge drugs and gene via electrostatic interaction with a nucleic acid. Several researchers formulate a nano-delivery system of polymerized Si-RNA to target Notch-1 or TNF-α which is conjugated with thiolated glycol chitosan for RA treatment (76). Si-RNA loaded chitosan nanoparticles markedly reduce tissue inflammation and erosion of bone in the CIA mouse model. Calcium phosphate coated with chitosan and encapsulated with bovine Lactoferrin which is on oral administration significantly reduces the rate of joint inflammation and expression of various inflammatory agents like IL-β, C-Jun N terminal kinase, nitric oxides, and MAPK, etc. In addition to these, it eliminates the crystal of calcium phosphate for mice joints and reduces chronicity of the inflammatory disease.

Alginate is a natural polysaccharides polymer that is used for RA treatment. Alginate is a copolymer of α-L-glucoronic acid (G) and β-D-mannuronic acid (M). IL-10 plasmid DNA loaded with Tuftsin functionally alginate nanoparticles efficacy repolarised pro-inflammatory macrophage (M1 type) into anti-inflammatory macrophage (M2 type) and protect joints from damage which is associated with adjuvant-induced arthritic (AIA) (77).

7.3.6 SOLID LIPID NANOPARTICLES (SLNS)

SLNS is a nanosized lipid-based colloidal carrier that used for targeted delivery with a wide range of therapeutical and domestic properties (78). SLNS is a nanocarrier for a large number of macromolecules like proteins, oligonucleotides, and DNA, SLNS loaded with actaric (4-acetyl aminophenylacetic acid) shows passive targeting and promising remises RA progression, decrease rate of inflammation, and cartilage degradation. It remarkably suppresses the production of cytokines (TNF α and IL-1β) and suppresses the expression of adhesive molecules CD44 receptors on the surface of fibroblast, macrophage, and synovial lymphocytes (79). Actaric-SLNS prolong circulation time, targeting efficacy, and suppress RA progression. Zhou et al. formulate HA conjugated SLNS loaded with PD (HA-PD-SLNS). HA-PD-SLNS have nanosized structure (≥200nm), higher drug encapsulating tendency, spherical structure, and greater uptake by LPS-activated RAW 264.7 cells, as compared to non-activated RAW 264.7 cell. It also leads to minimal bodyweight loss, minimal arthritic score, swelling of the paw, and release of pro-inflammatory cytokines in the animal serum administrated with HA-PD-SLNS (80).

7.3.7 Nanoemulsion

Nanoemulsion (NE) is a colloidal nanocarrier that tends to encapsulate both hydrophilic and hydrophobic therapeutical and imaging agents (79). It consists of two immiscible liquids and converts them into a solo phase isotropic system. It is stabilized by using an emulsifying agent like surfactants. NE has a significant pharmaceutical characteristic such as higher drug solubility, enhanced bioavailability, and protection payloads from biological and chemical degradation (79). NE has a similar resemblance with lipid structure having low density lipoprotein (LDL), which is extensively used as a targeted carrier, enhanced penetration rate, and higher accumulation in activated macrophage in synovial sites (81, 82). By using homogenizing technology at MTX is successfully loaded within NE for higher permeability and targeted delivery. Intravenous administration of MTX-NE to rabbits shows significant inhibition of leucocytes infiltration, higher accumulation in synovial fluid, reduce production of pro-inflammatory cytokines (TNFα, IL-6, IL-10, IL-7), and demonstrate anti-inflammatory action. Zhen et al. (83) encapsulate Curcumin within nanoemulsions which significantly enhance its solubility, bioavailability, therapeutical and pharmaceutical characteristics of Curcumin.

7.3.8 Carbon Nanotube

Carbon nanotube (CNT) is another attractive nanocarrier that has a distinct physiochemical characteristic that enable versatile encapsulating tendency for various therapeutical agents, higher target-specificity (83). CNT may act as an adjacent material or main carrier for RA treatment. An MTX-loaded multi-walled carbon tube (MWCNT) was formulated, which is further modified with folic acid (FA). Conjugation of FA over MWCNT/MTX promotes a specific target toward overexpressed FA on the surface of fibroblast, synovial macrophages, and monocytes. FA-MTX-MWCNTS shows sustain release profile, prolonged circulation time, enhanced penetration rate, and targetability through FA receptor endocytosis, greater aggregation of MTX in inflammable synovial sites, and improved anti-arthritis property as compared to FA non conjugated MTX-MWCNTS and commercial MTX (84).

7.3.9 Anti-Body Conjugated Nanomedicine

Another outstanding strategy to achieve targeted delivery of payloads is a conjugation of nanomedicine with anti-body (85). Recently, Lee et al. (86) develop a novel antibody conjugates nanomedicine i.e antibody (Tocilizumab), drug (alendronate, ALD) attached with actively targeted IL-6, and reduce the progression of RA. ALD is commonly administered for osteoporosis treatment as it acts as an anti-inflammatory agent, anti-osteoclastogenesis, and enhances bone density (87). TCZ-ALD conjugated nanoparticles significantly reduce arthritic score and production of pro-inflammatory cytokines (IL-6, TNF-α) in synovial fluid and serum. On other hand, TCZ is a kind of humanized monoclonal antibody that suppresses IL- in the inflammatory synovium (88). Scavenger receptor (SR) is upregulated on the macrophage surface of inflammable synovium is acts as a crucial biological target. Dextran sulfate (DS) (hydrophilic polysaccharides) conjugates with SR through a ligand-receptor conjugation (89). Nanoconjugation of DS, SR, and MTX (i.e. DS-g-MTX) shows sustained release profile, increased cell uptake, and targeted delivery to overexpressed SR on the activated macrophage, in comparison to non-targeted dextran-MTX nanomedicine. DS-g-MTX shows a higher reduction of paw inflammation, swelling, arthritic progression and decreases the expression of m-RNA, and significantly reduces cytokines like TNF-α, IL-6, and IL-1β (89).

7.3.10 ALBUMIN NANOPARTICLES

In inflammable joints, albumin is highly distributed which is an attractive target in inflammatory synovium. From various pre-clinical studies, it has been found that human serum albumin (HSA) is a promising drug carrier for inflammable joints (90). For instance, HSA conjugates with MTX (MTX-HSA) which suppresses synovial fibroblast and prevents cartilage degradation (91). To determine the pharmaceutical tendency of albumin nanoparticles (AL-NP), it is loaded with Tacrolimus (TAC). Nanoparticles of TAC-HSA demonstrate anti-arthritic action on intravenous administration and oral administration of TAC (41). Anakinra is a human recombinant IL-1 receptor antagonist (IL-1ra) that has an anti-RA property which enhanced on conjugation with HSA; HSA-IL-1ra considerably enhance plasma half-life and accumulation in the inflammatory joints of collagen-induced arthritic mouse model (92).

REFERENCES

1. Guo Q, Wang Y, Xu D, Nossent J, Pavlos NJ, Xu J. Rheumatoid arthritis: Pathological mechanisms and modern pharmacologic therapies. *Bone Res [Internet]*. 2018;6(1). Available from: http://dx.doi.org/10.1038/s41413-018-0016-9
2. Gorantla S, Singhvi G, Rapalli VK, Waghule T. Targeted drug-delivery systems in the treatment of rheumatoid arthritis: Recent advancement and clinical status. *Ther Deliv*. 2020;11:269–84.
3. McInnes IB, Schett G. The pathogenesis of rheumatoid arthritis. *N Engl J Med [Internet]*. 2011 Dec 8 [cited 2020 Dec 30];365(23):2205–19. Available from: www.nejm.org/doi/abs/10.1056/NEJMra1004965
4. Gómez-Bañuelos E, Mukherjee A, Darrah E, Andrade F. Clinical medicine rheumatoid arthritis-associated mechanisms of porphyromonas gingivalis and aggregatibacter actinomycetemcomitans. *J Clin Med*. 2019 [cited 2021 Feb 23];8(9):1309. Available from: www.mdpi.com/journal/jcm
5. McInnes IB, Schett G. Pathogenetic insights from the treatment of rheumatoid arthritis. *Lancet [Internet]*. 2017 [cited 2020 Nov 9];389: 2328–37. Lancet Publishing Group. Available from: https://pubmed.ncbi.nlm.nih.gov/28612747/
6. Alunno A, Carubbi F, Giacomelli R, Gerli R. Cytokines in the pathogenesis of rheumatoid arthritis: New players and therapeutic targets. *BMC Rheumatol [Internet]*. 2017 [cited 2020 Nov 9];1:1–13. BioMed Central Ltd. Available from: https://bmcrheumatol.biomedcentral.com/articles/10.1186/s41927-017-0001-8
7. Prosperi D, Colombo M, Zanoni I, Granucci F. Drug nanocarriers to treat autoimmunity and chronic inflammatory diseases. *Semin Immunol [Internet]*. 2017 [cited 2020 Nov 9];34:61–7. Academic Press. Available from: https://pubmed.ncbi.nlm.nih.gov/28855088/
8. Lin Y-J, Anzaghe M, Schülke S. Update on the pathomechanism, diagnosis, and treatment options for rheumatoid arthritis. *Cells [Internet]*. 2020 Apr 3 [cited 2021 Mar 7];9(4):880. Available from: www.ncbi.nlm.nih.gov/pmc/articles/PMC7226834/
9. Benjamin O, Bansal P, Goyal A, Lappin S. Disease modifying anti-rheumatic drugs (DMARD). *StatPearls [Internet]*. 2019 [Updated 2019 Jan 6; cited 2021 Feb 23]. StatPearls Publishing. Available from: www.ncbi.nlm.nih.gov/books/NBK507863/
10. Gunaydin C, Bilge SS. Effects of nonsteroidal anti-inflammatory drugs at the molecular level. *Eurasian J Med*. 2018;50(2):116–21.
11. Wongrakpanich S, Wongrakpanich A, Melhado K, Rangaswami J. A comprehensive review of non-steroidal anti-inflammatory drug use in the elderly. *Aging Dis [Internet]*. 2018 [cited 2020 Nov 10];9:143–50. International Society on Aging and Disease. Available from: https://pubmed.ncbi.nlm.nih.gov/29392089/
12. Fang G, Zhang Q, Pang Y, Thu HE, Hussain Z. Nanomedicines for improved targetability to inflamed synovium for treatment of rheumatoid arthritis: Multi-functionalization as an emerging strategy to optimize therapeutic efficacy. *J Control Release [Internet]*. 2019 [cited 2020 Dec 30];303:181–208. Elsevier B.V. Available from: https://pubmed.ncbi.nlm.nih.gov/31015032/
13. Chen M, Daddy KA, Xiao Y, Ping Q, Zong L. Advanced nanomedicine for rheumatoid arthritis treatment: Focus on active targeting. *Expert Opin Drug Deliv [Internet]*. 2017;14(10):1141–4. Available from: https://doi.org/10.1080/17425247.2017.1372746
14. Danhier F, Feron O, Préat V. To exploit the tumor microenvironment: Passive and active tumor targeting of nanocarriers for anti-cancer drug delivery. *J Control Release [Internet]*. 2010 [cited 2020 Nov 10];148:135–46. Available from: https://pubmed.ncbi.nlm.nih.gov/20797419/

15. Sultana F, Neog MK, Rasool MK. Targeted delivery of morin, a dietary bioflavanol encapsulated mannosylated liposomes to the macrophages of adjuvant-induced arthritis rats inhibits inflammatory immune response and osteoclastogenesis. *Eur J Pharm Biopharm [Internet].* 2017 Jun 1 [cited 2020 Nov 10];115:229–42. Available from: https://pubmed.ncbi.nlm.nih.gov/28315446/

16. Metselaar JM, Wauben MHM, Wagenaar-Hilbers JPA, Boerman OC, Storm G. Complete remission of experimental arthritis by joint targeting of glucocorticoids with long-circulating liposomes. *Arthritis Rheum.* 2003 Jul 1;48(7):2059–66.

17. Hofkens W, Grevers LC, Walgreen B, De Vries TJ, Leenen PJM, Everts V, et al. Intravenously delivered glucocorticoid liposomes inhibit osteoclast activity and bone erosion in murine antigen-induced arthritis. *J Control Release [Internet].* 2011 Jun 30 [cited 2021 Feb 27];152(3):363–9. Available from: https://pubmed.ncbi.nlm.nih.gov/21396411/

18. Nogueira E, Gomes AC, Preto A, Cavaco-Paulo A. Folate-targeted nanoparticles for rheumatoid arthritis therapy. *Nanomedicine: NBM [Internet].* 2016 [cited 2021 Jan 4];12:1113–26. Elsevier Inc. Available from: https://pubmed.ncbi.nlm.nih.gov/26733257/

19. Paulos CM, Turk MJ, Breur GJ, Low PS. Folate receptor-mediated targeting of therapeutic and imaging agents to activated macrophages in rheumatoid arthritis. *Adv Drug Deliv Rev [Internet].* 2004 Apr 29 [cited 2021 Feb 28];56(8):1205–17. Available from: https://pubmed.ncbi.nlm.nih.gov/15094216/

20. Srinath P, Vyas SP, Diwan PV. Preparation and pharmacodynamic evaluation of liposomes of indomethacin. *Drug Dev Ind Pharm [Internet].* 2000 [cited 2021 Feb 28];26(3):313–21. Available from: https://pubmed.ncbi.nlm.nih.gov/10738648/

21. Corvo ML, Boerman OC, Oyen WJG, Van Bloois L, Cruz MEM, Crommelin DJA, et al. Intravenous administration of superoxide dismutase entrapped in long circulating liposomesII. In vivo fate in a rat model of adjuvant arthritis. *Biochim Biophys Acta—Biomembr.* 1999 Jul 15;1419(2):325–34.

22. Dellinger AL, Cunin P, Lee D, Kung AL, Brooks DB, Zhou Z, et al. Inhibition of inflammatory arthritis using fullerene nanomaterials. Frey O, editor. *PLoS One [Internet].* 2015 Apr 16 [cited 2021 Feb 28];10(4):e0126290. Available from: https://dx.plos.org/10.1371/journal.pone.0126290

23. Highton J, Guévremont D, Thomson J, Carlisle B, Tucker I. A trial of clodronate-liposomes as anti-macrophage treatment in a sheep model of arthritis. *Clin Exp Rheumatol [Internet].* 1999 Jan 1 [cited 2021 Feb 28];17(1):43–8. Available from: https://europepmc.org/article/med/10084031

24. Hu L, Luo X, Zhou S, Zhu J, Xiao M, Li C, et al. Neutrophil-mediated delivery of dexamethasone palmitate-loaded liposomes decorated with a sialic acid conjugate for rheumatoid arthritis treatment. *Pharm Res [Internet].* 2019 Jul 1 [cited 2021 Feb 28];36(7):1–15. Available from: https://doi.org/10.1007/s11095-019-2609-4

25. Zhang N, Xu C, Li N, Zhang S, Fu L, Chu X, et al. Folate receptor-targeted mixed polysialic acid micelles for combating rheumatoid arthritis: In vitro and in vivo evaluation. *Drug Deliv [Internet].* 2018 [cited 2020 Nov 10];25(1):1182–91. Available from: www.ncbi.nlm.nih.gov/pmc/articles/PMC6060703/?report=abstract

26. Yang YH, Rajaiah R, Ruoslahti E, Moudgil KD. Peptides targeting inflamed synovial vasculature attenuate autoimmune arthritis. *Proc Natl Acad Sci U S A [Internet].* 2011 Aug 2 [cited 2021 Feb 28];108(31):12857–62. Available from: www.pnas.org/cgi/doi/10.1073/pnas.1103569108

27. Koo OMY, Rubinstein I, Önyüksel H. Actively targeted low-dose camptothecin as a safe, long-acting, disease-modifying nanomedicine for rheumatoid arthritis. *Pharm Res [Internet].* 2011 Apr [cited 2021 Feb 28];28(4):776–87. Available from: https://pubmed.ncbi.nlm.nih.gov/21132352/

28. Helmy HS, El-Sahar AE, Sayed RH, Shamma RN, Salama AH, Elbaz EM. Therapeutic effects of lornoxicam-loaded nanomicellar formula in experimental models of rheumatoid arthritis. *Int J Nanomedicine [Internet].* 2017 Sep 22 [cited 2021 Feb 28];12:7015–23. Available from: https://pubmed.ncbi.nlm.nih.gov/29026298/

29. Wang Y, Zhao R, Gu Z, Dong C, Guo G, Li L. Effects of glucocorticoids on osteoporosis in rheumatoid arthritis: A systematic review and meta-analysis. *Osteoporos Int.* 2020;31(8):1401–9.

30. Lee H, Lee MY, Bhang SH, Kim BS, Kim YS, Ju JH, et al. Hyaluronate-gold nanoparticle/tocilizumab complex for the treatment of rheumatoid arthritis. *ACS Nano [Internet].* 2014 May 27 [cited 2020 Nov 10];8(5):4790–8. Available from: https://pubmed.ncbi.nlm.nih.gov/24730974/

31. Lee SM, Kim HJ, Ha YJ, Park YN, Lee SK, Park YB, et al. Targeted chemo-photothermal treatments of rheumatoid arthritis using gold half-shell multifunctional nanoparticles. *ACS Nano [Internet].* 2013 Jan 22 [cited 2021 Feb 28];7(1):50–7. Available from: https://pubmed.ncbi.nlm.nih.gov/23194301/

32. Markides H, Kehoe O, Morris RH, El Haj AJ. Whole body tracking of superparamagnetic iron oxide nanoparticle-labelled cells—a rheumatoid arthritis mouse model. *Stem Cell Res Ther [Internet].* 2013 Oct 17 [cited 2021 Feb 28];4(5):126. Available from: http://stemcellres.com/content/4/5/126

33. Ishihara T, Kubota T, Choi T, Higaki M. Treatment of experimental arthritis with stealth-type polymeric nanoparticles encapsulating betamethasone phosphate. *J Pharmacol Exp Ther [Internet]*. 2009 May [cited 2021 Feb 28];329(2):412–7. Available from: https://pubmed.ncbi.nlm.nih.gov/19244548/

34. Gouveia VM, Lopes-De-Araújo J, Costa Lima SA, Nunes C, Reis S. Hyaluronic acid-conjugated pH-sensitive liposomes for targeted delivery of prednisolone on rheumatoid arthritis therapy. *Nanomedicine [Internet]*. 2018 May 1 [cited 2021 Feb 28];13(9):1037–49. Available from: https://pubmed.ncbi.nlm.nih.gov/29790395/

35. Yang M, Ding J, Zhang Y, Chang F, Wang J, Gao Z, et al. Activated macrophage-targeted dextran-methotrexate/folate conjugate prevents deterioration of collagen-induced arthritis in mice. *J Mater Chem B [Internet]*. 2016 Mar 28 [cited 2021 Feb 28];4(12):2102–13. Available from: https://pubs.rsc.org/en/content/articlehtml/2016/tb/c5tb02479j

36. Yu C, Li X, Hou Y, Meng X, Wang D, Liu J, et al. Hyaluronic acid coated acid-sensitive nanoparticles for targeted therapy of adjuvant-induced arthritis in rats. *Molecules [Internet]*. 2019 Jan 2 [cited 2021 Feb 28];24(1). Available from: www.ncbi.nlm.nih.gov/pmc/articles/PMC6337373/

37. Kumar V, Leekha A, Tyagi A, Kaul A, Mishra AK, Verma AK. Preparation and evaluation of biopolymeric nanoparticles as drug delivery system in effective treatment of rheumatoid arthritis. *Pharm Res [Internet]*. 2017 Mar 1 [cited 2021 Feb 28];34(3):654–67. Available from: https://pubmed.ncbi.nlm.nih.gov/28097508/

38. Ye J, Wang Q, Zhou X, Zhang N. Injectable actarit-loaded solid lipid nanoparticles as passive targeting therapeutic agents for rheumatoid arthritis. *Int J Pharm [Internet]*. 2008 Mar 20 [cited 2021 Feb 28];352(1–2):273–9. Available from: https://pubmed.ncbi.nlm.nih.gov/18054182/

39. Kishore N, Raja MD, Kumar CS, Dhanalekshmi U, Srinivasan R. Lipid carriers for delivery of celecoxib: In vitro, in vivo assessment of nanomedicine in rheumatoid arthritis. *Eur J Lipid Sci Technol [Internet]*. 2016 Jun 1 [cited 2021 Feb 28];118(6):949–58. Available from: http://doi.wiley.com/10.1002/ejlt.201400658

40. Bilthariya U, Jain N, Rajoriya V, Jain AK. Folate-conjugated albumin nanoparticles for rheumatoid arthritis-targeted delivery of etoricoxib. *Drug Dev Ind Pharm [Internet]*. 2015 Jan 1 [cited 2021 Feb 28];41(1):95–104. Available from: https://pubmed.ncbi.nlm.nih.gov/24164469/

41. Thao LQ, Byeon HJ, Lee C, Lee S, Lee ES, Choi HG, et al. Pharmaceutical potential of tacrolimus-loaded albumin nanoparticles having targetability to rheumatoid arthritis tissues. *Int J Pharm [Internet]*. 2016 Jan 30 [cited 2021 Feb 28];497(1–2):268–76. Available from: https://pubmed.ncbi.nlm.nih.gov/26657273/

42. Sanadgol N, Wackerlig J. Developments of smart drug-delivery systems based on magnetic molecularly imprinted polymers for targeted cancer therapy: A short review. *Pharmaceutics*. 2020;12(9):1–31.

43. Gonda A, Zhao N, Shah JV, Calvelli HR, Kantamneni H, Francis NL, et al. Engineering tumor-targeting nanoparticles as vehicles for precision nanomedicine HHS public access. *Med One*. 2019;4.

44. Hussain A, Singh S, Sharma D, Webster TJ, Shafaat K, Faruk A. IJN-138267-elastic-liposomes-as-novel-carriers-recent-advances-in-drug. *Int J Nanomedicine [Internet]*. 2017 [cited 2021 Feb 23];12:5087. Available from: http://dx.doi.org/10.2147/IJN.S138267

45. Olusanya TOB, Ahmad RRH, Ibegbu DM, Smith JR, Elkordy AA. Liposomal drug delivery systems and anticancer drugs. *Molecules [Internet]*. 2018 [cited 2021 Feb 23];23. MDPI AG. Available from: https://pubmed.ncbi.nlm.nih.gov/29662019/

46. Mufamadi MS, Pillay V, Choonara YE, Du Toit LC, Modi G, Naidoo D, et al. A review on composite liposomal technologies for specialized drug delivery. *J Drug Deliv*. 2011;2011:1–19.

47. Bozzuto G, Molinari A. Liposomes as nanomedical devices. *Int J Nanomed [Internet]*. 2015 [cited 2021 Feb 24];10:975–99. Dove Medical Press Ltd. Available from: www.ncbi.nlm.nih.gov/pmc/articles/PMC4324542/

48. Guo Y, Walsh AM, Fearon U, Smith MD, Wechalekar MD, Yin X, et al. CD40L-dependent pathway is active at various stages of rheumatoid arthritis disease progression. *J Immunol [Internet]*. 2017 Jun 1 [cited 2021 Feb 24];198(11):4490–501. Available from: https://pubmed.ncbi.nlm.nih.gov/28455435/

49. Andreakos E, Rauchhaus U, Stavropoulos A, Endert G, Wendisch V, Benahmed AS, et al. Amphoteric liposomes enable systemic antigen-presenting cell-directed delivery of CD40 antisense and are therapeutically effective in experimental arthritis. *Arthritis Rheum*. 2009 Apr;60(4):994–1005.

50. Homma A, Sato H, Okamachi A, Emura T, Ishizawa T, Kato T, et al. Novel hyaluronic acid–methotrexate conjugates for osteoarthritis treatment. *Bioorg Med Chem [Internet]*. 2009 Jul 1 [cited 2020 Nov 10];17(13):4647–56. Available from: https://linkinghub.elsevier.com/retrieve/pii/S0968089609004295

51. Yuba E, Fukaya Y, Yanagihara S, Kasho N, Harada A. Development of mannose-modified carboxylated curdlan-coated liposomes for antigen presenting cell targeted antigen delivery. *Pharmaceutics*. 2020;12(8):1–14.

52. Vanniasinghe AS, Manolios N, Schibeci S, Lakhiani C, Kamali-Sarvestani E, Sharma R, et al. Targeting fibroblast-like synovial cells at sites of inflammation with peptide targeted liposomes results in inhibition of experimental arthritis. *Clin Immunol [Internet]*. 2014 Mar [cited 2020 Nov 10];151(1):43–54. Available from: https://pubmed.ncbi.nlm.nih.gov/24513809/

53. Morshed A, Abbas AB, Hu J, Xu H. Shedding new light on the role of $\alpha v \beta 3$ and $\alpha 5 \beta 1$ integrins in rheumatoid arthritis. *Molecules [Internet]*. 2019 [cited 2021 Feb 24];24. MDPI AG. Available from: www.ncbi.nlm.nih.gov/pmc/articles/PMC6515208/

54. Tan Q, Chu Y, Bie M, Wang Z, Xu X. Preparation and investigation of amphiphilic block copolymers/fullerene nanocomposites as nanocarriers for hydrophobic drug. *Materials (Basel) [Internet]*. 2017 [cited 2021 Feb 24];10(2). Available from: www.ncbi.nlm.nih.gov/pmc/articles/PMC5459121/

55. C. Booth VMN. Critical micelle concentration block copolymers of ethylene oxide and 1, 2-butylene oxide. 2019; (Cmc). Available from: www.sciencedirect.com/topics/materials-science/critical-micelle-concentration/pdf

56. Simmonds RE, Foxwell BM. Signalling, inflammation and arthritis: NF-κB and its relevance to arthritis and inflammation. *Rheumatology [Internet]*. 2008 May [cited 2020 Nov 10];47(5):584–90. Available from: https://pubmed.ncbi.nlm.nih.gov/18234712/

57. Makarov SS. NF-vvB in rheumatoid arthritis: A pivotal regulator of inflammation, hyperplasia, and tissue destruction. *Arthritis Res [Internet]*. 2001 [cited 2020 Nov 10];3:200–6. BioMed Central. Available from: http://arthritis-research.biomedcentral.com/articles/10.1186/ar300

58. Lee SJ, Lee A, Hwang SR, Park JS, Jang J, Huh MS, et al. TNF-α gene silencing using polymerized siRNA/thiolated glycol chitosan nanoparticles for rheumatoid arthritis. *Mol Ther [Internet]*. 2014 [cited 2020 Nov 10];22(2):397–408. Available from: https://pubmed.ncbi.nlm.nih.gov/24145554/

59. Wang Q, Jiang H, Li Y, Chen W, Li H, Peng K, et al. Targeting NF-kB signaling with polymeric hybrid micelles that co-deliver siRNA and dexamethasone for arthritis therapy. *Biomaterials [Internet]*. 2017 Apr 1 [cited 2020 Nov 10];122:10–22. Available from: https://pubmed.ncbi.nlm.nih.gov/28107661/

60. Zhang N, Xu C, Li N, Zhang S, Fu L, Chu X, et al. Folate receptor-targeted mixed polysialic acid micelles for combating rheumatoid arthritis: In vitro and in vivo evaluation. *Drug Deliv*. 2018 [cited 2021 Feb 28];25(1):1182–91. Available from: https://doi.org/10.1080/10717544.2018.1472677

61. Xu XL, Li WS, Wang XJ, Du YL, Kang XQ, Hu JB, et al. Endogenous sialic acid-engineered micelles: A multifunctional platform for on-demand methotrexate delivery and bone repair of rheumatoid arthritis. *Nanoscale [Internet]*. 2018 Feb 14 [cited 2020 Nov 10];10(6):2923–35. Available from: https://pubmed.ncbi.nlm.nih.gov/29369319/

62. Li C, Li H, Wang Q, Zhou M, Li M, Gong T, et al. pH-sensitive polymeric micelles for targeted delivery to inflamed joints. *J Control Release [Internet]*. 2017 Jan 28 [cited 2020 Nov 10];246:133–41. Available from: https://pubmed.ncbi.nlm.nih.gov/28038947/

63. Lee MY, Yang JA, Jung HS, Beack S, Choi JE, Hur W, et al. Hyaluronic acid-gold nanoparticle/interferon α complex for targeted treatment of hepatitis C virus infection. *ACS Nano [Internet]*. 2012 Nov 27 [cited 2020 Nov 10];6(11):9522–31. Available from: https://pubmed.ncbi.nlm.nih.gov/23092111/

64. Sul OJ, Kim JC, Kyung TW, Kim HJ, Kim YY, Kim SH, et al. Gold nanoparticles inhibited the receptor activator of nuclear factor-κB ligand (RANKL)-induced osteoclast formation by acting as an antioxidant. *Biosci Biotechnol Biochem [Internet]*. 2010 [cited 2020 Nov 10];74(11):2209–13. Available from: https://pubmed.ncbi.nlm.nih.gov/21071867/

65. Lee H, Lee MY, Bhang SH, Kim BS, Kim YS, Ju JH, et al. Hyaluronate-gold nanoparticle/tocilizumab complex for the treatment of rheumatoid arthritis. *ACS Nano [Internet]*. 2014 May 27 [cited 2021 Feb 28];8(5):4790–8. Available from: https://pubmed.ncbi.nlm.nih.gov/24730974/

66. Assassi S, Michael H, Weisman M, MinJae Lee P, Laurie Savage M, Diekman L, et al. New population-based references values for spinal mobility measures based on the 2009–2010. *Life Sci J*. 2014;11(10):1–29.

67. Wahajuddin, Arora S. Superparamagnetic iron oxide nanoparticles: Magnetic nanoplatforms as drug carriers. *Int J Nanomedicine [Internet]*. 2012 [cited 2021 Mar 1];7:3445–71. Available from: https://pubmed.ncbi.nlm.nih.gov/22848170/

68. Wang EC, Wang AZ. Nanoparticles and their applications in cell and molecular biology. *Integr Biol (United Kingdom) [Internet]*. 2014 [cited 2021 Mar 1];6:9–26. NIH Public Access. Available from: www.ncbi.nlm.nih.gov/pmc/articles/PMC3865110/

69. Butoescu N, Seemayer CA, Foti M, Jordan O, Doelker E. Dexamethasone-containing PLGA superparamagnetic microparticles as carriers for the local treatment of arthritis. *Biomaterials [Internet]*. 2009 Mar [cited 2021 Mar 1];30(9):1772–80. Available from: https://pubmed.ncbi.nlm.nih.gov/19135244/

70. Karimi M, Ghasemi A, Sahandi Zangabad P, Rahighi R, Moosavi Basri SM, Mirshekari H, et al. Smart micro/nanoparticles in stimulus-responsive drug/gene delivery systems. *Chem Soc Rev [Internet]*. 2016 [cited 2021 Mar 1];45:1457–501. Royal Society of Chemistry. Available from: www.ncbi.nlm.nih.gov/pmc/articles/PMC4775468/

71. Shao M, Hussain Z, Thu HE, Khan S, Katas H, Ahmed TA, et al. Drug nanocarrier, the future of atopic diseases: Advanced drug delivery systems and smart management of disease. *Colloids Surf B: Biointerfaces [Internet]*. 2016 [cited 2020 Nov 10];147:475–91. Elsevier B.V. Available from: https://pubmed.ncbi.nlm.nih.gov/27592075/

72. Alam MM, Han HS, Sung S, Kang JH, Sa KH, Al Faruque H, et al. Endogenous inspired biomineral-installed hyaluronan nanoparticles as pH-responsive carrier of methotrexate for rheumatoid arthritis. *J Control Release [Internet]*. 2017 Apr 28 [cited 2020 Nov 10];252:62–72. Available from: https://pubmed.ncbi.nlm.nih.gov/28288894/

73. Moura CC, Segundo MA, das Neves J, Reis S, Sarmento B. Co-association of methotrexate and SPIONs into anti-CD64 antibody-conjugated PLGA nanoparticles for theranostic application. *Int J Nanomedicine [Internet]*. 2014 Oct 23 [cited 2020 Nov 10];9(1):4911–22. Available from: www.ncbi.nlm.nih.gov/pmc/articles/PMC4211909/?report=abstract

74. Van Roon JAG, Van Vuuren AJ, Wijngaarden S, Jacobs KMG, Bijlsma JWJ, Lafeber FPJG, et al. Selective elimination of synovial inflammatory macrophages in rheumatoid arthritis by an Fc? receptor I-directed immunotoxin. *Arthritis Rheum [Internet]*. 2003 May 1 [cited 2020 Nov 10];48(5):1229–38. Available from: http://doi.wiley.com/10.1002/art.10940

75. Heo R, Park JS, Jang HJ, Kim SH, Shin JM, Suh YD, et al. Hyaluronan nanoparticles bearing γ-secretase inhibitor: In vivo therapeutic effects on rheumatoid arthritis. *J Control Release [Internet]*. 2014 Oct 28 [cited 2020 Sep 18];192:295–300. Available from: https://pubmed.ncbi.nlm.nih.gov/25109660/

76. Kim MJ, Park JS, Lee SJ, Jang J, Park JS, Back SH, et al. Notch1 targeting siRNA delivery nanoparticles for rheumatoid arthritis therapy. *J Control Release [Internet]*. 2015 Oct 28 [cited 2020 Apr 11];216:140–8. Available from: www.ncbi.nlm.nih.gov/pubmed/26282098

77. Lau CS, Chia F, Harrison A, Hsieh TY, Jain R, Jung SM, et al. APLAR rheumatoid arthritis treatment recommendations. *Int J Rheum Dis*. 2015;18(7):685–713.

78. Mishra V, Bansal KK, Verma A, Yadav N, Thakur S, Sudhakar K, et al. Solid lipid nanoparticles: Emerging colloidal nano drug delivery systems. *Pharmaceutics [Internet]*. 2018 [cited 2020 Nov 10];10. MDPI AG. Available from: www.ncbi.nlm.nih.gov/pmc/articles/PMC6321253/?report=abstract

79. Singh Y, Meher JG, Raval K, Khan FA, Chaurasia M, Jain NK, et al. Nanoemulsion: Concepts, development and applications in drug delivery. *J Control Release*. 2017;252:28–49. Elsevier B.V.

80. Zhou M, Hou J, Zhong Z, Hao N, Lin Y, Li C. Targeted delivery of hyaluronic acid-coated solid lipid nanoparticles for rheumatoid arthritis therapy. *Drug Deliv [Internet]*. 2018 [cited 2021 Mar 1];25(1):716–22. Available from: https://pubmed.ncbi.nlm.nih.gov/29516758/

81. Ades A, Carvalho JP, Graziani SR, Amancio RF, Souen JS, Pinotti JA, et al. Uptake of a cholesterol-rich emulsion by neoplastic ovarian tissues. *Gynecol Oncol [Internet]*. 2001 [cited 2020 Nov 10];82(1):84–7. Available from: https://pubmed.ncbi.nlm.nih.gov/11426966/

82. Padoveze AF, Maniero F, Oliveira TV, Vitorio TS, Couto RD, Maranhão RC. Effect of a cholesterol-rich diet on the metabolism of the free and esterified cholesterol components of a nanoemulsion that resembles LDL in rabbits. *Brazilian J Med Biol Res [Internet]*. 2009 [cited 2020 Nov 10];42(2):172–8. Available from: https://pubmed.ncbi.nlm.nih.gov/19274345/

83. Zheng Z, Sun Y, Liu Z, Zhang M, Li C, Cai H. The effect of curcumin and its nanoformulation on adjuvant-induced arthritis in rats. *Drug Des Devel Ther [Internet]*. 2015 Aug 27 [cited 2020 Nov 10];9:4931–42. Available from: https://pubmed.ncbi.nlm.nih.gov/26345159/

84. Kayat J, Mehra NK, Gajbhiye V, Jain NK. Drug targeting to arthritic region via folic acid appended surface-engineered multi-walled carbon nanotubes. *J Drug Target [Internet]*. 2016 Apr 20 [cited 2020 Nov 10];24(4):318–27. Available from: https://pubmed.ncbi.nlm.nih.gov/26289435/

85. Lyon RP, Bovee TD, Doronina SO, Burke PJ, Hunter JH, Neff-Laford HD, et al. Reducing hydrophobicity of homogeneous antibody-drug conjugates improves pharmacokinetics and therapeutic index. *Nat Biotechnol [Internet]*. 2015 Jul 13 [cited 2020 Nov 10];33(7):733–5. Available from: https://pubmed.ncbi.nlm.nih.gov/26076429/

86. Lee H, Bhang SH, Lee JH, Kim H, Hahn SK. Tocilizumab-Alendronate conjugate for treatment of rheumatoid arthritis. *Bioconjug Chem [Internet]*. 2017 Apr 19 [cited 2021 Mar 1];28(4):1084–92. Available from: https://pubs.acs.org/doi/abs/10.1021/acs.bioconjchem.7b00008

87. Breuil V, Euller-Ziegler L. Bisphosphonate therapy in rheumatoid arthritis. *Joint Bone Spine [Internet]*. 2006 [cited 2020 Nov 10];73:349–54. Available from: https://pubmed.ncbi.nlm.nih.gov/16616575/

88. Shetty A, Hanson R, Korsten P, Shawagfeh M, Arami S, Volkov S, et al. Tocilizumab in the treatment of rheumatoid arthritis and beyond. *Drug Des Devel Ther [Internet]*. 2014 [cited 2020 Nov 10];8:349–64. DOVE Medical Press Ltd. Available from: https://pubmed.ncbi.nlm.nih.gov/24729685/

89. Yang M, Ding J, Feng X, Chang F, Wang Y, Gao Z, et al. Scavenger receptor-mediated targeted treatment of collagen-induced arthritis by dextran sulfate-methotrexate prodrug. *Theranostics [Internet]*. 2017 Jan 1 [cited 2020 Nov 10];7(1):97–105. Available from: www.thno.org

90. Yan F, Li H, Zhong Z, Zhou M, Lin Y, Tang C, et al. Co-delivery of prednisolone and curcumin in human serum albumin nanoparticles for effective treatment of rheumatoid arthritis. *Int J Nanomedicine [Internet]*. 2019 [cited 2021 Mar 1];14:9113–25. Available from: www.ncbi.nlm.nih.gov/pmc/articles/PMC6878998/

91. Duan J, Dong J, Zhang T, Su Z, Ding J, Zhang Y, et al. Polyethyleneimine-functionalized iron oxide nanoparticles for systemic siRNA delivery in experimental arthritis. *Nanomedicine [Internet]*. 2014 [cited 2021 Mar 1];9(6):789–801. Available from: https://pubmed.ncbi.nlm.nih.gov/24392891/

92. Liu M, Huang Y, Hu L, Liu G, Hu X, Liu D, et al. Selective delivery of interleukine-1 receptor antagonist to inflamed joint by albumin fusion. *BMC Biotechnol [Internet]*. 2012 Sep 25 [cited 2021 Mar 1];12(1):68. Available from: https://bmcbiotechnol.biomedcentral.com/articles/10.1186/1472-6750-12-68

8 Nanotechnology-Based Approaches for Cancer Therapeutics

8 Nanotechnology-Based Approaches for Cancer Therapeutics

Akash Chaurasiya, Sumeet Katke, and Kanan Panchal

ABBREVIATIONS

CMC	Chemistry, manufacturing and controls
DNA	Deoxyribonucleic acid
EPR	Enhanced permeation retention
MDR	Multidrug resistance
MLV	Multilamellar vesicles
MPS	Mononuclear phagocytic system
MWCNTs	Multi-walled carbon nanotubes
NHL	Non-Hodgkin lymphoma
NSCLC	Non-small cell lung cancer
PEG	Polyethylene glycol
PNPs	Polymeric nanoparticles
RES	Reticuloendothelial system
RNA	Ribonucleic acid
SLNs	Solid lipid nanoparticles
SWCNTs	Single-walled carbon nanotubes
ULVs	Unilamellar vesicles

8.1 INTRODUCTION

Cancer is a significant cause of mortality across the world. Cancers of the lungs, oral cavity, stomach, and esophagus are common among male populations, whereas cervical cancer and breast cancer cases are widespread in female populations suffering from cancer [1]. Conventional areas of cancer therapy include surgery, radiation, and chemotherapy. Radiotherapy and chemotherapy cause significant adverse effects, as these methods also non-specifically target other rapidly dividing non-malignant cells. The typical limitations associated with conventional cancer chemotherapy are:

- Low aqueous solubility: most chemotherapeutic candidates have poor aqueous solubility, and therefore these drugs are formulated in organic solvents, which contribute to severe toxicity.
- Multidrug resistance (MDR) and low permeability: Many anticancer agents are substrate for efflux pumps such as P-glycoprotein (Pgp) pumps in the cell membrane, which causes low permeability and MDR.
- Lack of selectivity: chemotherapeutic drugs are not selective towards cancerous cells and show significant toxicity to other normal rapidly proliferating cells.
- Low therapeutic index: almost all chemotherapeutic agents have a low therapeutic index. Thus, increasing the dose to improve antitumor efficacy can cause substantial adverse effects for the patient.

DOI: 10.1201/9781003130055-8

To overcome the limitations associated with conventional cancer chemotherapeutics, researchers have focused their attention on the application of novel nano-formulations like liposomes, nanoparticles, dendrimers, and nanocrystals. These carrier systems provide improved transport across biological barriers, enable selective targeting of cancer cells, and control drug release at the site of action [2]. Some of the common advantages associated with nanotherapeutic drug delivery systems are:

- The problem of the solubility of anticancer drugs is mitigated.
- Improve the in vivo stability of the drug molecules by preventing degradation from proteases and other biological enzymes, which leads to improved half-life in systemic circulation.
- Surface modification of the nanocarriers helps in achieving targeted drug delivery.
- Delivery of multiple drugs in a single formulation is possible, through which the problem of MDR is mitigated.
- Controlled drug delivery at the cancer site can be achieved.
- Improved therapeutic index.

The majority of commercially available cancer therapeutics show cytotoxicity because of their high pharmacokinetic volume of distribution. These chemotherapeutic agents have a higher excretion rate for which higher doses are required to meet the minimum effective concentration. When such drugs are administered using conventional drug delivery systems, they lack target specificity, and high doses cause significant damage to non-cancerous tissues. This results in unwanted side effects such as bone marrow depression, alopecia, shedding of the gut epithelial cells, neuropathies, neutropenia, and kidney failure.

Liposomes, as a potential carrier system for anticancer drug delivery, have drawn much attention in the last few decades. The major limitation associated with liposomes is active uptake by the reticuloendothelial system (RES) in the liver and spleen. These issues can be resolved by developing surface-modified liposomes using flexible hydrophilic polymers such as polyethylene glycol. These hydrophilic polymers create steric stabilization, which restricts RES uptake to a lower level. Surface-modified liposomes with PEG improve the liposomal surface's hydrophilicity, which reduces the non-specific interactions of liposomes with RES cells. PEG also causes steric hindrance, preventing opsonins' coating to the liposomes, resulting in reduced opsonization reaction and uptake by RES cells [3]. Researchers have also explored tumor-targeting possibilities by appending various ligands and antibodies for site-specific delivery of anticancer drugs [4]. The USFDA approved a doxorubicin-loaded long-circulating liposome product (Doxil) in 1995 to treat various cancers [5].

Multidrug resistance (MDR) is also a common problem associated with conventional chemotherapeutic drugs. MDR occurs due to various reasons like modifications in drug metabolism, drug targets, and cellular repair. Nanoparticulate carrier systems, including liposomes, nanoparticles, and dendrimers, reported being a valuable tool to overcome MDR issues [6]. The drug encapsulated in nanocarriers can overcome MDR, mainly because of two major reasons:

- reduced exposure of drug molecules for renal excretion, which results in more effective drug delivery to tumor cells
- decreased exposure to membrane pumps.

8.2 APPLICATION OF NANOTECHNOLOGY IN CANCER TREATMENT

Cancer therapy effectiveness is improved when an optimum dose of the chemotherapeutic agent is administered to achieve maximal cancer tissue concentration. Nanotechnology-based formulations allow chemotherapeutic agents to target cancer cells, thus reducing the side effects [7].

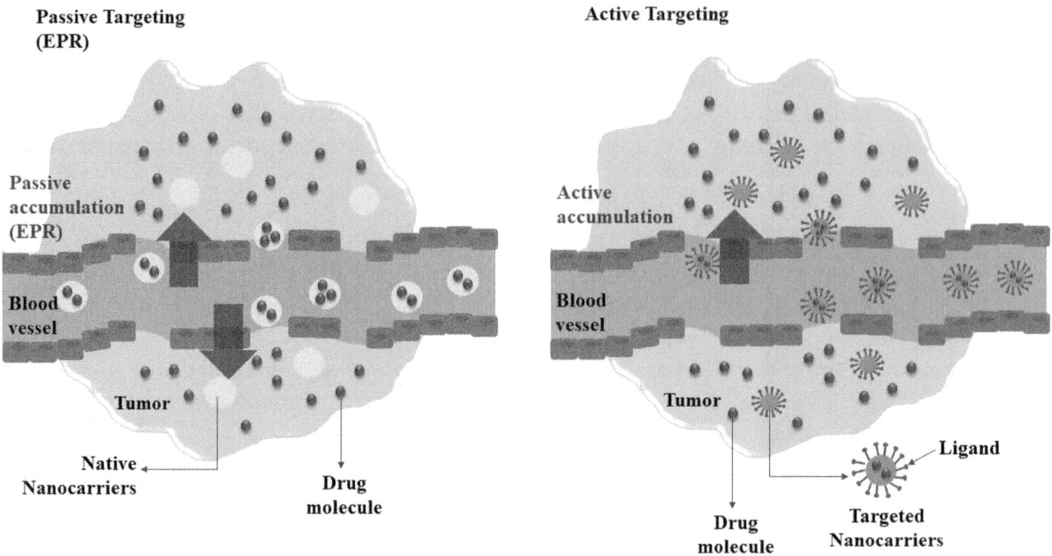

FIGURE 8.1 Nanotechnology-based approaches for drug targeting.

These formulations target drugs to specific sites in two ways: active targeting and passive targeting (Figure 8.1). Various challenges associated with targeting approaches are summarized in Table 8.1.

8.2.1 PASSIVE TARGETING

In passive targeting, chemotherapeutic drug delivery to tumor cells depends on carrier properties like size, circulation time, and tumor biology characteristics (vascularity, leakiness, etc.). Leaky tumor vasculature and the absence of lymphatic drainage enhance nanocarrier retention at the tumor site. Thus, these nanocarriers, when developed as formulations, provide improved pharmacokinetics, reduced side effects, and some tumor selectivity. Marketed formulations like Doxil/Caelyx are doxorubicin-loaded pegylated nanoliposomes that function on passive targeting principles through the EPR effect. The EPR effect is dependent on the extent of angiogenesis by the tumor, perivascular tumor growth, and intratumor pressure.

Physicochemical properties of nanotechnology-based formulations like size, surface chemistry, and charge govern the EPR effect and thus the effectiveness of the formulation. Size influences the permeation through blood vessels' fenestrations, renal excretion, and clearance through the reticuloendothelial system (RES). Surface chemistry and charge influence the opsonization of the carrier systems. Highly hydrophobic and charged particles are opsonized by the mononuclear phagocytic system (MPS). Alteration of surface chemistry by modification with polymers like polyethylene glycol induces hydrophilic and slightly anionic properties on the nanocarrier's surface. This surface modification thereby helps develop stealth drug delivery carriers that can improve in-vivo circulation time [8].

8.2.2 ACTIVE TARGETING

For active targeting, the nanocarrier surface is conjugated with molecules such as antibodies, ligands, aptamers, and peptides explicitly targeting the receptors over-expressed on the tumor cell surface [9]. Such tumor-targeted nanocarriers can be employed for tumor diagnosis and therapeutic

TABLE 8.1

Challenges Associated with Targeting Approaches

Targeting Approach	Challenges
Active	• Various biological barriers have to be crossed to reach and enter cancer cells. • Increased immunogenicity and plasma protein adsorption, consequently reducing bloodstream circulation time and ability to target tumors passively. • Nanocarriers internalized through pathways like endocytosis undergo degradation in lysosomes. • Factors such as nanocarrier-ligand conjugation chemistry and choice of ligand contribute to the efficiency of the delivery system. • Conjugation of targeting ligands to nanocarriers results in a complex manufacturing process compared to passive nanocarriers.
Passive	• The enhanced permeability and retention (EPR) effect is not produced in certain hypovascular tumors. • Variable endothelial gaps result in non-uniform extravasation of nanocarrier into tumors. • Physicochemical properties of nanocarrier such as size, elasticity, shape, and surface charge affect extravasation, accumulation of nanocarrier, and circulation time in vivo. • Lack of site-specific localization of drugs leads to suboptimal pharmacokinetics, which thereby compromises safety and efficacy.

or theranostic purposes. Various targets that can be exploited for active targeting are discussed subsequently and illustrated in Figure 8.2.

Antibody-based targeting: Targeting drugs to tumors can be achieved by identifying tumor-specific antigens or antigens that are overexpressed by the cancer cells and developing therapies that can specifically target these antigens [10]. Immunoconjugates employed for tumor targeting consist of an antibody and an effector moiety. The effector moiety is internalized in the cells by endocytosis while, the antibody binds to the surface-specific antigen.

Human epidermal growth factor receptor 2 (HER2 receptor): The HER2 receptor is responsible for cell signaling pathways that control cell division and survival and is thereby overexpressed in various cancer cells, including breast, ovarian, bladder, pancreatic, and stomach. Trastuzumab (humanized mAbs) shows anticancer activity against HER2-positive breast cancer cells and is very useful in treating breast cancer in cases where HER2 overexpression occurs.

Epidermal growth factor receptor (EGFR): EGFRs are significantly over-expressed in epithelial cancers. Mamot et al. developed EGFR-targeted liposomes that bind and internalize in EGFR-overexpressed tumor cells for intracellular delivery of doxorubicin, epirubicin, and vinorelbine [11]. These liposomes showed prolonged circulation and stable drug retention and superior efficacy compared to treatments with free and non-targeted liposomal drugs.

Aptamer based targeting: Aptamers are secondary or tertiary folded structures of short single-stranded DNA or RNA oligonucleotides. These are three-dimensional structures capable of binding to specific biological targets and are considered equivalent to antibodies in terms of their specificity and sensitivity to binding the target molecules [12].

Folate receptor targeted drug delivery: Overexpression of folate receptors is reported in various types of human cancers, including ovarian, lung, breast, brain, colon, and kidney. These overexpressed receptors can be targeted for anticancer drug uptake, thereby improving cancer treatment. Wang et al. developed a nanoparticle that consists of heparin-folate-paclitaxel (HFT) conjugate loaded with paclitaxel in the hydrophobic core of the nanoparticle. These nanoparticles were reported to improve paclitaxel delivery to the folate receptors' overexpressed cells [13].

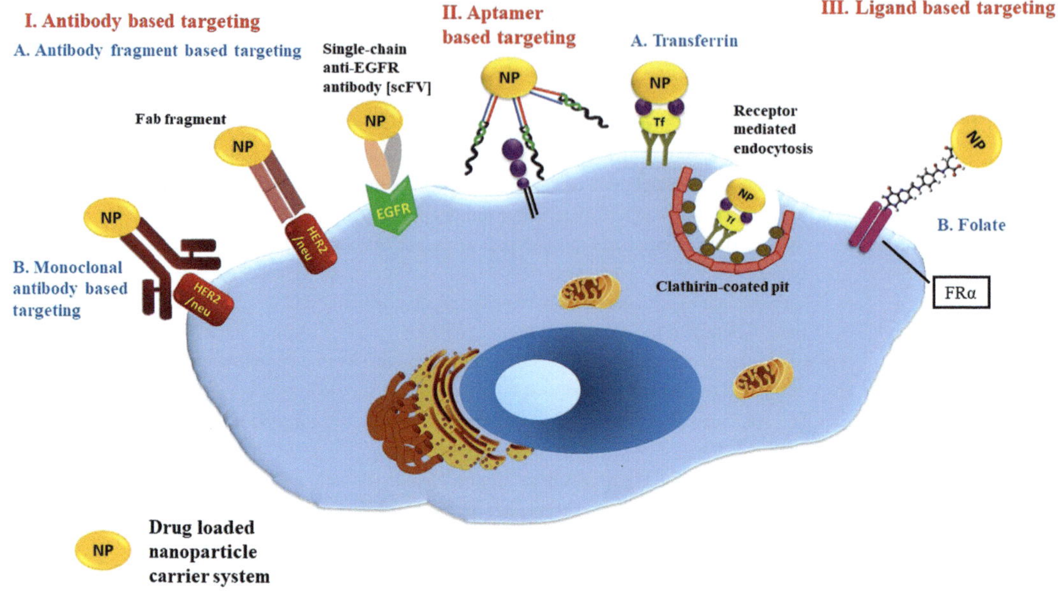

FIGURE 8.2 Various targets and approaches for active targeting.

8.3 VARIOUS NANOTECHNOLOGY-BASED APPROACHES FOR CANCER TREATMENT

With the advent of new technologies and a better understanding of nanotechnology-based carrier system preparation and evaluation, various approaches have evolved in the last few decades (Figure 8.3). These approaches have found application in drug delivery, diagnostics, and theranostics by virtue of unique physicochemical characteristics. In this section, we will discuss the potential role of these nanotechnology-based carrier systems in cancer therapeutics.

8.3.1 CARBON NANOTUBES

Carbon nanotubes (CNTs) are cylindrical molecules with a diameter as small as 1 nm consisting of a hexagonal arrangement of SP^2 hybridized carbon atoms. Carbon nanotubes obtained from rolling a single layer of graphene sheet are called single-walled carbon nanotubes (SWCNTs). Those obtained from rolling of multiple layers of graphene sheets are called multi-walled carbon nanotubes (MWCNTs). The difference between SWCNTs and MWCNTs is illustrated in Table 8.2. Surface modification of CNTs with various functional groups can lead to site-specific drug delivery, controlled drug release, improvement in aqueous dispersibility, biodistribution, and pharmacokinetics of anticancer drugs [14]. In one reported study, doxorubicin was loaded into branched polyethylene glycol (PEG)-functionalized SWCNTs and studied in vivo for cancer treatment. It was found that SWCNT-DOX significantly improved therapeutic efficacy and reduced toxicity compared to free DOX [15]. In another study, doxorubicin was conjugated with glycopolymer by non-covalent tethering, which was further coated on MWCNTs along with folic acid. This biocompatible hybrid-CNTS was a valuable strategy for dual receptor-mediated breast cancer therapy [16].

8.3.2 DENDRIMERS

Dendrimers are highly branched polymers with three-dimensional globular structures in the nanometric size range [17]. A dendrimer is derived from the Greek words *dendron*, meaning "tree", and

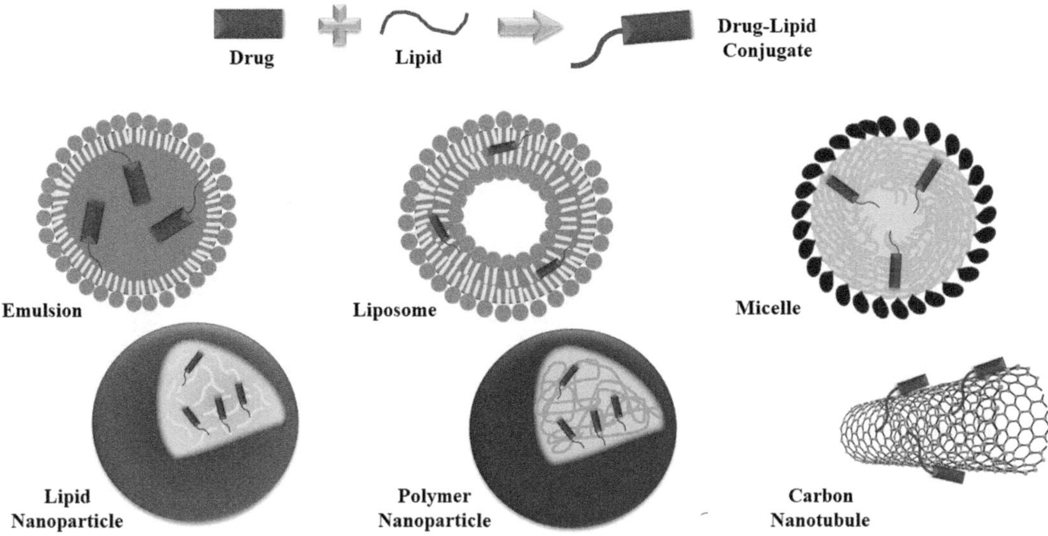

FIGURE 8.3   Various nanotechnology-based approaches.

meros, meaning "part". In comparison with linear, branched polymers, these are globular structures more controlled in shape and have a single molecular weight rather than a range of molecular weight and multiple peripheral functional groups. Structurally, dendrimers are composed of three components: a central core, an initiator layer (dendrons) comprising repeating units of the atom that emerge from the core, and outermost terminal functional groups that can be modified for optimum drug delivery [18].

Due to unique structures, shape, size, and drug loading capabilities, dendrimers possess several advantages:

- The presence of multivalent groups on the surface of dendrimers provides multiple interactions with biological receptor sites.
- Enhanced bioavailability due to improved solubility of drugs.
- Dendrimers have a higher renal threshold because of the larger size (up to several nanometers), limiting the renal clearance of the formulation.
- Enhanced permeation and retention is obtained owing to the nanometric size of dendrimers.

Dendrimers are proven to be a promising drug-delivery system due to exceptional drug interaction properties [19]. Three types of the mechanism of interactions between drug molecules and dendrimers have been explained:

- Simple encapsulation: the spherical properties of dendrimers and a hydrophobic core make them suitable for lipophilic molecules to encapsulate inside the interior cavity through hydrophobic interactions.
- Electrostatic interaction: functional groups such as carboxylic and amine groups on dendrimers' surface improve the solubility of hydrophobic drug molecules through electrostatic interactions.
- Covalent bond: in this type of interaction, functional groups on the surface of the dendrimer form covalent bonds with the drug molecule, and the release of the drug molecule depends on the cleavage of these covalent bonds by enzymatic or chemical reactions in vivo. This type of bond provides advantages like better release of the drug than simple encapsulation or electrostatic interaction.

TABLE 8.2

Differences between SWCNTs and MWCNTs

SWCNTs	MWCNTs
• Obtained from a single layer of graphene	• Obtained from multiple layers of graphene
• Catalyst is required during chemical synthesis	• Can be synthesized without a catalyst
• More defects obtained during functionalization	• Fewer defects were obtained, but optimization of the process is difficult
• Poor purity obtained during chemical synthesis	• High purity obtained during chemical synthesis
• Less accumulation in the body	• More accumulation in the body
• Easy to characterize and evaluate	• Difficult to characterize and evaluate

Several studies suggested the potential application of dendrimers for cancer treatment. Wang et al. developed fluorescein isothiocyanate (FI)– and folic acid (FA)–modified G5 PAMAM poly(amidoamine) dendrimers with acetyl terminal groups (G5.NHAc-FI-FA) to encapsulate the anticancer drug doxorubicin (DOX). These dendrimers showed target specific and controlled release of DOX [20]. Patri et al. synthesized anti–prostate surface membrane antigen (PSMA) antibody conjugated to dendrimers containing fluorochrome. They successfully developed dendrimers for potential prostate cancer–targeted therapy and imaging agents [21].

8.3.3 LIPOSOMES

Liposomes are vesicular carrier systems, generally ranging from 50 nm–100 μm in diameter, formed when phospholipids are hydrated in an aqueous media to form bilayers. They were first described by A.D. Bangham and colleagues and originally published a paper in 1965 [22]. Liposomes have an enclosed aqueous compartment enclosed by one or more layers of phospholipids. Drugs can be entrapped either in the aqueous compartment, in phospholipid bilayers, or at the interface between the aqueous compartment and lipid bilayers. The locus of entrapment depends on drug properties like solubility and log P value. Based on the size and number of phospholipid bilayers, liposomes are classified as multilamellar vesicles (MLVs) and unilamellar vesicles (ULVs). MLVs are concentric phospholipid spheres that enclose aqueous compartments forming an onion-like structure, while ULV has a single phospholipid bilayer enclosing the aqueous compartment [23].

Liposomes gained major attention among researchers as a successful drug delivery system due to the following advantages [24]:

- Drug loading capacity—hydrophilic and hydrophobic
- Sustained drug delivery
- Site-specific and targeted drug delivery
- Improvement in pharmacokinetic behavior like enhancement of half-life and therapeutic index of drugs
- Overcoming multidrug resistance
- Protection of drugs against the surrounding environment and preventing drug degradation

Liposomes as drug carrier systems played a pivotal role in controlled and targeted drug delivery, especially in cancer treatment [25]. Several anticancer drug-loaded liposomal formulations were successfully investigated and clinically tested for cancer treatment. Due to stable structure and controlled particle size in the nano range (100–200 nm), liposomes facilitate uptake by leaky tumor vasculature, which results in increased pharmacodynamics effects of encapsulated anticancer drugs. Additionally, they also prevent the uptake of anticancer drugs through tight junctions of normal tissues, which minimize the adverse effects of these drugs. Surface-modified liposomes have proven their potential for enhanced system circulation, drug retention, and drug loading. Liposomes provide adequate possibilities for formulation development based on characteristics required for drug localization at the site of action.

8.3.4 Nanoparticles

Nanoparticles are colloidal dispersions of polymers or lipid materials with drugs dispersed or dissolved in the matrix [26]. Nanoparticles range from approximately 10 to 1000 nm. Based on the material used for preparation, nanoparticles can be classified as polymer nanoparticles (PNPs) or solid lipid nanoparticles (SLNs). Lipid polymer nanoparticles (LPNs) are recent developments in nanoparticle development, which involve a combination of lipids and polymers. Like liposomes, nanoparticles also emerged as a potential carrier system for drug delivery due to advantages like:

- Easy modification of surface characteristics and surface charge can alter the pharmacokinetic behavior of the drug
- Controlled and sustained release of the drug
- Site-specific targeted drug delivery
- Drug delivery via receptor-mediated endocytosis
- The use of biocompatible lipids and polymers avoids systemic toxicity

Nanoparticles can be manufactured using various methods reported so far, like the emulsion-solvent evaporation method, double emulsification, evaporation method, salting out method, emulsion diffusion method, and precipitation method [27].

Due to inherent physicochemical properties, nanoparticles have been widely investigated for controlled and targeted delivery of anticancer drugs. Nanoparticles, due to control in size and surface modification possibilities, are proven to be a potential carrier system to enhance anticancer drugs' safety and efficacy. In one study, chimeric polypeptide doxorubicin (CP-Dox) nanoparticle formulation was investigated for IV administration. The formulation showed increased drug delivery to the tumor compared to a free drug [28]. Polymer-lipid nanoparticles of doxorubicin and mitomycin C were developed and tested in breast cancer cell lines. The results suggested the effective delivery of these drugs using polymer-lipid nanoparticles against multidrug-resistant breast cancer cell lines. They were found to be 20–30 times more effective than the free drug [29].

8.3.5 Drug Nanocrystals

Drug nanocrystals are crystalline structures with a nanometric size range. An important property of nanocrystalline drug formulation is that, unlike nanoparticles, nanocrystals do not possess any carrier material, and the particles are composed only of drug material. The particle size of nanocrystals ranges from 10 to 1000 nm [30]. Nanosuspension formulations are obtained by dispersing nanocrystals in aqueous or non-aqueous vehicles like low-molecular-weight polyethylene glycols or certain oils. The majority of new chemical entities possess poor water solubility, which creates a barrier in the development of suitable formulation. Commonly used approaches for solubility enhancement, that is, co-solvent or surfactant usage, have limitations due to their possible toxicity. To avoid toxicity and other limitations associated with available approaches, nanocrystal formulation is a preferred choice due to the following advantages [31]:

- Enhanced saturation solubility of poorly soluble drugs
- Improved dissolution rate due to increased surface area

- Improved adhesion to cell membranes/tissue surface
- Higher drug loading and steady in vivo dissolution can be achieved

Nanocrystals can be prepared using top-down and bottom-up techniques. In the top-down technique, larger particles' comminution is carried out with the application of high energy mechanical forces with methods like media milling and high-pressure homogenization. This technique is widely used in the commercial manufacturing of nanocrystals. In the bottom-up technique, nanocrystals are grown in a solution via the nucleation step, followed by the crystal growth step. In this technique, optimization of the process to control crystal growth is a critical step, as it directly affects the particle size.

Nanocrystals have also proven their application in cancer therapy through various means like enhancing solubilization of anticancer drugs, overcoming multidrug resistance and site-specific delivery of anticancer drugs. In one reported study, paclitaxel (PTX) nanocrystals were developed using D-R-tocopheryl polyethylene glycol-1000 succinate (TPGS), which showed the ability to overcome resistance in cancer therapy due to P-gp inhibition [32].

8.3.6 Nanoemulsions

Nanoemulsions are heterogeneous colloidal dispersions of nano-sized droplets. The formulation is a heterogeneous system consisting of two immiscible liquid components stabilized by incorporating excipients like surfactants or emulsifiers [33]. The droplet sizes range from 20 to 600 nm. Nanoemulsions are classified according to the dispersed and continuous phase as oil-in-water emulsions (O/W), water-in-oil emulsions (W/O), and double emulsions: water-in-oil-in-water (W/O/W) and oil-in-water-in-oil (O/W/O) emulsions [34]. In general, nanoemulsions can be prepared by various techniques like microfluidization, high-pressure homogenization, and sonication.

Nanoemulsions possess several advantages as a drug delivery tool:

- They improve bioavailability and reduce the toxicity of drugs.
- Lipophilic drug moieties can be formulated easily.
- The smaller size of nanoemulsion dispersion provides a greater surface area for drug absorption.
- A reduced amount of surfactants are required compared to the conventional emulsion, thus providing reduced toxicity.
- Formulations developed as double emulsions can be utilized as controlled drug delivery systems.

Nanoemulsions have been investigated for cancer therapy for various applications like oral bioavailability enhancement, adjuvant therapy, and theranostic applications. A multi-functional folate-targeted theranostic nanoemulsion was developed for doxorubicin and MRI contrast agent gadolinium (Gd) delivery. An MRI contrast agent was used to understand drug distribution and free drug–induced systemic toxicity [35]. Oral administration of anticancer drugs is a highly desirable attribute, but most anticancer drugs are either poorly soluble, poorly permeable, or both. Nanoemulsion has been studied extensively for oral delivery of anticancer drugs by virtue of enhanced solubility and membrane permeability [36].

8.3.7 Drug-Lipid Conjugates

Drug-lipid conjugates or lipidic prodrugs are drug delivery systems in which the active drug is bound to the lipid moiety through covalent or non-covalent interactions [37]. Conjugation of drugs with fatty acids, steroids, glycerides, and phospholipids is a commonly used technique for the preparation of drug-lipid conjugates [38]. Drug-lipid conjugates, due to inherent characteristics, possess several advantages as a potential drug delivery tool [39]:

- Low-toxicity biocompatible lipids can be used for the formulation of drug-lipid conjugates.
- Enhanced oral bioavailability.
- Hydrophilic drugs with a low therapeutic index can be loaded into drug-lipid conjugates.
- Improved stability of the drug molecule inside the gastrointestinal milieu.
- Controlled and targeted drug delivery systems can be formulated.

Several researchers have explored the potential of drug-lipid conjugates for anticancer drug delivery. Conjugation of 5-fluorouracil (5-FU) with cholesterol has resulted in higher cytotoxicity than that of 5-FU to the cancer cell expressing increased LDL receptors [40]. Doxorubicin conjugate with α-linolenic (LNA) and docosahexaenoic (DHA) acid showed higher cytotoxicity towards cancer cells than normal cells [41].

8.3.8 POLYMER DRUG CONJUGATES

Polymer drug conjugates, or polymeric prodrugs, are drug delivery systems where one or multiple therapeutic agents are attached to the functional groups of a polymer directly or through a spacer [42]. Helmut Ringsdorf proposed the concept of covalently bound polymer drug conjugates. This delivery system, also known as the Ringsdorf model, is composed of three unique components attached to a biocompatible polymer:

- Solubilizing unit: imparts hydrophilicity, thus improving solubility in aqueous systems.
- Therapeutic component.
- Targeting unit: induces target-specific delivery of the therapeutic component.

The advantages of polymer drug conjugates are solubility enhancement, controlled release of drug, improved pharmacokinetics, and site-targeted drug delivery. Polymer drug conjugates have shown significant success in cancer therapy in the form of commercially successful products like Abraxane (paclitaxel albumin nanoparticles) [43], discussed in detail in the latter part of this chapter. In other applications, polymer drug conjugates were reported to decrease systemic side effects associated with conventional therapy and improve the effectiveness of therapy via site-specific delivery of anticancer drugs [44, 45].

8.4 COMMERCIALLY SUCCESSFUL NANOTECHNOLOGY-BASED PRODUCTS

Nanotechnology-based pharmaceutical products have established their importance through clinical and commercial success (Table 8.3). There are numerous commercially successful products with proven clinical benefits in cancer treatment. Some of these nanoformulations are discussed in this section.

8.4.1 DOXIL

Doxil is an acronym of **Dox**orubicin **In** Liposomes. It is the first USFDA-approved PEGylated liposomal formulation and was developed by Janssen Pharmaceuticals, Inc., in the year 1995. It is available in a single-dose vial of 20 mg/10 mL and 50 mg/25 mL and indicated in ovarian cancer, AIDS-related Kaposi's sarcoma, and multiple myeloma [46]. The first human trials of doxorubicin-loaded oligolamellar vesicles were initiated in 1984. These liposomes are composed of fully hydrogenated soy phosphatidylcholine (HSPC), N-(carbonyl-methoxypolyethylene glycol 2000)-1,2-distearoyl-sn-glycero 3-phosphoethanolamine sodium salt (mPEG-DSPE), and cholesterol. Doxil is manufactured by an active drug loading process with an ammonium sulfate gradient [5]. Polyethylene glycol on the liposome surface provides steric stabilization to liposomes, thereby prolonging the circulation time of the intact liposomes in human blood plasma. The development of

TABLE 8.3

Clinical and Commercial Status of Nanotechnology-Based Products for Cancer Treatment

Product	Manufacturer/Clinical Trial Sponsor	Year of Approval/ Current Status	Formulation	Uses
Doxil	Janssen Pharmaceuticals	1995	PEGylated liposomal formulation of doxorubicin hydrochloride	Ovarian cancer, AIDS-related Kaposi's sarcoma, and multiple myeloma
Abraxane	Abraxis BioSciences	2005	Albumin-bound paclitaxel nanoparticle	Metastatic breast cancer and metastatic non-small cell lung cancer (NSCLC)
Marqibo	Acrotech Biopharma LLC	2012	Liposomal formulation of vincristine sulfate	Acute lymphoblastic leukemia (ALL)
Vyxeos	Jazz Pharmaceuticals	2017	Daunorubicin and cytarabine liposome for injection	Acute myeloid leukemia
ABBV-985	AbbVie	Phase 1	Antibody-drug conjugate	Advanced solid tumors
NKTR-102	Nektar Therapeutics	Phase 2	Polymer conjugate (pegylated irinotecan)	Relapsed small cell lung cancer
EphA2-targeting DOPC-encapsulated siRNA	M.D. Anderson Cancer Center	Phase 1	EphA2-targeting DOPC-encapsulated siRNA liposome	Advanced/recurrent malignancies

nano-sized liposomes (<100 nm) improved distribution of liposomes into tumor sites due to the EPR effect. Doxil significantly reduced the adverse effects caused by free doxorubicin, like cardiotoxicity, as encapsulated doxorubicin is not bioavailable to cardiac tissues [47].

8.4.2 Abraxane

Abraxane, also known as nanoparticle albumin-bound paclitaxel (nab-paclitaxel), is an injectable suspension formulation developed by Abraxis BioSciences that received USFDA approval in 2005. Abraxane is indicated to treat metastatic breast cancer and metastatic non-small cell lung cancer [43]. Nab-paclitaxel nanoparticles have a high negative zeta-potential, which provides steric stabilization by albumin and prevents agglomeration [48]. Abraxane is prepared by homogenization of human serum albumin at a 3–4% concentration with paclitaxel to obtain a nanoparticle with an average particle size of about 130 nm. This nanoparticle size range facilitates enhanced drug delivery at the tumor site through the EPR effect. Unlike taxol, a clear colorless injectable solution formulation of paclitaxel, abraxane is free of cremophor-EL and ethanol. Cremophor-EL is a solubilizing surfactant that may induce hypersensitivity in patients. This allows it to achieve a 50% higher maximum tolerated dose of paclitaxel. Based on the reported advantages, Abraxane constitutes an improvement in patient treatment and survival and a reduction in side-effects like neurotoxicity caused by paclitaxel [49].

8.4.3 Marqibo

Marqibo is a sphingomyelin and cholesterol-based liposomal formulation of vincristine sulfate to treat acute lymphoblastic leukemia (ALL). The formulation was developed and marketed by

Acrotech Biopharma LLC and got USFDA approval in 2012. Marqibo (vincristine-loaded liposomal injection) contains 5 mg/31 mL (0.16 mg/mL) vincristine sulfate per vial [50]. The extent of exposure to vincristine is a critical parameter to arrest cell division. Marqibo significantly increased the plasma exposure of vincristine compared to free circulating vincristine and achieved passive tumor-targeted drug delivery [51]. A phase 2, open-label, single-arm clinical trial was conducted to study the efficacy and tolerability of Marqibo in patients suffering from relapsed or refractory aggressive non-Hodgkin lymphoma (NHL). Marqibo showed a safety profile comparable to free vincristine at twice the dose intensity of standard free vincristine. It was concluded from the clinical trial that Marqibo is well tolerated in subjects, with improved efficacy and reduced side effects of vincristine [52].

8.5 FUTURE OF NANOMEDICINE FOR CANCER THERAPEUTICS

Various nano-drug delivery systems like nanoparticles, liposomes, nanoemulsions, dendrimers, nanocrystals, microspheres, carbon nanotubes, and quantum dots have been investigated to provide advantages over conventional formulations in cancer treatment. Nanotechnology provides opportunities to modify physicochemical properties of anticancer drugs like solubility and stability, improved bioavailability, reduced dose, and toxicity, thus improving the life expectancy of patients suffering from cancer, which is a leading cause of mortality [53].

Several nanotechnology-based approaches for cancer treatment under preclinical and clinical trials show promising results in better safety and efficacy [54]. Theranostic nanomedicines are next-generation drug products that allow molecular diagnosis and treatment to target novel cancer pathways for integrated simultaneous therapy and tracking. Efforts have also been put in to explore the commercial success of nanotechnology-based approaches for theranostic applications in cancer treatment [55]. Recent developments in nanomaterials and polymer chemistry have made significant development in the field of cancer drug delivery. Much progress has been achieved in this field. However, certain challenges related to understanding complex tumor biology; nanomaterial-biological tissue interactions; and chemistry, manufacturing, and controls (CMC) of nanoformulations are still to be overcome [2]. Considering the breakthroughs nanotechnology-based approaches have provided, the future of cancer treatment is looking very promising for disease management and patient survival.

REFERENCES

1. Moorthi, C., Manavalan, R., Kathiresan, K., Nanotherapeutics to overcome conventional cancer chemotherapy limitations, *Journal of Pharmacy and Pharmaceutical Sciences*, 14(1), 67–77, (2011).
2. Navya, P. N., Kaphale, A., Srinivas, S. P., Bhargava, S. K., Rotello, V. M., Daima, H. K., Current trends and challenges in cancer management and therapy using designer nanomaterials, *Nano Convergence*, 6, 29, (2019).
3. Klibanov, A. L., Maruyama, K., Torchilin, V. P., Huang, L., Amphipathic polyethyleneglycols effectively prolong the circulation time of liposomes, *FEBS Letters*, 268(1), 235–237, (1990).
4. Zamboni, W. C., Liposomal, nanoparticle, and conjugated formulations of anticancer agents, *Clinical Cancer Research*, 11(23), 8230–8234, (2005).
5. Barenholz, Y., Doxil®-the first FDA-approved nano-drug: Lessons learned, *Journal of Control Release*, 160(2), 117–134, (2012).
6. Sadava, D., Coleman, A., Kane, S. E., Liposomal daunorubicin overcomes drug resistance in human breast, ovarian and lung carcinoma cells, *Journal of Liposome Research*, 12(4), 301–309, (2002).
7. Attia, M. F., Anton, N., Wallyn, J., Omran, Z., Vandamme, T. F., An overview of active and passive targeting strategies to improve the nanocarriers efficiency to tumour sites, *The Journal of Pharmacy and Pharmacology*, 71(8), 1185–1198, (2019).
8. Avgoustakis, K., Beletsi, A., Panagi, Z., Klepetsanis, P., Karydas, A. G., Ithakissios, D. S., PLGA-mPEG nanoparticles of cisplatin: In vitro nanoparticle degradation, in vitro drug release and in vivo drug residence in blood properties, *Journal of Controlled Release*, 79(1–3), 123–135, (2002).

9. Bazak, R., Houri, M., El Achy, S., Kamel, S., Refaat, T., Cancer active targeting by nanoparticles: A comprehensive review of literature, *Journal of Cancer Research and Clinical Oncology*, 141(5), 769–784, (2015).

10. Attarwala H., Role of antibodies in cancer targeting, *Journal of Natural Science, Biology and Medicine*, 1(1), 53–56, (2010).

11. Mamot, C., Drummond, D. C., Noble, C. O., Kallab, V., Guo, Z., Hong, K., Kirpotin, D. B., Park, J. W., Epidermal growth factor receptor-targeted immunoliposomes significantly enhance the efficacy of multiple anticancer drugs in vivo, *Cancer Research*, 65(24), 11631–11638, (2005).

12. Zhang, L., Radovic-Moreno, A. F., Alexis, F., Gu, F. X., Basto, P. A., Bagalkot, V., Jon, S., Langer, R. S., Farokhzad, O. C., Co-delivery of hydrophobic and hydrophilic drugs from nanoparticle-aptamer bioconjugates, *ChemMedChem*, 2(9), 1268–1271, (2007).

13. Wang, X., Li, J., Wang, Y., Koenig, L., Gjyrezi, A., Giannakakou, P., Shin, E. H., Tighiouart, M., Chen, Z. G., Nie, S., Shin, D. M., A folate receptor-targeting nanoparticle minimizes drug resistance in a human cancer model, *ACS Nano*, 5(8), 6184–6194, (2011).

14. Zhang, W., Zhang, Z., Zhang, Y., The application of carbon nanotubes in target drug delivery systems for cancer therapies, *Nanoscale Research Letters*, 6(1), 555, (2011).

15. Liu, Z., Fan, A. C., Rakhra, K., Sherlock, S., Goodwin, A., Chen, X., Yang, Q., Felsher, D. W., Dai, H., Supramolecular stacking of doxorubicin on carbon nanotubes for in vivo cancer therapy, *Angewandte Chemie (International ed. in English)*, 48(41), 7668–7672, (2009).

16. Ozgen, P. S. O., Atasoy, S., Kurt, B. Z., Durmus, Z., Yigit, G., Dag, A., Glycopolymer decorated multi-wall carbon nanotubes for dual targeted breast cancer therapy, *Journal of Materials Chemistry B*, (8), 3123–3137, (2020).

17. Noriega-Luna, B., Godinez, L. A., Rodriguez, F. J., Rodriguez, A., Larrea, G. Z., Sossa-Frreyra, C. F., Mercado-Curiel, R. F., Manríquez, J., Bustos, E., Applications of dendrimers in drug delivery agents, diagnosis, therapy, and detection, *Journal of Nanomaterials*, 2014, (2014).

18. Abbasi, E., Aval, S. F., Akbarzadeh, A., Milani, M., Nasrabadi, H. T., Joo, S. W., Hanifehpour, Y., Nejati-Koshki, K., Pashaei-Asl, R., Dendrimers: Synthesis, applications, and properties, *Nanoscale Research Letters*, 9(1), 247, (2014).

19. Camminade, A. M., Turrin, C. E., Dendrimers for drug delivery, *Journal of Materials Chemistry B*, 2(26), 4055–4066, (2014).

20. Wang, Y., Cao, X., Guo, R., Shen, M., Zhang, M., Zhu, M., Shi, X., Targeted delivery of doxorubicin into cancer cells using a folic acid–dendrimer conjugate, *Polymer Chemistry*, 2, 1754–1760, (2011).

21. Patri, A. K., Myc, A., Beals, J., Thomas, T. P., Bander, N. H., Baker, J. R., Synthesis and in vitro testing of J591 antibody-dendrimer conjugates for targeted prostate cancer therapy, *Bioconjugate Chemistry*, 15(6), 1174–1181, (2004).

22. Sharma, A., Sharma, U. S., Liposomes in drug delivery: Progress and limitations, *International Journal of Pharmaceutics*, 154, 123–140, (1997).

23. Akbarzadeh, A., Rezaei-Sadabady, R., Davaran, S., Joo, S. W., Zarghami, N., Hanifehpour, Y., Samiei, M., Kouhi, M., Nejati-Koshki, K., Liposome: Classification, preparation, and applications, *Nanoscale Research Letters*, 8(1), 102, (2013).

24. Olusanya, T., Haj Ahmad, R. R., Ibegbu, D. M., Smith, J. R., Elkordy, A. A., Liposomal drug delivery systems and anticancer drugs, *Molecules (Basel, Switzerland)*, 23(4), 907, (2018).

25. Adlakha-Hutcheon, G., Bally, M. B., Shew, C. R., Madden, T. D., Controlled destabilization of a liposomal drug delivery system enhances mitoxantrone antitumor activity, *Nature Biotechnology*, 17(8), 775–779, (1999).

26. Li, Q., Cai, T., Huang, Y., Xia, X., Cole, S., Cai, Y., A review of the structure, preparation, and application of NLCs, PNPs, and PLNs, *Nanomaterials (Basel, Switzerland)*, 7(6), 122, (2017).

27. Pal, S. L., Jana, U., Manna, P. K., Mohanta, G. P., Manavalan, R., Nanoparticle: An overview of preparation and characterization, *Journal of Applied Pharmaceutical Science*, 1(6), 228–234, (2011).

28. Mastria, E. M., Cai, L. Y., Kan, M. J., Li, X., Schaal, J. L., Fiering, S., Gunn, M. D., Dewhirst, M. W., Nair, S. K., Chilkoti, A., Nanoparticle formulation improves doxorubicin efficacy by enhancing host antitumor immunity, *Journal of Controlled Release*, 269, 364–373, (2017).

29. Shuhendler, A. J., Cheung, R. Y., Manias, J., Connor, A., Rauth, A. M., Wu, X. Y., A novel doxorubicin-mitomycin C co-encapsulated nanoparticle formulation exhibits anti-cancer synergy in multidrug resistant human breast cancer cells, *Breast Cancer Research and Treatment*, 119(2), 255–269, (2010).

30. Junghanns, J. U., Müller, R. H., Nanocrystal technology, drug delivery and clinical applications, *International Journal of Nanomedicine*, 3(3), 295–309, (2008).

31. Miao, X., Yang, W., Feng, T., Lin, J., Huang, P., Drug nanocrystals for cancer therapy, *Nanomedicine and Nanobiotechnology*, 10(3), (2018).
32. Lu, Y., Li, Y., Wu, W., Injected nanocrystals for targeted drug delivery, *Acta Pharmaceutica Sinica B*, 6(2), 106–113, (2016).
33. Tayeb, H. H., Sainsbury, F., Nanoemulsions in drug delivery: Formulation to medical application, *Nanomedicine (London, England)*, 13(19), 2507–2525, (2018).
34. Jaiswal, M., Dudhe, R., Sharma, P. K., Nanoemulsion: An advanced mode of drug delivery system, *3 Biotech*, 5(2), 123–127, (2015).
35. Ganta, S., Singh, A., Rawal, Y., Cacaccio, J., Patel, N. R., Kulkarni, P., Ferris, C. F., Amiji, M. M., Coleman, T. P., Formulation development of a novel targeted theranostic nanoemulsion of docetaxel to overcome multidrug resistance in ovarian cancer, *Drug Delivery*, 23(3), 968–980, (2016).
36. Fofaria, N. M., Qhattal, H. S., Liu, X., Srivastava, S. K., Nanoemulsion formulations for anti-cancer agent Piplartine-characterization, toxicological, pharmacokinetics and efficacy studies, *International Journal of Pharmaceutics*, 498(1–2), 12–22, (2016).
37. Date, T., Paul, K., Singh, N., Jain, S., Drug-lipid conjugates for enhanced oral drug delivery, *AAPS Pharmaceutical Science and Technology*, 20(2), 41, (2019).
38. Irby, D., Du, C., Li, F., Lipid-drug conjugate for enhancing drug delivery, *Molecular Pharmaceutics*, 14(5), 1325–1338, (2017).
39. Banerjee, S., Kundu, A., Lipid-drug conjugates: A potential nanocarrier system for oral drug delivery applications, *Daru: Journal of Faculty of Pharmacy, Tehran University of Medical Sciences*, 26(1), 65–75, (2018).
40. Radwan, A. A., Alanazi, F. K., Design and synthesis of new cholesterol-conjugated 5-Fluorouracil: A novel potential delivery system for cancer treatment, *Molecules (Basel, Switzerland)*, 19(9), 13177–13187, (2014).
41. Mielczarek-Puta, M., Struga, M., Roszkowski, P., Synthesis and anticancer effects of conjugates of doxo-rubicin and unsaturated fatty acids (LNA and DHA), *Medicinal Chemistry Research*, 28, 2153–2164, (2019).
42. Alven, S., Nqoro, X., Buyana, B., Aderibigbe, B. A., Polymer-drug conjugate, a potential therapeutic to combat breast and lung cancer, *Pharmaceutics*, 12(5), 406, (2020).
43. Abraxane® USFDA Package Insert, www.accessdata.fda.gov/drugsatfda_docs/label/2020/021660s047lbl.pdf (Accessed on 30 Dec 2020)
44. Vasey, P. A., Kaye, S. B., Morrison, R., Twelves, C., Wilson, P., Duncan, R., Thomson, A. H., Murray, L. S., Hilditch, T. E., Murray, T., Burtles, S., Fraier, D., Frigerio, E., Cassidy, J., Phase I clinical and phar-macokinetic study of PK1 [N-(2-hydroxypropyl) methacrylamide copolymer doxorubicin]: First mem-ber of a new class of chemotherapeutic agents-drug-polymer conjugates, *Cancer Research Campaign Phase I/II Committee, Clinical Cancer Research*, 5(1), 83–94, (1999).
45. Ekladious, I., Colson, Y. L., Grinstaff, M. W., Polymer-drug conjugate therapeutics: Advances, insights and prospects, *Nature Reviews, Drug Discovery*, 18(4), 273–294, (2019).
46. Doxil® USFDA Package Insert, www.accessdata.fda.gov/drugsatfda_docs/label/2019/050718s055lbl.pdf (Accessed on 30 Dec 2020)
47. Gabizon, A., Shmeeda, H., Barenholz, Y., Pharmacokinetics of pegylated liposomal Doxorubicin: Review of animal and human studies, *Clinical Pharmacokinetics*, 42(5), 419–436, (2003).
48. Desai N., Challenges in development of nanoparticle-based therapeutics, *The AAPS Journal*, 14(2), 282–295, (2012).
49. Yared, J. A., Tkaczuk, K. H., Update on Taxane development: New analogs and new formulation, *Drug Design, Development and Therapy*, 6, 371–384, (2012).
50. Marqibo USFDA Package Insert, www.accessdata.fda.gov/drugsatfda_docs/label/2020/202497s011lbl.pdf (Accessed on 30 Dec 2020)
51. Silverman, J. A., Deitcher, S. R., Marqibo® (vincristine sulfate liposome injection) improves the phar-macokinetics and pharmacodynamics of vincristine, *Cancer Chemotherapy and Pharmacology*, 71(3), 555–564, (2013).
52. Rodriguez, M. A., Pytlik, R., Kozak, T., Chhanabhai, M., Gascoyne, R., Lu, B., Deitcher, S. R., Winter, J. N., Marqibo Investigators, Vincristine sulfate liposomes injection (Marqibo) in heavily pretreated patients with refractory aggressive non-Hodgkin lymphoma: Report of the pivotal phase 2 study, *Cancer*, 115(15), 3475–3482, (2009).
53. Gharpure, K. M., Wu, S. Y., Li, C., Lopez-Berestein, G., Sood, A. K., Nanotechnology: Future of onco-therapy, *Clinical Cancer Research*, 21(14), 3121–3130, (2015).

54. Shi, J., Kantoff, P. W., Wooster, R., Farokhzad, O. C., Cancer nanomedicine: Progress, challenges and opportunities, *Nature Reviews Cancer*, 17, 20–37, (2017).
55. Sonali, Viswanadh, M. K., Singh, R. P., Agrawal, P., Mehata, A. K., Pawde, D. M., Narendra, Sonkar, R., Muthu, M. S., Nanotheranostics: Emerging strategies for early diagnosis and therapy of brain cancer, *Nanotheranostics*, 2(1), 70–86, (2018).

9 Nanomedicine for MDR Reversal of Cancer Cells

Parth Patel and Keerti Jain

ACRONYMS

ABC   ATP binding cassette
Bcl-2   B-cell lymphoma-2
BIR   Baculovirus-IAP repeat
EPR   Enhanced permeation and retention
HIF   Hypoxia-inducing factor
IAP   Inhibitors of apoptosis protein
IFP   Interstitial fluid pressure
MAC   Membrane attack complexes
MDR   Multidrug resistant
MRP   MDR resistant protein
NPs   Nanoparticles
p-gp   Permeability glycoprotein

9.1 INTRODUCTION

The multidrug-resistant (MDR) phenomenon in mammalian cells is defined as the generation of cross-resistance to the large number of anti-tumor antibiotics and cytotoxic compounds, including natural alkaloids. In most of the cases, resistance that occurs during drug treatment is known as acquired drug resistance. This acquired drug resistance is a major problem in the treatment of cancer (1). Statistical data suggest that almost 90% of the mortality in cancer is due to the drug resistance developed by cancer cells (2). Thus, a deep understanding of the probable factors that produce resistance to anti-tumor drugs is very important for the development of new therapies and most importantly in preventing drug resistance in tumor cells. Additionally, these therapies can decrease the mortality rate by overcoming MDR in tumor cells (3, 4).

Anticancer drug resistance can be classified as acquired resistance and primary resistance. Primary resistance is due to natural immunity, while acquired resistance is developed during treatment. There are several reasons for the drug resistance such as accumulation of DNA targeting drugs in cytoplasm due to ATP binding cassette (ABC) transporter resulting in drug failure to target the nucleus of tumor cell. Long-term exposure of anticancer drugs also lead to development of resistance that is in severe cases produces cross resistance to other anticancer drugs and cause the MDR. In addition to this, drug resistance also involves alteration of transport pumps, mutation of oncogenes and tumor suppressor genes, and change in metabolism of drugs (5). To treat MDR cancers, various approaches are being investigated, and combination therapy is a widely researched approach. Combination therapy includes a chemotherapeutic agent and permeability glycoprotein (p-gp) inhibitor or an agent that produces an inhibitory effect on p-gp by some other mechanism (3, 6).

Nanotechnology is being investigated in diverse fields of science like wastewater treatment, the agriculture industry, and in biomedical applications. Nanomedicine shown ability to enhance the intracellular concentration of anticancer drugs and decreases the toxicity associated with the antineoplastic agents by passive or active targeting of tumor tissue. Nanosized particles have ability to quickly enter the highly permeable and leaky vasculature present in the tumor by using the

DOI: 10.1201/9781003130055-9

enhanced permeability and retention (EPR) effect. Moreover, tumor interstitium lacks established lymphatic system, so the chances of drug clearance through lymphatic vessels are minimum. This provides nanomedicines extra time in the interstitium of the tumor tissue. The EPR effect is much higher in tumor tissue compared to normal tissue (7–10).

9.2 CHARACTERISTICS OF CANCER TUMORS

MDR is the biggest challenge in the treatment of cancerous tumors using chemotherapy (12). Mechanisms hypothesized to be involved in the development of resistance to anticancer drugs in cancer cells are presented in Figure 9.1. The basic reasons behind the development of MDR are poor pharmacokinetic profile of chemotherapeutic agents; increased activity of the efflux pump; and tumor physiological conditions such as hypoxia, extracellular acidic milieu, high interstitial fluid pressure (IFP), and genetic modification. Moreover, these extrinsic and intrinsic factors interact with each other and make drug transportation more complicated (13).

9.2.1 Physiological Characteristic of Tumors

The physiological characteristic of cancerous tumors include abnormally organized blood vessels, acidic microenvironment, and high IFP. Tumor vasculatures have large inter-endothelial junctions, lack of lymphatic blood vessels inside the tumor, trifurcation with uneven diameter of branches, and heterogenous blood flow. The key contributor to disorganization of blood vessels is an imbalance between pro- and anti-angiogenic factors. These types of abnormalities will create a barrier for penetration of chemotherapeutic agents. Extravasation of therapeutic agents from blood vessels is mostly governed by diffusion; convection and transcytosis are also reasons for transvascular transport in tumors (14). Due to the presence of focal leaks in tumor blood vessels, downstream blood flow in tumors is compromised (15). Insufficient perfusion, uncontrolled proliferation, and deregulated metabolism lead to physicochemical changes such as hypoxia and decrease the pH of

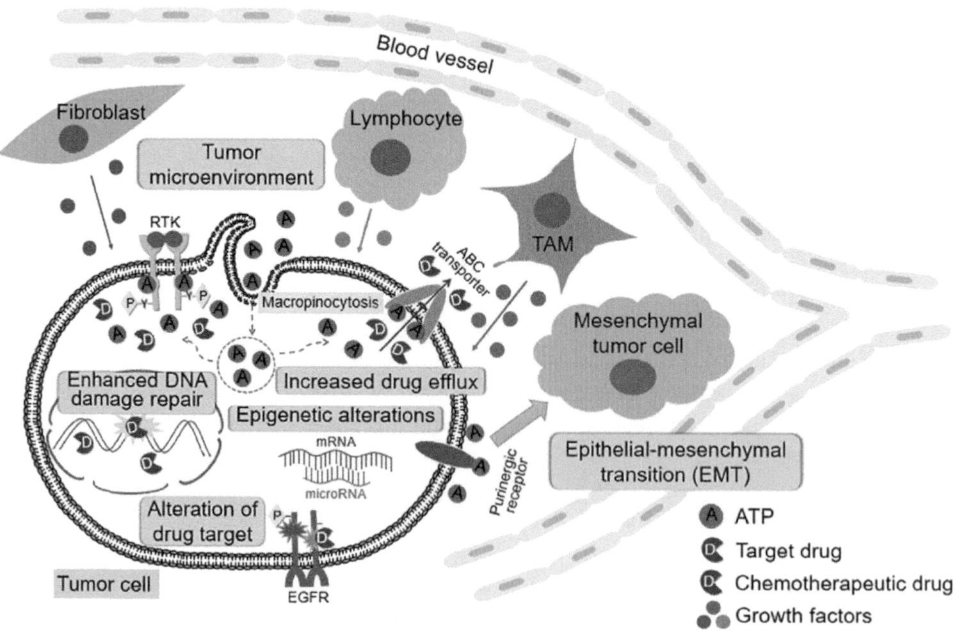

FIGURE 9.1 Mechanisms involved in drug resistance in cancer [reproduced with permission from (11)].

the tumor microenvironment; normally, pH lies between 6.5 and 6.8 in tumor tissue. One of the reasons behind acidic extracellular pH is that tumor cells use glycolytic pathways for energy production and thus produce lactic acid during glycolysis. This lactic acid is not cleared due to high IFP, so to maintain homeostasis, proton pumps are activated and make the extracellular microenvironment acidic. This acidic microenvironment might act as a barrier for weakly basic drugs (16).

9.2.2 Tumor IFP

Cancerous tumors have a lack of lymphatic blood vessels; thus interstitial fluid and soluble proteins are inefficiently removed and result in high IFP, which acts as a barrier in transcapillary transportation of therapeutic agents (17). Moreover, the extracellular matrix of tumor cells has a denser network of collagen fibers, which produces rigidity in connective tissues. Tumor cells also contain a high amount of fibroblast, which is directly bound to collagen fibers in an integrin-dependent manner and exerts increased IFP. Also, a high number of macrophages and inflammatory cells increase IFP by releasing cytokines and growth factors in the blood vessels and stroma fibroblasts (18). Due to the higher IFP, blood flow increases in the peri-tumor area, which causes peri-tumor hyperplasia. Generally, IFP is much higher in well-established stage 2 and stage 3 cancerous tumors compared to immature stage 1 tumors. IFP can be lowered by using angiotensin II, tumor necrosis factor-alpha (TNF-a), tumor necrosis factor-beta (TNF-β), dexamethasone, pentoxifylline, and taxol (19).

9.2.3 Role of Pro-Apoptotic Signals

Most chemotherapeutic drugs produce anticancer effects by inducing apoptosis by activation of caspases and Ca-channel nucleases. For instance, widely used anticancer drugs of the taxol family induce cell death by inhibiting the phosphorylation of apoptotic protein B-cell lymphoma-2 (Bcl-2). Similarly, glucocorticoids, extensively used in acute lymphoblastic leukaemia, trigger pro-apoptotic signals which produce cell cycle arrest and ultimately cell death. Human cancer cells show immortal characteristic because of downregulation of pro-apoptotic proteins such as Bax, Bak, Bad, and Bim and upregulation of anti-apoptotic proteins such as Bcl-2, Akt, and Mcl-1, which makes it difficult to form membrane attack complexes (MACs) and inhibit cytochrome-C, an apoptosis protein-activating factor from mitochondria (5). Generally, the Bcl-2 protein family is classified into two different functional groups, in which the first group (Bcl-2, Bcl-XL, Bcl-w, Mcl-1, Ced-9) will produce an inhibitory effect on apoptosis by hindering MAC formation, and the second group (Bax, Bak, Bik, Bid, and Harakiri) will produce apoptosis by promoting MAC formation (20).

9.2.4 Role of MDR Genes

MDR in human and rodents is normally associated with a decrease in cellular accumulation of anticancer drugs and overexpression of MDR genes. MDR genes like MDR1, MDR2, and MDR3 are responsible for membrane p-gp formation, a drug efflux protein of cells. Specifically, overexpression of a single human gene named MDR1 is responsible for MDR in humans. Mutation in MDR1 produces resistance to anticancer drugs in tumor cells. There are various mechanisms of amplification of the MDR1 gene, resulting in increased p-gp activity as a drug reflux pump. The MDR1 gene mostly appears in relapsing condition of tumors, which suggests that p-gp has a role in inducing the survival mechanism of tumor cells by expelling anticancer drugs. Studies in myeloma, leukaemia, and other childhood cancers suggests that the MDR1 gene has a very important role in the failure of chemotherapeutic treatment (17).

9.2.5 Role of Epigenetic Modification

The epigenetic modification, that is, change in the gene expression which is independent of DNA sequence and has known for its ability to produce non-genetic heterogeneity. This phenomenon can be studied as an abnormal pattern of DNA methylation, unusual histone modification, and unexpected change in chromatin composition. Epigenomes can survive in the presence of anticancer drugs due to abnormal transcription of efflux transporters, and production of DNA repair enzymes, resulting in drug resistant cells that are ineffective to cytotoxic drugs. By modulating the chromatin packaging, epigenetic changes will affect gene transcription. Thus, epigenetic changes are able to access DNA to produce sequence-specific transcription factors. Drug resistance in tumor cells is mostly produced by a combination of genetic and epigenetic markers (21).

9.2.6 Role of p-gp

p-gp belongs to a protein efflux pump of the ABC transport protein family and is widely present in human cancer cells such as gastrointestinal cancers like small and large intestine cancer, pancreatic cancer; genitourinary cancers like kidney, ovarian, and testicular cancers; childhood cancers like neuroblastoma and fibrosarcoma; and hematopoietic cancers like myeloma, lymphoma, and leukaemia. p-gp can immediately detect multiple drug moieties that enter the cell and make a complex with them. These drug moieties include not only natural anticancer molecules like vincristine, vinblastine, taxol, doxorubicin, and daunorubicin but also contain antihistaminic, anti-arrhythmic, statins (cholesterol lowering agents), and HIV protease inhibitors (22). Almost every resistant cell in human cancer shows over-expression of p-gp, an energy dependent drug efflux pump. The p-gp pump not only expels out the drug molecules, but it also involves in the transportation of nutrients and biologically important molecules from, into and out of the intracellular membrane (17). The binding of drug and p-gp, activates the ATP binding domain resulting in change in the shape of p-gp and expulsion of drug from the cell. Immediately, hydrolysis of the second molecule of ATP occurs, and p-gp reverts to its original shape. Now p-gp can bind and expel another lipophilic drug that enters the intracellular space. While the mechanism of other ABC transporter proteins is not known clearly, probably the ATP binding cassette plays an important role in initiation of drug transport in the extracellular medium. Drugs having neutral or positive charges are the substrate for p-gp and electrically bound to the protein.

To increase the accumulation of anticancer drugs in p-gp–overexpressing cells, various strategies have been applied. The competitive inhibition of p-gp with secondary substrate having comparative high affinity to p-gp than the anticancer drug molecule is the most acceptable strategy. More research is ongoing to find specific potent inhibitors of p-gp to reverse the resistance of tumor cells (23).

9.2.7 Role of Hypoxia

Hypoxia is a condition of significantly low concentration of oxygen inside the cells very. To overcome the hypoxia, tumor cells activate some reflex mechanisms such as angiogenesis, cell proliferation, glucose metabolism and activates hypoxia inducible factor (HIF) (12). HIF activity is mostly dependent on oxygen level inside the cell and hypoxic condition should be stabilized by the induction of α subunit. HIF-1α kept at low level during sufficient oxygen presence because of ubiquitination protein degradation (24). In normal cells HIF provoke the apoptosis and cell cycle arrest. Conversely, in drug resistant tumor cells anti-apoptotic genes such as Bcl-2, Bcl-xL, Mcl-1, NF-kB, survivin, etc. tend to be activated instead of apoptotic genes due to the activity of HIF. MDR1 gene, that is responsible for the overexpression of drug efflux protein p-gp was upregulated in hypoxic condition. That results in increase in drug resistance in tumor cells by enhancing drug's pumping out to extracellular region. Researchers have found significant role of HIF-1α in upregulation of MDR1 gene in colon cancer cells (25).

9.3 NANOMEDICINE IN MDR REVERSAL OF CANCER CELLS

Nanomedicines are composed of nano scale vehicle with striking biochemical and physical properties for designing of drug delivery system. Most used nanomaterials in nanomedicine are polymeric nanoparticles (NPs), dendrimers, micelles, liposomes, lipidic NPs, metallic NPs, carbon-based formulations like nanodiamonds, nanotubes, etc. NPs have particle size in nanometers that features that drug is not available as individual molecules alone. Nano-particulate system are emerging as an approach to overcome the lack of specificity of traditional drug delivery systems to reach at the solid tumor site. NPs due to its special structural properties and capacity to form conjugates with various polymers have shown ability to increase the therapeutic potential of drug, with decrease in side effects, extended drug release profile, etc. Some of the advantages of using nanomaterials as a drug delivery system are easy solubilization of poorly soluble drugs, high drug payload, provide protection from the external environment, low toxicity, prolonged circulation, controlled drug release, targeted drug delivery, etc (26).

Due to the EPR effect, nanomedicines can penetrate the tumor tissue by passing the biological membrane that is mostly impermeable to the large molecules. Due to the physicochemical properties of NP carriers and pathophysiological condition of tumor tissues passive targeting of NP happens. For transferring of nanomedicines in the tumor tissue by passive targeting some physico-chemical parameters such as particle size and surface chemistry played a very important role. Most desirable nanomedicines are the particles having longest blood circulation time. The pore size for extravasation through transvascular gaps is between 380 to 780 nm based on the type of tumor, the same way the pore size in tight endothelial cells is between 1 to 10 nm [11,83].

The mechanisms of nanomedicine mediated multi-drug resistance (MDR) reversal at different cellular and intracellular levels for MDR sensitive chemotherapeutic drug is shown graphically in Figure 9.2.

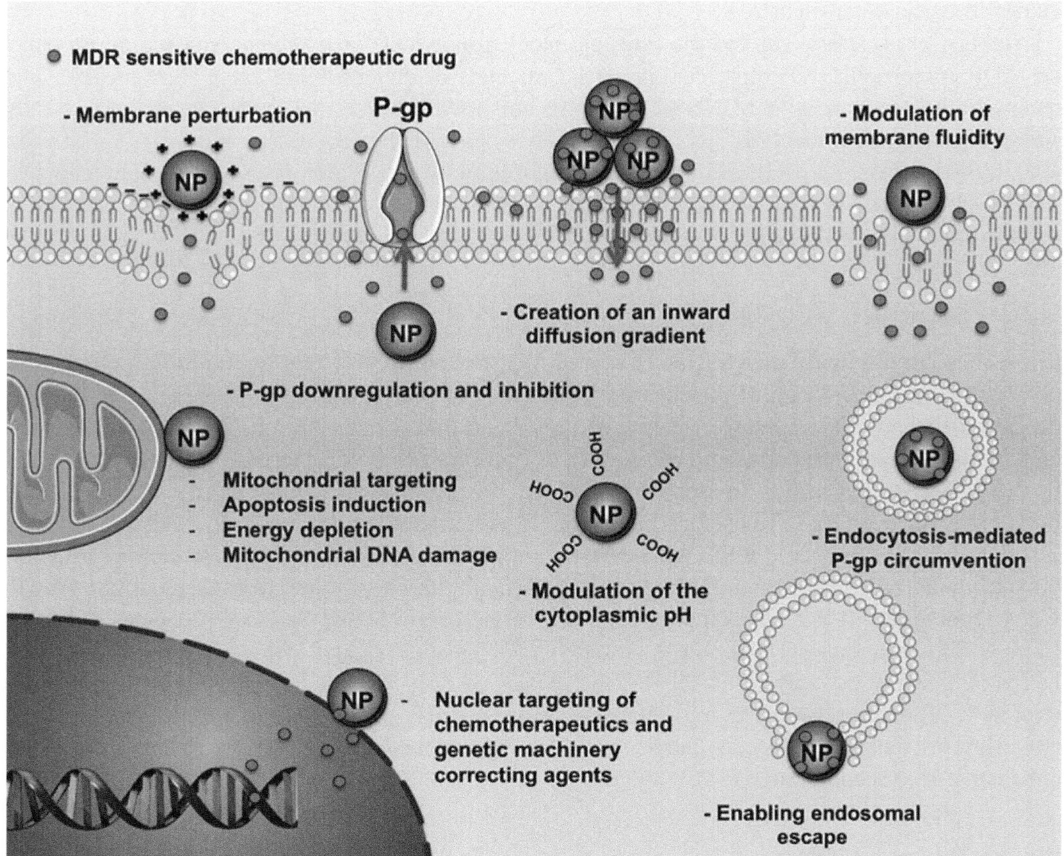

FIGURE 9.2 Graphical depiction of mechanisms of nanomedicine mediated MDR reversal at different cellular and intracellular levels for MDR sensitive chemotherapeutic drug [reproduced with permission from (27)].

Secondly, the plasma drug concentration should be high and long enough in the blood circulation for passively targeting the nanomedicines in tumor tissues. Most of the nanomedicines are administered via the intravenous route. In bloodstream, reticuloendothelial system (RES) is a major defence system of body that is also known as "mononuclear phagocytes system". RES can remove the nanomedicines from the blood and cause a major obstacle in blood circulation of nanomedicines for a longer period. Opsonization is the process where nanomedicines are identified as a foreign particle by phagocytic cell that results in withdrawal of nanomedicines from the bloodstream. The phagocytes present in Kupffer cells of liver and spleen are responsible for the elimination of nanomedicines (28).

9.3.1 MICELLES

Micelles are made up of the amphiphilic colloidal systems that form a self-assembly of molecules presenting the two different regions of opposite affinity in each solvent. Micelles can be classified as polymeric micelles and surfactant-based (mostly non-ionic) micelles. Micelles have ability to solubilize the poorly soluble drugs, particle size around 100 nm and, its surface protects it from phagocytic clearance and increase its blood circulation time. The effectiveness of micelles is dependent on critical micelle concentration (CMC) of surfactant and core viscosity (29). Polymeric micelles are highly versatile because of its ability to form a stable micelle, biodegradability, lower CMC and enhance the blood circulation time. Pluronic is a co-polymer and widely study for the delivery of drug in MDR tumor. Pluronic made up of poly-ethylene oxide (hydrophilic) and poly-propylene oxide (hydrophobic). So, the Pluronic forms a micelle that have hydrophobic inner core and hydrophilic outer surface.

Alakhov et al. (1996) studied the Pluronic block copolymer for its chemo sensitizing property on MDR tumor cells. Scientist have prepared micelles of daunorubicin using Pluronic P85 and compare its effectiveness on MDR-SKVLB cells and non MDR-SKVLB cells. Results of the study showed that IC_{50} dose of MDR cell is decreased because of the effect of Pluronic polymer (30). Jin et al. (2014) prepared a paclitaxel loaded amphiphilic graft copolymer, N-octyl-O-sulfate chitosan (NOSC) for reversal of p-gp mediated resistance of drug. NOSC was competitively inhibit the paclitaxel from binding with the p-gp and restrict the membrane fluidity (31).

9.3.2 LIPOSOMES

Liposomes are the lipid based vesicular system that has ability to carry hydrophilic molecules in core and hold the hydrophobic molecules between lipid bilayers. Liposome carrying anticancer drugs mostly shows the passive targeting to tumor and that is due to the EPR effect. Tumor cells containing a leaky vasculature are permeable to liposomes that will increase the drug accumulation (17). Second generation liposomes named as "Stealth liposome" has hold the PEG molecule in its outer surface. These liposomes have more blood circulation time and other advantages (32). Yang et al. (2007) prepared a PEGylated Immunoliposomes with the help of Herceptin, a recombinant humanized monoclonal antibody that specifically bound to the Human epidermal growth factor receptor-2 (HER-2). In comparative study of Herceptin bound Paclitaxel loaded PEGylated Immunoliposome versus Herceptin unbound liposomes showed that Herceptin bound liposomes had good penetrating capacity in HER-2 overexpressed breast tumor cells (33). Other approaches used in MDR reversal by Liposomes include formulating pH sensitive and charge reversal type carrier using pH sensitive polymers. Particularly this type of formulation uses lower pH of tumor for enhancing drug accumulation (34).

9.3.3 POLYMERIC NPS

Polymeric NPs are widely used because of its good bioavailability, ease of modification and broad structural varieties of polymer. Structurally these NPs are either reservoir type or matrix type formulations. Based on the source of origin natural or synthetic polymers are used in preparation (35). Sun et al. (2019) had developed a Doxorubicin and chloroquine based polymeric NPs using poly (lactic-co-glycolic acid) (PLGA) and TPGS as a carrier. These nanomedicines entered the MDR cancer cells by endocytosis and exerted a significant toxicity (36). Co-delivery of more than one therapeutic agent is an effective strategy for reversal of MDR. In co-delivery system one of the agents is chemosensitizer such as pyrrolidine dithiocarbamate (PDTC) that silence the effect of p-gp (37). Furthermore, Zhao et al. (2019) had prepared a core-shell type polymeric NPs of curcumin and paclitaxel using stearic acid and polyethyleneimine as polymer based for treatment of MDR ovarian cancer. Results of the study showed that this formulation produced significant cytotoxicity in cancer cells along with least side effect on normal cells (38).

9.3.4 Solid-lipid NPs (SLN)

SLNs are one of the therapeutic carriers which uses solid lipids and surfactant for vesicle formation. SLNs are mostly prepared by physiological lipids and have a particle size between 50 nm to 1000 nm. Resistance phenomenon mostly associated with the cell membrane in terms of blocking entry of drugs or expelling out the drugs that once entered the cell. This problem can be overcome by using lipids which has an inherent ability to produce cell membrane associated changes (39). Nanostructured lipid carriers (NLCs) are the second generation lipidic NPs that contains combination of solid and liquid lipids (40). Most of the research are based on co-delivery approach that includes addition of agent has the inhibitory effect on specific receptor of MDR tumor cells. Daddy J.C et al. (2020) have prepared Mitoxantrone and β-elemene containing Soya lecithin phospholipid based SLNs for the treatment of MDR in leukaemia. Due to using different lipids its blood circulation time increases and because of β-elemene its accumulation in tumor increases (41).

9.3.5 Nanocrystals

Nanocrystals are the nano sized crystals of drugs often combined with surfactant and co-surfactant to resolve the stability problem. Main advantage of nanocrystal is to enhance the solubility of poorly soluble drugs. Nanocrystals can be administered via various routes such as parenteral, oral, topical, transdermal, etc. (42, 43). Han et al. (2019) formulated a paclitaxel loaded nanocrystal and modified it using triphenyl phosphonium cation (TPP$^+$) conjugated Brij-98 for overcoming the MDR. Tumor penetration study showed that the conjugated nanocrystals gave high penetration in the paclitaxel resistant MCF-7 cells. Moreover, TPP$^+$was specifically used for the mitochondrial targeting; the cytotoxicity study showed efficient mitochondrial delivery of nanocrystals due to the conjugation TPP$^+$and Brij-98 (44).

9.3.6 Dendrimers

The word Dendrimers comes from the Greek word "Tree" that depicts the typical structure of dendrimer. Dendrimer can be defined as a highly branched structure of big synthetic molecules that has globular shape and size in nano meter range with large number of surface group. Unlike linear polymers dendrimers have well defined monodisperse molecular structure. Dendrimer as a carrier for drug delivery vehicle possesses many advantages such as ability to deliver the drug in intracellular environment, to cross the biological barrier, target specific structure, etc (2, 45–47). Zou et al. (2017) formulated a Paclitaxel loaded PEG-PAMAM nanoparticles for reversal of MDR ovarian cancer cells. Researchers also attached Borneol, a potent p-gp inhibitor in the conjugated system. Outcomes of the study showed enhanced anticancer activity compared to the free drug sample because of higher accumulation of paclitaxel in MDR cells (48).

9.3.7 NANOEMULSION

The Nanoemulsion can be defined as, Heterogeneous system composed of one immiscible liquid dispersed as droplets within the continuous phase, where the average droplet diameter is below 100 nm. Nanoemulsion should be transparent or translucent, in contrast to the opaque or milky white appearance of convectional emulsions. It is mostly used for enhancing the bioavailability of lipid drugs (49). Y. Ma et al. (2014) fabricated a nanoemulsion that carries the hydrophobic drug (paclitaxel) and hydrophilic drug (5-flurouracil) for overcoming the paclitaxel resistant in a MDR human epidermal carcinoma cells. This formulation exhibited improved anti-tumor activity and gave synergistic effect with decreased side effects (50).

9.3.8 METALLIC NPs

Metallic NPs are the colloidal particles that contains an inorganic metals or metal oxides with therapeutic agents either in the polymeric matrix or encapsulated into the polymeric shell. Metallic NPs are widely used for the contrast and tracking agents in diagnosis of cancer. Metallic NPs have significant cancer treatment due to its ability to deliver the drug to target specific tumor cell, high accumulation of therapeutic agent near to tumor cells and reduce the concentration of in healthy cells. Metallic NPs can be divided in two groups involving metals such as Ag, Cu, Au, and Pt and metal oxides such as Fe_3O_4, ZnO, CuO, Cu_2O, MgO, and TiO_2 (51). Kievit et al. (2011) fabricated doxorubicin that is covalently bound to polyethylene imine and conjugated to an iron oxide NPs coated with amine terminated polyethylene glycol for treatment of MDR tumor cells. Results suggested that conjugated doxorubicin have lower cell viability compared to the free drug treatment (52).

9.3.9 CARBON BASED NPs

Nanotubes, Nanodiamonds, etc are the allotropes of carbon-based NPs. Allotropes are differed from each other based on carbon arrangement. Carbon-based NPs are biocompatible and non-toxic. Its geometry does not fit with the tumor resistant efflux protein so can be used to deliver the anticancer drug in a MDR tumor. In addition to this, due to the various functional groups present on its surface, it is suitable for formulating the conjugated system (46, 53). Ghoneum et al. (2019) formulated a chemo sensitizing property of nanodiamond and nanoplatinum bounded daunorubicin against the MDR human myeloid leukaemia cells. Results of the study described that nanodiamond conjugation is act as an effective chemo sensitizer in reversal of HL60/AR cells (54).

Different nanomedicines investigated for anticancer drug delivery and to combat with the problem of resistance to chemotherapy in cancer cells is summarized in Table 9.1.

9.4 CONCLUSION

Successful treatment of MDR tumor is a big challenge but research in last few years opened a door for nanomedicines in MDR treatment. In past decades multiple attempts has been made to understand the mechanism behind developing the resistance in cancerous tumor. Comprehensive understanding of structural and functional features is required for designing of new technology based therapeutic system. Furthermore, heterogeneity in cancer tumor has made MDR more complex because some tumors are inherently resistance while some have developed a resistance during the treatment. Although, there are many strategies available for the treatment of MDR tumor but very few of them are clinically tested. In this regard nanomedicines are emerging as promising modalities to combat and reverse the problems of MDR in cancer treatment. Although significant research work is going on in this direction all over the world, yet systematic comprehensive studies are required to enhance efficacy and safety of these nanomedicines in MDR reversal of cancer cells.

TABLE 9.1

Summary of Nanomedicines Being Investigated for MDR Reversal of Cancer

Nanomedicine	Anticancer Drug	MDR reversing agent	Outcomes	Ref.
PLGA based NPs	Doxorubicin	Cyclosporine A	Survival rate of tumor bearing mice was increased	(55)
Hydrogels	Doxorubicin	Cyclosporin A	Improved cytotoxicity and increased retention of anticancer drug was observed in Bcll leukaemia cells	(56)
Polyethylene glycol and polycaprolactone based NPs	Doxorubicin + Paclitaxel	Verapamil	Enhanced drug concentration and retention of anticancer agents in MDR tumor cells	(57)
Self-micro emulsifying drug delivery system	Paclitaxel	Cyclosporin A	Increased bioavailability of anticancer drug due to co-administration of Cyclosporin A in Sprague dawley rats	(58)
Transferrin conjugated Micelles	Doxorubicin	Verapamil	Enhanced cytotoxicity of MDR tumor cells was observed	(59)
Nanoemulsion	Doxorubicin	Bromotetrandrine	Cytotoxicity was increased in the MCF7/ADR cells because of resistance modulating agent	(60)
Stealth liposomes	Topotecan	Amlodipine	Tumor size was significantly decreased due to the effective cytotoxicity of drug	(61)
Aerosol based Alginate based NPs	Doxorubicin	Verapamil	Increased cellular uptake of Doxorubicin and cytotoxicity	(62)
Lipid NPs	Paclitaxel	Verapamil	Improved cytotoxicity and tumor mass reduction in glioma mice model	(63)
Stealth liposomes	Doxorubicin	Verapamil	Enhanced cytotoxicity and improved pharmacokinetic profile of MDR tumor cells was noticed	(64)
Hydroxypropyl β-cyclodextrin conjugated SLN	Paclitaxel	Verapamil	Intracellular uptake of anticancer drug was increased	(65)
Cationic and anionic liposomes	Doxorubicin	VEGF siRNA and c-Myc siRNA	Down regulation of MDR expression and enhanced uptake of anticancer drug in NCI-ADR/RES resistant ovarian cancer cells	(66)
Antibody conjugated PLGA NPs	Paclitaxel	Anti P-gp antibody and curcumin (a chemosensitizing agent)	Because of antibodies significant enhancement in paclitaxel sensitivity was noticed both *in vitro* and *in vivo* in xenograft model of KB-V1 cells of mice	(67)

9.5 ACKNOWLEDGMENT

Authors are grateful to Department of Pharmaceuticals (DoP), Ministry of Chemicals and Fertilisers, Government of India for their support. NIPER Raebareli communication number for this manuscript is NIPER-R/Communication/193.

REFERENCES

1. IARC Publications Website—World Cancer Report 2008 [Internet]. [cited 2021 Feb 14]. Available from: https://publications.iarc.fr/Non-Series-Publications/World-Cancer-Reports/World-Cancer-Report-2008
2. Gauro R, Nandave M, Jain VK, Jain K. Advances in dendrimer-mediated targeted drug delivery to the brain. *Journal of Nanoparticle Research*. 2021 Mar;23(3):76.
3. Khan MA, Jain VK, Rizwanullah M, Ahmad J, Jain K. PI3K/AKT/mTOR pathway inhibitors in triple-negative breast cancer: A review on drug discovery and future challenges. *Drug Discovery Today*. 2019;24:2181–91. Elsevier Ltd.
4. Wilting RH, Dannenberg JH. Epigenetic mechanisms in tumorigenesis, tumor cell heterogeneity and drug resistance. *Drug Resistance Updates*. 2012 Feb 1;15(1–2):21–38.
5. Chen L, Zeng Y, Zhou SF. Role of apoptosis in cancer resistance to chemotherapy. In: *Current Understanding of Apoptosis—Programmed Cell Death*. InTechOpen, UK, 2018.
6. Wang S, Wang L, Chen M, Wang Y. Gambogic acid sensitizes resistant breast cancer cells to doxorubicin through inhibiting P-glycoprotein and suppressing surviving expression. *Chemico-Biological Interactions*. 2015 Jun 25;235:76–84.
7. Jain K, Shukla R, Yadav A, Ujjwal RR, Flora SJS. 3D Printing in development of nanomedicines. *Nanomaterials*. 2021;11(2):1–24.
8. Soni N, Jain K, Gupta U, Jain NK. Controlled delivery of gemcitabine hydrochloride using mannosylated poly(propyleneimine) dendrimers. *Journal of Nanoparticle Research*. 2015 Nov 1;17(11):1–17.
9. Jain A, Jain K, Mehra NK, Jain NK. Lipoproteins tethered dendrimeric nanoconstructs for effective targeting to cancer cells. *Journal of Nanoparticle Research*. 2013 Oct 1;15(10):1–18.
10. Afsana, Jain V, Haider N, Jain K. 3D printing in personalized drug delivery. *Current Pharmaceutical Design*. 2019 Mar 20;24(42):5062–71.
11. Wang X, Zhang H, Chen X. Drug resistance and combating drug resistance in cancer. *Cancer Drug Resistance*. 2019;2(2):141–60.
12. Pluen A, Boucher Y, Ramanujan S, McKee TD, Gohongi T, Di Tomaso E, et al. Role of tumor-host interactions in interstitial diffusion of macromolecules: Cranial vs. subcutaneous tumors. *Proceedings of the National Academy of Sciences of the United States of America*. 2001 Apr 10;98(8):4628–33.
13. Liao WL, Lin SC, Sunny Sun H, Tsai SJ. Hypoxia-induced tumor malignancy and drug resistance: Role of microRNAs, *Biomarkers and Genomic Medicine*. 2014;6:1–11. Elsevier Inc.
14. Jain RK. Transport of molecules across tumor vasculature. *Cancer and Metastasis Review*. 1987 Dec;6(4):559–93.
15. Fukumura D, Jain RK. Tumor microvasculature and microenvironment: Targets for anti-angiogenesis and normalization. *Microvascular Research*. 2007;74:72–84.
16. Boedtkjer E, Pedersen SF. The acidic tumor microenvironment as a driver of cancer., *Annual Review of Physiology*. 2020;82:103–26. Annual Reviews Inc.
17. Dong X. Nanomedicinal strategies to treat multidrug-resistant tumors: Current progress review. *Nanomedicine*. 2010;5:597–615.
18. Heldin CH, Rubin K, Pietras K, Östman A. High interstitial fluid pressure—an obstacle in cancer therapy. *Nature Reviews Cancer*. 2004;4(10):806–13.
19. Campbell R. Tumor physiology and delivery of nanopharmaceuticals. *Anti-Cancer Agents in Medicinal Chemistry*. 2008;6(6):503–12.
20. Bhola PD, Letai A. Mitochondria-judges and executioners of cell death sentences. *Molecular Cell*. 2016;61:695–704. Cell Press.
21. Gajda E, Godlewska M, Mariak Z, Nazaruk E, Gawel D. Combinatory treatment with mir-7-5p and drug-loaded cubosomes effectively impairs cancer cells. *International Journal of Molecular Sciences*. 2020;21(14):1–19.
22. Loo TW, Clarke DM. Recent progress in understanding the mechanism of P-glycoprotein-mediated drug efflux. *Journal of Membrane Biology*. 2005;206(3):173–85.
23. Gottesman MM. Mechanisms of cancer drug resistance Michael. Annual Review of Medicine. 2002;53:615–27.
24. Majmundar AJ, Wong WJ, Simon MC. Hypoxia-inducible factors and the response to hypoxic stress. *Molecular Cell*. 2010;40:294–309. Cell Press.
25. Ding Z, Yang L, Xie X, Xie F, Pan F, Li J, et al. Expression and significance of hypoxia-inducible factor-1 alpha and MDR1/P-glycoprotein in human colon carcinoma tissue and cells. *Journal of Cancer Research and Clinical Oncology*. 2010 Nov 9;136(11):1697–707.

26. Benny O, Fainaru O, Adini A, Cassiola F, Bazinet L, Adini I, et al. An orally delivered small-molecule formulation with antiangiogenic and anticancer activity. *Nature Biotechnology.* 2008 Jul;26(7):799–807.

27. Singh MS, Tammam SN, Shetab Boushehri MA, Lamprecht A. MDR in cancer: Addressing the underlying cellular alterations with the use of nanocarriers. *Pharmacological Research.* 2017;126:2–30. Academic Press.

28. Carrstensen H, Müller RH, Müller BW. Particle size, surface hydrophobicity and interaction with serum of parenteral fat emulsions and model drug carriers as parameters related to RES uptake. *Clinical Nutrition.* 1992 Oct 1;11(5):289–97.

29. Keskin D, Tezcaner A. Micelles as delivery system for cancer treatment. *Current Pharmaceutical Design.* 2017 May 29;23(35).

30. Alakhov VY, Moskaleva EY, Batrakova EV, Kabanov AV. Hypersensitization of multidrug resistant human ovarian carcinoma cells by pluronic P85 block copolymer. *Bioconjugate Chemistry.* 1996;7(2):209–16.

31. Jin X, Mo R, Ding Y, Zheng W, Zhang C. Paclitaxel-loaded N-octyl-O-sulfate chitosan micelles for superior cancer therapeutic efficacy and overcoming drug resistance. *Molecular Pharmaceutics.* 2014 Jan 6;11(1):145–57.

32. Immordino ML, Dosio F, Cattel L. Stealth liposomes: Review of the basic science, rationale, and clinical applications, existing and potential. *International Journal of Nanomedicine.* 2006;1:297–315.

33. Yang T, Choi MK, De Cui F, Lee SJ, Chung SJ, Shim CK, et al. Antitumor effect of paclitaxel-loaded PEGylated immunoliposomes against human breast cancer cells. *Pharmaceutical Research.* 2007 Dec;24(12):2402–11.

34. Chen M, Song F, Liu Y, Tian J, Liu C, Li R, et al. A dual pH-sensitive liposomal system with charge-reversal and NO generation for overcoming multidrug resistance in cancer. *Nanoscale.* 2019 Mar 7;11(9):3814–26.

35. El-Say KM, El-Sawy HS. Polymeric nanoparticles: Promising platform for drug delivery. *International Journal of Pharmaceutics.* 2017;528:675–91. Elsevier B.V.

36. Sun JH, Ye C, Bai EH, Zhang LL, Huo SJ, Yu HH, et al. Co-delivery nanoparticles of doxorubicin and chloroquine for improving the anti-cancer effect in vitro. *Nanotechnology.* 2019 Feb 22;30(8).

37. Cheng X, Li D, Sun M, He L, Zheng Y, Wang X, et al. Co-delivery of DOX and PDTC by pH-sensitive nanoparticles to overcome multidrug resistance in breast cancer. *Colloids and Surfaces B: Biointerfaces.* 2019 Sep 1;181:185–97.

38. Zhao MD, Li JQ, Chen FY, Dong W, Wen LJ, Fei WD, et al. Co-delivery of curcumin and paclitaxel by "core-shell" targeting amphiphilic copolymer to reverse resistance in the treatment of ovarian cancer. *International Journal of Nanomedicine.* 2019;14:9453–67.

39. Tammam SN. Lipid based nanoparticles as inherent reversing agents of multidrug resistance in cancer. *Current Pharmaceutical Design.* 2017 Nov 25;23(43):6714–29.

40. Paliwal R, Paliwal SR, Kenwat R, Das Kurmi B, Sahu MK. Solid lipid nanoparticles: A review on recent perspectives and patents. *Expert Opinion on Therapeutic Patents.* 2020;30:179–94. Taylor and Francis Ltd.

41. Kambere Amerigos Daddy JC, Chen M, Raza F, Xiao Y, Su Z, Ping Q. Co-encapsulation of mito-xantrone and β-Elemene in solid lipid nanoparticles to overcome multidrug resistance in Leukemia. *Pharmaceutics.* 2020 Feb 1;12(2).

42. Joshi K, Chandra A, Jain K, Talegaonkar S. Nanocrystalization: An emerging technology to enhance the bioavailability of poorly soluble drugs. *Pharmaceutical Nanotechnology.* 2019 Apr 9;7(4):259–78.

43. Pardhi VP, Verma T, Flora SJS, Chandasana H, Shukla R. Nanocrystals: An overview of fabrication, characterization and therapeutic applications in drug delivery. *Current Pharmaceutical Design.* 2019;24(43):5129–46.

44. Han X, Su R, Huang X, Wang Y, Kuang X, Zhou S, et al. Triphenylphosphonium-modified mitochondria-targeted paclitaxel nanocrystals for overcoming multidrug resistance. *Asian Journal of Pharmaceutical Sciences.* 2019 Sep 1;14(5):569–80.

45. Jain K. Dendrimers as nanobiopolymers in cancer chemotherapy. In: *NanoBioMedicine* (Volume I–VI). Studium Press, 2017.

46. Jain K. Dendrimers: Smart nanoengineered polymers for bioinspired applications in drug delivery. In: *Biopolymer-Based Composites: Drug Delivery and Biomedical Applications.* Elsevier, 2017, pp. 169–220.

47. Pardhi VP, Jain K. Impact of binary/ternary solid dispersion utilizing poloxamer 188 and TPGS to improve pharmaceutical attributes of Bedaquiline fumarate. *Journal of Drug Delivery Science and Technology.* 2021 Apr 1;62.

48. Zou L, Di Wang, Hu Y, Fu C, Li W, Dai L, et al. Drug resistance reversal in ovarian cancer cells of paclitaxel and borneol combination therapy mediated by PEG-PAMAM nanoparticles. *Oncotarget.* 2017;8(36):60453–68.

49. Singh Y, Meher JG, Raval K, Khan FA, Chaurasia M, Jain NK, et al. Nanoemulsion: Concepts, development and applications in drug delivery. *Journal of Controlled Release.* 2017;252:28–49. Elsevier B.V.

50. Ma Y, Liu D, Wang D, Wang Y, Fu Q, Fallon JK, et al. Combinational delivery of hydrophobic and hydrophilic anticancer drugs in single nanoemulsions to treat MDR in cancer. *Molecular Pharmaceutics.* 2014 Aug 4;11(8):2623–30.

51. Alavi M, Rai M. Recent advances in antibacterial applications of metal nanoparticles (MNPs) and metal nanocomposites (MNCs) against multidrug-resistant (MDR) bacteria. *Expert Review of Anti-Infective Therapy.* 2019;17:419–28. Taylor and Francis Ltd.

52. Kievit FM, Wang FY, Fang C, Mok H, Wang K, Silber JR, et al. Doxorubicin loaded iron oxide nanoparticles overcome multidrug resistance in cancer in vitro. *Journal of Controlled Release.* 2011 May 30;152(1):76–83.

53. Chauhan S, Jain N, Nagaich U. Nanodiamonds with powerful ability for drug delivery and biomedical applications: Recent updates on in vivo study and patents. *Journal of Pharmaceutical Analysis.* 2020;10(1):1–12.

54. Ghoneum A, Sharma S, Gimzewski J. Nano-hole induction by nanodiamond and nanoplatinum liquid, DPV576, reverses multidrug resistance in human myeloid leukemia (HL60/AR). *International Journal of Nanomedicine.* 2013 Jul 18;8:2567–73.

55. Xu L, Li H, Wang Y, Dong F, Wang H, Zhang S. Enhanced activity of doxorubicin in drug resistant A549 tumor cells by encapsulation of P-glycoprotein inhibitor in PLGA-based nanovectors. *Oncology Letters.* 2014 Feb 1;7(2):387–92.

56. Šťastný M, Plocová D, Etrych T, Kovář M, Ulbrich K, Íhová B. HPMA-hydrogels containing cytostatic drugs: Kinetics of the drug release and in vivo efficacy. *Journal of Controlled Release.* 2002 May 17;81(1–2):101–11.

57. Elamanchili P, McEachern C, Burt H. Reversal of multidrug resistance by Methoxypolyethylene glycol-block-polycaprolactone diblock copolymers through the inhibition of P-glycoprotein function. *Journal of Pharmaceutical Sciences.* 2009 Mar 1;98(3):945–58.

58. Yang S, Gursoy RN, Lambert G, Benita S. Enhanced oral absorption of paclitaxel in a novel self-microemulsifying drug delivery system with or without concomitant use of P-glycoprotein inhibitors. *Pharmaceutical Research.* 2004 Feb;21(2):261–70.

59. Wu J, Lu Y, Lee A, Pan X, Yang X, Zhao X, et al. Reversal of multidrug resistance by transferrin-conjugated liposomes co-encapsulating doxorubicin and verapamil. *Journal of Pharmacy and Pharmaceutical Sciences.* 2007 Jul 21;10(3):350–7.

60. Cao X, Luo J, Gong T, Zhang ZR, Sun X, Fu Y. Coencapsulated doxorubicin and bromotetrandrine lipid nanoemulsions in reversing multidrug resistance in breast cancer in vitro and in vivo. *Molecular Pharmaceutics.* 2015 Jan 5;12(1):274–86.

61. Li B, Zhang R, Xiu X, Tao Z, Chen L, Xie Z, et al. Ferromagnetism of Ni-doped ZnO powders prepared by sol-gel method above room temperature. *Journal of Rare Earths.* 2006;24(SUPPL.):186–8.

62. Chavanpatil MD, Khdair A, Gerard B, Bachmeier C, Miller DW, Shekhar MPV, et al. Surfactant-polymer nanoparticles overcome P-glycoprotein-mediated drug efflux. *Molecular Pharmaceutics.* 2007 Sep;4(5):730–8.

63. Lamprecht A, Benoit JP. Etoposide nanocarriers suppress glioma cell growth by intracellular drug delivery and simultaneous P-glycoprotein inhibition. *Journal of Controlled Release.* 2006;112(2):208–13.

64. Wang JC, Goh BC, Lu WL, Zhang Q, Chang A, Liu XY, et al. In vitro cytotoxicity of stealth liposomes co-encapsulating doxorubicin and verapamil on doxorubicin-resistant tumor cells. *Biological and Pharmaceutical Bulletin.* 2005 May;28(5):822–8.

65. Bang KH, Na YG, Huh HW, Hwang SJ, Kim MS, Kim M, et al. The delivery strategy of paclitaxel nanostructured lipid carrier coated with platelet membrane. *Cancers (Basel).* 2019;11(6):11.

66. Chen Y, Bathula SR, Li J, Huang L. Multifunctional nanoparticles delivering small interfering RNA and doxorubicin overcome drug resistance in cancer. *Journal of Biological Chemistry.* 2010 Jul 16;285(29):22639–50.

67. Punfa W, Suzuki S, Pitchakarn P, Yodkeeree S, Naiki T, Takahashi S, et al. Curcumin-loaded PLGA nanoparticles conjugated with anti-P-glycoprotein antibody to overcome multidrug resistance. *Asian Pacific Journal of Cancer Prevention.* 2014;15(21):9249–58.

10 Progress in Nanocarrier-Mediated Intracellular Drug Delivery

Sabyasachi Maiti, Rishi Paliwal, and Harsh Yadav

10.1 INTRODUCTION

Drug delivery is difficult since different biologically active compounds must be transported intracellularly. It is better to get therapeutic effects inside the cytoplasm; on the nucleus; or on other cell organelles such as mitochondria, lysosomes, or the endoplasmic reticulum. Drug delivery can be done by injecting drugs, proteins, enzymes, antibodies, or nanocarriers loaded with drugs inside the cell. Drug delivery methods are being worked on at the nanoscale level to solve the problems of non-specificity, poor pharmacokinetics, insufficient treatment efficacy, and high systemic toxicity [1]. Drug delivery systems must also get past several biological barriers to get therapeutic compounds to a specific pathological site. The vehicles must exhibit high stability and prolonged circulation in the bloodstream to overcome extracellular obstacles [2]. So far, the intracellular barrier has been shown to impede drug release by preventing endocytosis, endosomal escape, and controlled drug release [3]. Due to the enhanced permeability and retention (EPR) effect, nanoparticles may be able to get through biological barriers. In order to release therapeutic molecules at the targeted site, an effective drug reservoir must be created with the flexibility of modification. For this, various nanostructures, such as micelles, liposomes, polymer-drug conjugates, dendrimers, and metal-based nanoparticles, have been investigated. The delivery of anticancer medicines inside cells is particularly important. The EPR effect can attract the right-sized nanoparticles to the tumor site [4, 5].

Various nanostructures, such as micelles, liposomes, polymer-drug conjugates, dendrimers, and metal-based nanoparticles, have been investigated for this. The delivery of anticancer medicines inside the cells is particularly important. The EPR effect can attract the right-sized nanoparticles to the tumor site [4, 5].

When compared to typical tissue, tumor tissue has distinct intracellular microenvironments, including high levels of GSH (2–10 mM) and a low pH (4.5–6.5) [6]. These biological characteristics can be used to create nanocarriers for intracellular drug release that are pH, temperature, and redox sensitive.

In the past 10 years, there has been a lot of importance in crafting stimuli-triggered nanocarriers that release therapeutic chemicals in reaction to intracellular signals from tumors, particularly those with high pH and redox potential. To deliver anticancer drugs intracellularly, reduction-responsive polymeric carriers that are stable enough in external environments but quickly destabilize in response to intracellular pH, enzymes, and redox have been created and tested. These stimuli-responsive nanocarriers have shown good blood stability and redox-triggered drug release in the cell nucleus and cytosol. This has led to a significant increase in antitumor activity compared to the reduction-insensitive counterparts.

The pH-sensitive nanovehicles are intended to interfere with transportation mechanisms and release medications into endosomal and/or lysosomal compartments (pH 5.5 and 4.5, respectively). It is very well known that the therapeutic efficacy of nanocarriers depends critically on the successful escape of nanocarriers from the intracellular endosomes or lysosomes [7]. The nanocarriers are

DOI: 10.1201/9781003130055-10

taken up by the cells by the process of cellular uptake and then trapped by endosomes and lysosomes [8, 9]. The drug is then quickly released from the endosome/lysosome as a result of low pH of the endosome/lysosome breaking the chemical links that are responsible for labile acidity [10]. In this chapter, the research findings in the field of pH- and glutathione (GSH)-sensitive nanocarriers for intracellular drug delivery are discussed.

10.2 APPROACHES FOR INTRACELLULAR DRUG DELIVERY

10.2.1 REDOX-RESPONSIVE POLYMERIC MICELLES

Researchers are considering making redox-sensitive nanocarriers to deliver anticancer drugs inside cancer cells, owing to higher levels of GSH than normal cells (about 2–10 mM) [11]. In animal cells, GSH/glutathione disulfide is a crucial redox pair that controls their antioxidative potency [12]. Nicotinamide adenine dinucleotide phosphate hydrogen (NADPH) and glutathione reductase keep GSH/GSSG from being decreased. Also, the endosomal compartment is redox active. Arunachalam et al. [13] found that the redox potential is controlled by the gamma-interferon-inducible lysosomalthiol reductase (GILT) enzyme when cysteine is co-present but not when GSH is present. This change in GSH concentration has made it possible to make GSH-responsive nanocarriers for accurate drug delivery inside cells. The glutathione-responsive nanocarriers can release the entrapped bioactive molecules at a faster rate, resulting in an appreciable therapeutic effect. The mechanism of glutathione responsive intracellular drug delivery is depicted in Figure 10.1.

Kamimura et al. [14] found that pH-sensitive nanoparticles made of poly(ethylene glycol) (PEG)-*b*-poly(4-vinylbenzylphosphonate) block copolymers could hold 320 mg doxorubicin (DOX)/g. The nanoparticles entered the cells through the endocytic pathway and settled in the late endosome or lysosome. The DOX then moved through the cytoplasm and into nuclei because the acidic pH caused the phosphonate groups on the polymer chains to become protonated. So, the nanoparticles

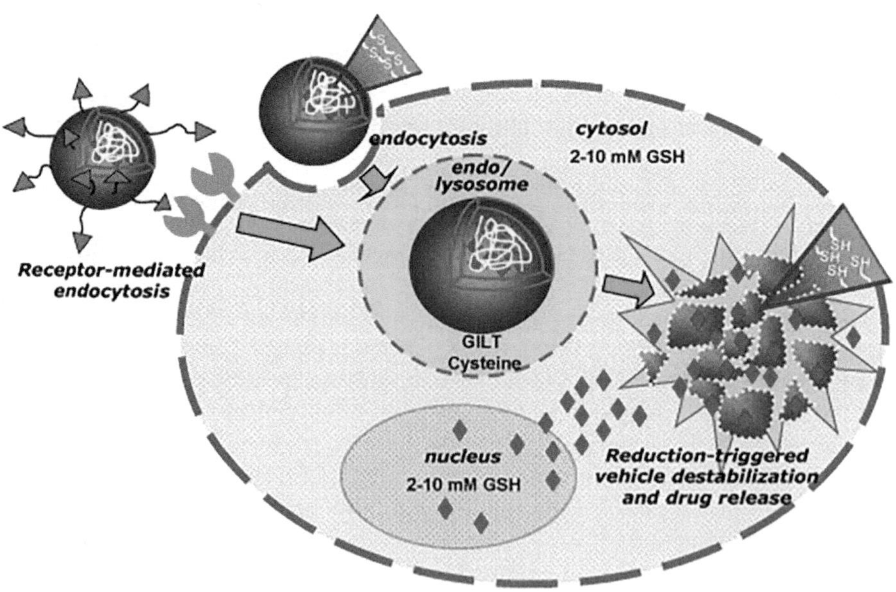

FIGURE 10.1 Intracellular trafficking pathway of GSH-responsive nano-vehicles showing cellular internalization, endosomal escape, reduction-triggered vehicle degradation, and drug release phases. Reproduced with permission from [6].

could get rid of the efflux mechanisms of P-gp overexpressed KB/MRP cancer cells and entered the nuclei of cancer cells, making them effective chemotherapy for MDR cancer cells. Khorsand et al. [15] looked into how well an amphiphilic poly(ethylene oxide) (PEO)-*b*-disulfide-labeled polymethacrylate copolymer could carry DOX inside cells. Within 5 hours of being exposed to GSH, more than 70% of the DOX that had been encapsulated was released due to the breaking of disulfide bonds of micellar cores. GSH caused the micelles to become less stable and DOX to be released faster from HeLa cancer cells. This system shows a lot of promise for delivering drugs inside cells. Zhang and his group [16] made poly (ɤ-benzyl-L-glutamate)-*b*-dextran copolymer micelles whose dextran shells were crosslinked with 3,3-dithiodipropionic acid. In phosphate-buffered saline (PBS), the disulfide-crosslinked micelles were stable, but they broke apart in a reducing environment that mimicked the conditions inside cells. In 12 hours, about 75% of the doxorubicin was quickly released in PBS with 0.01M GSH. The redox response was also tested *in vitro* on cervical cancer cells after they were treated with glutathione monoester, which raises the level of GSH inside the cell. HeLa and HepG2 cells previously treated with glutathione monoester were much less likely to multiply than control cells. Wang and his colleagues [17] added hydrophobic groups and pH-sensitive urocanic acid to pullulan. Doxorubicin was successfully loaded with the help of urocanyl and cholesterol succinylpullulan. As the degree of substitution of the cholesterol moiety went from 3.5 to 8.7, the pH-sensitive drug release property got worse. This may be because the cholesterol moiety forms a dense hydrophobic core. The nanoparticles with DS values of 6.8% and 3.5% for urocanyl and cholesterol, respectively, showed the strongest response to pH-induced drug release. The best drug release was seen at endosomal pH. This could be because the protonation of urocanyl moieties causes endosomes to swell and burst. After being taken in by MCF-7 cells, the nanoparticles delivered DOX to the cell nucleus. Cao et al. [18] made pH- and redox-sensitive methoxy polyethylene glycol (mPEG)-benzoic-imine linked-poly (ɛ-caprolactone)-S-S-poly(ɛ-caprolactone) that could self-assemble into doxorubicin-filled nanoparticles. At pH 5.0 with GSH (10 mM), the amount of drug release was double what it was at pH 7.4 without GSH. Under an acidic condition, the benzoic-imine linkers were broken. Under a redox condition, the disulfide bonds in the copolymer were changed into thiols. The carriers enhanced drug release in HeLa cells in higher GSH concentrations. Both pH and redox sensitivity made it easier for the drug to be released in a simulated tumor environment and for drug molecules to enter the nuclei of cells to have a better effect against cancer.

Chen et al. [19] crafted a diselenide core-crosslinked mPEGylated starch copolymer by reacting 3,3'-diselanediyldipropanoic acid with starch and loaded DOX in the micellar core by the dialysis method. In a normal physiological environment, the crosslinked micelles were very stable. The low energy of diselenide bonds enabled micelles to release the drug more quickly and completely at 10 mM GSH, which is similar to the microenvironment inside a tumor cell. About 84% of DOX was discharged from the diselenide core, but only 60% was released from the disulfide core in 120 h in presence of 10 mM GSH. Cellular uptake studies in mouse TC1 lung cells showed that high GSH quickly broke the diselenide bonds in the cytoplasm, resulting in intracellular drug release from the micelles and the entry of doxorubicin into the cell nucleus, where it could interact with DNA and stop the growth of tumors. Song and his colleagues [20] made paclitaxel-loaded hyaluronic acid-S-S-vitamin E succinate nanoconjugates. The nanocarriers showed significantly higher cytotoxicity and apoptosis-inducing activity on CD44 overexpressed A549 tumor cells than insensitive nanoparticles and Taxol. When mice with A549 tumors were given the nanoparticles, they showed the best antitumor effect (75.4% tumor inhibition) with the least side effects.

Block copolymer nanomicelles can be engineered to have micelle cores that are responsive to reduction and cores that are sensitive to acid at the core/corona contact. This type of stimulus-responsive degradation can enable synergistic/accelerated drug release at two different sites [21]. In line with this, Jazani et al. [22] reported a diblock copolymer made of a hydrophilic PEG block connected by a acid-cleavable ketal linkage to a hydrophobic methacrylate block with hanging disulfide linkages. They thought that the ketal linkages would cleave at the core/shell interface in endosomal or lysosomal pH, and then the pendant disulfides would break under the action of glutathione in the cell. This would throw off balance between hydrophobic and hydrophilic groups in the micelle cores and speed up the release of doxorubicin, which would stop the growth of HeLa cells. As a consequence of sluggish and insufficient drug release, non-pH-responsive micelles may establish ineffective drug levels inside the target cells [23]. To effectively kill tumor cells, smart micelles must be created with the capacity for endosomal escape and quick drug release. The fundamental changes in acidity of solid tumors and normal tissues made the pH-sensitive polymeric particles seem to be very attractive. Yang et al. [24] found that paclitaxel-loaded poly (ethylene glycol)-phenylhydrazone-dilaurate micelles were pH-sensitive and biocompatible. More drug was released than was seen at pH 7.4 as a result of the copolymer's hydrazone bond breakdown at pH 5.5. The dissociation of the micelles from the endosome was accelerated by the hydrolysis of the copolymer in A549 cells. The effective endo/lysosomal escape of pH-sensitive carriers dictated an improved anticancer impact. Luo et al. [25] noticed the formation of chitosan-cystamine-retinoic acid conjugate micelles in water. Disulfide bonds disrupted when the micelles were exposed to PBS (pH 7.4) containing GSH (10 mM) for 48 hours. This caused 63.7% of the paclitaxel to be released quickly. Up to 200 g/ml, the blank micelles did not kill LO-2 cells when they carried drugs. HepG2 cells were killed much more by the drug-loaded micelles than by the drug alone. By simultaneously releasing retinoic acid and paclitaxel, the two agents activated receptor-mediated apoptosis, thereby exerting synergistic anticancer effects through RA-mediated sensitization. HepG2 cells ingested micellar particles in a time- and concentration-dependent way via clathrin-mediated endocytosis and macropinocytosis. The micelles allowed paclitaxel to reach the cell nucleus of HepG2 cells and made it easier for paclitaxel to work by preventing natural microtubule depolymerization.

In mammals, heparosan serves as a natural precursor to producing heparin. In vivo, glucuronidase and hexosaminidase degrade this into N-acetylglucosamine and glucuronic acid in lysosomes. The cells then recycle the monosaccharides so they don't accumulate in tissues [26]. This indicated that heparosan is biocompatible [27]. Qiu et al. [28] developed redox-sensitive heparosan-cystamine-vitamin E succinate micelles to administer doxorubicin intracellularly. The disulfide bond was in charge of the copolymer's redox sensitivity. In a simulated tumor microenvironment, the device delivered roughly 77–82% of the medication with reasonable serum stability (PBS containing GSH, pH 5.0). The redox-sensitive micelles showed more toxicity than non-sensitive heparosan-adipic acid dihydrazide-tocopherol succinate micelles in human gastric cancer cell lines due to enhanced cellular uptake and drug release.

The linear polysaccharide hyaluronic acid, which is non-toxic, biocompatible, and biodegradable, has affinity towards CD44 receptors overexpressed on the surface of many cancer cells. Liu et al. [29] connected hexadecanol-modified hyaluronic acid with mPEG-S-S-COOH via ester linkage. The micellar carriers released 74.3% paclitaxel after 24 hours in media supplemented with GSH. Compared to Taxol, the developed paclitaxel formulations showed better antitumor effectiveness and cytotoxicity on MCF-7 cells in a dose-dependent manner. This can happen because paclitaxel is quickly released from the micelles and gets into the cells well. In Kunming mice carrying the H22 tumor, the micelles exhibited about 65% tumor inhibition.

Zheng et al. [30] developed polyion complex micelles of cyclic arginyl-glycyl-aspartic acid peptide (cRGD)-modified PEG-*b*-poly(L-lysine) and dimethylmaleic anhydride-modified doxorubicin for intracellular transport of doxorubicin. The purpose of attaching the cRGD was to improve the cell uptake of micelles by specifically recognizing the αvβ3 integrin on the tumor cell membranes. With the dissolution of the micelles, the intracellular acidic microenvironment assumed effective drug release. Furthermore, compared to insensitive controls, the targeted micelles showed improved inhibitory efficacies toward hepatoma. The intelligent, multipurpose micelles offered a potential base for targeted cancer therapy.

The properties of the stimuli-responsive polymeric micelles are shown in Table 10.1.

TABLE 10.1

Properties and Mechanisms of Intracellular Drug Release from Polymeric Micelles

Polymeric Micellar System	Particle Size (nm)	Drug Loading Content	Drug Entrapment Efficiency	CAC (mg/L)	Mechanism of Intracellular Drug Release	Reference
Poly(ethylene glycol)-*b*-poly(4-vinylbenzylphosphonate)	42	–	32%	–	• Endocytosis revealed pH-sensitive drug release. • MDR cancer cells lack the efflux mechanism and are localized in the nuclei.	[14]
PEO-b-polymethacrylate copolymer having pendant disulfide linkage	174	0.44%	–	49	• Redox-cleavage of disulfide core assisted intracellular release of DOX.	[15]
Poly(γ-benzyl-L-glutamate)-block-dextran (PBLG-b-dextran) copolymers	158	12.6%	75.6%	–	• Endocytosis is followed by GSH-accelerated breakdown of the disulfide crosslinker and intracellular drug release, followed by localization in the cell nucleus.	[16]
Urocanyl and cholesterol succinylpullulan	198	17.2%	57.3%	24.2	• Endocytosis, endosomal localization, and swelling at the acidic pH of the endosome as a result of protonation of urcanyl moieties. • Water and ion influx, endosome bursting, and medication release into the cytoplasm before being transported to the cell nucleus to exert its therapeutic effect.	[17]
Methoxy PEG-benzoic-imine—poly(ε-caprolactone—SS-poly (ε-caprolactone-Hy-mPEG) and triblock copolymer	93–118	4.2%	58–84%	10	• Redox-sensitive breakage of disulfide bonds.	[18]
Diselenide core-crosslinked PEGylated starch copolymer	160	3.5%	22.3%.	23	• Release of DOX from micelles inside the cell and subsequent localization of DOX in the cell nucleus are the results of diselenide bonds breaking under conditions of high GSH concentration in the cytoplasm.	[19]
Hyaluronic acid-disulfide-vitamin E succinate	175	33.5%	90.6%	36.3	• Cellular uptake initiated by CD44 receptor-mediated endocytosis. • Breakage of redox-sensitive disulfide bond by reducing agents.	[20]

(Continued)

TABLE 10.1   (Continued)

Properties and Mechanisms of Intracellular Drug Release from Polymeric Micelles

Polymeric Micellar System	Particle Size (nm)	Drug Loading Content	Drug Entrapment Efficiency	CAC (mg/L)	Mechanism of Intracellular Drug Release	Reference
PEG-*b*-methacrylate having pendant disulfide linkages	116	2.5%	–	8.2	• Disulfide pendant cleavage is degraded by an acidic pH and a reduction-responsive mechanism.	[22]
Poly (ethylene glycol)-phenylhydrazone-dilaurate	135	3.2%	65–68%	7.5	• Endocytosis pathway and endo/lysosomal escape. • The chemical bond that is acid-labile hydrolyzes when the pH changes.	[24]
Chitosan-cystamine-retinoic acid conjugate	128	13.9%	91.3%	26	• Clathrin-mediated endocytosis and macropinocytosis. • Drug release from intracellular storage and accumulation in the tumor via the EPR effect.	[25]
Heparosan-cystamine-vitamin E succinate	90–120	13%–15%	88%–90%	16.5–18.5	• Clathrin-mediated endocytosis. • GSH-responsive drug release in tumor cell environment (pH 5.0).	[28]
mPEG-S-S-hyaluronic acid-C10	168	14.7%	86%	10.5	• Fast absorption of micelles by cells. • EPR effect and receptor-mediated endocytosis lead to accumulation in the tumor. • Disulfide linkages in mPEG-SS-HA-C16 are broken in the presence of GSH.	[29]
cRGD-modified poly(ethylene glycol)-*block*-poly(L-lysine)	80–110	10.0%	95.0%	–	• Enhanced cell uptake caused by internalization of the ligand receptor.	[30]

10.2.2 pH-Sensitive Liposomes

Under very acidic conditions, pH-sensitive liposomes can help endosomes fuse or become less stable, which moves their cargo into the cell. In Salmonella-, Listeria-, and Mycobacteria-caused intracellular infections, antibiotics must get into the site of infection inside the cell to reach the right therapeutic concentration. Even though many antibiotics work in the lab, they often don't work against bacterial infections inside cells. This is because they don't get into cells well below the maximum tolerable dose or because lysosomal enzymes break them down [31] (Kumana & Yuen 1994). For gentamicin intracellular delivery, Lutwyche et al. [32] created dioleoylphosphatidyl ethanolamine-based liposomes, enhancing the drug's therapeutic effectiveness against intracellular infections. The liposomes eradicated intracellular infections and killed more than 75% of the intracellular *Salmonella typhimurium*. In conclusion, the study hypothesized that treating intracellular infections would benefit from encapsulating membrane-impermeable antibiotics in suitable lipid-based carriers. Due to their capacity for endo/lysosome escape, pH-sensitive liposomes are particularly promising nanocarriers; nevertheless, PEG coating reduces their pH responsiveness. Kanamala et al. [33] created PEG-cleavable pH-sensitive liposomes emphasizing the intracellular PEG-detachment technique. They used a hydrazide–hydrazone bond to conjugate PEG2000 with a phospholipid. When compared to control pH-sensitive liposomes, the liposomes significantly accumulated in the MIA PaCa-2 xenograft model and demonstrated quick endo/lysosome escape capability in cancer cells. Hyaluronic acid (HA) that is pH-sensitive, CD44-targeted, and 2-carboxycyclohexane-1-carboxylated was created by Miyazaki and his research team [34]. To do this, the carboxyl groups of the modified and unmodified hyaluronic acid polymers were coupled with 1-aminodecane. This allowed the polymers to adhere to the membranes of liposomes. These phosphatidylcholine liposomes from egg yolks treated with polymers demonstrated their durability at neutral pH but discharged the load in mildly acidic circumstances. The delivery of the actives into CD44-expressing cells was more effective with 2-carboxycyclohexane-1-carboxylated HA-modified liposomes than with HA-modified, 3-methyl-glutarylated HA-modified or untreated liposomes. The doxorubicin encapsulation efficiency ranged from 70 to 80% for 3-methyl-glutarylated HA-C10-modified liposomes (150 nm) and 2-carboxycyclohexane-1-carboxylated HA-C10-modified liposomes but was >95% for unmodified liposomes and HA-C10-modified liposomes (140 nm). This might be because the drug-loaded modified liposomes were made in a pH 6.0 aqueous solution, which slightly destabilized the liposomal membrane. Yet, even after drug loading, the liposomes retained their nanoscale size and surface charge. These liposomes used the endo/lysosomes' pH-responsive membrane disruption capabilities to transfer anticancer drugs to the inside cells. Therefore, as a CD44-positive cell-specific intracellular drug delivery system, the pH-sensitive HA derivative-modified liposomes showed potential. Tang and colleagues [35] tested pH-sensitive liposomes functionalized with hyaluronic acid to overcome gemcitabine resistance in pancreatic cancer. Using a carbodiimide reaction, the polymer carboxylic acid was conjugated with the amines of 1,2-dioleoyl-sn-glycero-3-phosphoethanolamine to decorate a liposomal system with a polymeric surface. The capacity of liposomes to escape endosomes was unaffected by HA's facilitation of cellular uptake and cytotoxic nature. However, the ability of HA to partially resensitize cancer cells to gemcitabine therapy was recognized because the tumor cells continued to grow following treatment. Overall, there was just a slight improvement in overcoming gemcitabine resistance. A combination of pressure and temperature-mediated intracellular drug delivery method was put out by Yudina et al. [36] At 37°C, temperature-sensitive liposomes were loaded with a cell-permeable TO-PRO-3 dye capable of displaying intense fluorescence upon binding to nucleic acids. The dye can be released when exposed to mild hyperthermia at 42°C. After the ultrasound cavitated the microbubbles to make the cell membrane more permeable, the dye was sent to the cytosol and the nucleus. This method seemed to work well for the intracellular distribution of drugs that can't get into cells and are quickly broken down or cleared out of the bloodstream. Dhawan and colleagues [37] reported redox-responsive, self-assembled cystine-tryptophan dipeptide vesicles for doxorubicin intracellular release. The vesicles entered HeLa and MDA-MB-231 cells, where they released their cargo in response to GSH levels. Because of the high cytosolic GSH concentration, these naturally occurring peptide-based carriers disintegrated inside cells, creating new opportunities for targeted drug delivery.

10.2.3 METAL-BASED NANOPARTICLES

Banerjee and Chen [38] proposed adipic dihydrazide-grafted gum arabic-modified magnetic nanoparticles (34.2 nm) for targeted release of doxorubicin to tumor cells. The gum arabic modified magnetic nanoparticles displayed near-infrared fluorescence characteristics. Around 6.52 mg/g of doxorubicin was paired. The hydrolysis of the C=N bond caused the nanoparticles to release 74% of the medication after 5 hours at pH 5.0. This system demonstrated synchronous imaging, sensing, and pH-sensitive drug targeting. Gum arabic surface modification of nanoparticles opens up a new route for developing hepatocyte-specific diagnostic or therapeutic agents for treating liver malignancies and other hepatocytic disorders since gum arabic can interact with asialoglycoprotein receptors of hepatocytes. With a pore diameter of 2.3 nm, Moghaddam et al. [39] developed GSH-responsive mesoporous silica nanoparticles of 130 nm size. Due to the substantial voids in the hollow architectures, the particles demonstrated a high DOX loading capacity of 9%. In simulating the intracellular tumor microenvironment (PBS, pH 6.0 supplemented with 10 mM GSH), over 60% DOX release was noticed within 14 days. It's possible that the presence of lysosomal thiol-reductase enzyme caused the nanoparticles to lose their hollow form and undergo destruction in endocytic compartments [13, 40]. Almost 50% of the cells in endolysosomal environments of MCF-7 cancer cells were destroyed by the DOX-loaded nanospheres (6 µg/ml). Chen et al. [41] created dual-pH-sensitive mesoporous silica nanoparticles for the intracellular release of doxorubicin. Benzoboric acid–functionalized nanoparticles were produced by interacting amine-functionalized silica nanoparticles with 3-(bromomethyl)phenylboronic acid. Mono-6-deoxy-6-EDA-cyclodextrin (β-CD-NH$_2$) was added after DOX loading to fill the pores by forming a pH-sensitive boronate ester bond, resulting in DOX-loaded β-CD-NH$_2$ capped nanoparticles. Another pH-sensitive benzoic imine link was also introduced on subsequent reaction of the nanoparticles with methoxypoly(ethylene glycol) benzaldehyde. The generated nanoparticles had a drug entrapment effectiveness of 56.8% and an average diameter of roughly 292 nm. At pH 5.0, the boronate ester linkages were broken, causing the DOX to be released quickly (65.3% in 8 hours). The hydrolysis of imine bonds caused the detachment of mPEG and the release of positively charged amino groups at the extracellular matrix pH of tumor tissues (pH 6.5), which resulted in approximately 3.4-fold higher uptake of the drug carriers in HeLa cell than that observed at pH 7.4. The drug carriers that were left blank showed good cell biocompatibility. The mesoporous nanoparticles with dual pH sensitivity may increase cancer cell medication uptake. In a different study, intracellular delivery of DOX was achieved using 150 nm-sized calcium carbonate ($CaCO_3$) core crosslinked mPEG-*b*-poly(L-glutamic acid) nanoparticles [42]. The nanoparticles had a 14.6% drug loading capacity and a 52.3% drug loading efficiency, respectively. Due to decomposition of the $CaCO_3$ mineral under acidic conditions, the nanoparticles released 76.2% more DOX at pH 5.5 than at pH 7.4. The nanoparticles showed superior cell uptake by murine osteosarcoma K7 cells after prolonged incubation and acid-responsive sustained DOX release via mineralization of $CaCO_3$.

10.2.4 OTHER NANOSYSTEMS

Lee and his colleagues [43] produced nanogels via polyionic complexation of poly (diethylene-triaminepentaacetic dianhydride-co-cystamine) and mPEG-*b*-poly(L-lysine), followed by genipin cross-linking. The loading capacity and drug loading efficiency were 33.6% and 8.4%, respectively. Disulfide bond breakage caused the nanogels to disintegrate in acidic and reductive environments. Under the impact of the acidic and reductive environment of the endosome/lysosome after endocytosis by the U-87 MG cells, the nanogels released the compounds into the cytoplasm. As a result, against U-87 MG cells, the curcumin nanogels demonstrated a significantly higher level of cellular growth inhibition than free curcumin. Short cationic peptides (cell penetrating peptides) are effective at moving cargo across cell membranes [44]. In terms of intracellular drug delivery, Tat has been used the most extensively. Li and colleagues [45] created nanoparticles by coupling dendrigraft poly-L-lysine (DGL) with Tat-KK peptide that has been PEG-grafted. In order to minimize the cationic toxicity caused by electrostatic interaction between the nanoparticles and normal cell membrane, dimethylmaleic anhydride was reacted to amidatelysine in Tat-KK peptide. This created pH-sensitive β-carboxylic amide which was sensitive to hydrolysis at an acidic environment. Due to highly dendritic structure and the electrostatic interaction between the positively charged DOX and the negatively charged DGL-PEG-Tat-KK-DMA, the loading efficiencies and DOX loading content were 74.6% and 29.5%, respectively. The release rate was around three times higher at acidic pH 5.0 than it was at neutral pH. Under the acidic pH, HepG2 cells significantly increased cellular uptake and cytotoxicity. Due to the nanoparticles' selective internalization and pH-sensitive intracellular drug release, they demonstrated superior anticancer activity in tumor-bearing animals, with tumor inhibition 1.48 times higher than with free drug.

The anti-inflammatory and antioxidant compound N-acetyl-L-cysteine has much potential for treating conditions including stroke and neuroinflammation. Navath et al. [46] developed GSH-sensitive poly(amidoamine) dendrimer-cysteine conjugates for intracellular delivery. The dendrimer conjugates increased the cysteine concentration inside the cells, and consequently GSH-sensitive cleavage allowed effective and quick cellular drug release. Surfactants based on lysine were added to tripolyphosphate-chitosan nanoparticles [47]. At pH 7.4, the nanostructures (170–328 nm) barely generated any membrane permeabilization, but at the acidic pH of endosomes, the membrane-destabilizing activity was visible. Few cytotoxic effects were seen when these pH-responsive NPs were used to treat 3T3 fibroblasts. Lysine-based amphiphiles were incorporated into chitosan carriers to create pH-sensitive membranolytic and maybe endosomolytic nanocarriers, which appeared to be the best choice for intracellular drug delivery. TPP-crosslinked folic-thiolated chitosan (FTC) nanoparticles of 250–360 nm size were developed by Mazzotta et al. [48] for the purpose of delivering methotrexate to cervical cancer cells. The drug entrapment varied from 18 to 56%. In vitro, the particles demonstrated redox-responsive drug release. Also, compared to non-target particles, functionalized nanoparticles had a greater inhibitory effect on cell proliferation. Via folate receptors, nanoparticles were selectively taken up by cells. The carriers overall demonstrated promise for effective intracellular anticancer medication delivery. After the Schiff-base reaction between 4,4-dihydrazide diphenyl disulfide and benzene-1,3,5-tricarbaldehyde, Wang and colleagues [49] created a crystalline porous polymer. After ultrasonication of hydrazone, an acid-cleavable material, and a porous polymer having redox-responsive disulfide links, along with co-assembly with Poloxamer 188, nanoparticles were created. A drug loading percentage of around 18% was achieved thanks to the potent hydrophobic contacts and pi–pi stacking interactions between the aromatic rings of nanocarriers and doxorubicin. Under a simulated tumor cell microenvironment, the carriers dissolved and quickly released doxorubicin (approximately 50% in 4 hours). The adsorption of Poloxamer 188 PEG chains onto the surface of nanocarriers increased the water dispersibility and long-circulating property of nanoparticles. The medication was released from the nanocarriers in response to an acidic pH and GSH. HepG2 cells ingested the nanocarriers through an endocytosis process. The dual-sensitive acid and redox nanocarriers assumed exceptionally high drug concentration within HepG2 tumor cells when compared to free drugs and, as a result, are anticipated to realize improved anticancer efficacy.

10.3 CONCLUSION

In this chapter, recent progress in intracellular delivery of drugs was assessed. It was noted that pH- and glutathione-responsive polymeric micelles had enormous potential for intracellular delivery of anticancer agents. The rapid instability of nanocarriers inside cells to release drugs into the cell nucleus and cytosol is known to be caused by the acidic endosomal/lysosomal pH and greater glutathione content. The potential for effective intracellular drug administration using pH- and GSH-responsive nanocarriers, such as polymeric nanomicelles, modified liposomes, metal-based nanoparticles, nanogels, and dendrimers, could maximize drug efficacy and/or decrease drug and drug carrier-associated side effects. Uncertainty still exists regarding the precise intracellular fate of reduction-sensitive nanocarriers. Future clinical use of these new devices would be enabled by a deeper understanding of intracellular trafficking and the outcomes of nanocarriers.

REFERENCES

1. Ge Z, Liu S. Functional block copolymer assemblies responsive to tumor and intracellular microenvironments for site-specific drug delivery and enhanced imaging performance. *Chem Soc Rev.* 2013 Apr;42:7289–325.
2. Elsabahy M, Wooley KL. Design of polymeric nanoparticles for biomedical delivery applications. *Chem Soc Rev.* 2012 Apr 7;41(7):2545–61.
3. Nie S. Understanding and overcoming major barriers in cancer nanomedicine. *Nanomedicine (London).* 2010 Jun;5(4):523–8.
4. Park JH, Lee S, Kim JH, Park K, Kim K, Kwon IC. Polymeric nanomedicine for cancer therapy. *Prog Polym Sci.* 2008 Jan;33(1):113–37.
5. Maeda H, Nakamura H, Fang J. The EPR effect for macromolecular drug delivery to solid tumors: Improvement of tumor uptake, lowering of systemic toxicity, and distinct tumor imaging in vivo. *Adv Drug Deliv Rev.* 2013 Jan;65(1):71–9.
6. Cheng R, Feng F, Meng F, Deng C, Feijen J, Zhong Z. Glutathione-responsive nano-vehicles as a promising platform for targeted intracellular drug and gene delivery. *J Control Release.* 2011 May;152(1):2–12.
7. Qiu L, Zhu M, Gong K. pH-triggered degradable polymeric micelles for targeted anti-tumor drug delivery. *Mater Sci Eng C.* 2017 Sept;78:912–22.
8. Chou LY, Ming K, Chan WC. Strategies for the intracellular delivery of nanoparticles. *Chem Soc Rev.* 2011 Jan;40(1):233–45.
9. Varkouhi AK, Scholte M, Storm G, Haisma HJ. Endosomal escape pathways for delivery of biologicals. *J Control Release.* 2011 May;151(3):220–28.
10. Fang XB, Zhang JM, Xie X, Liu D, He C-W, Wan J-B, Chen M-W. pH-sensitive micelles based on acid-labile pluronic F68-curcumin conjugates for improved tumor intracellular drug delivery. *Int J Pharm.* 2016 Apr 11;502(1–2):28–37.
11. Schafer FQ, Buettner GR. Redox environment of the cell as viewed through the redox state of the glutathione disulfide/glutathione couple. *Free Radic Biol Med.* 2001 Jun;30(11):1191–212.
12. Wu G, Fang Y-Z, Yang S, Lupton JR, Turner ND. Glutathione metabolism and its implications for health. *J Nutr.* 2004 Mar;134(3):489–92.
13. Arunachalam B, Phan UT, Geuze HJ, Cresswell P. Enzymatic reduction of disulfide bonds in lysosomes: Characterization of a gamma-interferon-inducible lysosomal thiol reductase (GILT). *Proc. Natl Acad Sci USA.* 2000 Jan;97(2):745–50.
14. Kamimura M, Furukawa T, Akiyama S, Nagasaki Y. Enhanced intracellular drug delivery of pH-sensitive doxorubicin/poly(ethylene glycol)-block-poly-(4-vinylbenzyl phosphonate) nanoparticles in multi-drug resistant human epidermoid KB carcinoma cells. *Biomater Sci.* 2013 Jan;1:361–67.
15. Khorsand B, Lapointe G, Brett C, Oh JK. Intracellular drug delivery nanocarriers of glutathione-responsive degradable block copolymers having pendant disulfide linkages. *Biomacromolecules.* 2013 Jun;14(6):2103–11.
16. Zhang A, Zhang Z, Shi F, Xiao C, Ding J, Zhuang X, He C, Chen L, Chen X. Redox-sensitive shell-crosslinked polypeptide block-polysaccharide micelles for efficient intracellular anticancer drug delivery. *Macromol Biosci.* 2013 Sep;13(9):1249–58.
17. Wang Y, Liu Y, Liu Y, Wang Y, Wu J, Li R, Yang J, Zhang N. pH-sensitive pullulan-based nanoparticles for intracellular drug delivery. *Polym Chem.* 2014 Aug;5:423–32.
18. Cao Y, Zhao J, Zhang, Y, Liu J, Liu J, Dong A, Deng L. pH/redox dual-sensitive nanoparticles based on PCL/PEG triblock copolymer for enhanced intracellular doxorubicin release. *RSC Adv.* 2015 Mar;5:28060–69.
19. Chen M, Gao C, Lu S, Chen Y, Mingzhu L. Preparation of redox-sensitive, core-crosslinked micelles selfassembled from mPEGylated starch conjugates: Remarkable extracellular stability and rapid intracellular drug release. *RSC Adv.* 2016 Apr;6:46159–69.

20. Song Y, Cai H, Yin T, Huo M, Ma P, Zhou J, Lai W. Paclitaxel-loaded redox-sensitive nanoparticles based on hyaluronic acid-vitamin Esuccinate conjugates for improved lung cancer treatment. *Int J Nanomedicine*. 2018 Mar;13:1585–1600.

21. Sun T, Li P, Oh JK. Dual location dual reduction/photoresponsive block copolymer micelles: Disassembly and synergistic release. *Macromol Rapid Commun*. 2015 Oct;36(19):1742–48.

22. Jazani AM, Arezi N, Shetty C, Hong SH, Li H, Wang X, Oh JK. Tumor-targeting intracellular drug delivery based on dual acid/reduction-degradable nanoassemblies with ketal interface and disulfide core locations. *Polym Chem*. 2019 May;10:2840–53.

23. Wu H, Zhu L, Torchilin VP. pH-sensitive poly(histidine)-PEG/DSPE-PEG co-polymer micelles for cytosolic drug delivery. *Biomaterials*. 2013 Jan;34(4):1213–22.

24. Yang Y, Wang Z, Peng Y, Ding J, Zhou W. A smart pH-sensitive delivery system for enhanced anticancer efficacy via paclitaxel endosomal escape. *Front Pharmacol*. 2019 Jan;24(10):10.

25. Luo T, Han J, Zhao F, Pan X, Tian B, Ding X, Zhang J. Redox-sensitive micelles based on retinoic acid modified chitosan conjugate for intracellular drug delivery and smart drug release in cancer therapy. *Carbohydr Polym*. 2019 Jul 1;215:8–19.

26. Deangelis PL. HEPtune: A process of conjugating a naturally occurring sugar molecule, heparosan, to a drug for enhanced drug delivery. *Drug Dev Del*. 2013 Jan;3:1–5.

27. Jing W, Roberts JW, Green DE, Almond A, Deangelis PL. Synthesis and characterization of heparosan-granulocyte-colony stimulating factor conjugates: A natural sugar-based drug delivery system to treat neutropenia. *Glycobiology*. 2017 Nov;27(11):1052–61.

28. Qiu L, Ge L, Long M, Mao J, Ahmed KS, Shan X, Zhang H, Qin L, Lv G, Chen J. Redox-responsive biocompatible nanocarriers based on novel heparosan polysaccharides for intracellular anticancer drug delivery. *Asian J Pharm Sci*. 2020 Jan;15(1):83–94.

29. Liu J, Liang N, Li S, Han Y, Yan P, Kawashima Y, Cui F, Sun S. Tumor-targeting and redox-sensitive micelles based on hyaluronic acid conjugate for delivery of paclitaxel. *J Biomater Appl*. 2020 May;34(10):1458–69.

30. Zheng P, Liu Y, Chen J, Xu W, Li G, Ding J. Targeted pH-responsive polyion complex micelle for controlled intracellular drug delivery. *Chinese Chem Lett*. 2020 May;31(5):1178–82.

31. Kumana CR, Yuen KY. Parenteral aminoglycoside therapy: Selection, administration, and monitoring. *Drugs*. 1994 Jun;47(6):902–13.

32. Lutwyche P, Cordeiro C, Wiseman DJ, St-Louis M, Uh M, Hope MJ, Webb MS, Finlay BB. Intracellular delivery and antibacterial activity of gentamicin encapsulated in pH-sensitive liposomes. *Antimicrob Agents Chemother*. 1998 Oct;42(10):2511–20.

33. Kanamala M, Palmer BD, Jamieson SMF, Wilson WR, Wu Z. Dual pH-sensitive liposomes with low pH-triggered sheddable PEG for enhanced tumor-targeted drug delivery. *Nanomedicine*. 2019 Jul;14(15):1971–89.

34. Miyazaki M, Yuba E, Hayashi H, Harada A, Kono K. Hyaluronic acid-based pH-sensitive polymer-modified liposomes for cell-specific intracellular drug delivery systems. *Bioconjug Chem*. 2018 Jan;29(1):44–55.

35. Tang M, Svirskis D, Leung E, Kanamala M, Wang H, Zimei W. Can intracellular drug delivery using hyaluronic acid functionalised pH-sensitive liposomes overcome gemcitabine resistance in pancreatic cancer? *J Control Release*. 2019 Jul;305:89–100.

36. Yudina A, de Smet M, Lepetit-Coiffé M, Langereis S, Ruijssevelt LV, Smirnov P, Bouchaud V, Voisin P, Grüll H, Moonen CTW. Ultrasound-mediated intracellular drug delivery using microbubbles and temperature-sensitive liposomes. *J Control Release*. 2011 Nov;155(3):442–48.

37. Dhawan S, Ghosh S, Ravinder R, Bais SS, Basak S, Krishnan NMA, Agarwal M, Banerjee M, Haridas V. Redox sensitive self-assembling dipeptide for sustained intracellular drug delivery. *Bioconjug Chem*. 2019 Sep 18;30(9):2458–68.

38. Banerjee SS, Chen D-H. Multifunctional pH-sensitive magnetic nanoparticles for simultaneous imaging, sensing and targeted intracellular anticancer drug delivery. *Nanotechnology*. 2008 Dec;19(50):505104.

39. Moghaddam SPH, Yazdimamaghani M, Ghandehari H. Glutathione-sensitive hollow mesoporous silica nanoparticles for controlled drug delivery. *J Control Release*. 2018 Jul;282:62–75.

40. Hastings KT, Cresswell P. Disulfide reduction in the endocytic pathway: Immunological functions of gamma-interferon-inducible lysosomal thiol reductase. *Antioxid Redox Signal*. 2011 Aug;15(3):657–668.

41. Chen H, Kuang Y, Liu R, Chen Z, Chen Z, Jiang B, Sun Z, Chen X, Li C. Dual-pH-sensitive mesoporous silica nanoparticle-based drug delivery system for tumor-triggered intracellular drug release. *J Mater Sci*. 2018 May;53:10653–65.

42. Li K, Li D, Zhao L, Chang Y, Zhang Y, Cui Y, Zhang Z. Calcium-mineralized polypeptide nanoparticle for intracellular drug delivery in osteosarcoma chemotherapy. *Bioact Mater.* 2020 Jun;5(3):721–31.

43. Lee P-Y, Tuan-Mu H-Y, Hsiao L-W, Hu JJ, Jan JS. Nanogels comprising reduction-cleavable polymers for glutathione-induced intracellular curcumin delivery. *J Polym Res.* 2017 Apr;24:66–75.

44. Wang H, Yang X, Sun C, Mao C, Zhu Y, Wang J. Matrix metalloproteinase 2-responsive micelle for siRNA delivery. *Biomaterials.* 2014 Aug;35(26):7622–34.

45. Li X-X, Chen J, Shen J-M, Zhuang R, Zhang S-Q, Zhu Z-Y, Ma J-B. pH-sensitive nanoparticles as smart carriers for selective intracellular drug delivery to tumor. *Int J Pharm.* 2018 Jul;545(1–2):274–85.

46. Navath RS, Kurtoglu YE, Wang B, Kannan S, Romero R, Kannan RM. Dendrimer-drug conjugates for tailored intracellular drug release based on glutathione levels. *Bioconjug Chem.* 2008 Dec;19(12):2446–55.

47. Nogueira DR, Scheeren LE, Pilar Vinardell M, Mitjans M, Infante MR, Rolim CMB. Nanoparticles incorporating pH-responsive surfactants as a viable approach to improve the intracellular drug delivery. *Mater Sci Eng C Mater Biol Appl.* 2015 Dec;57:100–6.

48. Mazzotta E, Benedittis SD, Qualtieri A, Muzzalupo R. Actively targeted and redox responsive delivery of anticancer drug by chitosan nanoparticles. *Pharmaceutics.* 2019 Dec 26;12(1):26.

49. Wang C, Liu H, Liu S, Wang Z, Zhang J. pH and Redox dual-sensitive covalent organic framework nanocarriers to resolve the dilemma between extracellular drug loading and intracellular drug release. *Front Chem.* 2020 Jun;8:1–11.

11 Nanomedicine-Based Approaches for Management of Psoriasis

Shaik Rahana Parveen, Sheetu Wadhwa,
Sachin Kumar Singh, and Rajesh Kumar

11.1 INTRODUCTION

Psoriasis is a chronic autoimmune skin disease [1], and as per the WHO, it affects 1.5–5% of the natives of developing countries and 0.9–11.4% worldwide [2]. It appears as red scaly lesions on the skin due to the invasion of T helper type 1 and Th17 immune cells in the epidermis, dermis, resulting to vascular regeneration and atypical keratinocyte distinction [3]. The etiology of psoriasis results from a complex interaction of genetic factors, environmental factors, and exaggeration includes skin trauma, stress, streptococcal infections, drugs, etc. Psoriasis-associated comorbidities are cardiovascular diseases, psoriatic arthritis, diabetes mellitus type 2, dyslipidemia, obesity, ankylosing spondylitis (AS), rheumatoid arthritis, Behcet disease, systemic lupus erythematosus (SLE), systemic sclerosis (SSc), and dermatomyositis (DM) [4].

11.2 TYPES OF PSORIASIS

Psoriasis can be divided into mild, moderate, and severe based on the severity of the disease. Different types of psoriasis are plaque, pustular, inverse, guttate, and nail psoriasis [5], and 80–90% of people are affected with plaque psoriasis only [6].

11.2.1 FEATURES OF PSORIATIC SKIN

Disturbance of the barrier function of skin was studied by Ghadially et al. by using the transepithelial water loss method [7]. In 2014, Takahashi et al. reported that psoriatic skin contains a low proportion of water, natural moisturizing factor, and free fatty acids in comparison to normal skin [8]. In 2015, Sano described lower levels of ceramide in psoriatic skin [9]. Unusual thickening of the stratum corneum does not allow the penetration of conventional formulations. Hence the problems associated with penetration can be reduced by utilizing nanotechnology-based approaches for topical administration [10, 11].

11.3 PATHOGENESIS OF PSORIASIS

The underlying mechanism of the pathogenesis of psoriasis is hyperactivity of the immune system. This was confirmed by the administration of immune-suppressing drugs. Sustained inflammation causes psoriasis. Certain factors which trigger psoriasis include injury of skin, drugs, trauma, stress, leaky gut, and skin infections (increased *Staphylococcus, Coryne bacterium, Propiono bacterium,* and *Streptococcus aureus*). This leads to synthesis of antimicrobial peptides (LL37, β-defensins, and S100) from the damaged keratinocytes of the skin. LL37 complexes with self-DNA, which is produced from damaged cells, and this complex stimulates the toll-like receptors (TLR-9) of plasmacytoid dendritic cells (plasmacytoid DCs). Activated plasmacytoid DCs produce type-1 interferon-α,β (INF-α and β). Type-1 interferon nodding aids the establishment of myeloid dendritic cells (mDCs) phenotype, differentiation function of IFN-γ in T-helper cell one (Th1) and T-helper cell 17 (Th17). It leads to production of interleukin 17 (IL-17), tumor necrosis factor (TNF-α), interleukin-1(IL-1), and interleukin 6 (IL-6). LL37 also binds with RNA and stimulates pDC of TLR7. The complex of LL37-RNA acts on the myeloid dendritic cells of TLR-8 and activates myeloid dendritic cells. Activated myeloid dendritic cells migrate into lymph nodes and secretes more TNF-α, IL-23, and IL-12, then modulates differentiation and proliferation of Th17 and Th1. T-helper cell 17 (Th17), interleukin-21, and interleukin-22 activate keratinocyte multiplication in the epidermis. The overexpression of TNF-α, IL-23, and Th-17 causes inflammation, which leads to plaque psoriasis. The IL-17 cytokine family is composed of interleukin-17A, 17B, 17C, 17D, 17E, and IL17F. IL17A binds to trimeric receptor and forms the adaptor protein ACT1. The extracellular signal-regulated kinase (ERK), [12] transforming growth factor β activated kinase 1 binding protein 1 (TAK1), transforming growth factor beta (TGF-β), p38 mitogen activated protein kinases (MAPKs), glycogen synthase kinase 3 β (GSK-3 β) and I-kappa B kinase (IKK) are all activated when ACT1 binds with IL17. These kinases enable the nuclear factor kappa light chain enhancer of activated B-cells (NFkB) [13], activator protein 1 (AP-1) and CCAAT enhancer proteins [14] transcription factor, cytokines, chemokines, and antimicrobial peptides. T helper type 1 and T helper 2 cytokines act via the Janus kinase signal transducer and activator of transcription proteins (JAK-STAT pathway), and T helper 17 cells are transmitted by Act1 and NFkB. Drugs that target the tumor necrosis factor −α (TNF-α), interleukin-23, interleukin-17 [15], and JAK/STAT pathways are effective in the treatment of plaque psoriasis. The key role in psoriasis is triggered by NF-κ B, which provides maximum transcription of those cytokines, so the primary objective of the treatment of psoriasis is inhibition of TNF-α, NF-kB, and IL-17A, which may ultimately prevent the remission of the disease [16]. Another cause of psoriasis is the absence of interleukin 10 (IL-10), or dysregulation of regulatory T cells leads to psoriasis. Interleukin 10 can be induced by the use of probiotics. In several types of psoriasis, different kinds of inflammatory mediators are released. In plaque psoriasis, TNF-α, IL-23, and T-helper 17 cells (Th17) are released.

In nail psoriasis and psoriatic arthritis, the tumor necrosis factor alpha (TNF-α) [17] nuclear factor kappa B (NFkB), IL6 and IL8 were over-expressed. However, interleukin 1β, interleukin-36α and interleukin 36γ transcripts were expressed in pustular psoriasis. Upregulation of T cells in guttate psoriasis occurs by streptococcal stimulation [18–21].

11.4 CONVENTIONAL APPROACHES FOR PSORIASIS

Conventional psoriasis approaches are topical treatment, phototherapy, and biological systemic treatment. Topical treatment is employed for mild to moderate conditions, along with phototherapy, which includes corticosteroids, dithranol, vitamin D analogs, tacrolimus, and retinoids. Several studies reported that topical therapy does not remove lesions completely [22–26]. Ultraviolet radiation in combination with psoralen used earlier due to their less remission rate and high effectiveness, but this combination is not preferred nowadays as it is associated with severe side effects such as photoaging, carcinoma, and melanoma [27, 28]. Methotrexate, cyclosporine, acitretin, and fumaric acid ester drugs have been administered systemically. Methotrexate, a folic acid inhibitor has greater efficacy, but it has severe hepatotoxicity, admonished in pregnancy, thrombocytopenia and leukemia. Cyclosporin is an immunosuppressant, however it has risk of glomerulosclerosis, lymphoma, renal impairment, and hypertension. Acitretin induces a teratogenic effect and dyslipidemia [29–32]. Biologicals specifically target TNF-α, IL-17, and IL-23. Etanercept, adalimumab, infliximab, and certolizumab are TNF-α inhibitors. Ustekinumab, guselkumab, tildrakizumab, and risankizumab inhibit interleukin 23, and secukinumab, ixekizumab, and brodalumab diminish the activity of IL-17. Natural agents like curcumin, capsaicin, fish oil, green tea, berries, and aloe vera extract have potential effects on psoriasis [33–36]. The selection of therapy is based on the severity of the disease. Most researchers are focusing on topical route due to its lower cyto-toxicity, safety, better patient compliance, site-specific effects, and lack of immune suppression when compared with systemic routes [37, 38].

11.5 NANOMEDICINE FOR PSORIASIS

Nanotechnology-based drug delivery systems have been explored in the last few decades as novel strategies to overcome the existing limitations of drugs and delivery systems. They increase the solubility of hydrophobic drugs and provide controlled or sustained drug release; site-specific delivery; and a safe, effective and stable dosage form with reduced side effects. Various polymer-, lipid-, and metallic-based nanocarriers have been explored for the management of psoriasis and are discussed in the current chapter [39].

Polymeric nanoparticles are colloidal nanoparticles prepared by the dispersion, encapsulation, or adsorption of a drug into a polymer. Their size is in the range of 10–1000 nm [40]. There are different types of polymeric nanoparticles: nanospheres, nanocapsules, dendrimers, polymeric micelles, and nanogels [41]. Suitable natural or synthetic polymers are selected based on their properties as well as drugs.

Ishihara and co-workers in 2005 formulated polylactic acid polymer-based nanoparticles loaded with betamethasone along with zinc and reported an increase in the efficacy of the drug and a sustained release effect [42]. Cyclosporine loaded in a polylactic co-glycolic acid polymeric matrix developed by Jain and co-workers in 2011 exhibit increased drug concentration in psoriatic skin and higher efficacy [43]. Hydrocortisone containing poly caprolactone nanoparticles formulated by Rosado et al. reported increased drug permeability [44]. Singa et al. in 2010 developed methotrexate-loaded polymeric nanogel [45] and reported improved accumulation in the skin. Sun et al. formulated hydrogels of curcumin-loaded PLGA [46]. Mao and team developed a hydrogel of RRR-tocopheryl succinate polylysin (VES-g-PLL)-loaded with curcumin nanoparticles and the developed formulation showed potential effect in a sustained manner [47]. Several polymeric and metallic-based nanoparticles for topical delivery are listed in Table 11.1.

TABLE 11.1

Polymeric or Metallic Nanoparticle-Based Approaches for the Management of Psoriasis

Drug	Polymeric/Metallic Nanoparticles	Significance	References
Betamethasone + Zn	Polylactic acid	Increases efficacy	[42]
Cyclosporine	Polylactic co-glycolic acid polymeric matrix	Increases the concentration of the drug in psoriatic skin	[43]
Hydrocortisone	Poly caprolactone	Permeability increased	[44]
Curcumin	Polylactic co-glycolic acid PLGA	Accumulation of drug increased in stratum corneum	[46]
Curcumin	RRR-tocopheryl succinate polylysin (VES-g-PLL)	Increases potential effect	[47]
Methotrexate	Gold nanoparticles	Inhibits cell growth and enhances penetration of methotrexate in psoriatic skin	[48]
Corneal cherry	Silver and gold nanoparticles	Targets macrophages of psoriatic skin	[49, 50]
Poly phenols and anthocyanins	Silver nanoparticles	Improves anti-inflammatory effect and reduces cytokine production	[51]

Metallic nanoparticles are prepared in the form of nanotubes, nanopores, nanorods, nanoclusters, and nanostars by using gold, silver, zirconium, copper, palladium, iron, selenium, and strontium [49, 52, 53]. Bessar et al. formulated methotrexate gold nano particles, which inhibit the cell growth and enhance the penetration of methotrexate in psoriatic skin [48]. Crisan developed corneal cherry silver and gold nanoparticles extracted from the cornus mas. These nanoparticles targeted the macrophages of psoriatic skin [49, 50]. David et al. developed poly-phenol- and anthocyanin-loaded silver nanoparticles by using a green synthesis method and reported that it has a greater anti-inflammatory effect and reduces cytokine production [51].

Lipid-based nanoparticles are synthesized by natural lipids, which include liposomes, polyamphiphiles, solid lipid nanoparticles, nanostructured lipid-based carriers, and nanoemulsions [54, 55]. Lipid-based nanoparticle approaches are listed in Table 11.2.

Solid lipid nanoparticles are spherical lipids with a size in the range of 10–1000 nm. They are synthesized by solid lipids and surfactants. A single surfactant or a mixture of surfactants is utilized based on their properties and route of administration. Cold and hot homogenization techniques, micro-emulsion [75, 76], emulsification-ultrasonication, solvent emulsification diffusion/

TABLE 11.2

Lipid-Based Nanoparticles for Topical Treatment of Psoriasis

Drug	Delivery System	Action	References
Tacrolimus	Solid lipid nanoparticles (SLNs)	Showed enhanced permeation	[56]
Methotrexate + etanercept	SLNs	Insignificant permeation	[57]
Momentasone furoate	SLNs	Increased drug permeation	[58]
Thymol	Nanostructured lipid-based carriers	Thymol	[59]
Momentasone furaoate	NLCs	Elevated levels of drug deposited in the membrane	[60]
Methotrexate	NLCs	Increased skin permeation of drug	[61]
Clobetasol propionate	NLCs	Drug deposition increased	[62]
Tacrolimus	NLCs	Permeability of drug increased	[63]
Fluticasonepropionate	NLCs	Increased the stability of drug	[64]
Fusidic acid	Liposomes	Substantial effect and increased stability	[65]
Tretinoin	Liposomes	Increased permeability of drug in to the skin	[66]
Anthralin	Emulsomes	Increased the efficacy of the drug and improved stability of product	[66]
Methotrexate	Liposomes	Increased drug permeability	[67]
Anthocyanins	Niosomes	Extended the release of drug	[68]
Capsaicin	Emulsomes	Increased permeability in psoriatic skin	[69]
Methotrexate	Nanoemulsion	Eminent anti-psoriatic effect	[70]
Tacrolimus	Nanoemulsion	Increased penetration of drug	[71]
Clobetasol propionate	Nanoemulsion	Eminent effectiveness	[72]
Dihranol	SLNs	Showed prominent effect	[73]
Tacrolimus + curcumin	Lipospheres	Significant anti-psoriatic effect	[74]

evaporation, the film-ultrasonication method, hot-melt extrusion, and supercritical fluid methods were used for the manufacturing of solid lipid nanoparticles. Ruihua et al. in 2012 loaded tacrolimus in solid lipid nanoparticles by using a modified emulsification method; it showed greater permeability [56]. Ferreira et al. reported that a combination drug in solid lipid nanoparticle form decreased psoriatic skin permeability when developed using a hot ultrasonication method [57]. Madan et al. developed momentasone furoate solid lipid nanoparticles by the solvent injection method and found that it releases a drug in a sustained manner and exhibits significant permeability [58]. Zhang and Smith used a pre-emulsion ultrasonication method for the development of dithranol solid lipid nanoparticles, which showed greater efficacy.

Nanostructured lipid-based carriers are an advanced type of lipid carrier for topical delivery, fabricated by the mixture of liquid, solid lipids, and surfactants. Types of NLCs include the imperfect type, amorphous type, and multiple oil in solid fat in water type (O/F/W) [77–79]. Many methods are employed for the preparation of NLCs, such as homogenization [80–83], micro-emulsion [84, 85], emulsification solvent evaporation method [86, 87], emulsification solvent diffusion [88], solvent injection method [89], phase inversion [90], multiple emulsion [91], ultrasonication [92], and membrane contractor techniques [93]. Pivetta et al. loaded thymol in nanostructured lipid-based carriers by using a hot emulsion sonication method. It showed greater potential effect on psoriasis plaques [59]. Kaur, Sharma, and Bedi in 2018 formulated and evaluated momentasone furaoate NLCs by a micro-emulsion method and reported that a higher amount of drug was deposited on skin [60]. Pinto et al. explored methotrexate containing NLCs by a homogenization technique, and they increased the skin permeability in psoriatic skin [61]. Silva et al. reported that a clobetasol propionate-loaded nanostructured lipid-based carrier enhanced the deposition of drugs in psoriatic skin [62] Nam et al. formulated and evaluated tacrolimus containing NLCs reported as it increases the penetration of drug compared with commercial product [63]. Doktorovova et al. employed a modified micro-emulsion method for fluticasone propionate NLC preparation and reported it increased the stability of the drug [64]. Lipospheres are spherical lipid-based nanoparticles manufactured by using different methods such as melting methods, cosolvent methods, spray drying, spray congealing, multiple microemulsion, and supercritical fluid methods [94].

Vesicular-based lipid systems: Liposomes are bilayered, amphiphilic, self-assembling vesicular nanosystems placed in an aqueous system. In this system, both hydrophilic and hydrophobic drugs can be incorporated [95]. Various methods employed for the preparation of liposomes are sonication, extrusion, freeze thawing, lipid film hydration, micro-emulsification, extrusion or drying reconstitution, ether injection, ethanol injection, reverse phase evaporation, and detergent removal methods [96]. Wadhwa et al. loaded fusidic acid in liposomes by a thin film hydration method and reported the liposomes showed greater efficacy and were more stable [65]. Raza et al. explored tretinoin liposomes using a thin film hydration method and described that this system increased the stability and permeability of drugs into the skin [66]. Srisuk et al. formulated and evaluated methotrexate liposomes and reported that they increased the permeability of drugs into psoriatic skin [67].

Niosomes are bi-layered, amphiphilic, non-ionic surfactant-based uni- or multilamellar vesicles [97, 98]. Anthocyanins containing niosomes were prepared by Manconi et al., who reported that they extended the release of drugs from niosomes [68] in a sustained manner.

Emulsomes are bi-layered phospholipid nanovesicular systems consisting of an internal solid lipid core [99]. Gupta et al. developed capsaicin-containing emulsomes and described that they increased the permeability of drugs into psoriatic skin [69] Raza et al. developed and evaluated anthralin-containing emulsomes and reported that they enhanced stability, improved the efficacy of the drug compared with commercial ones, and showed a better anti-psoriatic effect under evaluation in an imiquimode-induced psoriasis tail model [100].

Nanoemulsions are nano-sized emulsions, Rajitha et al. formulated a chaulmoogra oil nanoemulsion containing methotrexate as an active agent and described that it has an anti-psoriatic effect [70]. Sahu et al. explored a tacrolimus-loaded nanoemulsion and reported that it increases penetration of drugs [71]. Alam et al. explored clobetasol propionate nanoemulsions and described that they increased the efficacy of drugs in psoriatic skin [72].

11.6 CONCLUSION

Even though the prevalence rate of psoriasis is effectively lower than that of other chronic skin conditions, the psychological effect on the quality of life of psoriatic patients is unbearable. Due to its underlying mechanism and complex pathogenesis, the main factors that cause psoriasis are still unclear. Several treatment options available are emollients, corticosteroid therapy, phototherapy, and biologics, but none of them provide effective treatment and prevent recurrence. Recently various nanomedicine-based approaches have been explored for existing therapeutic agents for topical application. These strategies provide targeted drug delivery, improved drug permeation, fewer adverse effects, and lower recurrence chances, which can provide new insights into the management of psoriasis.

REFERENCES

1. Sala M, Elaissari A, Fessi H. Advances in psoriasis physiopathology and treatments: Up to date of mechanistic insights and perspectives of novel therapies based on innovative skin drug delivery systems (ISDDS). *Journal of Controlled Release.* 2016 Oct 10;239:182–202.
2. Michalek IM, Loring B, John SM. A systematic review of worldwide epidemiology of psoriasis. *Journal of the European Academy of Dermatology and Venereology.* 2017 Feb;31(2):205–12.
3. Das RP, Jain AK, Ramesh V. Current concepts in the pathogenesis of psoriasis. *Indian Journal of Dermatology.* 2009 Jan;54(1):7.
4. Ju HJ, Kim KJ, Kim DS, Lee JH, Kim GM, Park CJ, Bae JM. Increased risks of autoimmune rheumatic diseases in patients with psoriasis: A nationwide population-based study. *Journal of the American Academy of Dermatology.* 2018 Oct 1;79(4):778–81.
5. Sarac G, Koca TT, Baglan T. A brief summary of clinical types of psoriasis. *Northern Clinics of Istanbul.* 2016;3(1):79.
6. Sticherling M. Psoriasis and autoimmunity. *Autoimmunity Reviews.* 2016 Dec 1;15(12):1167–70.
7. Ghadially R, Reed JT, Elias PM. Stratum corneum structure and function correlates with phenotype in psoriasis. *Journal of Investigative Dermatology.* 1996 Oct 1;107(4):558–64.
8. Takahashi H, Tsuji H, Minami-Hori M, Miyauchi Y, Iizuka H. Defective barrier function accompanied by structural changes of psoriatic stratum corneum. *The Journal of Dermatology.* 2014 Feb;41(2):144–8.
9. Sano S. Psoriasis as a barrier disease. *Dermatologica Sinica.* 2015 Jun 1;33(2):64–9.
10. Pradhan M, Alexander A, Singh MR, Singh D, Saraf S, Saraf S. Understanding the prospective of nano-formulations towards the treatment of psoriasis. *Biomedicine & Pharmacotherapy.* 2018 Nov 1;107:447–63.
11. Singhvi G, Hejmady S, Rapalli VK, Dubey SK, Dubey S. Nanocarriers for topical delivery in psoriasis. In *Delivery of Drugs.* 2020 Jan 1 (pp. 75–96). Elsevier.
12. Rendon A, Schäkel K. Psoriasis pathogenesis and treatment. *International Journal of Molecular Sciences.* 2019 Mar 23;20(6):1475.
13. Di Meglio P, Villanova F, Nestle FO. Psoriasis. *Cold Spring Harbor Perspectives in Medicine.* 2014 Aug 1;4(8):a015354. doi: 10.1101/cshperspect.a015354. PMID: 25085957; PMCID: PMC4109580.
14. Liang Y, Sarkar MK, Tsoi LC, Gudjonsson JE. Psoriasis: A mixed autoimmune and autoinflammatory disease. *Current Opinion in Immunology.* 2017 Dec 1;49:1–8.
15. Harden JL, Krueger JG, Bowcock AM. The immunogenetics of psoriasis: A comprehensive review. *Journal of Autoimmunity.* 2015 Nov 1;64:66–73.
16. Huang TH, Lin CF, Alalaiwe A, Yang SC, Fang JY. Apoptotic or antiproliferative activity of natural products against keratinocytes for the treatment of psoriasis. *International Journal of Molecular Sciences.* 2019 May 24;20(10):2558.
17. Morizane S, Gallo RL. Antimicrobial peptides in the pathogenesis of psoriasis. *The Journal of Dermatology.* 2012 Mar;39(3):225–30.
18. Boutet MA, Nerviani A, Gallo Afflitto G, Pitzalis C. Role of the IL-23/IL-17 axis in psoriasis and psoriatic arthritis: The clinical importance of its divergence in skin and joints. *International Journal of Molecular Sciences.* 2018 Feb 9;19(2):530.

19. Sakkas LI, Bogdanos DP. Are psoriasis and psoriatic arthritis the same disease? The IL-23/IL-17 axis data. *Autoimmunity Reviews.* 2017 Jan 1;16(1):10–5.

20. Bissonnette R, Fuentes-Duculan J, Mashiko S, Li X, Bonifacio KM, Cueto I, Suárez-Fariñas M, Maari C, Bolduc C, Nigen S, Sarfati M. Palmoplantar pustular psoriasis (PPPP) is characterized by activation of the IL-17A pathway. *Journal of Dermatological Science.* 2017 Jan 1;85(1):20–6.

21. Wilsmann-Theis D, Schnell LM, Ralser-Isselstein V, Bieber T, Schön MP, Hüffmeier U, Mössner R. Successful treatment with interleukin-17A antagonists of generalized pustular psoriasis in patients without IL36RN mutations. *The Journal of Dermatology.* 2018 Jul;45(7):850–4.

22. Kragballe K. Topical corticosteroids: Mechanisms of action. *Acta Dermato-Venereologica. Supplementum.* 1989 Jan 1;151:7–10.

23. Kemény L, Ruzicka T, Braun-Falco O. Dithranol: A review of the mechanism of action in the treatment of psoriasis vulgaris. *Skin Pharmacology and Physiology.* 1990 Mar 31;3(1):1–20.

24. Saurat JH. Retinoids and psoriasis: Novel issues in retinoid pharmacology and implications for psoriasis treatment. *Journal of the American Academy of Dermatology.* 1999 Sep 1;41(3):S2–6.

25. Kim GK. The rationale behind topical vitamin d analogs in the treatment of psoriasis: Where does topical calcitriol fit in? *The Journal of Clinical and Aesthetic Dermatology.* 2010 Aug;3(8):46.

26. Higgins E. Psoriasis. *Medicine.* 2017 Mar 10:1–11.

27. Parrish JA, Jaenicke KF. Action spectrum for phototherapy of psoriasis. *Journal of Investigative Dermatology.* 1981 May 1;76(5):359–62.

28. Menter A, Gottlieb A, Feldman SR, Van Voorhees AS, Leonardi CL, Gordon KB, Lebwohl M, Koo JY, Elmets CA, Korman NJ, Beutner KR. Guidelines of care for the management of psoriasis and psoriatic arthritis: Section 1. Overview of psoriasis and guidelines of care for the treatment of psoriasis with biologics. *Journal of the American Academy of Dermatology.* 2008 May 1;58(5):826–50.

29. Silverman AK, Ellis CN, Voorhees JJ. Hypervitaminosis A syndrome: A paradigm of retinoid side effects. *Journal of the American Academy of Dermatology.* 1987 May 1;16(5):1027–39.

30. Buchman AL. Side effects of corticosteroid therapy. *Journal of Clinical Gastroenterology.* 2001 Oct 1;33(4):289–94.

31. Czarnecka-Operacz M, Sadowska-Przytocka A. The possibilities and principles of methotrexate treatment of psoriasis–the updated knowledge. *Advances in Dermatology and Allergology/Postępy Dermatologii i Alergologii.* 2014 Dec 3;31(6):392–400.

32. Balak DM. Fumaric acid esters in the management of psoriasis. *Psoriasis: Targets and Therapy.* 2015 Jan 5:9–23.

33. Agarwal R, Katare OP, Vyas SP. Preparation and in vitro evaluation of liposomal/niosomal delivery systems for antipsoriatic drug dithranol. *International Journal of Pharmaceutics.* 2001 Oct 9;228(1–2):43–52.

34. Crisan D, Scharffetter-Kochanek K, Crisan M, Schatz S, Hainzl A, Olenic L, Filip A, Schneider LA, Sindrilaru A. Topical silver and gold nanoparticles complexed with Cornus mas suppress inflammation in human psoriasis plaques by inhibiting NF-κB activity. *Experimental Dermatology.* 2018 Oct;27(10):1166–9.

35. Murphy EC, Schaffter SW, Friedman AJ. Nanotechnology for psoriasis therapy. *Current Dermatology Reports.* 2019 Mar;8:14–25.

36. Chen X, Hong S, Sun X, Xu W, Li H, Ma T, Zheng Q, Zhao H, Zhou Y, Qiang Y, Li B. Efficacy of fish oil and its components in the management of psoriasis: A systematic review of 18 randomized controlled trials. *Nutrition Reviews.* 2020 Oct;78(10):827–40.

37. Harden JL, Krueger JG, Bowcock AM. The immunogenetics of psoriasis: A comprehensive review. *Journal of Autoimmunity.* 2015 Nov 1;64:66–73.

38. Musa SH, Basri M, Fard Masoumi HR, Shamsudin N, Salim N. Enhancement of physicochemical properties of nanocolloidal carrier loaded with cyclosporine for topical treatment of psoriasis: In vitro diffusion and in vivo hydrating action. *International Journal of Nanomedicine.* 2017 Mar 28:2427–41.

39. Rahman M, Akhter S, Beg S. Nanomedicine advances in topical infective and non-infective skin diseases therapy. *Recent Patents on Anti-Infective Drug Discovery.* 2018 Aug 1;13(2):104.

40. Garg T, Rath G, Goyal AK. Nanotechnological approaches for the effective management of psoriasis. *Artificial Cells, Nanomedicine, and Biotechnology.* 2016 Aug 17;44(6):1374–82.

41. Soni KS, Desale SS, Bronich TK. Nanogels: An overview of properties, biomedical applications and obstacles to clinical translation. *Journal of Controlled Release.* 2016 Oct 28;240:109–26.

42. Ishihara T, Izumo N, Higaki M, Shimada E, Hagi T, Mine L, Ogawa Y, Mizushima Y. Role of zinc in formulation of PLGA/PLA nanoparticles encapsulating betamethasone phosphate and its release profile. *Journal of Controlled Release.* 2005 Jun 20;105(1–2):68–76.

43. Jain S, Mittal A, Jain KA. Enhanced topical delivery of cyclosporin-A using PLGA nanoparticles as carrier. *Current Nanoscience.* 2011 Aug 1;7(4):524–30.

44. Rosado C, Silva C, Reis CP. Hydrocortisone-loaded poly (ε-caprolactone) nanoparticles for atopic dermatitis treatment. *Pharmaceutical Development and Technology.* 2013 Jun 1;18(3):710–8.

45. Singka GS, Samah NA, Zulfakar MH, Yurdasiper A, Heard CM. Enhanced topical delivery and anti-inflammatory activity of methotrexate from an activated nanogel. *European Journal of Pharmaceutics and Biopharmaceutics.* 2010 Oct 1;76(2):275–81.

46. Sun L, Liu Z, Wang L, Cun D, Tong HH, Yan R, Chen X, Wang R, Zheng Y. Enhanced topical penetration, system exposure and anti-psoriasis activity of two particle-sized, curcumin-loaded PLGA nanoparticles in hydrogel. *Journal of Controlled Release.* 2017 May 28;254:44–54.

47. Mao KL, Fan ZL, Yuan JD, Chen PP, Yang JJ, Xu J, ZhuGe DL, Jin BH, Zhu QY, Shen BX, Sohawon Y. Skin-penetrating polymeric nanoparticles incorporated in silk fibroin hydrogel for topical delivery of curcumin to improve its therapeutic effect on psoriasis mouse model. *Colloids and Surfaces B: Biointerfaces.* 2017 Dec 1;160:704–14.

48. Bessar H, Venditti I, Benassi L, Vaschieri C, Azzoni P, Pellacani G, Magnoni C, Botti E, Casagrande V, Federici M, Costanzo A. Functionalized gold nanoparticles for topical delivery of methotrexate for the possible treatment of psoriasis. *Colloids and Surfaces B: Biointerfaces.* 2016 May 1;141:141–7.

49. Crisan D. Anti-inflammatory effect of metallic silver and gold nanoparticles complexed with polyphenolic compounds in human chronic stationary plaque psoriasis (Doctoral dissertation, Universität Ulm).

50. Crisan D, Scharffetter-Kochanek K, Crisan M, Schatz S, Hainzl A, Olenic L, Filip A, Schneider LA, Sindrilaru A. Topical silver and gold nanoparticles complexed with Cornus mas suppress inflammation in human psoriasis plaques by inhibiting NF-κB activity. *Experimental Dermatology.* 2018 Oct;27(10):1166–9.

51. David L, Moldovan B, Vulcu A, Olenic L, Perde-Schrepler M, Fischer-Fodor E, Florea A, Crisan M, Chiorean I, Clichici S, Filip GA. Green synthesis, characterization and anti-inflammatory activity of silver nanoparticles using European black elderberry fruits extract. *Colloids and Surfaces B: Biointerfaces.* 2014 Oct 1;122:767–77.

52. Shankar PD, Shobana S, Karuppusamy I, Pugazhendhi A, Ramkumar VS, Arvindnarayan S, Kumar G. A review on the biosynthesis of metallic nanoparticles (gold and silver) using bio-components of microalgae: Formation mechanism and applications. *Enzyme and Microbial Technology.* 2016 Dec 1;95:28–44.

53. Ali I, Mukhtar SD, Lone MN, Ali HS, Aboul-Enein HY. Recent advances in mesoporous silica and gold based nanovectors in anticancer drug delivery system. *Current Organic Chemistry.* 2017 Oct 1;21(23):2400–15.

54. Puri A, Loomis K, Smith B, Lee JH, Yavlovich A, Heldman E, Blumenthal R. Lipid-based nanoparticles as pharmaceutical drug carriers: From concepts to clinic. *Critical Reviews™ in Therapeutic Drug Carrier Systems.* 2009;26(6).

55. Bhatia S, Bhatia S. Nanoparticles types, classification, characterization, fabrication methods and drug delivery applications. *Natural Polymer Drug Delivery Systems: Nanoparticles, Plants, and Algae.* 2016:33–93.

56. Wang R, Li L, Wang B, Zhang T, Sun L. FK506-loaded solid lipid nanoparticles: Preparation, characterization and in vitro transdermal drug delivery. *African Journal of Pharmacy and Pharmacology.* 2012 Mar 29;6(12):904–13.

57. Ferreira M, Barreiros L, Segundo MA, Torres T, Selores M, Lima SA, Reis S. Topical co-delivery of methotrexate and etanercept using lipid nanoparticles: A targeted approach for psoriasis management. *Colloids and Surfaces B: Biointerfaces.* 2017 Nov 1;159:23–9.

58. Madan JR, Khude PA, Dua K. Development and evaluation of solid lipid nanoparticles of mometasone furoate for topical delivery. *International Journal of Pharmaceutical Investigation.* 2014 Apr;4(2):60.

59. Pivetta TP, Simões S, Araújo MM, Carvalho T, Arruda C, Marcato PD. Development of nanoparticles from natural lipids for topical delivery of thymol: Investigation of its anti-inflammatory properties. *Colloids and Surfaces B: Biointerfaces.* 2018 Apr 1;164:281–90.

60. Kaur N, Sharma K, Bedi N. Topical nanostructured lipid carrier based hydrogel of mometasone furoate for the treatment of psoriasis. *Pharmaceutical Nanotechnology.* 2018 Jun 1;6(2):133–43.

61. Pinto MF, Moura CC, Nunes C, Segundo MA, Lima SA, Reis S. A new topical formulation for psoriasis: Development of methotrexate-loaded nanostructured lipid carriers. *International Journal of Pharmaceutics.* 2014 Dec 30;477(1–2):519–26.

62. Silva LA, Taveira SF, Lima EM, Marreto RN. In vitro skin penetration of clobetasol from lipid nanoparticles: Drug extraction and quantitation in different skin layers. *Brazilian Journal of Pharmaceutical Sciences.* 2012;48:811–7.

63. Nam SH, Ji XY, Park JS. Investigation of tacrolimus loaded nanostructured lipid carriers for topical drug delivery. *Bulletin of the Korean Chemical Society.* 2011;32(3):956–60.

64. Doktorovová S, Araújo J, Garcia ML, Rakovský E, Souto EB. Formulating fluticasone propionate in novel PEG-containing nanostructured lipid carriers (PEG-NLC). *Colloids and Surfaces B: Biointerfaces.* 2010 Feb 1;75(2):538–42.

65. Wadhwa S, Singh B, Sharma G, Raza K, Katare OP. Liposomal Fusidic acid as a potential delivery system: A new paradigm in the treatment of chronic plaque psoriasis. *Drug Delivery.* 2016 May 3;23(4):1204–13.

66. Raza K, Singh B, Lohan S, Sharma G, Negi P, Yachha Y, Katare OP. Nano-lipoidal carriers of tretinoin with enhanced percutaneous absorption, photostability, biocompatibility and anti-psoriatic activity. *International Journal of Pharmaceutics.* 2013 Nov 1;456(1):65–72.

67. Srisuk P, Thongnopnua P, Raktanonchai U, Kanokpanont S. Physico-chemical characteristics of methotrexate-entrapped oleic acid-containing deformable liposomes for in vitro transepidermal delivery targeting psoriasis treatment. *International Journal of Pharmaceutics.* 2012 May 10;427(2):426–34.

68. Manconi M, Sinico C, Caddeo C, Vila AO, Valenti D, Fadda AM. Penetration enhancer containing vesicles as carriers for dermal delivery of tretinoin. *International Journal of Pharmaceutics.* 2011 Jun 30;412(1–2):37–46.

69. Gupta R, Gupta M, Mangal S, Agrawal U, Vyas SP. Capsaicin-loaded vesicular systems designed for enhancing localized delivery for psoriasis therapy. *Artificial Cells, Nanomedicine, and Biotechnology.* 2016 Apr 2;44(3):825–34.

70. Rajitha P, Shammika P, Aiswarya S, Gopikrishnan A, Jayakumar R, Sabitha M. Chaulmoogra oil based methotrexate loaded topical nanoemulsion for the treatment of psoriasis. *Journal of Drug Delivery Science and Technology.* 2019 Feb 1;49:463–76.

71. Sahu S, Katiyar SS, Kushwah V, Jain S. Active natural oil-based nanoemulsion containing tacrolimus for synergistic antipsoriatic efficacy. *Nanomedicine.* 2018 Aug;13(16):1985–98.

72. Alam MS, Ali MS, Zakir F, Alam N, Alam MI, Ahmad F, Siddiqui MR, Ali MD, Ansari MS, Ahmad S, Ali M. Enhancement of anti-dermatitis potential of clobetasol propionate by DHA [docosahexaenoic acid] rich algal oil nanoemulsion gel. *Iranian Journal of Pharmaceutical Research: IJPR.* 2016;15(1):35.

73. Zhang J, Smith E. Percutaneous permeation of betamethasone 17-valerate incorporated in lipid nanoparticles. *Journal of Pharmaceutical Sciences.* 2011 Mar 1;100(3):896–903.

74. Jain A, Doppalapudi S, Domb AJ, Khan W. Tacrolimus and curcumin co-loaded liposphere gel: Synergistic combination towards management of psoriasis. *Journal of Controlled Release.* 2016 Dec 10;243:132–45.

75. Gupta S, Kesarla R, Chotai N, Misra A, Omri A. Systematic approach for the formulation and optimization of solid lipid nanoparticles of efavirenz by high pressure homogenization using design of experiments for brain targeting and enhanced bioavailability. *Biomed Research International.* 2017 Jan 23;2017.

76. Müller RH, Mäder K, Gohla S. Solid lipid nanoparticles (SLN) for controlled drug delivery–a review of the state of the art. *European Journal of Pharmaceutics and Biopharmaceutics.* 2000 Jul 3;50(1):161–77.

77. Müller RH, Radtke M, Wissing S. Nanostructured lipid matrices for improved microencapsulation of drugs. *International Journal of Pharmaceutics.* 2002 Aug 21;242(1–2):121–8.

78. Üner M. Preparation, characterization and physico-chemical properties of solid lipid nanoparticles (SLN) and nanostructured lipid carriers (NLC): Their benefits as colloidal drug carrier systems. *Die Pharmazie-An International Journal of Pharmaceutical Sciences.* 2006 May 1;61(5):375–86.

79. Jaiswal P, Gidwani B, Vyas A. Nanostructured lipid carriers and their current application in targeted drug delivery. *Artificial Cells, Nanomedicine, and Biotechnology.* 2016 Jan 2;44(1):27–40.

80. Kasongo KW, Müller RH, Walker RB. The use of hot and cold high pressure homogenization to enhance the loading capacity and encapsulation efficiency of nanostructured lipid carriers for the hydrophilic antiretroviral drug, didanosine for potential administration to paediatric patients. *Pharmaceutical Development and Technology.* 2012 Jun 1;17(3):353–62.

81. Souto EB, Müller RH. Investigation of the factors influencing the incorporation of clotrimazole in SLN and NLC prepared by hot high-pressure homogenization. *Journal of Microencapsulation.* 2006 Jan 1;23(4):377–88.

82. Zhuang CY, Li N, Wang M, Zhang XN, Pan WS, Peng JJ, Pan YS, Tang X. Preparation and characterization of vinpocetine loaded nanostructured lipid carriers (NLC) for improved oral bioavailability. *International Journal of Pharmaceutics.* 2010 Jul 15;394(1–2):179–85.

83. Gaba B, Fazil M, Khan S, Ali A, Baboota S, Ali J. Nanostructured lipid carrier system for topical delivery of terbinafine hydrochloride. *Bulletin of Faculty of Pharmacy, Cairo University.* 2015 Dec 1;53(2):147–59.

84. Ghate VM, Lewis SA, Prabhu P, Dubey A, Patel N. Nanostructured lipid carriers for the topical delivery of tretinoin. *European Journal of Pharmaceutics and Biopharmaceutics*. 2016 Nov 1;108:253–61.

85. Ugazio E, Cavalli R, Gasco MR. Incorporation of cyclosporin A in solid lipid nanoparticles (SLN). *International Journal of Pharmaceutics*. 2002 Jul 25;241(2):341–4.

86. Mendes AI, Silva AC, Catita JA, Cerqueira F, Gabriel C, Lopes CM. Miconazole-loaded nanostructured lipid carriers (NLC) for local delivery to the oral mucosa: Improving antifungal activity. *Colloids and Surfaces B: Biointerfaces*. 2013 Nov 1;111:755–63.

87. Ranpise NS, Korabu SS, Ghodake VN. Second generation lipid nanoparticles (NLC) as an oral drug carrier for delivery of lercanidipine hydrochloride. *Colloids and Surfaces B: Biointerfaces*. 2014 Apr 1;116:81–7.

88. Shah NV, Seth AK, Balaraman R, Aundhia CJ, Maheshwari RA, Parmar GR. Nanostructured lipid carriers for oral bioavailability enhancement of raloxifene: Design and in vivo study. *Journal of Advanced Research*. 2016 May 1;7(3):423–34.

89. Schubert MA, Müller-Goymann CC. Solvent injection as a new approach for manufacturing lipid nanoparticles–evaluation of the method and process parameters. *European Journal of Pharmaceutics and Biopharmaceutics*. 2003 Jan 1;55(1):125–31.

90. Sun M, Nie S, Pan X, Zhang R, Fan Z, Wang S. Quercetin-nanostructured lipid carriers: Characteristics and anti-breast cancer activities in vitro. *Colloids and Surfaces B: Biointerfaces*. 2014 Jan 1;113:15–24.

91. Fangueiro JF, Andreani T, Egea MA, Garcia ML, Souto SB, Souto EB. Experimental factorial design applied to mucoadhesive lipid nanoparticles via multiple emulsion process. *Colloids and Surfaces B: Biointerfaces*. 2012 Dec 1;100:84–9.

92. Tan SW, Billa N, Roberts CR, Burley JC. Surfactant effects on the physical characteristics of Amphotericin B-containing nanostructured lipid carriers. *Colloids and Surfaces A: Physicochemical and Engineering Aspects*. 2010 Dec 3;372(1–3):73–9.

93. Charcosset C, El-Harati A, Fessi H. Preparation of solid lipid nanoparticles using a membrane contactor. *Journal of Controlled Release*. 2005 Nov 2;108(1):112–20.

94. Dudala TB, Yalavarthi PR, Vadlamudi HC, Thanniru J, Yaga G, Mudumala NL, Pasupati VK. A perspective overview on lipospheres as lipid carrier systems. *International Journal of Pharmaceutical Investigation*. 2014 Oct;4(4):149.

95. Jain S, Jain V, Mahajan SC. Lipid based vesicular drug delivery systems. *Advances in Pharmaceutics*. 2014 Sep 2;2014:1–2.

96. Akbarzadeh A, Rezaei-Sadabady R, Davaran S, Joo SW, Zarghami N, Hanifehpour Y, Samiei M, Kouhi M, Nejati-Koshki K. Liposome: Classification, preparation, and applications. *Nanoscale Research Letters*. 2013 Dec;8:1–9.

97. Bansal S, Kashyap CP, Aggarwal G, Harikumar SL. A comparative review on vesicular drug delivery system and stability issues. *International Journal of Research in Pharmacy and Chemistry*. 2012;2(3):704–13.

98. Jain S, Jain V, Mahajan SC. Lipid based vesicular drug delivery systems. *Advances in Pharmaceutics*. 2014 Sep 2;2014:1–2.

99. Zhou X, Chen Z. Preparation and performance evaluation of emulsomes as a drug delivery system for silybin. *Archives of Pharmacal Research*. 2015 Dec;38:2193–200.

100. Raza K, Katare OP, Setia A, Bhatia A, Singh B. Improved therapeutic performance of dithranol against psoriasis employing systematically optimized nanoemulsomes. *Journal of Microencapsulation*. 2013 May 1;30(3):225–36.

12 Ethical and Regulatory Aspects of Nanomedicine

Disha Kesharwani, Ashish Baldi,
Shivani Rai Paliwal, and Rishi Paliwal

12.1 INTRODUCTION

Nanotechnology in medical science covers the study, preparation, research, marketing, and application of nanomedicines. Nanomedicines are formulations containing drugs in the nanoscale range (1–100 nm) in one dimension. Nanopharmaceuticals are preparations containing nanomaterials for therapeutic treatment, reduction, or prevention of any disorder [1, 2]. Nanotechnology is a vast field and developing every second. Nanomedicine can be considered a vital part of every field including diagnosis, monitoring, and treatment. Nanotechnology has the potential to transform most industries. It has a great impact on medical and health care systems. Nanomedicine could have an enormous impact on society in the future. Nanomedicine is very efficient to improve patient quality of life, reduce societal and economic costs associated with healthcare, offer early detection of pathological conditions, reduce the severity of therapy, and result in improved clinical outcomes for the patient [3].

Developing medical technologies and scientific discoveries bring up many questions relating to the role of human dignity in medical research and in the society of the future. Nanomedicines have been found to improve human potential and empower the healthy professionals to miniscule the time of diagnosis and treatment. The area of nanotechnology covers the use of nanoparticulate molecules, diagnostic nanodevices and targeted drug delivery to different organs as well as production of new therapeutic materials like nanoprotheses, nanorobots and biosensing [3]. A strong focus on extremes of nanoethics is highly imperative as the ethical assessment tend to diverge radically. A more updated, balanced and knowledgeable ethical assessment is needed. There are a lot of loopholes of nanoethics: (1) Reduction of ethics to cost/benefit analysis. (2) Non-prudent description of ethics as risk management tool. (3) Puzzlement of technique with technology and human nature with human condition. These points need to be clarified to step up progressively towards development of nanotechnology [4].

European group of ethics (EGE) have been issued a draft report on 17 January 2007 that concedes the potential of nanomedicine for developing new diagnostic tools and therapies. The group put forward some statements that some measures will essentially be taken to verify the safety of nanomaterials. A website on ethics and nanomedicine was also recommended as an open platform for public to question and to find information from researchers. They have also recommended public discussions on the matters put up by nanomedicine development. The ethical, legal and social implications (ELSI) of nanomedicines were also prominently emphasized in the report. They recommended that upto 3% of the research budget be conserved for ELSI research. The report have also suggested to upgrade the education of the field and to encourage the researchers to make ethics an inextricable part in research [4].

12.2 SAFETY CONCERN/COMPATIBILITY OF NANOMEDICINE TO THE BIOLOGIC SYSTEM

Nanotechnology is successful because of the smaller particle size which felicitates the particles entry into various body parts. The smaller particles size multiples its potency, sometimes toxic. It is

DOI: 10.1201/9781003130055-12

essential to control the degree of particle's toxicity. So that this toxicity can be used at certain desirable conditions, such as treatment of cancer. However, the nanoparticles used in in-vitro diagnostics are free from this concern [5]. Ethical aspects in nano-drug delivery system arises from the step of nanomaterials selection. As a broad range of materials either natural, synthetic, hydrophilic or hydrophobic in nature can be used to deliver the active drug molecule. The nature of the material has a great impact on the risk associated with using them in delivery system. This shows that, it is very difficult to determine the safety of nanomaterials due to their diverse chemical configuration.

Also the physical characteristics of ingredients affect the basic physicochemical properties of the nanomedicine. These properties which make the nanomedicine unique and effective can also cause risks. For example, the nanomedicines have the ability to cross the blood brain barrier unintentionally, can activate a severe immune response, unintentional accumulation and toxicity in certain tissues. These properties raises questions about risks associated with the nanomedicines which are generally not observed with the conventional dosage form of drug. As the nano-based therapies are growing enormously, the specifications of clinical trials are the matter of great concern. As with the clinical trial there are chances of risk and benefits for human research subjects. The human research subjects should first informed about the complexity of nano-technological study and their consent should be taken, as an ethical step [6]. It is an important topic for the subjects involved, to understand carefully. Along with this the long term effects of nanomedicines are unknown. The study period can be of many years. So it is the responsibility of R & D scientists to do long term follows up of subjects under clinical trial study. The subjects must be clearly informed that there must be some unpredictable and prospective effects of study.

The targeted drug delivery is the most developed and popular domain of nanomedicine. Due to these properties the nano-sized particles of active drug molecule can be delivered directly to the diseased tissues of the body. The nanomedicines behavior is very unpredictable in-vivo. They behave differently than in vitro condition. Nanoparticles can disintegrate to tiny particles or aggregate to lumps that can be toxic to the biological system. These possibilities cause a mandatory ethical step of short term and long term clinical studies to prove that the nanomaterials are really more important and safer than other delivery systems. The long term studies followed by post marketing surveillance or phase IV study should be a compulsory step by the nanomedicine companies to ensure the safe use of nanomedicine. This practice is poorly practiced as the current laws do not enforce them. Although some regulatory steps should be taken to make these steps mandatory. FDA should make it a mandatory step for the nanomedicine companies [7, 8].

12.3 ETHICS IN MEDICAL APPLICATION

The nanotechnology development also causes long term justice and access issues. As the nanotherapy is very expensive initially when introduced in the market due to patent protection. The prices drop when the competitors work to develop similar therapies or after the term of the patent when generics start to flow in the market. During the term of the patent, these expensive therapies are out of reach for the middle class status people. Nano-technological therapies exacerbated the problems associated with socioeconomic differences [9]. Therefore the fair distributions of benefits of nanomedicines to all the classes of society at affordable prices are also of great ethical consideration. The availability of novel nano-therapies at affordable prices to all segments of society is directly related to the control over the patent rights. So in order to make it fair for lower socio-economic class, the national and international patent laws should ensure that the patentees do not have immoderate control on market [10, 11].

12.4 ETHICAL ISSUES RAISED BY NANOTECHNOLOGY

Although nanotechnology offers a lot of improvement in medical system but it also negatively affects the health system. As the unknown adverse effects are still the matter of study. We have

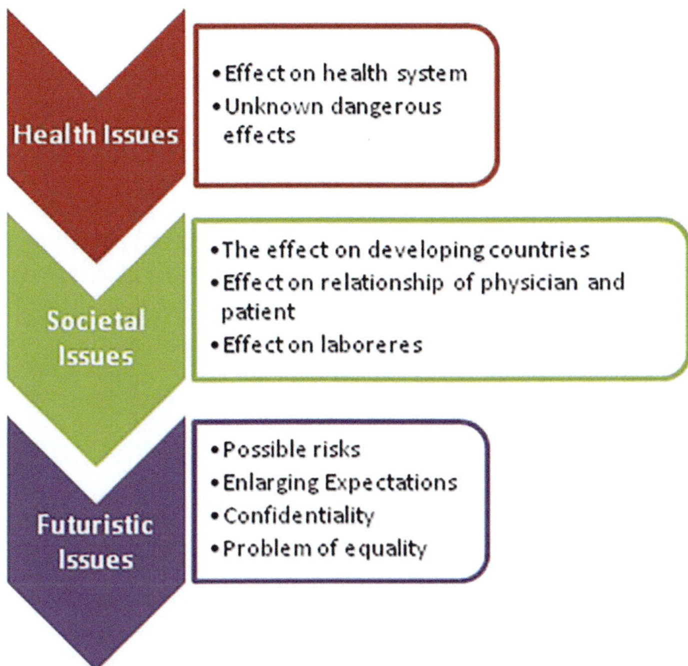

FIGURE 12.1 Issues related to nanomedicine.

already discussed that the nanomedicine can behave in completely different way in-vivo as compared to the effects observed in in-vitro study. Figure 12.1 represents the issues raised by nanomedicines. It causes competition between the developed and developing countries. As the developed countries consider nanotechnological industries as a powerful global tool [12, 13]. Another societal and ethical impact is on the relationship of physician and patient. As the progression of technology caused the replacement of humanitarian relationship with the machineries. The art of execution is completely transformed to a team and technology service. It is also very important to discuss the unknown toxic effects of nanoparticles that is dangerous for the workers and researchers [14, 15].

The nanotechnology also have some futuristic issues. As the power of expanding nanotechnology may cause to nourish false hopes. It can be a cause of waste of time and money. It is very important to stay and give a deep thought on practicable part of it. Today the risks linked with nano-technological treatment are not certain. But it should not be more impactful as compared to the benefit offered by it. Otherwise the treatment would not be meaningful. The ethical issues related to confidentiality of nano-technological databases also exist in the field. The reason behind this confidentiality is the exiting competition between the countries. The developing countries are still struggling in this aspect. Even the developed technology is limited to rich flora of people. It is not available to all the levels general public of the country [16, 17].

12.5 ETHICAL ISSUES RAISED BY APPLICATION OF NANOMEDICINES

With the expansion of science and technology of nanomedicines the consideration of ethical issues and laws are also important. Nanoethicists believed that consideration of ethics should be an important part of research and development process [18]. So it is very important to particularly address all the aspects of nanomedicines to minimize its adverse effects on the environment and to avoid the public reaction. Without regulation, unexpected and unwanted adverse events due to applied nanotechnology in nanomedicine can be expected and also it can be a way to make profit of some unethical persons [11, 19].

Practice of ethics is mandatory for application of nanotechnology at any step. Like during diagnosis, approval of diagnostic tool and privacy consent of patient is important [20].

Likewise use of nanomedicine without approval for safety and efficacy in the treatment, must be a breach of informed consent principle [21]. Along with this practitioners protection is also needed who has to come in contact with the newly used nanomatertial. Development of new nanosubstances, should also avoid misconduct during researc, publication and patenting. As noted by Allon *et al.*, "Some scientists agree that advancements in nanotechnology may give rise to various new ethical challenges, whilst others proclaim that these challenges are not new and that nanotechnology basically facsimiles recurrent bioethical dilemmas" [22].

Internationally, alliance and implementation of local and international law for control of the use of nanotechnology in nanomedicine is an important requirement against the possible emerging misconduct and unethical practice in medicine.

12.6 PERSPECTIVE OF PRACTITIONER ABOUT ETHICAL ISSUES RELATED TO NANOMEDICINE

Many industrial and developing countries have assigned remarkable amounts of funding for nanotechnological research. However, to now there has been little formal study regarding ethical and social issues of nanomedicines all over the world. Therefore it seems that we need to consider ethics training assessment and scholarship in nanomedicines. Preliminary proposals for research ethics, and medical ethics training for scientists and clinicians are also need [23].

12.7 REGULATORY ASPECTS OF NANOMATERIALS

Nanotechnology is the study of materials in nano range. When the material is converted to nano-scale the physicochemical, mechanical, biological, electronic, optical and various other properties are altered, which can be very useful in different fields including food, agriculture, health, energy, chemicals, environment and industries. Also this technology is expanding exponentially in Pharmaceutical sector. This nano-scale conversion may also change the pharmacokinetic and

---

TABLE 12.1

Ethical Issues Generated from Different Fields of Nanomedicine

S. No.	Different Fields	Ethical issus
1.	Diagnosis	Conflict of interest
		Approval of Diagnostic tool
		Privacy of Patient's Data
2.	Treatment	Conflict of interest
		Nanodrug and nanotherapy technique approval
		Informed consent and Do no harm principle
3.	Prevention	Conflict of interest
		Nanovaccine technique approval
		Informed consent and Environmental and ecotoxicology
4.	Research	Intellectual property rights related
		Delinquency in research
		Delinquency in publication

toxicokinetic and biotransformation properties of drug molecules which raise various quality, safety and efficacy issues.

The fast development of nanotechnology has given speed to the industrial sector. Many countries all over the world have been active in examining the appropriateness of their regulatory frameworks for dealing with nanotechnologies. These developed products completely change the results of treatment or therapy in terms of efficacy, bioavailability, intensity, packaging, time duration etc. At the same time these technology also pose risk to human health and environment due to their properties [24].

The development of nanomedicines enforced the efforts worldwide to regulate the production and safe use of these materials either by legislation or guidance. As currently there is no legislation that is completely dedicated to the regulation of nanomedicines. The available legislation is accepted by many countries, considering it specific enough to regulate the technology. But many amendments have been suggested by some non-governmental NGOs and European parliament. By noticing potential risks in this field many experts are working for preparing a strong law completely dedicated to NMs. The list includes European scientific countries and agencies, the Organization of Economic Cooperation and Development (OECD) and United State Food and Drug Administration. The EU and Switzerland were the only world region where the provisions specific to nanomaterials were incorporated in the running legislation [25, 26].

In India, there is also no specific concrete guideline for the development and evaluation of nano-pharmaceuticals. So it has been felt obligatory to construct an exhaustive guideline specific for quality, safety and efficacy of nano-pharmaceuticals. So that, the therapeutic applications of nano-pharmaceuticals can be transparent, compatible and foreseeable in India.

The guideline is applicable to nano-pharmaceuticals in finished form as well as to the API of new molecule or of an approved molecule with altered dimensions or properties associated with nanotechnology application in diagnosis, treatment, or prevention of disease in human (New Drugs and Clinical Trials Rules 2019).

The guideline does not applicable to-

  (i)   Incidental presence of nanoparticles.
 (ii)   Drug products containing microbes or proteins naturally in nanoscale range
(iii)   Medical devices and in vitro diagnostics using nano particle modified cell based therapy.

The guidelines evaluations of nanopharmaceuticals in India were prepared by a joint contribution of Central Drug Standard Control Organization (CDSCO), Department of Biotechnology under the Ministry of Science and Technology, and the Indian Council of Medical Research (ICMR) under the Ministry of Health and Family Welfare. These guidelines have been issued as there is no guideline worldwide that is globally accepted.

12.7.1 REGULATION OF EVALUATION OF NANO-PHARMACEUTICALS WITH CONTEXT OF SCHEDULE Y OF DRUGS AND COSMETICS RULES 1945

The guideline for the evaluation of nano-pharmaceuticals have been constructed in line with the provision of schedule Y of D &C 1945 with special consideration of NPs. Schedule Y provides requirements and guidelines for manufacturing and import of new drugs to perform clinical trial, to manufacture and import new drug, specific requirements of chemicals and pharmaceutical information as well as non-clinical and clinical data related to nano-technological based products. The general requirements of schedule Y are similar for new drug weather it belongs to nano-pharmaceutical class or not. But because of complexity of nano-technological products it is considered on a case by case approach for evaluation of quality, safety and efficacy.

For the safety studies the guidelines specified in second schedule of New Drugs and Clinical Trial Rules, 2019 should be followed. However if there is no specific study included, the principles of USFDA, ICH or OECD guideline can be followed. These guidelines have a close adherence to the provisions of Drugs and Clinical trial Rules, 2019 with special reference to quality, safety and efficacy of nano-pharmaceuticals.

Following documents have been considered for the construction of these guidelines:

1. Schedule Y of D & C Rules 1945
2. New Drugs and Clinical Trials Rules, 2019
3. Second Regulatory Review on Nanopharmaceuticals, European Union, 2012
4. EU-NCL survey with the "Nanomedicine"
5. working group of the international pharmaceutical regulators
6. Regulatory Aspects of the Nanopharmaceuticals in the EU, 2017

12.8 STABILITY TESTING OF NANOPHARMACEUTICALS

Stability testing of nano-pharmaceuticals should be designed according to requirements specified in appendix IX of schedule Y of D & C Rules 1945. A systemic and extensive stability study should be designed for developmental nano-pharmaceutical products after loading of drug its stability should be tested timely. The properties to be focused on are size of nanoparticles, functionality, stability, intensity, degradation products, size distribution, poly-dispersity index, zeta potential, surface chemistry etc. Small angle X-ray diffraction and microscopy should be used for determining layer thickness and morphology.

12.9 ANIMAL STUDY DATA

The animal study should be according to the guideline specified in appendix IV of schedule Y of Drugs and Cosmetics Rule 1945. This study is very essential to gather the knowledge of activity and toxicity of free drug, delivery system behavior, and influence of drug release rate on target and selection of appropriate range of nano-pharmaceutical. For evaluating nano-pharmaceuticals efficacy pre-clinical research should generate data sets that explain the properties of product behavior. Such properties include-accumulation of drug at disease site, its distribution to other non-diseased

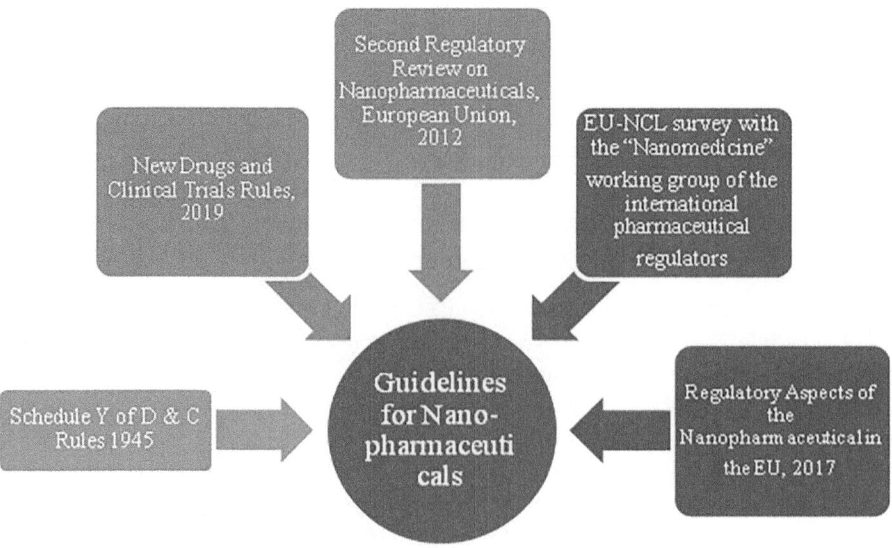

FIGURE 12.2 Guidelines for nanopharmaceuticals.

TABLE 12.2

General Information Required to Be Submitted

S. No.	Titles		Subtitles
1.	Introduction	a.	Brief of nanopharmaceutical
		b.	Justification for its development
		c.	Indication
		d.	Category
2.	Drug and Formulation related Information	a.	Ingredients Information
		(i)	Drugs brief
		(ii)	Nano-material and excipients information
		(iii)	Nano-formulations brief
		b.	Physicochemical Characterization
		(i)	Individual components
		(ii)	Chemical name and structure
		(iii)	Empirical formula
		(iv)	Molecular structure
		(v)	Product Description
			Size distribution
			Particle size, shape and texture
			pH
			Viscosity
			Surface charge
		c.	Analytical Analysis
		(i)	UV spectra
		(ii)	FTIR spectra
		(iii)	Mass spectra
		(iv)	NMR spectra
		d.	Monograph specification
		(i)	Identity
		(ii)	Impurity profile
		(iii)	Assay
		(iv)	Drug release kinetics
		(v)	Degradation kinetics
		e.	Stability Study
		f.	Pharmaceutical data
		(i)	Justification for nanoformulation
		(ii)	Dosage form
		(iii)	Route of administration
		(iv)	Composition
		(v)	Frequency of administration
		(vi)	Drug excipient compatibility
		(vii)	Validation
		(viii)	Finished product specification
		i.	Comparison of the product with innovator's product, if applicable
		j.	Packaging specification
3.	Animal Pharmacology Study	a.	Pharmacokinetics
		b.	Pharmacodynamics
		c.	Special pharmacological actions

(*Continued*)

TABLE 12.2   (Continued)
General Information Required to Be Submitted

S. No.	Titles	Subtitles	
4.	Animal Toxicology Study	a.	General toxicity study
		b.	Genotoxicity
		c.	Systemic toxicity
		d.	Hypersensitivity
		e.	Carcinogenicity
5.	Human Clinical Study	a.	Summary
		b.	General pharmacological effects
		c.	Specific pharmacological effects
		d.	Pharmacokinetics
		e.	Pharmacodynamics
6.	Therapeutic exploratory trial	a.	Summary
		b.	Report
7.	Therapeutic confirmatory trial	a.	Summary
		b.	Report
8.	Bioavailability and Bioequivalence test	a.	Summary
		b.	Protocol
		c.	Report
9.	Regulatory status in countries	a.	Marketed
		b.	Restricted
10.	Prescribing Information	a.	Label

organs etc. From the data sets the bioavailable drug, free drug and the concentration of drug at the site of action can be calculated. The peripheral pharmacokinetics of the nano-pharmaceuticals should also be assessed. All these features contribute to determine the potential efficacy. On the basis of results obtained the dominant feature can influence the choice of delivery system and desired release kinetics [27–33].

12.10   INFORMATIONS REQUIRED FOR EVALUATION OF NANOPHARMACEUTICALS

The information required for evaluation of nano-pharmaceuticals is generally based on case by case approach. Table 12.2 shows the general informations that should be submitted to the regulatory authority with application form to manufacture nano-pharmaceutical for marketing and to conduct clinical trials in India.

To regulate the appropriate use of nanotechnological products, a regulatory policy has been framed FDA. The policy is science based and completely focused on products. The legal standards are product specific. Nanotechnology products will be regulated by FDA through existing statutory authorities, following the specific standards applicable to each and every type of product under its jurisdiction. The Agency is taking a prudent scientific approach to assess each product on its own merits, and does not make broad, general assumptions about the safety of nanotechnology products.

12.11   CONCLUSION AND FUTURE PROSPECTS

Translational nanomedicine perspective requires scrutiny of each and every newly developed nano-medicine product before their approval per required regulatory guidelines. Although, it has been a challenging task for regulatory agencies too for establishing clear general guidelines for nanomedicine class of therapeutics. However, recently significant attempts have been made by these agencies to frame some regulations for upcoming nanomedicine based products. In future, more appropriate and clearer regulations will be required for next generation nanotheranognsitcs, personal medicines, 3-D generated products and AI-driven nanomedicine product.

REFERENCES

1. Fatehi L, Wolf SM, McCullough J. Recommendations for nanomedicine human subjects research oversight: An evolutionary approach for an emerging field. *Journal of Law, Medicine & Ethics.* 2012;40(4):716–750.
2. Ragelle H, Danhier F, Preat V. Nanoparticle-based drug delivery systems: A commercial and regulatory outlook as the field matures. *Expert Opinion on Drug Delivery.* 2017 Jul;14(7):851–864.
3. Mack TC, editor. Hopes and visions for the 21st century. *World Future Society.* 2007.
4. Gordijn B. Nanoethics: From utopian dreams and apocalyptic nightmares towards a more balanced view. *Science and Engineering Ethics.* 2005 Dec;11:521–33.
5. Jain KK, Jain KK. *The Handbook of Nanomedicine.* Totowa: Humana Press; 2008 Feb 24.
6. Oberdörster G, Oberdörster E, Oberdörster J. Nanotoxicology: An emerging discipline evolving from studies of ultrafine particles. *Environmental Health Perspectives.* 2005 Jul;113(7):823–39.
7. Gökçay B, Berna AR. Nanotechnology, nanomedicine; ethical aspects. *Revista romana de bioetica.* 2015 Jul;13(3).
8. Strom BL. How the US drug safety system should be changed. *JAMA.* 2006 May 3;295(17):2072–5.
9. Grewal AS, Lather V, Sharma N, Singh S, Narang RS, Narang JK, Pandita D. Recent updates on nanomedicine based products: current scenario and future opportunities. *Applied Clinical Research, Clinical Trials and Regulatory Affairs.* 2018 Aug 1;5(2):132–44.
10. Resnik, David B. Symposium: Drugs for the developing world: Developing drugs for the developing world: An economic, legal, moral, and political dilemma. In *AIDS: Society, Ethics and Law.* Routledge, UK; 2018:491–512.
11. Resnik DB. Fair drug prices and the patent system. *Health Care Analysis.* 2004 Jun;12:91–115.
12. Ebbesen M, Andersen S, Besenbacher F. Ethics in nanotechnology: Starting from scratch? *Bulletin of Science, Technology & Society.* 2006;26:451–462.
13. Sparrow R. The social impacts of nanotechnology, an ethical and political analysis. *Bioethical Inquiry.* 2009;6:13–23.
14. UNESCO. Universal Declaration on Bioethics and Human Rights. 2005:7.
15. UNESCO. The Ethics and Politics of Nanotechnology. 2006:13.
16. Cameron N. Nanotechnology, medicine and the human condition: A perspective from U.S. European commission: Group on ethics in science and new technologies. *Ethical Aspects of Nanomedicine.* 2006:31–37.
17. Hogle L. Science, ethics and the "problems" of governing nanotechnologies. *Journal of Law, Medicine & Ethics.* 2009:749–758.
18. Tremblay JF. Drug patent struggles in Asia. *Chemical & Engineering News.* 2007;85(6):11.
19. Resnik DB, Tinkle SS. Ethical issues in clinical trials involving nanomedicine. *Contemporary Clinical Trials.* 2007;28(4):433–441.
20. Satalkar P, Elger BS, Shaw DM. Stakeholder views on participant selection for first-in-human trials in cancer nanomedicine. *Current Oncology.* 2016;23:e530–7.
21. King NM. Nanomedicine first-in-human research: Challenges for informed consent. *Journal of Law, Medicine & Ethics.* 2012;40:823–30.
22. Allon I, Ben-Yehudah A, Dekel R, Solbakk JH, Weltring KM, Siegal G. Ethical issues in nanomedicine: Tempest in a teapot? *Medicine, Health Care and Philosophy.* 2017;20:3–11.
23. Manchikanti P, Uppala S, Bonta RK. Patents in nanobiotechnology: A cross jurisdictional approach. *Recent Patents on Biotechnology.* 2017;11:5270.
24. Harea JI, Lammers T, Ashford MB, Purie S, Barry ST. Challenges and strategies in anti-cancer nanomedicine development: An industry perspective. *Advanced Drug Delivery Reviews.* 2017;108:25–38.
25. Stern ST, Hall JB, Yu LL. Translational considerations for cancer nanomedicine. *Journal of Controlled Release.* 2010;146:164–74.
26. Ai J, Biazar E, Jafarpour M et al. Nanotoxicology and nanoparticle safety in biomedical designs. *International Journal of Nanomedicine.* 2011;6:1117–1127.

27. Sainz V, Conniot J, Matos AI. Regulatory aspects on nanomedicines. *Biochemical and Biophysical Research Communications*. 2015;468:504–10.
28. Emily M, Ioanna N, Scott B, Beat F. Reflections on FDA draft guidance for products containing nanomaterials: Is the abbreviated new drug application (ANDA) a suitable pathway for nanomedicines? *The AAPS Journal*. 2018;20:92.
29. Patel P, Shah J. Safety and toxicological considerations of nanomedicines: The future directions. *Current Clinical Pharmacology*. 2017;12:73–82.
30. Troiano G, Nolan J, Parsons D. A quality by design approach to developing and manufacturing polymeric nanoparticle drug products. *The AAPS Journal*. 2016;18:1354–65.
31. Giannakou C, Park MV, de Jong WH. A comparison of immunotoxic effects of nanomedicinal products with regulatory immunotoxicity testing requirements. *International Journal of Nanomedicine*. 2016;11:2935–52.
32. Miernicki M, Hofmann T, Eisenberger I. Legal and practical challenges in classifying nanomaterials according to regulatory definitions. *Nature Nanotechnology*. 2019;14:208–16.
33. Soares S, Sousa J, Pais A, Vitorino C. Nanomedicine: Principles, properties, and regulatory issues. *Frontiers in Chemistry*. 2018;6:360.

13 Regulatory Toxicological Assessment of Nanomedicines

Kunjbihari Sulakhiya, Ramu Singh, and Rishi Paliwal

13.1 INTRODUCTION

Nanomedicine is a branch of medicine that utilizes tools and techniques of nanotechnology to develop nanomaterials at their nano-size (ranging from 1–1000 nm) for the diagnosis, prevention and treatment of various diseases as well as for repairing impaired biological systems (1). It covers all three prominent areas of nanotechnology such as diagnostics, imaging agents and drug delivery with nanoparticles, more concisely known as theranostics used for both diagnosis and therapy (2, 3). Simply, nanomedicines are nanomaterials prepared by nanotechnology used for medical purposes. Nanomaterials are natural or synthetic materials with >50% particles of 1–100-nm size with unique physiochemical characteristics compared to conventional materials used in the dosage formulations (4, 5). Size, particle size distribution and surface area are fundamental parameters for the identification of nanomaterials in the nanomedicines. These unique physiochemical properties of nanomaterials including high surface area to volume ratio and controlled release have great advantages in nanoformulations, thereby altering pharmacokinetics (absorption, distribution, metabolism, excretion), pharmacodynamics (crossing of biological barriers, specific tissue/organ targeting, efficacy) and safety parameters (6). According to the US National Nanotechnology Initiative, nanoproducts may be divided into four different categories: passive nanostructures, active nanostructures, systems of nanosystems and molecular nanosystems (7). Nanomedicines are the passive nanostructures that include nanoparticles, liposomes, dendrimers, micelles, quantum dots, nanorods, nanorobots, nanoshells, nanotubes, nanofibers, fullerenes, nanowires, nanodiamonds, nanohorns, c-dots and nanocrystals (8–10). Nanoparticles (NPs) are of different types, for example, gold NPs, iron oxide NPs, RNA NPs and plasmonic NPs, and are important components of nanomedicines.

The Food and Drug Administration (FDA) advises investigating the safety, efficacy, environmental hazards and regulatory aspects of nanomaterials due to their novel characteristics (11). In a few decades, nanomedicines gained great attention in clinical practice as theragnostics to deliver toxic agents, to address multiple targets, to improve efficacy by reducing dose and toxicity, to target specific sites in a controlled release manner and to enhance transport across biological barriers of the body (12). Nanomedicines consist of nanomaterials which are commonly used as *in vivo* and *in vitro* diagnostic agents, *in vivo* therapeutic agents, implantable nanomaterials and regenerative medicines. Biomedical applications of nanomedicines may be classified into different categories. First as *in vivo* diagnostic agents (smart imaging) in computed tomography (CT), magnetic resonance imaging (MRI), positron emission tomography (ET), single-photon emission computed tomography (SPECT), fluorescence imaging and photoacoustic imaging for the imaging of the anatomy and physiology of the human body. Second as *in vitro* diagnostic agents (high-throughput screening) in quantum dot (QD)–based fluorescence polarization immunoassays, high-throughput multiplex detection technology assays (microfluidic chips, chemical nose sensors), luminescent transducers, C-dot (carbon dot)–based fluorescence resonance energy transfer (FRET), C-dot–based fluorescent pH sensors, surface plasmon resonance-based screening (chiroplasmonic assay), surface-enhanced Raman scattering (SERS), nanowire field-effect transistors (FETs), biomechanical assays (ultrasensitive cell traction force microscopy) for the identification

TABLE 13.1

Toxicity Assessment Tests for Nanomedicines as per Regulatory Authorities

Type of Study	Organism/ Animal Used	Dose	Route of Administration or Exposure	Duration of Treatment/ Exposure	Observations/ Parameters to Study	References
Acute or single-dose toxicity study—median lethal dose 50 (LD50) test	• Two rodent species (rat and mice) • 5 female animals/group	2000 mg/kg BW	Oral, inhalation, dermal or as intended for humans	• Single or several doses within 24 hours by oral gavage, and animals should be observed for 14 days	• Signs of intoxication, effect on body weight, gross pathological changes, mode of death • Minimum lethal dose (MLD) • Maximum tolerated dose (MTD) • Target organ toxicity • Mortality • LD_{50}, no observed adverse effect level (NOAEL), no observed effect level (NOEL), and low observed adverse effect level (LOAEL) determination	(16)
Acute or single-dose toxicity study—fixed dose procedure (FDP)	Female rat	• An initial dose level that causes some signs of toxicity but does not produce severe toxic effects or mortality is chosen based on the sighting study • Starting dose should be selected from suggested fixed doses, that is, 5, 50, 300 and 2000 mg/kg BW • If no sighting study, then starting dose should be 300 mg/kg	Oral	• Single or several doses within 24 hours by oral gavage and animals should be observed for 14 days	• Animals are observed for 30 min, 4 and 24 hours and a total of 14 days. • Changes in skin and fur; eyes; respiratory, circulatory and nervous systems; and behavior of animals. • Observations of convulsion, salivation, diarrhea, lethargy, sleep and coma. • Gross necroscopy, microscopic examination of organs	(16)

Subacute or sub-chronic toxicity study	• One rodent (rat or mice) and one non-rodent • One non-rodent species (2–3/sex/group for 14 days) (4–6/sex/group for 90 and 180 days)	At least three graded doses	As intended for humans	• Given in 14, 28, 90 or 180 days (duration depends on therapeutic indication) • One rodent (6–10/sex/group for 14 days) (15–30/sex/group for 90 and 180 days)	• Gross examination of the site of injection. • ECG and fundus examination in non-rodent. • Cage-side observations, body weight changes, food/water intake, blood biochemistry, hematology, gross and microscopic studies of all viscera and tissues. • Maximum tolerated dose (MTD) • Target organ toxicity	(16)
Chronic toxicity/ carcinogenicity study	• One rodent (rat or mice) and one non-rodent • Ten animals/group	At least three graded doses, a limit of 1000 mg/kg BW/day	Oral/inhalational/ dermal	• Six to 12 months (chronic phase) to 2 years duration (carcinogenicity phase) in rodents • One year or longer duration in non-rodent	• Gross examination of the site of injection • ECG and fundus examination in non-rodent • Cage-side observations, body weight changes, food/water intake, blood biochemistry, hematology, gross and microscopic studies of all viscera and tissues at 3, 6 and 12 months • Maximum tolerated dose (MTD) • No observed adverse effect level (NOAEL)	(16)
Dermal toxicity study	• One rat or rabbit/group	Three different concentrations of the formulation or 0.5 ml or 0.5 g in moistened form	Applied on a small area of skin, that is, 6 cm^2 using a gauze patch on the shaved skin of the animals	The exposure period may be 4 hours or 7 to 90 days depending on the clinical duration of use	• Nature and degree of irritation or corrosion • Signs of erythema, oedema and eschar formation • Gross examination of the site of application including histological examination	(17, 18)

(*Continued*)

TABLE 13.1 (Continued)

Toxicity Assessment Tests for Nanomedicines per Regulatory Authorities

Type of Study	Organism/ Animal Used	Dose	Route of Administration or Exposure	Duration of Treatment/ Exposure	Observations/ Parameters to Study	References
Photo-allergy/ dermal photo-toxicity study	Pre-test: 8 guinea pig Main test: 10 guinea pig for test compounds + 5 animals for controls	Pretest: 4 concentrations (patch application for 2 hr ± 15 min.) with and without UV exposure (10 J/cm^2) Main test: Highest non-irritant dose selected in pretest (0.3 ml/patch application for 2 hr ± 15 min.) with UV exposure (10 J/cm^2)	Topically on skin	• Patch application of test compounds for 2 hr ± 15 min. on day 0, 2, 4, 7, 9 and 11 • Repeat the exposure of the test substance between days 20 to 24	• Gross examination and grading of erythema and oedema formation at the site of application after 24 and 48 hours of exposure	(18)
Vaginal toxicity study	Rabbit or dog; 6–10 animals/dose group	Higher conc. or multiple daily doses as intended for human use	Vaginal mucosa (topically)	Seven to 30 days	• Swelling, closure of introitus and histopathological examination of the vaginal wall or mucosa	(18)
Rectal tolerance test	Rabbit or dog; 6–10 animals/dose group	Maximum dose in volume than proposed human dose or multiple daily dose as intended for human use	Rectal administration	Seven to 30 days	• Sliding on the backside, pain, blood and/or mucus in feces, condition of anal region/ sphincter, gross histological examination of rectal mucosa	(18)
Ocular toxicity study	2 species including rabbits;	2 different concentrations exceeding the human dose based on initial single-dose application or 0.1 ml liquid and 100 mg solids	Conjunctival sac or cornea	Twenty-one days and not more than 90 days	• Signs of pain, repeated pawing or rubbing of the eye, excessive blinking and tearing • Slit-lamp examination to observe the changes in the cornea, iris and aqueous humor • Gross examination of the surface epithelium of the cornea and conjunctiva by fluorescent dyes • Intra-ocular tension changes monitoring by tonometer • Histopathological examination of eyes after fixation in Davidson's or Zenker's fluid to observe vascularization, pannus formation, adhesions, staining etc.	(16, 17, 19)

Inhalational toxicity study	One rodent and one non-rodent; 10 male and 10 female rodents	Five mg/ml limit dose; three dose groups and negative control (filtered air) or vehicle control (vehicle)	Aerosols by nose-only method	Six hr/day and 5 days a week up to 90 days (13 weeks); water and food should not be given during the exposure of test substance	• Temperature, humidity and flow rate of the exposure chamber should be recorded • Regular parameters of systemic toxicity studies • Test substance effects on respiratory rate, bronchoalveolar lavage fluid (BAL) examination, histological examination of respiratory tract and lung tissue	(18, 20)
Allergenicity/ hypersensitivity test 1. Guinea pig maximization test (GPMT) 2. Local lymph node assay	For determination of maximum dose: Four guinea pig/sex (two of each sex is given Freund's adjuvant) For determination of minimum irritant dose: Two animals/sex For min study: Six animals/group/sex (test and control group) Six mice/group of either sex (male or female only)	Four dose levels Three graded doses (highest—nonirritant dose + vehicle control)	Intradermal/topical topical (ear skin)	Day 1 (intradermal induction) to day 21 (topical challenge), re-challenge for 7–30 days if no response observed after the primary challenge Topically applied on ear skin for 3 consecutive days and on day 5	• Individual animal scores and maximization grading of erythema and oedema • Increase in ^{3}H-thymidine or bromo-deoxy-uridine (BrdU) level in draining auricular lymph node is measured (lymph node is collected after 5 hrs of ^{3}H-thymidine or BrdU IV injection)	(18) (18)
Male fertility study	Rat; six animals/group	Three doses were selected from 14- or 28-day toxicity studies conducted in the rats; the highest dose is one that shows minimal toxicity in systemic studies	Intended route of clinical use	28–70 days before mating with the female in a ratio of 1:2 and continue until the confirmation of pregnancy or 10 days post-pairing or mating, whichever is earlier	• The fertility index of a pregnant female is examined after 13 days of gestation • Male animals are sacrificed and then the weights of each testis and epididymis are measured • Sperm motility and morphology examination from one epididymis • Histopathological examination of both testis and other epididymis	(18)

(Continued)

TABLE 13.1   (Continued)

Toxicity Assessment Tests for Nanomedicines per Regulatory Authorities

Type of Study	Organism/ Animal Used	Dose	Route of Administration or Exposure	Duration of Treatment/ Exposure	Observations/ Parameters to Study	References
Female reproduction and developmental toxicity studies 1. Female fertility study 2. Teratogenicity 3. Perinatal study	Rat; 15 animals/sex/dose group One rodent (rat) and one non-rodent (rabbit); 20 pregnant rats or mice and 12 rabbits/dose group (control and treated group) Rodent (pregnant rat, dams); 15 dams/dose/ group (control and treated group; total four groups), F1 litters including 15 males and 15 females/ group	• Three graded doses, the highest dose is the maximum tolerated dose (MTD) obtained from systemic toxicity studies • The test drug is administered for 14 days in females and 28 days in males before mating Three doses; the highest dose causes minimum maternal toxicity, and the lowest dose is supposed to be used in humans for clinical purposes or its multiplication Three dose levels comparable to multiples of human dose	Intended route of therapeutic use As intended for human clinical use Intended route for clinical use	Drug treatment continues from mating to the gestation period to weaning of pups The drug is treated throughout the organogenesis period Administration of the test drug is started from day 15 of gestation (last trimester of pregnancy) and the dose causing low fetal damage is continued throughout lactation and weaning	• Body weight, food intake, signs of toxicity, mating behavior, progress of gestation/ parturition periods, length of gestation, parturition, post-partum health and gross pathology and histopathology of affected organs of dams should be recorded • The pups are also subjected to observe the sex-wise distribution in litters, body weight, signs of toxicity, survival and growth parameters, gross examination, histopathology of the organs • Gross examination of all fetuses • Skeletal and visceral abnormalities examination should be done in one fetus and its half • Dams should be observed for signs of intoxication, body weight and food intake; uterus examination; ovaries and uterine contents; number of corpora lutea; implantation sites • Fetuses should be observed for their total number, gender, and body weight as well as gross skeletal and visceral abnormalities • Dams are sacrificed to examine body weight, food intake, signs of intoxication, progress of gestation/parturition periods, gross pathology • Pups are observed for clinical signs, sex-wise distribution in a group, body weight, growth parameters, gross examination, survival, autopsy and histopathology • F1 generation's mating performance and fertility and F2 generation growth parameters are also examined	(18)

Genotoxicity	*S. typhimurium* strains	Five log dose levels, each set	*In-vitro* exposure	The test compound is injected in	A 2.5-fold or more increase in the number of	(18)
In-vitro studies	such as TA98, TA100,	of three replicates	*In-vitro* exposure	the Petri dish containing a culture	tester strains causing reverse mutation as	
1. Ames' test	TA102, TA1535, TA97	Three log dose levels plus	Route of	of tester strains with or without	compared to spontaneous revertant is considered	
(reverse	or *Escherichia coli*	'solvent' and 'positive'	administration is	metabolic activator, s9 mix.	positive	
mutation assay	WP2uvrA or *E. coli*	control group, each set of	as intended for	Positive control may use	Increased the number of chromosomal aberrations	
in Salmonella)	WP2 uvrA (pKM101)	three replicates	human use	9-aminoacridine, 2-nitrofluorine,	in the metaphase of cell division is observed and	
2. *In-vitro*	CHO cells or on human	Three log dose levels plus	Route of	sodium azide and mitomycin C	compared with the normal control	
cytogenetic	lymphocytes in culture	'solvent' and 'positive'	administration is	Test compounds are administered	Increased the number of chromosomal aberrations	
assay	One rodent (rat); five	control group	as intended for	in the vessels containing CHO	(breaks, gaps, sister chromatid exchange etc.) in	
(chromosomal	animals/sex/dose groups	Three log dose levels plus	human use	cell lines or human lymphocyte	the metaphase of cell division (minimum 100	
aberration	One rodent (mouse); five	'solvent' and 'positive'		culture with or without metabolic	cells) is observed and compared with the normal	
assay)	animals/sex/dose groups	control group		activator, S9 mix. Positive control	control	
In-vivo studies				like cyclophosphamide with S9	Increased the number of micronuclei in	
1. *In-vivo*				mix and mitomycin C without	polychromatic erythrocytes (minimum 1000) is	
cytogenetic				metabolic activation used to	observed and compared with the normal control	
assay				detect and reproduce the		
(chromosomal				clastogenic effects		
aberration				•Cyclophosphamide is used as		
assay)				positive control		
2. *In-vivo*				•Test compound is administered to		
micronucleus				animals on day 1, then colchicine		
assay				administration (i.p.) at 22 hours		
				•After 2 hours of colchicine		
				injection, animals are sacrificed to		
				aspirate bone marrow from the		
				femur and flush with hypotonic		
				saline for 20 min., then pelleted		
				and resuspended in Carnoy's fluid		

(*Continued*)

TABLE 13.1 (Continued)
Toxicity Assessment Tests for Nanomedicines per Regulatory Authorities

Type of Study	Organism/ Animal Used	Dose	Route of Administration or Exposure	Duration of Treatment/ Exposure	Observations/ Parameters to Study	References
				• Again, the cells are pelleted and a drop is put on the glass slide, stained with Giemsa • Cyclophosphamide and mitomycin C are used as a positive control • Test compound is administered on days 1 and 2 followed by the sacrifice of animals after 6 hours of the last injection • Take out femur bone marrow, flush with fetal bovine serum for 20 min., make pellet and make a smear on a glass slide • Stain with Giemsa-MayGruenwald staining		
Mutagenicity/ carcinogenicity	Rodent (rat), mice may be used if required with scientific justification • Not subjected to sacrifice—50 animals/ sex/dose group • High-dose group—20 animals/sex/dose group • Control group—Ten animals/sex/dose group	Three dose levels plus control and vehicle control group, highest dose (sub-lethal dose) and lowest dose (intended human therapeutic dose or multiple of it)	Route of administration— as intended for human use	• Test drug is administered every day (7 days a week) over the recommended therapeutic duration (24 months for rats and 18 months for mice)	• General observations like signs of toxicity, body weight and food intake, clinical chemistry parameters, hematology parameters, urine analysis, organ weight, gross pathology and histopathology • Macroscopic changes at autopsy and histopathology of organs and tissues are observed • Detailed descriptions of benign and malignant tumor development, time of detection, site, dimensions and histological typing should be done • Short-term bioassay, neonatal mouse assay and tests using transgenic animals may be done in addition, if required	(18)

| **Immunogenicity/ immunotoxicity** (T-cell–dependent antibody response; TDAR assay, immunotyping, natural killer cell activity assays, host resistance studies, macrophage/neutrophil function, and assays to measure cell-mediated immunity) | • As mentioned in standard toxicity studies (acute, subacute and chronic), the highest dose (above NOAEL) | At least three graded doses | As intended for humans | • Test drugs or substances given daily for 28 days | • It is performed in case of signs of immunotoxic potential as observed in standard toxicity studies (STSs), anti-inflammatory drugs, drugs for immunocompromised patients, high disposition of drugs in the immune system, signs of immunotoxicity during clinical trials
• Additional immunotoxicity testing is done when sufficient data of risk is not there
• Evaluation parameters include total and absolute differential leukocyte counts, globulin and A/G ratios, lymphoid organs/tissues gross pathology, thymus, spleen and lymph nodes weight, histopathology of thymus, spleen, lymph node, bone marrow, Peyer's patch, BALT and NALT etc. | (21) |

of biological components such as molecules, cells and tissues in biological fluids outside of the human body as diagnostic markers. Third as *in vivo* therapeutic agents (particle-based delivery) in NP-based anticancer drug delivery for solid tumors (dendrimers), nanoparticulate delivery vehicles (liposomes, micelles, chitosan, nanodiamonds, mesoporous silica NPs, carbon nanotubes, graphenes), specific cell and tissue targeting (passive, active and magnetic targeting), non-invasive delivery of macromolecular biopharmaceuticals (polypeptides, proteins) across biological barriers, controlled release delivery systems (stimuli-responsive drug-loaded NPs, thermo-responsive drug nanocarriers) for the diagnosis and treatment of various diseases including cancer, cardiovascular and neurodegenerative diseases and photothermal cancer therapy is promising way to treat cancer. Fourth as biodegradable implants (implantable nanomaterials) in the form of carbon nanostructures such as single/multiwall carbon nanotubes (SWCNTs/MWCNTs), carbon nanohorns, nanodiamonds, fullerenes, graphenes for the drug delivery, biological response and biodegradation inside the body, biologically derived implants are also used as regenerative medicines to regenerate injured tissues, development of artificial organs and organs-on-a-chip applications. Fifth as theranostic agents (combination of *in vivo* diagnosis and treatment) in image-guided tumor resection and drug delivery tracing uses NPs for the diagnosis, removal and treatment of tumors after surgery as well as monitoring of drug delivery into tumor cells (9). The beneficial clinical outcomes of nanomedicine depend on the physiochemical properties of nanomaterials; the pathophysiology of diseases; and the interaction of nanomaterials with biological components, including proteins, phospholipids and membrane-bound substances (12).

Nanomedicines are highly regulated by the regulatory authorities of each country as nanotechnological products to ensure their safety and efficacy before their market authorization. Since the need for nanomedicines is increasing day by day due to their added advantages over conventional medicines, critical safety assessment is of the utmost importance per various regulatory agencies (6). Typically, nanomedicines are rapidly accommodated by the cells of the reticuloendothelial system (RES) and accumulate in the liver and spleen tissues, leading to toxicity. Toxicological evaluation of nanomedicines is important to ensure their safety; however, there is a lack of concise and clear methodology to perform toxicity studies systematically. This chapter deals with various toxicological studies required to be performed per different regulatory authorities to ensure the safety of nanomedicines. Further, a detailed methodology of each toxicity test is discussed and compared with different regulatory agencies such as International Council for Harmonisation, OECD and Schedule Y. It also deals with the role of various physiochemical properties of nanomedicines and biological systems in nanomedicine toxicity.

13.2 REGULATORY TOXICOLOGY AND ITS IMPORTANCE

Regulatory toxicology deals with the collection, processing and evaluation of epidemiological and experimental toxicology data for the protection of health from chemical substances based on their toxicological assessment. It enables to development of new protocols and methods for the improvement of the scientific domain to decide a particular product's market authorization (13). With the increased demand for nanomedicine in the healthcare system, ensuring safety per the guidelines of regulatory bodies is essential to maintain the trust of consumers as well as to avoid confusion among users about safety concerns. Rigorous regulatory toxicological assessments are an important part of the development of safer nanomedicines; therefore, the 'safer-by-design' initiative was launched by the European authorities. Regulatory bodies have framed guidelines for the assessment of the toxicity of nanomedicines on humans and the environment to minimize the risk and to improve the therapeutic index (14). These regulatory agencies have definitive guidelines which include various *in vitro, in situ, in silico* and *in vivo* toxicity tests with detailed study protocol and methodology to ensure the optimum safety of nanomedicines before marketing approval. Authorities also emphasize the role of physicochemical properties, route of administration, interaction with biological systems and elimination of nanomedicines and their toxicity (15). Therefore, regulatory bodies play a significant role in the minimization of toxicity, thereby improving efficacy. Table 13.1 lists important toxicity assessment tests for nanomedicines per regulatory authorities.

13.3 SAFE-BY-DESIGN AND NANOMEDICINE

With increasing applications of nanomedicines, more attention is being paid to the safety and efficacy of these medicines in patients. The basic concept of safe-by-design is to identify the risks and prevent or reduce them at an early stage of drug development to avoid potentially harmful effects of nanomaterials on human health and the surrounding environment as well as to develop efficacious nanomedicines. Safe-by-design (SbD) is a new concept to ensure safety at the initial stage of the innovation process and coexists with the quality by design (QbD) approach, which utilizes critical quality attributes (CQAs) for the development of nanomedicines of desired and optimum characteristics (22, 23). SbD is not yet included in the regulatory guidelines of various regulatory bodies including the ICH, EMA and FDA. The complex nature of nanomaterials and the interaction of nanomedicines with biological systems play significant roles in the prediction of adverse effects and subsequently market authorization. The lack of guidelines, tools and standards for assessing the toxicities of nanomedicines are a profound concern to fully utilize the advantages of nanomedicines in the health care system. Therefore, it is of the utmost importance to develop safe and effective medicines, and it could be made possible by employing the SbD approach in the drug development process (24).

13.4 TOXICITY ASSESSMENT OF NANOMEDICINES

Nanotoxicology is the branch of toxicology that deals with toxicity studies of nanotechnological-derived products, including nanomedicines. The main objective of these studies is to identify the potential toxic or harmful effects of nanopharmaceuticals on human beings and the environment (16). The toxic effects associated with nanomedicines, especially nanoparticles, include dermatitis, urticaria, asthma, hypertension, arrhythmia, auto-immune diseases and cancer and brain disorders, and these may be due to the novel characteristics of nanomedicines (25). Figure 13.1 represents the prooxidant pathway for nanoparticle-induced toxicities for quick reference of the mechanism. There are no clear guidelines for toxicity evaluation of nanomedicines; however, basic *in vitro*, *in silico* and *in vivo* tests are used to investigate the toxic effects per standard testing protocols. It is vital to ensure the safety as well as efficacy of nano-enabled products including nanomedicines due to their increased biomedical applications as theranostics. Safety assessment through applying different toxicological tests is essential to observe possible adverse effects of nanomedicines due to their physicochemical properties, biokinetics and interaction with human body systems. Nanopharmaceuticals have smaller sizes, large surface-area-to-volume ratios and unique shapes, which sometimes may be the reason for the toxic effects of nanomedicine. There are various steps involved in the toxicological assessment of nanomaterials in which a systemic approach is applied to assess the potential adverse effects of nanomaterials on the human body with strict regulatory compliance. The steps of toxicological risk assessment include hazard identification, dose-response assessment, exposure assessment, risk characterization, toxicological risk assessment of nanomaterials, *in vitro* toxicity tests and *in vivo* toxicity tests. Therefore, it is necessary to apply both traditional and new known toxicity tests to identify the potential risks associated with the use of nanomedicines. Further, these toxicological data might be useful for both patient safety and regulatory authorities to commercialize nanopharmaceuticals.

According to Limaye and co-workers (25), nanomedicine-related toxicity issues may be managed by adopting certain measures, including (1) identification of safety problems unique to nanomedicines through a battery of *in vitro* and *in vivo* toxicity testing and quantitative nanostructure-activity relationship (QNAR) modeling; (2) establishment of correlation between physicochemical properties and pharmacokinetic and pharmacodynamic behaviors; (3) improved understanding of

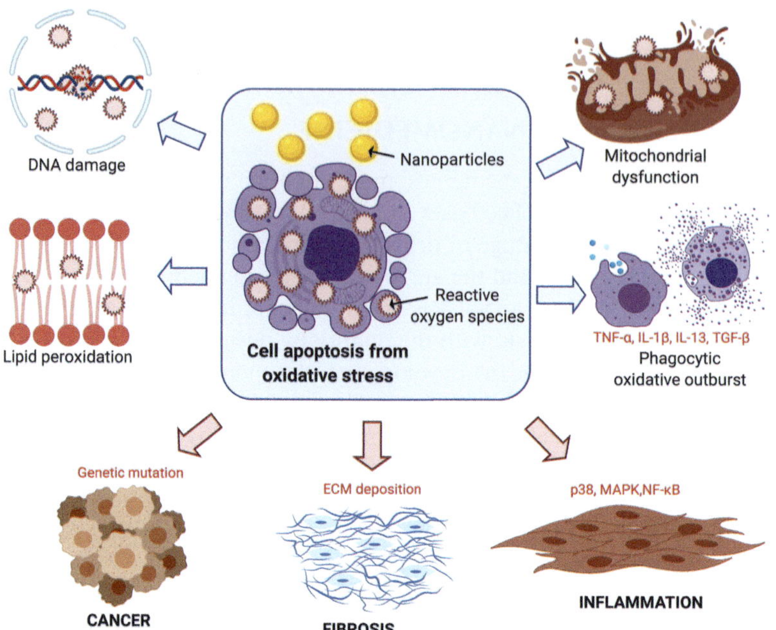

FIGURE 13.1 Prooxidant pathway for nanoparticle-induced toxicities. Upon nanoparticle exposure, ROS generation induces oxidative DNA damage, strand breaks, protein denaturation and lipid peroxidation. Mitochondrial membrane damage results from excess free radical production, leading to necrosis and cell death. Phagocytes (i.e., neutrophils and macrophages) generate massive ROS upon incomplete phagocytosis of nanoparticles, triggering an inflammatory cascade of chemokine and cytokine expression via activation of cell signaling pathways.

(Adopted from Damasco and co-workers) (26).

transport mechanisms across cell membrane and other biological compartments through permeability assays; (4) availability of complete pharmacokinetic information of the products; (5) development of standardized correlation of bio-distribution with safety and efficacy; (6) creation of robust data bank about interactions between nanomaterials and biological systems; (7) standardization of nanomaterials, protocols, refinement of definition and classification and exploration of international harmonization and treaties; and (8) specifications for regulatory submissions. Here we discuss various toxicity tests that are and/or may be used to ensure the safety of nanomedicines before their market authorization per the regulatory guidelines of the OECD, ICH, USFDA and Schedule Y.

13.5 ROLE OF PHYSICOCHEMICAL PROPERTIES IN NANOMEDICINE TOXICITY

The physicochemical characteristics of nanoparticles are major contributing factors in the development of toxicity. These properties include particle size, morphology (shape), overall surface area, availability of active functional groups, surface charge and catalytic potential. Particle size in the case of nanomedicine has been considered the first and foremost important criterion for evaluation of therapeutic performance as well as toxicity. Small-sized particles usually enter via penetration to epithelial cells and can cross endothelial barriers to enter the blood and lymphatic system, and from there they reach various organs/tissues. Such nanoparticles could be accessed via transcytosis mechanisms or by a simple diffusion process through the cell membrane and get deposited into vital organs like the brain, liver, heart, kidney and spleen and even into deeper biological locations like the bone marrow and nervous system. Nanoparticles may also reach blood circulation via body cavities through ingestion and via skin. If more flexible particles are developed, even large-size nanoparticles could enter through the skin. Size-based unique features of nanoparticles make them suitable to enter inflamed tissues, the epithelium lining of GIT and liver, leaky vasculature of tumors and also microcapillaries. The major toxic effects of deposited nanoparticles include the generation of platelet aggregation, leading to the development of thrombosis, inflammation in the respiratory tract, stroke and myocardial infarction and neurological diseases. Being tiny in size, nanoparticles enter the cell cytosol and reach intracellular locations and could generate damage to cell metabolism, nuclei and mitochondria functioning, leading to mutation and even cell death (27).

13.6 CONCLUSION AND FUTURE PERSPECTIVES

Nanomedicine is full of advantages but still has some limitations, especially related to toxicological aspects. Nanoparticles in medicine should be dealt with by using careful observations of their safety and toxicity. Regulatory agencies are much concerned about the safety of this new but efficacious class of therapeutics, which is otherwise not looked into conventional body distribution patterns. Henceforth, for every new nanomedicine introduced, its toxicological considerations should be well addressed before efficacy is claimed. In the future, more elaborate plans will be required to develop safe-by-design nanomedicines.

REFERENCES

1. Paliwal, S. R., Kenwat, R., Maiti, S., & Paliwal, R. (2020 Nov 1). Nanotheranostics for cancer therapy and detection: State of the art. *Current Pharmaceutical Design*, 26(42), 5503–17.
2. Paliwal, R., Chaurasiya, A., Panchal, K., Nayak, P., Parveen, N., & Paliwal, S. R. (2022 Jan 1). Engineering and functionalization of nanomaterials for theranostic applications in infectious diseases. In *Nanotheranostics for Treatment and Diagnosis of Infectious Diseases* (pp. 45–71). Academic Press.
3. Astruc, D. (2016). Introduction to nanomedicine. *Molecules*, 21(1), 4. https://doi.org/10.3390/molecules21010004
4. Nayak, V., Singh, K. R., Paliwal, R., Singh, J., Pandey, M. D., & Singh, R. P. (2023 Jan 1). Introduction to nanotechnological utility in the pharmaceutical industry. In *Nanotechnology for Drug Delivery and Pharmaceuticals* (pp. 337–355). Academic Press.
5. Soares, S., Sousa, J., Pais, A., & Vitorino, C. (2018). Nanomedicine: Principles, properties, and regulatory issues. *Frontiers in Chemistry*, 6, 360.
6. Paliwal, R., Kumar, P., Chaurasiya, A., Kenwat, R., Katke, S., & Paliwal, S. R. (2022 Jan 1). Development of nanomedicines and nano-similars: Recent advances in regulatory landscape. *Current Pharmaceutical Design*, 28(2), 165–77.
7. Yao, C., & Lu, J. (2012). Introduction to nanomedicine. *Nanomedicine*, 3–19. https://doi.org/10.1533/9780857096449.1.1
8. Patra, J. K., Das, G., Fraceto, L. F., Campos, E. V. R., del Pilar Rodriguez-Torres, M., Acosta-Torres, L. S., . . . Shin, H. S. (2018). Nano based drug delivery systems: Recent developments and future prospects. *Journal of Nanobiotechnology*, 16(1), 1–33.
9. Pelaz, B., Alexiou, C., Alvarez-Puebla, R. A., Alves, F., Andrews, A. M., Ashraf, S., . . . Parak, W. J. (2017). Diverse applications of nanomedicine. *ACS Nano*, 11(3), 2313–81.
10. Paliwal, R., Babu, R. J., & Palakurthi, S. (2014 Dec). Nanomedicine scale-up technologies: Feasibilities and challenges. *AAPS Pharmaceutical Science and Technology*, 15(6), 1527–34.
11. FDA (2014). *Guidance for Industry Considering Whether an FDA-Regulated Product Involves the Application of Nanotechnology*. Food and Drug Administration. www.fda.gov/downloads/RegulatoryInformation/Guidances/UCM401695.pdf
12. Hua, S., & Wu, S. Y. (2018). Advances and challenges in nanomedicine. *Frontiers in Pharmacology*, 9, 1397.

13. Schwenk, M., Werner, M., & Younes, M. (2002). Regulatory toxicology: Objectives and tasks defined by the working group of the German society of experimental and clinical pharmacology and toxicology. *Toxicology Letters*, 126(3), 145–53.

14. Accomasso, L., Cristallini, C., & Giachino, C. (2018). Risk assessment and risk minimization in nanomedicine: A need for predictive, alternative, and 3Rs strategies. *Frontiers in Pharmacology*, 9, 228.

15. Foulkes, R., Man, E., Thind, J., Yeung, S., Joy, A., & Hoskins, C. (2020). The regulation of nanomaterials and nanomedicines for clinical application: Current and future perspectives. *Biomaterials Science*, 8(17), 4653–64.

16. Erkekoglu, P., & Kocer-Gumusel, B. (2018). Toxicity assessment of nanopharmaceuticals. In *Inorganic Frameworks as Smart Nanomedicines* (pp. 565–603). William Andrew Publishing.

17. www.oecd-ilibrary.org/docserver/9789264070585-en.pdf?expires=1701787314&id=id&accname=guest&checksum=C0AAEA7677CD58B5F7E0E5B4EF10E90C/ accessed on 22.08.2023

18. https://cdsco.gov.in/opencms/export/sites/CDSCO_WEB/Pdf-documents/acts_rules/2016DrugsandCosmeticsAct1940Rules1945.pdf/ accessed on 24.08.2023

19. www.oecd-ilibrary.org/environment/test-no-405-acute-eye-irritation-corrosion_9789264185333-en/ accessed on 24.08.2023

20. OECD (2018). *Test No. 413: Subchronic Inhalation Toxicity: 90-day Study, OECD Guidelines for the Testing of Chemicals, Section 4*. OECD Publishing. https://doi.org/10.1787/9789264070806-en

21. www.fda.gov/media/72047/download/ accessed on 20.11.2021

22. Kesharwani, D., Paul, S. D., Paliwal, R., & Satapathy, T. (2023 Jun 1). Development, QbD based optimization and in vitro characterization of Diacerein loaded nanostructured lipid carriers for topical applications. *Journal of Radiation Research and Applied Sciences*, 16(2), 100565.

23. Kesharwani, D., Paul, S. D., Paliwal, R., & Satapathy T. (2023 Mar 1). Exploring potential of diacerin nanogel for topical application in arthritis: Formulation development, QbD based optimization and preclinical evaluation. *Colloids and Surfaces B: Biointerfaces*, 223, 113160.

24. Schmutz, M., Borges, O., Jesus, S., Borchard, G., Perale, G., Zinn, M., . . . Som, C. (2020). A methodological safe-by-design approach for the development of nanomedicines. *Frontiers in Bioengineering and Biotechnology*, 8, 258.

25. Limaye, V., Fortwengel, G., & Limaye, D. (2014). Regulatory roadmap for nanotechnology based medicines. *International Journal of Drug Regulatory Affairs*, 2014(2 (4)), 33–41.

26. Damasco, J. A., Ravi, S., Perez, J. D., Hagaman, D. E., & Melancon, M. P. (2020 Nov 2). Understanding nanoparticle toxicity to direct a safe-by-design approach in cancer nanomedicine. *Nanomaterials*, 10(11), 2186.

27. Manke, A., Wang, L., & Rojanasakul, Y. (2013 Oct). Mechanisms of nanoparticle-induced oxidative stress and toxicity. *BioMed Research International*, 2013.

14 Synthesis of Targeted Nanoparticles

Routes and Applications

Vijay Kumar Singh, Veena Devi Singh, and Swati Verma

14.1 INTRODUCTION

Nanomedicines, like conventional medicine, provide breakthroughs in the diagnosis and treatment of a wide range of medical issues. Nanotechnology employed in health care research has enormous human health advantages while avoiding adverse effects [1]. As drug carriers have been thoroughly investigated, there are numerous strategies for drug delivery among these nanostructures. Several variables influence a medication's effectiveness, including intrinsic drug properties, solubility in biological fluids, specificity of action, penetration through biological membranes, and cellular absorption [2]. Several difficulties with systemic drug administration have been identified by researchers. To access the intended tissues, the drug should first bypass many enzyme barriers. It has been discovered that drug administration with no target specificity generates toxicity due to random dispersion into normal healthy tissues [3]. Several research investigations have demonstrated that the use of nanotechnology in medicine delivery has the promise of delivering pharmaceuticals to precise areas. Target-specific nanoparticles (NPs) for drug delivery have the potential to improve treatment by boosting drug safety and decreasing the dosage of novel medicines [4]. In addition to enhancing physicochemical qualities, surface modification of NPs with biological ligands may help in drug binding to a specific receptor on the surface of target cells. Furthermore, ligand-based targeted medicines may enhance selectivity and increase drug distribution to sick cells. Passive or active targeting tactics are used in targeted drug delivery systems. Free nanocarriers circulate in the circulation for a longer period than free medicines in passive targeting. Nanoparticles with passive targeting penetrate deeper into the illness site, resulting in much greater medication accumulation through the enhanced permeability and retention (EPR) effect [5, 6]. The interaction between surface-modified NPs and the targeted cell is essential for active targeting. These devices have the benefit of delivering medications into the most resistant cells with sustained circulation [7]. Proteins, peptides, nucleic acids, polysaccharides, antibodies, tiny molecules, and aptamers have all been identified and exploited as biological ligands for drug targeting success. Following NP production, these ligands are functionalized on the surface of nanoparticles by chemical conjugation or physical adsorption [8, 9]. Polymeric nanoparticles, lipid nanoparticles, liposomes, nanoemulsions, nanogels, and dendrimers are now being studied extensively, and the majority of them are in clinical trials for imaging and drug administration [10]. This chapter discusses synthetic techniques for biological ligand conjugation and their application to NP-mediated medication delivery. The contents of this chapter are meant to provide evidence-based knowledge for designing NPs for desired targeted drug delivery system.

14.2 CONJUGATION OF LIGANDS AND NANOCARRIERS

Ligand selection is a critical parameter for the well-defined morphology and appropriate function of NPs. These ligands influence the solubility and availability of active components in the produced NPs [11]. Small organic chemicals like oleic acid and trisodium citrate are utilized as ligands, as are big polymers such as polyethylene glycols and functional biomolecules such as oligonucleotides, peptides, and proteins, which offer additional features to NPs [12, 13]. As a result, the proper ligand selection and technique for functionalizing the NP's surface will increase the NP quality. NPS must be functionalized for targeted drug administration by putting reactive moieties on the surface, and supplying a functional group may aid in conjugating the ligands using relevant chemistry. The conjugated ligand on NPS will enable tailored medication delivery [14]. Covalent and noncovalent conjugation are two ways of linking ligands on the surface of nanocarriers. Covalent conjugation methods, on the other hand, are most typically utilized to functionalize NPs [15]. In the conjugation of ligands to NPs, the reactions between amine and carboxylate to form an amide bond, the carbonyl group, hydrazide or alkoxy amine to form an oxime bond, and the reaction between thiols and haloacetyl or maleimide to form disulfide or thioester bonds are commonly used reactions [16–18].

14.2.1 Conjugation of Ligands to Nanocarriers by Amide Bonds

There are two phases involved in the creation of an amide bond. Figure 14.1 depicts the whole reaction and its process. The carboxylic group is activated by (DCC/EDC) carbodiimide in the first stage. An intermediate O-acylisourea is produced during carboxylic group activation. The activated group then interacts with the amine to produce an amide bond [17]. When DCC is used to activate a molecule with an excess of carboxylate groups that do not have an amine target, the activated carboxylate may create an anhydride when it combines with another carboxylic group under anhydrous circumstances. An amide bond is formed when this anhydride intermediate interacts with an amine. Furthermore, when activated carboxylate combines with an amino acid, it may form an azlactone. This azlactone can establish a covalent amide bond with the amine [19]. The benefit of this strategy is that originally chosen ligands do not need to be modified. Furthermore, activation of peptide-derived carboxylic groups of amino acids may be challenging. As a result, these carboxylic groups must be connected with NHS (N-hydroxysuccinimide) before the reaction [20]. In another study, Blume *et al.* established amide bond formation between PEG-COOH–coated liposomes and ligands. The designed product was utilized to distribute certain medications [21]. Another study bonded biocompatible polyamidoamine dendrimers (PAMAM) to the surface of carbon nanotubes. The substance dispersed and stabilized well in aqueous media and was proven to be effective for gene therapy [22]. The information presented previously was connected to the production of an amide bond on the nanocarrier surface through carboxylic group activation. Several additional techniques for activating the main amine group and forming amide bonds on the surface of the nanocarrier have also been disclosed. Chou and colleagues [23] described the use of dithiobis (succinimidyl propionate) (DSP) in the manufacture of nanocarriers and activated amino groups. Furthermore, NHS is employed to create ester bonds with the monoclonal antibody trastuzumab. The created substance was discovered to be effective for cancer gene therapy [24].

14.2.2 Conjugation of Ligands to Nanocarriers by Thioether Bonds

The interaction between the thiol and the maleimide group produces the thioester bond. Figure 14.2 depicts the whole reaction and its mechanism. At ambient temperature, the reaction is exceedingly effective and creates a stable bond in an aqueous solution [25, 26]. However, because of accompanying side reactions such as disulfide production and intermolecular rearrangement, selectivity toward the creation of thioether bonds is rather poor. Furthermore, natural thiol groups are not found in all proteins [27, 28]. As a result, it must be introduced either by the use of crosslinking agents or by lowering the existing disulfide bonds. Crosslinkers that are often employed include succinimidyl-S-acetylthioacetate (SATA) and N-hydroxysuccinimidyl 3-(2-pyridyldithio) propionate (SPDP), both of which provide a primary amine group for coupling with ligands. The thiol group is not easily accessible in the case of SPDP. To decrease the disulfide link to the thiol group, dithiothreitol (DTT)-reducing agents are utilized. After deacetylation with hydroxylamine, the thiol

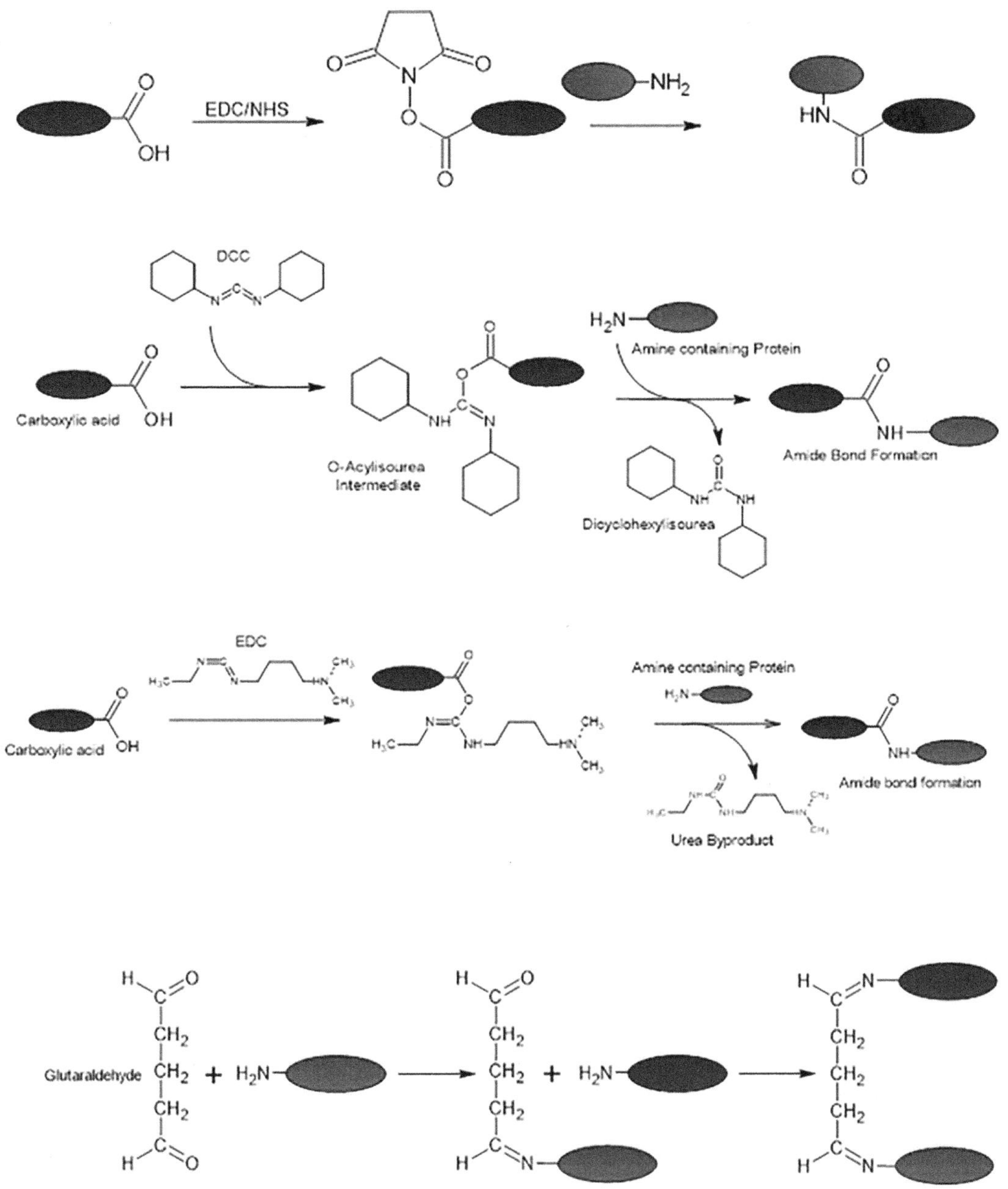

FIGURE 14.1 Formation of amide bond crosslinking between two primary amine.

group in SATA may be accessible for the process. For drug delivery, a system comprising thioester linkages demonstrated good selectivity and sustained circulation [17, 29]. Kirpotin *et al.* developed a liposome-based drug delivery system including cholesterol and PEG-modified phosphatidyletha-nolamine (DSPE). A thioester bond was used to attach antibodies to the nanocarrier. Two separate processes were used to produce the synthesis. The first antibody was coupled with a liposome double layer. The ligand was conjugated to the distal end of PEG chains in the other approach. The new approach demonstrated anti-HER2-immunoliposome uptake on malignant cells, resulting in

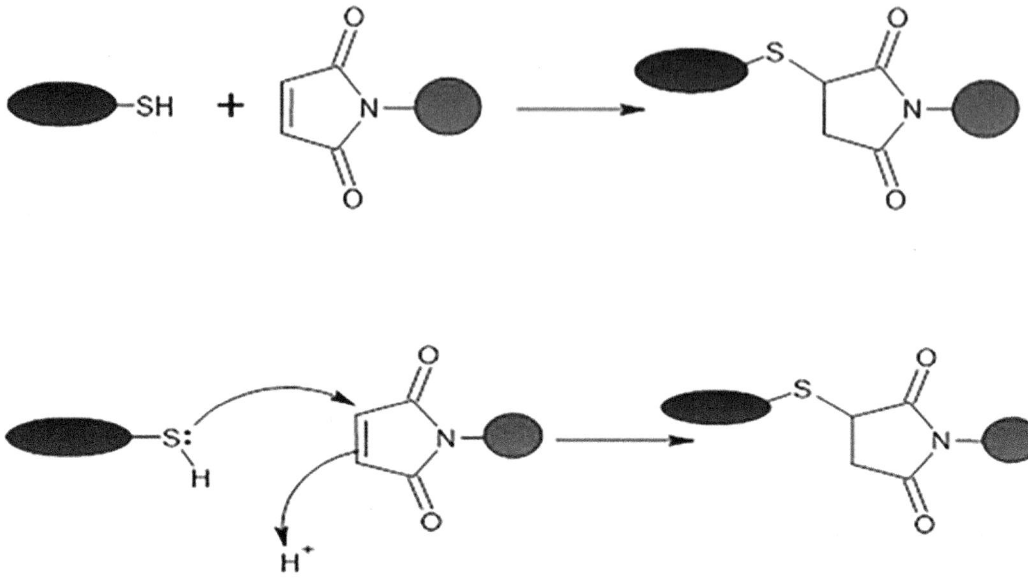

FIGURE 14.2 Formation of thioether bonds.

tumor shrinkage. The system's targeting effectiveness was related to the concentration of encapsulated antibodies [30]. Furthermore, numerous studies proved the efficacy of the devised technique for the successful delivery of doxorubicin [31]. Lu *et al.* created functionalized carbon nanotubes with folic acid through a thioether link for targeted DOX administration. The created approach has been proven effective in cancer medication targeting [32]. As a result, amide and thioether linkages are often utilized to functionalize nano-carrier systems.

14.2.3 Conjugation of Ligands to Nanocarriers by Disulfide Linkage

The formation of a disulfide bond by the conjugation of two thiol groups is one of the simplest and quickest coupling processes. Figure 14.3 depicts the whole reaction and its mechanism. The nanocarrier provides the first thiol group, whereas the ligand provides the second. However, disulfide bonds in serum have been demonstrated to be particularly weak throughout the oxidation-reduction phase [33]. As a consequence, the disulfide bond has been gradually replaced by more stable bonds. It has previously been shown that thiolated ligands may be synthesized by weakening the disulfide link or using SATA or SPDP [34, 35]. Disulfide linkages may also be formed by reacting thiolated ligands with the pyridyldithiomoiety of the anchor (PE-PDP, PDP-PEG-DSPE, and PDPSA) [6]. A disulfide link has been discovered between liposomes and the monoclonal antibody anti-My9. The liposome surface was anchored with PDP-SA, and SPDP was employed to activate the ligand, which was held for its immune reactive activity. The established strategy is effective against promyelocytic leukemia (HL-60) [36].

14.2.4 Conjugation of Ligands to Nanocarriers by Acetyl-Hydrazone Group

Hydrazide bonds may also be used to conjugate antibodies to the surfaces of nanocarriers. Figure 14.4 depicts the whole reaction and its mechanism. In this mechanism, aldehyde moieties of antibodies (ligands) may be covalently linked to hydrazide groups attached to the surface of liposomes in this mechanism [21]. Typically, ligands lack aldehyde groups. They should be generated by moderate oxidation of carbohydrate groups and then react with the linker's hydrazide

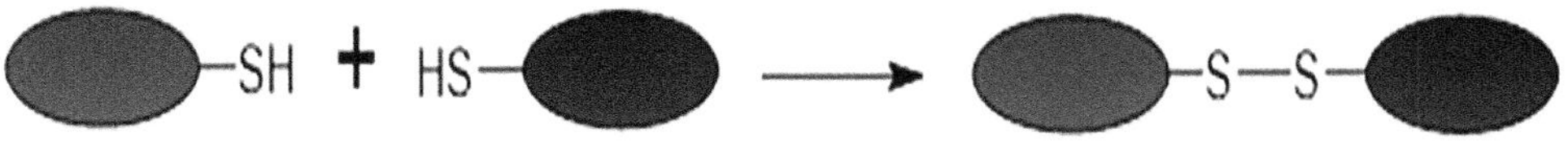

FIGURE 14.3 Formation of disulfide bonds.

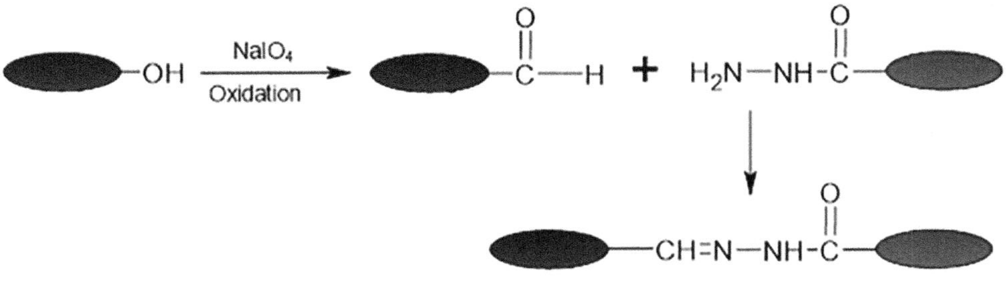

FIGURE 14.4 Formation of acetyl-hydrazone.

group. Galactoseoxidase and sodium periodate are the oxidizing agents employed in the oxidation of carbohydrates. To safeguard the antibody activity, the reaction should be carried out under mild circumstances. After aldehyde moieties develop on antibodies, they may directly bind to a nanocarrier using a hydrazide-hydrophobic linker or be associated with functionalized PEG–lipid hydrazide liposomes. The main benefit of this process is that ligands are correctly organized following attachment to the liposome surface. The total yield of the reaction in this technique, however, was poor [24]. Harding *et al.* established the creation of acetyl-hydrazone bonds on the liposome surface to conjugate C225 antibodies. In vivo testing revealed that PEG-grafted immunoliposomes are more immunogenic than free IgG [37].

14.2.5 CONJUGATION OF LIGANDS TO NANOCARRIERS BY POLYCYCLIC GROUP

The Diels-Alder (DA) reaction is the addition reaction between diene and dienophile that results in the creation of a bicyclic molecule. The high yield of this reaction, when used to bind specific ligands to the surface of nanocarriers, is a benefit (near 100%). Under moderate circumstances, the reaction is readily triggered [38–40]. The DA reaction produces a ligan-conjugated nanocarrier system that forms a particular interaction with cancer cells. Shi *et al.* used a DA reaction to produce an antibody anti-HER2 conjugation on a nanocarrier. The nanoparticles were created via a DA cycloaddition process in which the furan group on the carrier's surface was the diene and the antibody modified with a maleimide group was the dienophile. The authors developed a method for producing bioactive immunonanoparticles [41]. According to the researchers, Diels-Alder cycloadditions were also used to generate peptide–oligonucleotide conjugates.

14.2.6 CONJUGATION OF LIGANDS TO NANOCARRIERS BY CLICK CHEMISTRY

Chemistry reactions have certain advantages over traditional reactions. In an aqueous medium, they react quickly and produce fewer hazardous byproducts. Click chemistry is often used to attach ligands to the surface of nanoparticles. The most frequent ligands utilized to increase nanocarrier binding efficiency and specificity on cell lines are antibodies [42–45]. Colombo *et al.* demonstrated anti-HER2 antibody binding to nanoparticle surfaces via azide-nitrone cycloaddition. They employed genetic modification to add the amino acid serine to the scFv N terminus of the anti-HER2 antibody.

Serine was oxidized to the aldehyde using sodium periodate, and the aldehyde was subsequently transformed to nitrone using N-methylhydroxylamine. Finally, the nitrone group of scFv was coupled to dibenzocyclooctene-modified hybrid multifunctional nanoparticles using click chemistry. When the nanoparticles were overexpressed in MCF7 cells, they showed better binding to HER2. According to the previous studies, advances in click chemistry did not influence antibody binding affinity [46]. In another paper, Chen *et al.* demonstrated the production of DOX-loaded nanogels to address multi-drug resistance. A nanogel was created using poly (hydroxyethyl methacrylamide-co-N-(2-azidoethyl) methacrylamide. Following gel formation, copper-free click chemistry was employed to bind folic acid (FA)-polyethylene glycol (PEG)-BCN to the azide groups on the surface of the nanogel. The pH-sensitive hydrazine connection boosted DOX release from the nanogel in cancer cells. The produced nanogel was evaluated for cellular absorption on FA receptor-positive and -negative cell lines, B16F10 and A549, respectively. FA receptor-positive cell lines demonstrated increased cellular absorption due to receptor-mediated endocytosis. Furthermore, the FA-functionalized DOX-loaded nanogel was resistant to DOX and successfully killed DOX-tolerant 4T1 cells [47].

14.3 BIOLOGICAL LIGANDS AND THEIR APPLICATION IN TARGETED NANOPARTICLES

14.3.1 MONOCLONAL ANTIBODIES

Monoclonal antibodies may be employed in immunology investigations and as a medication carrier to assist pharmaceuticals in targeting certain receptors. Wang *et al.* developed an immunomagnetic nanosensor based on the interaction of antigen CD133 with its anti-CD133 monoclonal antibody (mAb) of glioblastoma CSCs [48]. As nanosensor cores, nanoparticles were created by crosslinking carboxymethyl chitosan (CMCS) with sodium tripolyphosphate (TPP) and then chemically modified with polyethyleneimine (PEI). The nanoparticle was coupled with Anti-CD133 mAb to construct an immunomagnetic nanosensor, which was tested for cellular toxicity before being administered to the targeted CSCs for imaging. The nanosensor demonstrated good specificity while being less harmful. As a consequence of these findings, manufactured anti-CD133 mAb-nano-MSN might be employed for molecular imaging of targeted CSCs in cancer diagnosis and treatment [49]. Cho *et al.* created a tailored anticancer formulation for visualizing and targeting colon cancer using cetuximab as a ligand in a study. Cetuximab-conjugated magneto-fluorescent silica nanoparticles (MFSN-Ctx) were created by the author to preferentially target colon cancer cells, generate visible fluorescence signals, and increase MRI signals. A magnetic field was used to boost the concentration of MFSN-Ctx in a tumor. Finally, MFSNCtx provides a clinically acceptable noninvasive imaging technique for diagnosis and is promising for measuring therapy response in EGFR-expressing malignancies [50].

14.3.2 PEPTIDES

Peptides are smaller than antibodies and offer benefits in targeting ligands such as high stability and ease of conjugation on the surface of nanoparticles. Using a peptide-conjugated drug delivery approach, medicines may be effectively administered via peptide receptors produced on specific cells. In another investigation, Chi *et al.* created doxorubicin (DOX)-loaded liposomes tagged with IL4RPep-1 (IL4RPep-1-L-Dox). IL4RPep-1 [51]. Furthermore, as compared to free DOX, intra-venous treatment of IL4RPep-1-L-Dox boosted DOX aggregation and antitumor development in H226 tumor-bearing mice. Immunofluorescence microscopy confirmed the presence of IL4RPep-1 coding liposomes in vascular endothelial cells from tumor tissue [52].

14.3.3 APTAMERS

Aptamers are small single-stranded DNA or RNA oligonucleotides with the ability to bind a wide range of biological substrates [53]. They may interact with receptors and biomarkers, particularly through hydrogen bonding, electrostatic force, and van der Waals forces [53]. Aptamer-medicated medication delivery has shown promise in cancer therapy. Li *et al.* created EGFR aptamer-chitosan conjugated liposomes for erlotinib administration to lung cancer patients. When compared to the usual delivery strategy, aptamer-functionalized liposomes demonstrated great toxicity and effective drug transport to EGFR mutant cancer cells. As a result, aptamer-coupled liposomes may be employed to deliver drugs to highly resistant tumor cells. Additionally, adopting an aptamer-functionalized liposome-based drug delivery system improved the targeted distribution of cabazitaxel to tumor cells. The accumulation of cabazitaxel-loaded liposomes within tumor cells is enabled by the target-specific binding of aptamer (TLS1c) to tumor cells (MEAR) in this work [54]. Functionalization of NPs with aptamers is another frequent drug delivery approach used to improve the efficacy of anticancer medicines. Chen *et al.* created aptamer-mediated docetaxel-loaded polymeric NPs for prostate cancer treatments. An in vitro investigation found that anti-PSMA aptamer-mediated drug delivery improves cellular uptake and anticancer efficacy of DTX-apt-NPS over conventional NPs [55].

14.3.4 FOLATES

Folic acid (FA) is a nutrient with a low molecular weight that is necessary for nucleotide production. It is commonly utilized as a drug delivery targeting ligand [56]. FA exhibited a high affinity for the endogenous folate receptor, which has been identified as a cancer marker in a variety of human malignancies. Many therapeutic drugs have been conjugated with FA for targeted medication delivery to tumors [56]. Lv *et al.* created FA functionalized mesoporous silica NPs (MSNs) for targeted drug administration and adorned them with gas-filled microbubbles (MBs). Ultrasound irradiation bursts the MB, releasing the prepared MSNs in specific tissues [57]. Tanshinone IIA (TAN)-loaded MSNs with high loading capacity and the ability to cause apoptosis in tumor cells were created. Furthermore, FA-modified MSNs and MB without TAM showed no cytotoxicity in HeLa or A549 cells. MSN-FA-TAN-MB, on the other hand, boosted cellular absorption through the folate receptor and accelerated apoptosis in HeLa cells. The findings imply that a medication delivery method based on ultrasound-guided release and FA-functionalized NPs may be employed successfully. Ma *et al.* created graphene oxide GO-NPs for DOX delivery in another investigation. FA-BSAs (FA-grafted bovine serum albumins) were employed as GO-NP surface targeting agents. Furthermore, DOX was connected to GO-NPs through hydrogen-bond interactions, resulting in a significant drug loading in a DOX to FA-BSA/GO mass ratio of 3:1. pH-sensitive and long-lasting drug release patterns were found in the produced NPs [58]. An alkaline precipitation approach in the presence of sodium alginate was recently used to create alginate-coated magnetic NPs (co-MIONs). PEGylation was accomplished by attaching PEG to the carboxylic group of alginates. The produced NPs were further functionalized with folate by attaching the folic acid to the PEG's terminal OH group (Mag-Alg-PEG-FA). FA-functionalized DOX-loaded NPs were examined for cellular absorption and anticancer effectiveness in the MDA-MB-231 cell line, which expresses the folate receptor. The results suggested that folate-functionalized, pegylated co-MIONS might effectively transport DOX to cancer cells in solid tumors [59].

14.3.5 LECTINS

Lectins are ligands that may adhere to glycosylated membranes and are utilized to deliver drugs to particular sites. Glyconanoparticles and glycodendrimers, two forms of targeted drug delivery systems, were shown to be lectin receptor C specific. Furthermore, by selecting appropriate lectins, cell-specific targeting may be achieved [60]. Dube *et al.* created galactosylated liposomes for silibinin administration by targeting hepatocyte lectin receptors. The produced liposomal vesicles were covalently bonded with P-aminophenyl–D-galactopyranoside. In albino rats, the intrahepatic distribution of galactosylated liposomal-loaded silibinin was investigated. The findings indicate that galactosylated liposomes are more efficient and appropriate for delivering silibinin to hepatocytes [61].

TABLE 14.1

Application of Ligands in Functionalization of Nanocarriers for Drug Delivery and Localization in Targeted Sites

Ligand	Linker/Anchor	Target	API/Active Targeting Molecule	Nanoparticles	Conjugation Chemistry
Monoclonal antibody AR-3	N-succinimidyl-3-(2-pyridyldithio) propionate (SPDP)/ MPB-PE	HT-29 human colon adenocarcinoma cell line	5-fluorouridine (5-FUR)	Liposomes and immunoliposomes	Thiol/maleimide
Fab fragments	Succinimidyl-S-acetyl thioacetate (SATA)/ MPB-PE	–	–	Liposomes	Sulfhydryl-maleimide
Monoclonal antibodies OVTL3 and RIVI000	MPB-PE	OVCAR-4 human ovarian tumor cell line	–	Liposomes and immunoliposomes	Sulfhydryl-maleimide
Monoclonal antibody CC52 (IgG1)	MPB-PE and mPEG-DSPE	Colon carcinoma CC531	5-fuorodeoxyuridine (FUdR)	Liposomes and immunoliposomes	Sulfhydryl-maleimide coupling
Monoclonal antibody OV-TL3,	MPB-PE	Human ovarian cancer cell line NIH:OVCAR-3 originated	Doxorubicin	Liposomes and immunoliposomes	Sulfhydryl-maleimide coupling
Reticuloendothelial system (RES) and anisamide (AA)	DSPE-PEG$_{2000}$	Sigma receptor over-expressed in H460 human lung cancer cells	ACE inhibitor (EV peptide	LPH nanoparticles	Amine/carboxyl
Mannosylated lipoarabinomannan (ManLAM)	–	Human DC-specific C-type lectin receptor DC-SIGN	Vaccine components	Nanoparticles	Biotin/streptavidin
Myristic acid (MC)	Polyethylenimine	Gene therapy of U87 glioblastoma	–	MC-PEI/DNA Nanoparticle	Amine/carboxyl
Monoclonal antibody IgG	Carbohydrates	C-type lectin receptor DC-SIGN	MHC class I or II-restricted Ags	PLGA nanoparticle (NP) vaccine carriers	Biotin/streptavidin
EpCAM antibody	–	Colon cancer cells (colo205, sw480, and NCM460)	–	Silica nanoparticle	NaIO$_4$ oxidation
Monoclonal antibody anti-CD44	–	Hepatocellular carcinoma cells	Doxorubicin (Dox)	Liposomal nanoparticles	Thiol/maleimide
Cetuximab antibody	PLGA-ZnS:Mn2+	EGF receptor overexpressing cells with antibody	Camptothecin	Nanoparticle	Amine/carboxylate

Monoclonal antibody	–	IL-6, IFN-γ and AFP (alpha-fetoprotein)	–	Silicon nanoparticles	Amide/ glutaraldehyde
Monoclonal antibody IgG2a	–	Beta(7) integrin	Cyclin D1 (CyD1)-small interfering RNA (siRNA)	Liposomes	Amine/carboxylate
Monoclonal antibody	–	Prostate-specific antigen (PSA)	–	Iron oxide nanoparticles	Glutaraldehyde/ amine
Monoclonal humanized mouse IgG1 trastuzumab	Succinic anhydride	Her2+ breast and ovarian cancers	Doxorubicin	Chitosan nanoparticles	Thiol/maleimide
Monoclonal humanized IgG2b (anti-DR5)	–	DR5-overexpressing malignant melanoma cells	Dacarbazine	Polylactic acid (PLA) nanoparticles	Amine/carboxylate
Monoclonal mouse IgG1 (anti-Her2 antibody)	–	Her2-expressing tumor	–	Iron oxide nanoparticles	Amine/carboxylate
Monoclonal antibodies (EGFR)	–	EGFR expressed on BcaCD885 cells oral squamous cell carcinoma (OSCC)	–	Quantum dots	Thiol/maleimide
Anti-EGFR antibody (ScFvEGFR)	Heparin	EGFR-expressing lung cancer H292 cells	Cis-diamminedichloroplatinum(II) (DDP, cisplatin)	Heparin-DDP (EHDDP) nanoparticles	Amine/carboxylate
IL-4R binding peptides I4R	–	Interleukin-4 receptor (IL-4R)	–	Glycol chitosan (HGC) nanoparticles	Amine/carboxylate
AH1, TRP2, PAn DR epitope (PADRE), and HA1 peptides	–	MHC Class II ECD	DNA vaccines	Polyamidoamine (G5-PAMAM) dendrimers	Thiol/maleimide
iRGD peptides	–	αvβ3, αvβ5 integrins	siRNA	PLGA-PLL-PEG nanoparticles	Thiol/maleimide
LRP ligand (angiopep-2 and/or aprotinin)	–	Brain capillary endothelial cells (BCECs)	Rhodamine B isothiocyanate (RBITC)	Angiopep-conjugated poly(ethylene glycol)-co-poly(ε-caprolactone) nanoparticles	Thiol/maleimide
TNF-related apoptosis-inducing ligand (TRAIL) and transferrin	Dimethylmaleic anhydride (DMMA) and sulfosuccinimidyl-4-(N-maleimidomethyl) cyclohexane-1-carboxylate (sulfo-SMCC)	HCT 116, doxorubicin-resistant MCF-7, and CAPAN-1	Doxorubicin	Human serum albumin (HSA) nanoparticles	Thiol-maleimide

TABLE 14.1 (Continued)

Application of Ligands in Functionalization of Nanocarriers for Drug Delivery and Localization in Targeted Sites

Ligand	Linker/Anchor	Target	API/Active Targeting Molecule	Nanoparticles	Conjugation Chemistry
Nucleic acid ligands (aptamers)	–	Prostate LNCaP epithelial cells	Rhodamine-labeled dextran	PLA-PEG-COOH nanoparticles	Amine/carboxylate
Folate	–	Bel-7402 hepatoma cell line	10-Hydroxycamptothecin	N-succinyl-N′-octyl chitosan micelle	Amine/carboxylate
Folic acid (FA)	Sodium dodecyl sulfate (SDS) N-isopropylacrylamide (NIPAAm)	A549 and OVCAR-3	Tyrosine kinase inhibitor erlotinib (ETB)	Chitosan nanoparticles	Amine/carboxylate, thiol/maleimide
Folic acid	–	C6 glioma cells	Doxorubicin	PAMAM G5 dendrimers	Thiol/maleimide
Folic acid	–	FAR-expressing colorectal cancer cells (SW480 and MSC)	Oxaliplatin	PEG-PAMAM G4 dendrimers	Thiol/maleimide
Folic acid	–	Lung cancer cells A549	Resveratrol (RSV)	Dextran stearate (DF) polymeric micelle nanoparticles	Amine/carboxyl
Folic acid	–	MDA-MB-231 breast cancer cells, human prostate cancer PC3 cells, colon cancer HT29 cells	Methotrexate	Lipid-polymer hybrid nanoparticles (LPHNPs)	Amine/carboxyl
Anti-EGFR aptamer (Apt)	–	Epidermal growth factor receptor (EGFR)	Tyrosine kinase inhibitor (TKI) erlotinib	Liposomes	Thiol/maleimide
5TR1 aptamer	–	MUC1þC26 cell line	Doxorubicin	PEGylated liposomal	Thiol/maleimide
Anti-PSMA aptamer	–	Prostate cancer	Docetaxel (DTX)	Polymeric NPs	Amine/carboxylate
AS1411 aptamer		miR-21-inhibited ovarian cancer cells	Cisplatin	Poly(lactic-co-glycolic acid) nanoparticles	Amine/carboxylate
Anti-MUC1 aptamer	–	MCF-7 cells	Doxorubicin/KLA peptide	DNA nanoparticles	Amine/carboxylate
EGFR aptamer	–	Osteosarcoma cells and CSCs	Salinomycin	Polymer-lipid hybrid nanoparticles	Thiol/maleimide
PSMA aptamer	–	PSMA-overexpressing LNCaP and PSMA(-) PC3 cancer cells	Cisplatin	PLGA-b-PEG nanoparticles	Amine/carboxylate
Affibody ligands		Human epidermal growth factor receptor 2 (HER-2)	Paclitaxel	Polymeric nanoparticles	Thiol/maleimide

14.3.6 TRANSFERRIN

Transferrin is a kind of glycoprotein. Transferrin is routinely utilized for targeted medication delivery. The benefits of drug-transferrin conjugates include increased plasma half-life, regulated drug tissue distribution, and better stability [62, 63]. Transferrin-modified targeted DOX-loaded mesoporous silica nanoparticles were created by Zhou *et al.* (HMSNs). After an intravenous injection to nude mouse models, the produced NPs demonstrated the longest mouse survival duration. The findings showed that NPs are biocompatible and may lower the toxicity of DOX [64]. In a separate study, the researchers created temozolomide (TMZ)-loaded transferrin (Tf)-functionalized poly (lactic-co-glycolic acid) (PLGA) nanoparticles for drug delivery to glioma U87MG cells. Tf-PLGA-TMZ was tested for anti-glioma effectiveness in nude mice. Tf-targeted nanoparticles improved cellular uptake and decreased cell viability in U87MG cells. Chemotherapy also reduced tumor volume and improved survival in nude mice injected with U87MG cells. The findings imply that Tf-modified PLGA nanoparticles have the potential for efficient TMZ administration for glioma therapy [65, 66].

14.3.7 LACTOFERRIN

Lactoferrin (Lf) is a transferrin family glycoprotein. Several studies have shown that Lf receptors regulate its biological activities, and it has been employed effectively as a ligand in targeted drug delivery [67]. Lactoferrin-functionalized magnetic polydiacetylene nanocarriers were prepared by Fang *et al.* (PDNCs). In glioblastoma, Lf receptors are overexpressed, which improves the ability of the LF functionalized nanocarrier to traverse the BBB. Huang *et al.* created a non-viral gene vector based on Lf-modified polyamidoamine with polyethyleneglycol as a spacer. Lf uptake in the brain was observed to be greater in brain-adjusted PAMAM-PEG-Lf. According to these results, Lf may be a potential ligand for brain-targeted gene delivery systems [68].

The application of the previously mentioned ligands in the functionalization of different nanocarriers for drug delivery and localization in targeted sites is summarized in Table 14.1.

14.4 CONCLUSION

In this chapter, we have covered synthetic techniques and the use of biological ligands in the production of NPs focused on the targeted delivery of drugs. It was shown that ligands may increase therapeutic effectiveness by increasing the selective binding of drug-loaded NPs to sick tissues. The availability of ligands and their conjugation with NPS for targeting will have significant uses in disease imaging, diagnosis, and therapy. Furthermore, ligand-based targeted drug delivery provided flexibility in the selection of ligands for drug delivery optimization until the required effectiveness was attained. These advancements in ligand-targeted drug delivery lower drug toxic effects while increasing potency and effectiveness. Though these systems are far from flawless at the moment, it can be concluded that the ligand-based approach to targeted drug delivery is well established and seems to be promising.

REFERENCES

1. Mishra, B., B.B. Patel, and S. Tiwari. 2010. Colloidal nanocarriers: a review on formulation technology, types and applications toward targeted drug delivery. *Nanomedicine: Nanotechnology, Biology, and Medicine*, 6, no. 1: 9–24. https://doi.org/10.1016/j.nano.2009.04.008
2. Dingemanse, J., and S. Appel-Dingemanse. 2007. Integrated pharmacokinetics and pharmacodynamics in drug development. *Clinical Pharmacokinetics*, 46, no. 9: 713–37. https://doi.org/10.2165/00003088-200746090-00001
3. Kanduluru, A.K., and P.S. Low. 2017. Development of a ligand-targeted therapeutic agent for neurokinin-1 receptor expressing cancers. *Molecular Pharmaceutics*, 14, no. 11: 3859–65. https://doi.org/10.1021/acs.molpharmaceut.7b00583

4. Flynn, T., and C. Wei. 2005. The pathway to commercialization for nanomedicine. *Nanomedicine: Nanotechnology, Biology, and Medicine*, 1, no. 1: 47–51. https://doi.org/10.1016/j.nano.2004.11.010

5. Torchilin, V.P. 2006. Multifunctional nanocarriers. *Advanced Drug Delivery Reviews*, 58, no. 14: 1532–55. https://doi.org/10.1016/j.addr.2012.09.031

6. Parveen, S., R. Misra, and S.K. Sahoo. 2012. Nanoparticles: a boon to drug delivery, therapeutics, diagnostics and imaging. *Nanomedicine: Nanotechnology, Biology, and Medicine*, 8, no. 2: 147–66. https://doi.org/10.1117/12.547922

7. Mehra, N.K., V. Mishra, and N.K. Jain. 2014. A review of ligand tethered surface engineered carbon nanotubes. *Biomaterials*, 35, no. 4: 1267–83. https://doi.org/10.1016/j.biomaterials.2013.10.032

8. Liu, Y., Y. Hui, R. Ran, et al. 2018. Synergetic combinations of dual-targeting ligands for enhanced in vitro and in vivo tumor targeting. *Advance Healthcare Material*, 7.

9. Ran, R., H. Wang, Y. Liu, et al. 2018. Microfluidic self-assembly of a combinatorial library of single- and dual-ligand liposomes for in vitro and in vivo tumor targeting. *European Journal of Pharmaceutics and Biopharmaceutics*, 130: 1–10. https://doi.org/10.1016/j.ejpb.2018.06.017

10. Koo, O.M., I. Rubinstein, and H. Onyuksel. 2005. Role of nanotechnology in targeted drug delivery and imaging: a concise review. *Nanomedicine*, 1, no. 3: 193–212. https://doi.org/10.1016/j.nano.2005.06.004

11. Chakraborty, I., D. Jimenez de Aberasturi, N. Pazos-Perez, et al. 2018. Ion-selective ligands: How colloidal nano- and micro-particles can introduce new functionalities. *Physical Chemistry*, 232: 1307–1317.

12. Liu, W.Y., M. Tagawa, H.L.L. Xin, et al. 2016. Diamond family of nanoparticle superlattices. *Science*, 351: 582–586. https://doi.org/10.1126/science.aad2080

13. Kyriazi, M.-E., D. Giust, A.H. El-Sagheer, et al. 2018. Multiplexed mRna sensing and combinatorial-targeted drug delivery using DNA-gold nanoparticle dimers. *ACS Nanotechnology*, 12: 3333–3340. https://doi.org/10.1021/acsnano.7b08620

14. Johnson, J.A., Y.Y. Lu, J.A. Van Deventer, and D.A. Tirrell. 2010. Residue-specific incorporation of non-canonical amino acids into proteins: recent developments and applications. *Current Opinion in Chemical Biology*, 14, no. 6: 774–80. https://doi.org/10.1016/j.cbpa.2010.09.013

15. Hermanson, G.H. 2008. *Bioconjugate Techniques*. Academic Press, San Diego, California USA. https://doi.org/10.1021/jm9608319

16. Friedman, A.D., S.E. Claypool, and R. Liu. 2013. The smart targeting of nanoparticles. *Current Pharmaceutical Design*, 19, no. 35: 6315–29. https://doi.org/10.2174/13816128113199990375

17. Liu, C.C., A.V. Mack, M.L. Tsao, et al. 2008. Protein evolution with an expanded genetic code. *Proceedings of the National Academy of Sciences of the United States of America*, 105, no. 46:17688–93. PubMed: 19004806

18. Wei, C. 2005. The valuable and significant role of nanomedicine. *Nanomedicine: Nanotechnology, Biology, and Medicine*, 1, no. 4: 285. https://doi.org/10.1016/j.nano.2005.10.010

19. Nobs, L., F. Buchegger, R. Gurny, and E. All'emann. 2004. Current methods for attaching targeting ligands to liposomes and nanoparticles. *Journal of Pharmaceutical Sciences*, 93, no. 8: 1980–92. https://doi.org/10.1002/jps.20098

20. Kocbek, P., N. Obermajer, M. Cegnar, and J. Kos. 2007. Targeting cancer cells using PLGA nanoparticles surface modified with monoclonal antibody. *Journal of Controlled Release*, 120, no. 1–2: 18–26. https://doi.org/10.1016/j.jconrel.2007.03.012

21. Blume, G., M.D.J.A. Crommelin, I.A.J.M. Bakker-Woudenberg, C. Kluft, and G. Storm. 1993. Specific targeting with poly (ethylene glycol)-modified liposomes: coupling of homing devices to the ends of the polymeric chains combines effective target binding with long circulation times. *Biochimica et Biophysica Acta—Biomembranes*, 1149, no. 1: 180–84.

22. Zhang, B., Q. Chen, H. Tang, et al. 2010. Characterization of and biomolecule immobilization on the biocompatiblemulti-walled carbon nanotubes generated by functionalization with polyamidoamine dendrimers. *Colloids and Surfaces B: Biointerfaces*, 80, no. 1: 18–25.

23. Chou, H.-T., T.-P. Wang, C.-Y. Lee, N.-H. Tai, and H.-Y. Chang. 2013. Photothermal effects of multi-walled carbon nanotubes on the viability of BT-474 cancer cells. *Materials Science and Engineering*, 33, no. 2: 989–95. https://doi.org/10.1016/j.msec.2012.11.035

24. Chiu, S.J., N.T. Ueno, and R.J. Lee. 2004. Tumor-targeted gene delivery via anti-HER2 antibody (trastuzumab, Herceptin) conjugated polyethylenimine. *Journal of Controlled Release*, 97, no. 2: 357–69. https://doi.org/10.1016/j.jconrel.2004.03.019

25. Crosasso, P., P. Brusa, F. Dosio, et al. 1997. Antitumoral activity of liposomes and immunoliposomes containing 5-fluorouridine prodrugs. *Journal of Pharmaceutical Science*, 86: 832–9. https://doi.org/10.1021/js9604467

26. Liu, Y., H. Miyoshi, and M. Nakamura. 2007. Nanomedicine for drug delivery and imaging: a promising avenue for cancer therapy and diagnosis using targeted functional nanoparticles. *International Journal of Cancer*, 120, no. 12: 2527–37. https://doi.org/10.1002/ijc.22709

27. Derksen, J.T., and G.L. Scherphof. 1985. An improved method for the covalent coupling of proteins to liposomes. *Biochimia et Biophysica Acta*, 814: 151–5. https://doi.org/10.1016/0005-2736(85)90430-4

28. Derksen, J.T., H.W. Morselt, and G.L. Scherphof. 1988. Uptake and processing of immunoglobulin-coated liposomes by subpopulations of rat liver macrophages. *Biochimia et Biophysica Acta*, 971: 127–36. https://doi.org/10.1016/0167-4889(88)90184-X

29. Martin, F.J., and D. Papahadjopoulos. 1982. Irreversible coupling of immunoglobulin fragments to pre-formed vesicles. An improved method for liposome targeting. *The Journal of Biological Chemistry*, 257, no. 1: 286–88. https://doi.org/10.1016/S0021-9258(19)68359-6

30. Kirpotin, D., J.W. Park, and K. Hong. 1997. Sterically stabilized anti-HER2 immunoliposomes: design and targeting to human breast cancer cells in vitro. *Biochemistry*, 36, no. 1: 66–75. https://doi.org/10.1021/bi962148u

31. Ren, J., S. Shen, D. Wang, et al. 2012. The targeted delivery of anticancer drugs to brain glioma by PEGylated oxidized multiwalled carbon nanotubes modified with angiopep-2. *Biomaterials*, 33, no. 11: 3324–33. https://doi.org/10.1016/j.biomaterials.2012.01.025

32. Lu, Y.J., K.C. Wei, C.C.M. Ma, S.Y. Yang, and J.P. Chen. 2012. Dual targeted delivery of doxorubicin to cancer cells using folate conjugated magnetic multi-walled carbon nanotubes. *Colloids and Surfaces B: Biointerfaces*, 89, no. 1: 1–9. https://doi.org/10.1016/j.colsurfb.2011.08.001

33. Martin, F.J., W.L. Hubbell, and D. Papahadjopoulos. 1981. Immuno specific targeting of liposomes to cells: a novel and efficient method for covalent attachment of Fab0 fragments via disulfide bonds. *Biochemistry*, 20: 4229–38. https://doi.org/10.1021/bi00517a043

34. Ivanov, V.O., S.N. Preobrazhensky, V.P. Tsibulsky, V.R. Babaev, V.S. Repin, and V.N. Smirnov. 1985. Liposome uptake by cultured macrophages mediated by modified low-density lipoproteins. *Biochimica et Biophysica Acta*, 846, no. 1: 76–84. https://doi.org/10.1016/0167-4889(85)90112-0

35. Shaik, M.S., N. Kanikkannan, and M. Singh. 2001. Conjugation of anti-My9 antibody to stealth monensin liposomes and the effect of conjugated liposomes on the cytotoxicity of immunotoxin. *Journal of Controlled Release*, 76, no. 3: 285–95. https://doi.org/10.1016/S0168-3659(01)00450-3

36. Hansen, C.B., G.Y. Kao, E.H. Moase, S. Zalipsky, and T.M. Allen. 1995. Attachment of antibodies to sterically stabilized liposomes: evaluation, comparison and optimization of coupling procedures. *Biochimia et Biophysicia Acta*, 1239: 133–44.

37. Harding, J.A., C.M. Engbers, M.S. Newman, N.I. Goldstein, and S. Zalipsky. 1997. Immunogenicity and pharmacokinetic attributes of poly (ethylene glycol)-grafted immunoliposomes. *Biochimia et Biophysicia Acta*, 1327: 181–92.

38. DeMenezes, D.E.L., L.M. Pilarski, and T.M. Allen. 1998. In vitro and in vivo targeting of immunoliposomal doxorubicin to human Bcell lymphoma. *Cancer Research*, 58, no. 15: 3320–30. https://cancerres.aacrjournals.org/content/canres/58/15/3320.full.pdf

39. Chua, M.M., S.T. Fan, and F. Karush. 1984. Attachment of immunoglobulin to liposomal membrane via protein carbohydrate. *Biochimica et Biophysica Acta*, 800, no. 3: 291–300. https://doi.org/10.1016/0304-4165(84)90408-2

40. Chamow, S.M., T.P. Kogan, D.H. Peers, R.C. Hastings, R.A. Byrn, and A. Ashkenazi. 1992. Conjugation of soluble CD4 without loss of biological activity via a novel carbohydrate-directed cross-linking reagent. *The Journal of Biological Chemistry*, 267, no. 22: 15916–22. https://doi.org/10.1016/S0021-9258(19)49621-X

41. Shi, M., J.H. Wosnick, K. Ho, A. Keating, and M.S. Shoichet. 2007. Immuno-polymeric nanoparticles by Diels-Alder chemistry. *Angewandte Chemie*, 46, no. 32: 6126–31. https://doi.org/10.1002/anie.200701032

42. De Araújo, A.D., J.M. Palomo, J. Cramer, et al. 2005. Diels-Alder ligation and surface immobilization of proteins. *Angewandte Chemie, International Edition*, 45, no. 2: 296–301. https://doi.org/10.1002/anie.200502266

43. Marchan, V., S. Ortega, D. Pulido, E. Pedroso, and A. Grandas. 2006. Diels-Alder cycloadditions in water for the straightforward preparation of peptide–oligonucleotide conjugates. *Nucleic Acids Research*, 34, no. 3: 1–24. https://doi.org/10.1093/nar/gnj020

44. Kolb, H.C., M.G. Finn, and K.B. Sharpless. 2004. Click chemistry: diverse chemical function from a few good reactions. *Angewandte Chemie International Edition*, 40: 1–21. https://doi.org/10.1002/1521-3773(20010601)40:11<2004::AID-ANIE2004>3.0.CO;2-5

45. Yoon, H.Y., H. Koo, K. Kim, and I.C. Kwon. 2017. Molecular imaging based on metabolic glycoengineering and bioorthogonal click chemistry. *Biomaterials*, 132: 28–36. https://doi.org/10.1016/j.biomaterials.2017.04.003

46. Colombo, M., S. Sommaruga, and S. Mazzucchelli. 2012. Site-specific conjugation of ScFvs antibodies to nanoparticles by bioorthogonal strain-promoted alkyne–Nitrone cycloaddition. *Angewandte Chemie International Edition*, 51: 496–9. https://doi.org/10.1002/anie.201106775

47. Chen, Y., O. Tezcan, and D. Li. 2017. Overcoming multidrug resistance using folate receptor-targeted and pH-responsive polymeric nanogels containing covalently entrapped doxorubicin. *Nanotechnology*, 9: 10404–19. Overcoming multidrug resistance using folate receptor-targeted and pH-responsive polymeric nanogels containing covalently entrapped doxorubicin—Nanoscale (RSC Publishing).

48. Wang, X., B. Li, R. Li, et al. 2018. Anti-CD133 monoclonal antibody conjugated immunomagnetic nanosensor for molecular imaging of targeted cancer stem cells. *Sensors Actuators B: Chemistry*, 255: 3447–57. https://doi.org/10.1016/j.snb.2017.09.175

49. Cho, Y.-S., T.-J. Yoon, E.-S. Jang, and K.S. Hong. 2010. Cetuximab-conjugated magnetofluorescent silica nanoparticles for in vivo colon cancer targeting and imaging. *Cancer Letters*, 299, no. 1: 63–71. https://doi.org/10.1016/j.canlet.2010.08.004

50. Sewald, N., and H.-D. Jakubke. 2015. *Peptides: Chemistry and Biology*. John Wiley & Sons, Verlag GmbH.

51. Chi, L., M.-H. Na, H.-K. Jung, et al. 2015. Enhanced delivery of liposomes to lung tumor through targeting interleukin-4 receptor on both tumor cells and tumor endothelial cells. *Journal of Control Release*, 209: 327–36. https://doi.org/10.1016/j.jconrel.2015.05.260

52. Chushak, Y.G., J.A. Martin, J.L. Chavez, N. Kelley-Loughnane, and M.O. Stone. 2014. Computational design of RNA libraries for in vitro selection of aptamers. *Methods of Molecular Biology*, 1111: 1–15. https://doi.org/10.1007/978-1-62703-755-6_1

53. Hayashi, T., H. Oshima, T. Mashima, T. Nagata, and M. Kinoshita. 2014. Molecular binding of an RNA aptamer and a partial peptide of a prion protein: crucial importance of water entropy in molecular recognition. *Nucleic Acids Research*, 42, no. 11: 6861–75. https://doi.org/10.1093/nar/gku382

54. Li, F., H. Mei, X. Xie, et al. 2017. Aptamer-conjugated chitosan-anchored liposomal complexes for targeted delivery of erlotinib to EGFR-mutated lung cancer cells. *AAPS Journal*, 19, no. 3: 814–26. https://doi.org/10.1208/s12248-017-0057-9

55. Chen, Z., Z. Tai, F. Gu, C. Hu, Q. Zhu, and S. Gao. 2016. Aptamer-mediated delivery of docetaxel to prostate cancer through polymeric nanoparticles for enhancement of antitumor efficacy. *European Journal of Pharmaceutics& Biopharmaceutics*, 107: 130–41. https://doi.org/10.1016/j.ejpb.2016.07.007

56. Low, P., W. Henne, and D. Doorneweerd. 2008. Discovery and development of folic-acid-based receptor targeting for imaging and therapy of cancer and inflammatory diseases. *Accounts of Chemical Research*, 41, no. 1: 120–9.

57. Lv, Y., Y. Cao, P. Li, et al. 2017. Ultrasound-triggered destruction of folate-functionalized mesoporous silica nanoparticle-loaded microbubble for targeted tumor therapy. *Advance Healthcare Mater*, 6.

58. Ma, N., J. Liu, and W. He. 2017. Folic acid-grafted bovine serum albumin decorated graphene oxide: an efficient drug carrier for targeted cancer therapy. *Journal of Colloid and Interface Science*, 15: 598–607. https://doi.org/10.1016/j.jcis.2016.11.097

59. Angelopoulou, A., A. Kolokithas-Ntoukas, F. Christos, and A. Konstantinos. 2019. Folic acid-functionalized, condensed magnetic nanoparticles for targeted delivery of doxorubicin to tumor cancer cells overexpressing the folate receptor. *ACS Omega*, 4, no. 26: 22214–27. https://doi.org/10.1021/acsomega.9b03594

60. Kurmi, B.D., J. Kayat, V. Gajbhiye, R.K. Tekade, and N.K. Jain. 2010. Micro- and nanocarrier-mediated lung targeting. *Expert Opinion in Drug Delivery*, 7: 781–94. https://doi.org/10.1517/17425247.2010.492212

61. Dube, D., K. Khatri, A.K. Goyal, N. Mishra, and S.P. Vyas. 2010. Preparation and evaluation of galactosylated vesicular carrier for hepatic targeting of silibinin. *Drug Development and Industrial Pharmacy*, 36, no. 5: 547–55. https://doi.org/10.3109/03639040903325560

62. Kim, C.S., R. Mout, Y. Zhao, et al. 2015. Co-delivery of protein and small molecule therapeutics using nanoparticle-stabilized nanocapsules. *Bioconjugate Chemistry*, 26, no. 5: 950–4. https://doi.org/10.1021/acs.bioconjchem.5b00146

63. Pattni, B.S., V.V. Chupin, and V.P. Torchilin. 2015. New developments in liposomal drug delivery. *Chemical Review*, 115, no. 19: 10938–66. https://doi.org/10.1021/acs.chemrev.5b00046

64. Zhou, J., M. Li, W.Q. Lim, et al. 2018. A transferrin-conjugated hollow nanoplatform for redox-controlled and targeted chemotherapy of tumor with reduced inflammatory reactions. *Theranostics*, 8, no. 2: 518–25. https://doi.org/10.7150/thno.21194

65. Jinning, M., M. Xiangfu, C. Zhao, Y. Yang, and L. Guodong. 2019 Jul. Development of transferrin-modified poly (lactic-co-glycolic acid) nanoparticles for glioma therapy. *Anticancer Drugs*, 30, no. 6: 604–10. https://doi.org/10.1097/CAD.0000000000000754
66. Hu, K., Y. Shi, W. Jiang, J. Han, S. Huang, and X. Jiang. 2011. Lactoferrin conjugated PEG-PLGA nanoparticles for brain delivery: preparation, characterization and efficacy in Parkinson's disease. *International Journal of Pharmacy*, 415, no. 12: 273–83. https://doi.org/10.1016/j.ijpharm.2011.05.062
67. Fang, J.H., T.L. Chiu, W.C. Huang, et al. 2016. Dual-targeting lactoferrin-conjugated polymerized magnetic polydiacetylene-assembled nanocarriers with self-responsive fluorescence/magnetic resonance imaging for in vivo brain tumor therapy. *Advanced Healthcare Materials*, 5, no. 6: 688–95. https://doi.org/10.1002/adhm.201500750
68. Huang, R., K. Weilun, Y. Liu, C. Jiang, and Y. Pei. 2008. The use of lactoferrin as a ligand for targeting the polyamidoamine-based gene delivery system to the brain. *Biomaterials*, 29, no. 2: 238–46. https://doi.org/10.1016/j.biomaterials.2007.09.024

15 Exploring the Realm of Nanotechnology in HIV and COVID-19

Priyanka Salunkhe, Susmit Mhatre, Tishya Srivastava, Shivraj Naik, and Vandana Patravale

15.1 INTRODUCTION

15.1.1 VIRAL DISEASES

With our landscapes and environments changing rapidly, there is a lot at stake. Viruses with RNA as their genetic material adapt to and exploit these varying conditions. It comes as no surprise that several prominent recent examples of emerging or re-emerging diseases are caused by RNA viruses, such as severe acute respiratory syndrome-related coronavirus (SARS-CoV-2). A complex interplay of factors can influence and play important roles in disease emergence, such as virus genetic variation (mutation, recombination, and reassortment) and environmental factors (including ecological, social, health care, and behavioral influences). Such factors, coupled with the enormous increase in the human population and urbanization during the last 50 years, have greatly expanded the number of sampling events testing the fitness of RNA virus variants in different human cell backgrounds and potential transmission modes. This change, together with advances in the speed and volume of global transportation, creates increased opportunities for the emergence and re-emergence of viral diseases. We need to look for newer technologies and targeted solutions to handle these viral strains and their growing speed.

15.1.2 HIV AND COVID-19

The human immunodeficiency virus (HIV) belongs to the family retroviridae, which causes acquired immunodeficiency syndrome (AIDS), destroys CD4+ T cells, and weakens the immune system, making an individual vulnerable to other opportunistic infections, and therefore illustrates the world's profound challenge in dealing with it since 1981 (3). In acute HIV infection, people generally show normal flu-like symptoms. As the disease progresses to a chronic stage, one may not feel sick or have any symptoms. But if viral load is detectable, one can transmit the disease even when symptoms are absent. The late stage of infection, known as AIDS, weakens the body's immune system and causes a high chance of opportunistic infection (4).

Apart from this, the virus that has gained much attention recently and caused a global lockdown is the SARS-CoV-2. It belongs to the coronaviridae family and was named a coronavirus because of characteristic crown-like spikes on its outer surface. Coronaviruses are smaller in size (65–125 nm in diameter) and contain a single-stranded RNA as a nucleic material of size ranging from 26 to 32 kbs in length. SARS-CoV-2 causes coronavirus disease-19 (COVID-19), which has created havoc in the entire world (5). The majority of patients with COVID-19 show mild to moderate symptoms, but approximately 15% progress to severe pneumonia, and about 5% in due course develop acute respiratory distress syndrome (ARDS), septic shock, or multiple organ failure. In patients with severe COVID-19, lymphopenia is commonly seen, with drastically reduced numbers of CD4+ T

DOI: 10.1201/9781003130055-15

TABLE 15.1

Some Examples of Nanomedicines for Viral Diseases (1, 2)

Therapeutic Agent	Drug Category	Nanosystem	Application
Enviroxime	Anti-rhinoviral	Liposomes	Increase solubility and reduce toxicity
Ganciclovir	Anti-cytomegaloviral	Liposomes	Increase in bioavailability
3D8 scFv	Monoclonal antibody (mAb) with nucleic acid hydrolyzing activity	PLGA NPs	Improved cellular uptake and sustained release
Curcumin	Anti-HIV	Curcumin-loaded apotransferrin NP	Increase in activity
Adefovir dipivoxil	Anti-hepatitis A and B	SLNs	Increase in activity
Rilpivirine	Anti-HIV	Nanosuspension	Increase in bioavailability
Silver	Anti-HSV	NPs	Reduce the risk of resistance
Saquinavir	Anti-HIV	Nanoemulsion	Enhanced oral bioavailability and brain disposition
Ribavirin	Anti-RSV	Niosomes	Liver targeting
Lamivudine	Anti-HIV	Poly(lactic acid)/chitosan NPs	Controlled delivery
Ritonavir	Anti-HIV	SNEDDS	Increase in bioavailability

cells, CD8+ T cells, B cells, and natural killer (NK) cells and a decreased percentage of monocytes, eosinophils, and basophils. An upsurge in neutrophil count and the neutrophil-to-lymphocyte ratio usually indicates higher disease severity and poor clinical outcome (6).

15.1.3 HIV: Current Status and Statistics

According to the Joint United Nations Programme on HIV/AIDS (UNAIDS) reports 2019, there were nearly 38 million people all across the globe with HIV. Approximately 1.7 million people were newly infected with HIV, which implies a 23% decline in new HIV infections since 2010. These figures represent slow progress in HIV transmission prevention strategies. Improvement in testing and access to treatment represents the key to manage this deadly disease. In 2019, around 81% of people with HIV knew about their HIV status. Around 67% of individuals have access to anti-retroviral therapy (ART), and 59% of all receiving ART had a viral load of an undetectable amount. These figures represents a hope of accomplishing UNAIDS's set goal targets of 90–90–90: 90% of all people with HIV know about their HIV status, 90% of all those who know about their HIV status will be on ART, and 90% of all people receiving ART will have viral suppression to a negligible amount by 2020 (7). Around 6.9 lakhs of people died in 2019 because of AIDS-related illnesses (8). Though there has been a noteworthy decrease in the death rate due to HIV, more research is necessary in this field to get rid of it entirely. With a detailed understanding of HIV-1, various drugs for specific viral proteins are developed. Different classes of anti-HIV drugs are shown in Figure 15.1.

ART is ideally initiated early in the course of HIV and continues throughout the life of an HIV patient. It can reduce HIV-associated morbidity, prolong life expectancy, suppress viral load, and further prevent HIV transmission. But some limitations accompany it, like frequent dosing to keep the viral load suppressed, pill burden and hence patient non-compliance, potential drug–drug interactions and adverse effects associated with the regimen, drug resistance developed, and lower tolerability. As an efficacious vaccine for HIV is not available to date, research efforts to develop novel formulations to overcome the current treatment limitations are necessary to curb this global epidemic (10–13).

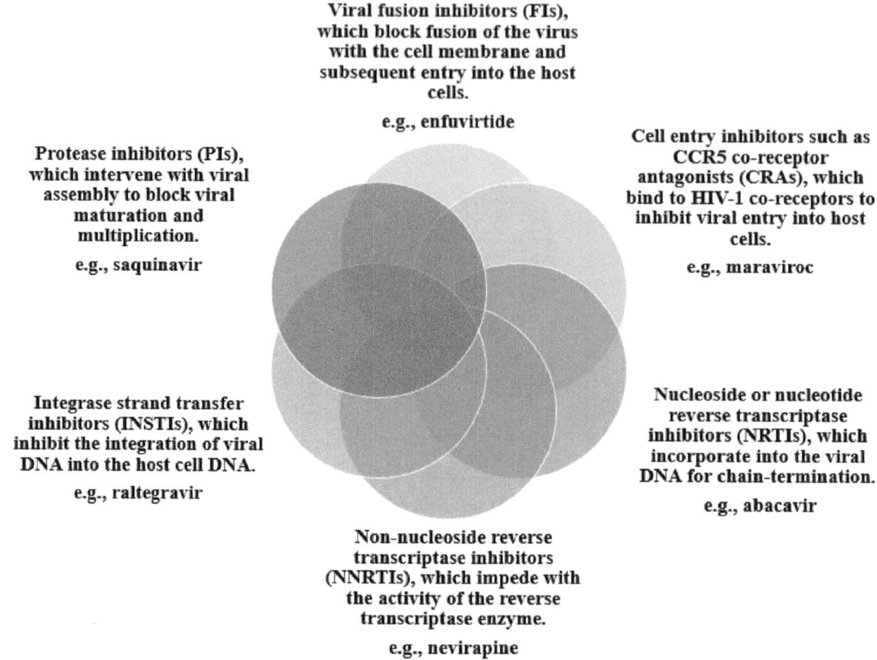

FIGURE 15.1   Classification of anti-HIV drugs (9).

15.1.4 COVID-19: CURRENT STATUS AND STATISTICS

The COVID-19 infection has rapidly spread across the globe and infected millions of people in a short period. According to the WHO, more than 70 million confirmed cases and 1.6 million deaths were reported globally as of mid-December 2020 (14). The USA, India, and Brazil are the three nations with the most cases reported. The mortality rate varied across different nations, with the highest being 9.4% in Mexico and 4.9% in Iran (15). Management of COVID-19 has been a challenge for all healthcare workers because of the rapid rate of viral infection with no approved treatment methods. To develop effective treatment methods in a shorter period, drug repurposing has been employed widely by researchers globally. Drug repurposing is a technique of finding new therapeutic applications of previously approved drugs (16). Several antiviral drugs, corticosteroids, antiparasitic, monoclonal antibodies, and herbal drugs are being repurposed to identify their applications in the treatment of COVID-19 (17). All these drugs are in different phases of clinical trials. Previously, hydroxychloroquine, as a sole drug or in combination with chloroquine and azithromycin, was used in clinical practice. Lopinavir/ritonavir was also widely used in drug therapy. However, these treatments are now discontinued (18). The US FDA approved the use of remdesivir in adults and pediatric patients of age 12 or higher and weighing at least 40 kilograms in October 2020. Earlier, in May 2020, remdesivir had received an emergency use authorization in adults and children with severe infection. The US FDA has also granted emergency use authorization for the drug barcitinib, a drug originally approved for rheumatoid arthritis. Other leading drugs in clinical trials are favipiravir, umifenovir, dexamethasone, ivermectin, niclosamide, and tocilizumab (19).

15.1.5 LIMITATIONS OF CURRENT TREATMENT APPROACHES

As remdesivir is the only drug currently approved for the treatment of COVID-19, there are still a lot of research and trials being conducted to find more effective therapies. Some clinical trials have reported side effects like anemia, constipation, thrombocytopenia, and increased bilirubin concentrations in 12% of the patients (20). Hydroxychloroquine was found to give inconsistent results between *in vitro* and *in vivo* studies (21). A study also reported ototoxicity associated with the administration of chloroquine and hydroxychloroquine, of which the exact pathophysiology is yet to be discovered (22). A recent study reported that hydroxychloroquine exhibits retinal toxicity, cardiac toxicity, macular degeneration, and systemic lupus erythematosus (18). Some therapies involving only one antiviral drug like lopinavir or ritonavir have been seen to be ineffective in the treatment of COVID-19 (23). Moreover, lopinavir/ritonavir therapy has been associated with acute kidney injury in patients with COVID-19 (24). A major issue with other therapies is the dose requirement of the antiviral drug. With a higher dose, there are higher chances of observing side effects in patients. When formulating dosage forms for COVID-19, there is a need to validate the physicochemical properties, stability, and therapeutic efficacy of the repurposed drugs.

15.2 NANOMEDICINE FOR VIRAL DISEASES

A new paradigm for enhancing the efficacy of bioactive molecules with the use of nanotechnology in medicine has attracted increasing attention and has been largely exploited in many medical fields (25). Various organic-based nanodelivery systems for antiviral agents, including liposomes, polymeric nanoparticles (NPs), solid lipid NPs (SLNs), hybrid NPs, dendrimers, nanoemulsions, micellar systems, and self-assembled nanostructures, have been proposed. Factors such as safety, biocompatibility, biodegradability, and compatibility with the drug should be considered to develop efficient nanocarrier platforms. It is worth noting that the main parameters that determine NP functionality are particle size, size distribution, shape, and surface characteristics (e.g. chemistry, charge) (26). Additionally, NP features should be fine-tuned to optimize the pharmacokinetic profile, *in vivo* biodistribution, and viral interactions.

Nanosystems help overcome the limitations of antiviral therapy in multiple methods. To overcome the blood-brain barrier (BBB), there is extensive use of polymeric nanosystems crossing the BBB. They are capable of delivering more dosages of drugs at the targeted sites specifically, and some are even stimuli-responsive nanosystems that can be triggered via magnetic fields (27). Viral medicines do not easily target the liver. Nanosystems can be designed to possess target specificity by conjugating ligands to their surface to target lymph nodes, lymphoid tissue, and macrophages (28). Some of the major challenges faced in antiviral therapy are gastric degradation, poor aqueous solubility, low mucosal permeability, and short residence time of the drug administered. With the advancement of nanosystems in antiviral therapy, gastroretentive nanosystems can be developed. Polymeric nanosystems with high drug loading and better bioavailability cater to the limitations of poor solubility. Further, nanosystems with sustained drug release, mucoadhesiveness, and mucopenetrating features can also provide effective drug administration (29).

15.3 NANOMEDICINE FOR HIV

Nanomedicine has encouraged new treatment and prevention approaches to HIV-1 infection. Most nanomedical applications toward HIV are preclinical or have failed at the clinical stage. However, clinical trials investigating the controlled and sustained release of ART drugs via nanoformulations have shown immense promise (30).

15.3.1 NANOTECHNOLOGY FOR HIV TREATMENT

With advances in nanotechnology, numerous nanosystems including liposomes, various NPs like inorganic, polymeric, and lipid-based dendrimers, nanosuspensions, nanoemulsions, micelles, and self-assembled nanostructures have been suggested for antiretroviral drugs (31).

Liposomes, which are lipidic vesicles, have gained much attention, as they are rapidly taken up by the reticuloendothelial system, get cleared from circulation, and hence are suitable for targeting macrophages (3). One study reported that elastic liposomal formulation of zidovudine shows increased skin permeation, sustained drug release, stability, and lymphatic uptake (32). To improve transdermal flux, ethanol can be incorporated into liposomal structures to form ethosomes. The ethanolic liposomal solution of lamivudine has been proved effective in *in vitro* and *ex vivo* studies compared to an ethanolic drug solution by Jain et al. (32).

Antiretroviral drugs or their prodrugs, either alone or in combination with other molecules, such as targeting moieties, can be attached covalently onto dendrimer (repeatedly branched macromolecules) surfaces. Dendrimers are perfect for targeted drug delivery, as one can control their physicochemical properties by modifying the core groups, the extent of branching, and the nature and number of functional groups on the surface (3). Dutta et al. formulated efavirenz (EFV)-loaded tuftsin (a natural macrophage activator tetrapeptide (Thr-Lys-Pro-Arg))-conjugated poly(propyleneimine) dendrimers, which offer targeted delivery to macrophages with improved phagocytic and anti-HIV activity (33).

Because of their unique size, shape, and surface characteristics, NPs have gained much attention for treating various diseases. Furthermore, because NPs have a large surface area-to-volume ratio, varied molecules such as drug molecules, immunological adjuvants, and ligands can be conjugated to their surface, which can then be targeted to sites of latent HIV reservoirs. Antiretroviral drug NP-loaded films represent a new option for developing vaginal microbicide (34). Inorganic and polymeric NPs also have been employed in delivering antiretroviral drug molecules. Cunha-Reis et al. developed EFV loaded poly(lactic-co-glycolic acid) NPs, which were then incorporated alongside free tenofovir (TFV) into fast-dissolving films. This film offers higher and more prolonged local drug levels as compared to the administration of TFV and EFV in aqueous vehicles (35). Various biomimetic approaches like coating NPs with a cellular membrane represent a unique strategy to target drugs to a particular site. Wei et al. coated PLGA NPs with T-cell membrane, which selectively binds with gp120 of HIV and neutralizes the viral infection of peripheral mononuclear blood cells and elicits antibodies with broadly neutralizing activity (36).

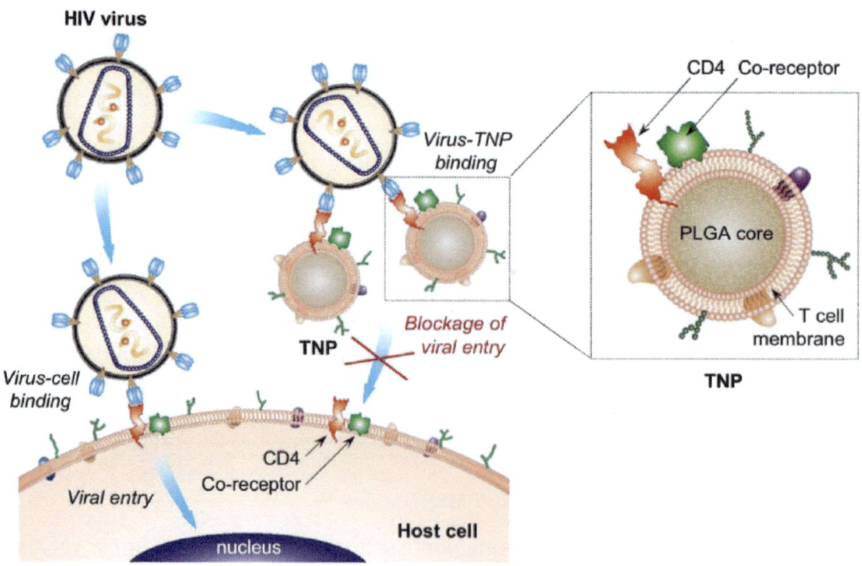

FIGURE 15.2   T-cell-membrane-coated nanoparticles designed for attenuating HIV infectivity (36).

To control HIV-1 in microglial cells, which are the central nervous system (CNS) resident macrophages, a unique drug delivery system is required to cross the BBB. Roy et al. developed EFV nanodiamonds (NDs), which are ~10 nm in size and improve the bioavailability of EFV, which suffers from low bioavailability due to ~99.5% blood plasma protein binding. The small size, natural biocompatibility, and minimal toxicity of functionalized NDs aid in the transport of anti-HIV-1 drugs across the BBB, making it one of the best candidate systems for improving drug delivery to the CNS (37).

A nanosuspension, which is a biphasic system containing antiviral agents, can be taken up quickly by primary macrophages and show time-dependent kinetics. These systems can cross the cellular barrier and enable fast entry into the cell because of their nano size (1). Baert et al. formulated a nanosuspension using rilpivirine (TMC278), a single 20 mg/kg dose of which served as a long-acting, once-a-month injectable formulation (38). Vyas et al. formulated a novel nanoemulsion, another biphasic system loaded with saquinavir (SQV), using edible oils rich in essential polyunsaturated fatty acids (PUFA) as an internal phase and egg phosphatidylcholine (Lipoid-E80) and deoxycholic acid as the external phase. The Cmax (brain) was five-fold, and AUC was three-fold higher in comparison to SQV suspension, suggesting the enhanced rate and extent of SQV uptake following oral administration (39).

15.3.2 Nanotechnology for HIV Diagnosis

An early diagnosis of a disease is vital to increase an individual's life span and control the further spread of the disease. Methods based on detecting antibodies are not reliable, as at the beginning of the infection, no antibodies are produced, and hence early detection of the disease is not possible. In the case of neonates, maternal antibodies will persist for around 12 months, which makes it difficult to diagnose conditions. Current methods like PCR-based detection of the viral genome, specific primers, and probes in plasma and viral culture with normal donor lymphocytes can conflict with the use of nanotechnology. Glyconanoparticle (GNP)-based assays have shown HIV-1 p24 antigen at levels as low as 0.1 pg/mL and give 100–150-fold enhancement to the detection limit, enabling detection of HIV-1 infection three days earlier than traditional colorimetric ELISA. Therefore, quicker detection times and enhanced sensitivity can be achieved by nanotechnology-based diagnostics (3). Carbon nanostructures, quantum dots, nanoclusters, and metallic and metal oxide NPs are being employed to develop highly sensitive HIV biosensors that can lower detection limits by several orders of magnitude (40).

15.3.3 Nanotechnology for HIV Prevention

Approaches for preventing an infection play an essential role in the fight against global epidemics like HIV. Despite the continuous effort to evade this global challenge, the number of new infections has been reducing over recent years but at a slower pace than required. This alarming challenge highlights that more effort needs to be invested, particularly in the field of prevention.

15.3.3.1 Vaccines

The development of a vaccine to prevent or control HIV-1 infection has been an elusive goal since the virus was first found. Remarkably, NPs play a role as adjuvants and vaccine delivery systems. Also, NP-encapsulated antigens are protected from body fluids such as lymph, serum, and mucus, increasing their half-life and leading to prolonged and more robust immune response initiation (3). Several vaccines entered clinical trials, but no effective vaccine is yet available because of the complex nature of disease mechanism and their interaction with the immune system. Due to the high genetic variability of the virus, the immune system is unable to stimulate reactive neutralizing antibodies and hence immune escape (30). Nevertheless, efforts are ongoing to overcome these and other limiting issues in effective vaccine development.

15.3.3.2 Vaginal Microbicide for Prevention of Sexual Transmission of HIV

In the absence of an effective vaccine for HIV, microbicides have gained much attention as a recent preventive strategy (3). A microbicide is defined as an anti-infective for vaginal or rectal application that protects against sexually transmitted infections (STIs), including HIV (41). The classification of microbicides, depending on their mechanism of action, are membrane disruptive agents, attachment or fusion or entry (AFE) inhibitors, reverse transcriptase inhibitors, and dendritic cell uptake inhibitors (42). Nanotechnology plays a noteworthy role in the development of microbicidal formulations. Nanosystems intended for microbicide development may either have inherent antiviral activity or act as carriers for a microbicide. The surface chemical functionalization of nanosystems can be helpful for the inactivation of a virus (43). One of the first developed nanosystem-based microbicides was Starpharma'sVivaGel, which contains SPL7013 dendrimer as an active ingredient, mainly owing to its anti-HIV activity by direct interaction of terminal naphthalene disulfonate groups with gp120 of HIV, a viral surface glycoprotein essential for cell infection (44). Apart from dendrimers, polymeric NP-based microbicides have also been explored for efficient transport of a drug across barriers and better cellular uptake. Poly (D, L-lactide-co-glycolide) NPs delivering a highly potent anti-HIV protein, PSC-RANTES, were shown to offer more significant antiviral activity over an extended period, thus confirming the prospects of achieving long-acting microbicide action when active drugs are presented in NP carrier systems (41). Another nanomicrobicide containing tetra-hydrocurcumin (THC) in o/w microemulsion-based gel was also shown to possess significant anti-HIV activity in *in silico* and *in vitro* studies (45). With the application of nanotechnology, the area of microbicidal development will flourish in the coming years.

15.4 NANOMEDICINE FOR COVID-19

Nanotechnology can offer effective solutions to tackle COVID-19 because of the numerous advantages offered by these techniques. Formulating nanotechnology-based drug delivery systems for repurposed drugs can help in reducing the dose and hence eliminating the associated side-effects (46). Nanotechnology-based therapies can be developed to target various stages in the viral replication cycle, including the attachment of the virus to the host cell (47). Surface-modified NPs can target structural proteins, especially the spike protein of SARS-CoV-2, and hence prevent the entry of the virus in the host cell (48). The S2 subunit of the spike protein has three domains named HR1, HR2, and fusion peptides.

In a study, PEGylated gold nanorods were loaded with a synthetic peptide (49). This assembly was seen to inhibit HR1 activity ten times more than peptide alone, thus inactivating the membrane fusion mechanism of MERS-CoV. A similar approach can be adopted for SARS-CoV-2 too due to the structural similarities between the two viruses. Han et al. developed peptide inhibitors from the protease domain of ACE2, which binds to the receptor-binding domain of the SARS-CoV-2. The stability of these inhibitors functionalized on NPs on the host receptor was validated using a computational approach, thus blocking viral infection (50).

Apart from treatment methods, nanotechnology has also been employed in vaccines and for diagnostic purposes. NPs exhibit several mechanisms like protection, regulation, and controlled delivery of antigens that help in enhancing the efficiency of vaccines (51). Nanovaccines for a coronavirus are commonly developed using structure-based assembly (47). Virus-like particles, which lack the viral genome but are structurally similar to the virus, are developed by expressing the structural proteins of the virus in suitable organisms (52). These NPs displaying structural proteins by undergoing self-assembly and surface modification can effectively attach to the ACE2 receptors and alert the immune system (53). NPs, especially metallic NPs exhibiting magnetic and electronic properties, have wide applications in the diagnosis of COVID-19. A study reported the development of magnetic NPs modified with proteins to bind to the viral RNA and extract nucleic acids (54). Additionally, silver NPs, superparamagnetic NPs, and gold NPs have also found applications in the diagnosis of coronaviruses (55–57).

15.5 FUTURE PERSPECTIVES

The occurrence of new viruses and their heterogeneity have demanded innovative therapies. With several countries under lockdown, the need of the hour is nanomedicine drug delivery. Considering specific targeting, nanotechnology opens a new avenue for antiviral therapy. The strategy of using NPs to combat COVID-19 viral infection could involve mechanisms that affect the entry of the virus into the host cells until their inactivation. Blockage of the viral surface proteins may lead to virus inactivation, so targeted NPs specific to virus-expressed proteins could reduce viral internalization (48).

The similarity between HIV and COVID-19 is significant. Metal NPs have shown the ability to block viral attachment to the cell surface, leading to the inhibition of viral internalization and thereby impairing viral replication during viral entry. NPs composed of titanium, silver, gold, and zinc have already shown results against HIV, influenza virus, herpes simplex virus, respiratory syncytial virus, transmissible gastroenteritis virus, monkey pox virus, and zika virus (58).

Organic NPs have been used for delivering antivirals such as zidovudine, acyclovir, dapivirine, and EFV to improve drug bioavailability and promote efficient and targeted drug delivery (59). The main limitations of antivirals are the lack of specific targeting, resulting in cytotoxicity of the host cell, which can be addressed by organic NPs.

The versatility of NPs makes them tunable vectors for virus targeting and specific drug delivery. Antimicrobial drugs have been tested in clinical trials for COVID-19, such as chloroquine, lopinavir, ritonavir, ribavirin, and remdesivir, and have demonstrated promising results against SARS-CoV-2 (60). Nanoencapsulation of antimicrobial drugs will contribute to the development of effective treatments for COVID-19 and other viral diseases.

Although it is well established that nanotechnology-based systems improve existing therapeutics in medicine, their application in viral diseases is underexplored and underused, as observed in the SARS-CoV-2 pandemic.

Nanostructured systems can impact diagnosis since they can improve detection and sensitivity and increase signal amplification specificity in polymerase chain reaction analysis and prophylaxis as adjuvants for vaccines, as well as therapeutics for COVID-19 through the targeting of antiviral

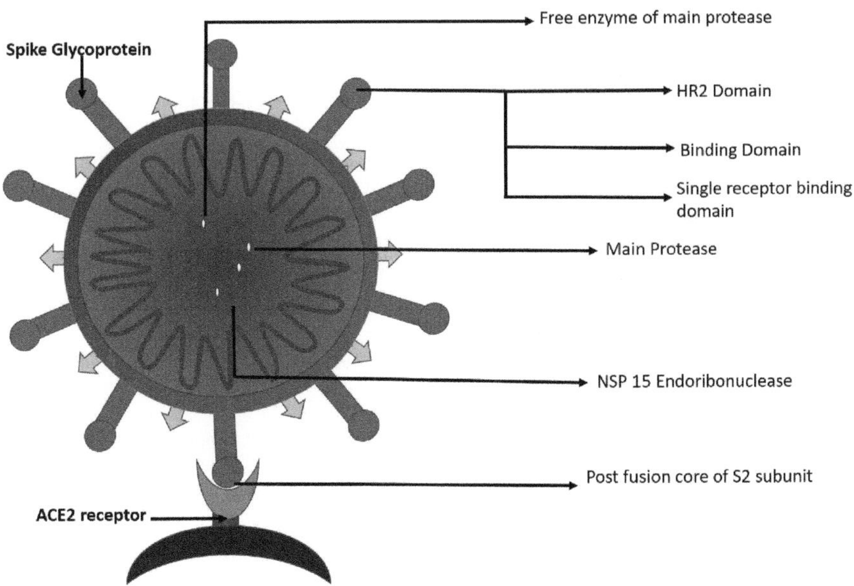

FIGURE 15.3 Structural targets of SARS-CoV-2 (61).

drugs. In summary, NPs may play an important role at different stages of COVID-19 pathogenesis, considering their inhibition potential in the initial attachment and membrane fusion during viral entry and infected cell protein fusion. Furthermore, nanoencapsulated drugs may be more efficient in activating intracellular mechanisms to cause irreversible damage to viruses and inhibition of viral transcription, translation, and replication.

15.6 CONCLUSION

The implications of both viral diseases on human health are significant, and effective strategies have to be developed for their management. Several reports present the advantages of nanotechnology-based treatments and vaccines. However, their approval in clinical practice remains a challenge. More studies are required to understand the interface between NPs and SARS-CoV-2 to trace a rational design of targeted therapeutics. Certainly, in a pandemic involving all the health organizations trying to elucidate the pathogenesis of SARS-CoV-2, nanotechnology could represent a convenient strategy in addition to other approaches to provide positive outcomes for COVID-19 treatment.

Highlights

- HIV and COVID-19 management are a challenge for researchers and medical workers
- The limitations with current treatments need to be overcome
- Nanotechnology-based approaches are promising to better tackle viral diseases
- Studies in diagnosis, prevention, and treatment of HIV have been reported
- Nanomedicine in COVID-19 is unexplored but has tremendous potential

REFERENCES

1. Mehendale R, Joshi M, Patravale V. Nanomedicines for treatment of viral diseases. *Critical Reviews in Therapeutic Drug Carrier Systems*. 2013;30(1):1–49.
2. Lembo D, Donalisio M, Civra A, Argenziano M, Lembo D, Donalisio M, et al. Expert opinion on drug delivery nanomedicine formulations for the delivery of antiviral drugs: a promising solution for the treatment of viral infections. *Expert Opinion on Drug Delivery*. 2018;15(1):93–114.
3. Saravanan M, Asmalash T, Gebrekidan A, Gebreegziabiher D, Araya T, Hilekiros H, et al. Nano-medicine as a newly emerging approach to combat Human Immunodeficiency Virus (HIV). *Pharmaceutical Nanotechnology*. 2018;06:17–27.
4. Symptoms of HIV | HIV.gov [Internet]. [cited 2020 Dec 9]. Available from: www.hiv.gov/hiv-basics/overview/about-hiv-and-aids/symptoms-of-hiv
5. Adnan M, Khan S, Kazmi A, Bashir N, Siddique R. COVID-19 infection: origin, transmission, and characteristics of human coronaviruses. *Journal of Advanced Research*. 2020;24:91–8.
6. Cao X. COVID-19: immunopathology and its implications for therapy. *Nature Reviews Immunology*. 2019;2019.
7. Global Statistics | HIV.gov [Internet]. [cited 2020 Oct 3]. Available from: www.hiv.gov/hiv-basics/overview/data-and-trends/global-statistics
8. WHO | *Data and Statistics*. WHO. 2020.
9. Gao Y, Kraft JC, Yu D, Ho RJY. Recent developments of nanotherapeutics for targeted and long-acting, combination HIV chemotherapy. *European Journal of Pharmaceutics and Biopharmaceutics*. 2019;138:75–91.
10. Siccardi M, Martin P, McDonald TO, Liptrott NJ, Giardiello M, Rannard S, et al. Nanomedicines for HIV therapy. *Therapeutic Delivery*. 2013;4(2):153–6.
11. Cihlar T, Fordyce M. Current status and prospects of HIV treatment. *Current Opinion in Virology*. 2016;18:50–6.
12. Hobson JJ, Owen A, Rannard SP. The potential value of nanomedicine and novel oral dosage forms in the treatment of HIV. *Nanomedicine*. 2018;13(16):1963–5.
13. Kutscher HL, Prasad PN, Morse GD, Reynolds JL. Emerging nanomedicine approaches to targeting HIV-1 and antiretroviral therapy. *Future Virology*. 2016;11(2):101–4.

14. WHO Coronavirus Disease (COVID-19) Dashboard [Internet]. [cited 2020 Dec 20]. Available from: https://covid19.who.int

15. Johns Hopkins Coronavirus Resource Center [Internet]. [cited 2020 Dec 7]. *Mortality Analyses.* Available from: https://coronavirus.jhu.edu/data/mortality

16. Pushpakom S, Iorio F, Eyers PA, Escott KJ, Hopper S, Wells A, et al. Drug repurposing: progress, challenges and recommendations. *Nature Reviews Drug Discovery.* 2019 Jan;18(1):41–58.

17. Shende P, Khanolkar B, Gaud RS. Drug repurposing: new strategies for addressing COVID-19 outbreak. *Expert Review of Anti-Infective Therapy.* 2020 Nov 13;0(ja):null.

18. Fernandez-Ruiz R, Bornkamp N, Kim MY, Askanase A, Zezon A, Tseng CE, et al. Discontinuation of hydroxychloroquine in older patients with systemic lupus erythematosus: a multicenter retrospective study. *Arthritis Research & Therapy.* 2020 Aug 17;22(1):191.

19. Siemieniuk RA, Bartoszko JJ, Ge L, Zeraatkar D, Izcovich A, Kum E, et al. Drug treatments for covid-19: living systematic review and network meta-analysis. *BMJ [Internet].* 2020 Jul 30 [cited 2020 Nov 26];370. Available from: www.bmj.com/content/370/bmj.m2980

20. Beigel JH, Tomashek KM, Dodd LE, Mehta AK, Zingman BS, Kalil AC, et al. Remdesivir for the treatment of Covid-19—final report. *New England Journal of Medicine [Internet].* 2020 May 22 [cited 2020 Dec 7]; Available from: www.nejm.org/doi/10.1056/NEJMoa2007764

21. Schluenz LA, Ramos-Otero GP, Nawarskas JJ. Chloroquine or hydroxychloroquine for management of Coronavirus disease 2019: friend or foe? *Cardiology in Review.* 2020 Jun 29;28(5):266–71.

22. De Luca P, Scarpa A, De Bonis E, Cavaliere M, Viola P, Gioacchini FM, et al. Chloroquine and hydroxychloroquine ototoxicity; potential implications for SARS-CoV-2 treatment. A brief review of the literature. *American Journal of Otolaryngology.* 2020 Jul 8;102640.

23. Hussain N, Yoganathan A, Hewage S, Alom S, Harky A. The effect of antivirals on COVID-19: a systematic review. *Expert Review of Anti-infective Therapy.* 2020 Sep 12;0(0):1–14.

24. Binois Y, Hachad H, Salem JE, Charpentier J, Lebrun-Vignes B, Pène F, et al. Acute kidney injury associated with lopinavir/ritonavir combined therapy in patients with COVID-19. *Kidney International Reports.* 2020 Oct;5(10):1787–90.

25. Patra JK, Das G, Fraceto LF, Campos EVR, Rodriguez-Torres M del P, Acosta-Torres LS, et al. Nano based drug delivery systems: recent developments and future prospects. *Journal of Nanobiotechnology [Internet].* 2018 Sep 19 [cited 2020 Dec 13];16. Available from: www.ncbi.nlm.nih.gov/pmc/articles/PMC6145203/

26. Zazo H, Colino CI, Lanao JM. Current applications of nanoparticles in infectious diseases. *Journal of Controlled Release.* 2016 Feb 28;224:86–102.

27. Dufort S, Sancey L, Coll JL. Physico-chemical parameters that govern nanoparticles fate also dictate rules for their molecular evolution. *Advanced Drug Delivery Reviews.* 2012 Feb;64(2):179–89.

28. Liu D, Yang F, Xiong F, Gu N. The smart drug delivery system and its clinical potential. *Theranostics.* 2016;6(9):1306–23.

29. Li J, Mao H, Kawazoe N, Chen G. Insight into the interactions between nanoparticles and cells. *Biomaterials Science.* 2017 Jan 31;5(2):173–89.

30. Roy U, Rodríguez J, Barber P, Das Neves J, Sarmento B, Nair M. The potential of HIV-1 nanotherapeutics: from in vitro studies to clinical trials. *Nanomedicine.* 2015;10(24):3597–609.

31. Lembo D, Donalisio M, Civra A, Argenziano M, Cavalli R. Nanomedicine formulations for the delivery of antiviral drugs: a promising solution for the treatment of viral infections. *Expert Opinion on Drug Delivery.* 2018;15(1):93–114.

32. Jain S, Tiwary AK, Jain NK. PEGylated elastic liposomal formulation for lymphatic targeting of zidovudine. *Current Drug Delivery.* 2008;5(4):275–81.

33. Dutta T, Garg M, Jain NK. Targeting of efavirenz loaded tuftsin conjugated poly (propyleneimine) dendrimers to HIV infected macrophages in vitro. *European Journal of Pharmaceutical Sciences.* 2008;4:181–9.

34. das Neves J, Sarmento B. Antiretroviral drug-loaded nanoparticles-in-films: a new option for developing vaginal microbicides? *Expert Opinion on Drug Delivery.* 2017;14(4):449–52.

35. Cunha-Reis C, Machado A, Barreiros L, Araújo F, Nunes R, Seabra V, et al. Nanoparticles-in-film for the combined vaginal delivery of anti-HIV microbicide drugs. *Journal of Controlled Release.* 2016;243:43–53.

36. Wei X, Zhang G, Ran D, Krishnan N, Fang RH, Gao W, et al. T-Cell-mimicking nanoparticles can neutralize HIV infectivity. *Advanced Materials.* 2018;30(45):1–9.

37. Roy U, Drozd V, Durygin A, Rodriguez J, Barber P, Atluri V, et al. Characterization of nanodiamond-based anti-HIV drug delivery to the brain. *Scientific Reports.* 2018;8(1):1–12.

38. Baert L, van't Klooster G, Dries W, François M, Wouters A, Basstanie E, et al. Development of a long-acting injectable formulation with nanoparticles of rilpivirine (TMC278) for HIV treatment. *European Journal of Pharmaceutics and Biopharmaceutics.* 2009;72(3):502–8.

39. Vyas TK, Shahiwala A, Amiji MM. Improved oral bioavailability and brain transport of Saquinavir upon administration in novel nanoemulsion formulations. *International Journal of Pharmaceutics.* 2008;347:93–101.

40. Farzin L, Shamsipur M, Samandari L, Sheibani S. HIV biosensors for early diagnosis of infection: the intertwine of nanotechnology with sensing strategies. *Talanta.* 2020;206(June 2019):120201.

41. Brako F, Mahalingam S, Rami-Abraham B, Craig DQM, Edirisinghe M. Application of nanotechnology for the development of microbicides. *Nanotechnology.* 2017;28(5).

42. Rosenberg ZF, Mitchnick M, Coplan P. Vaginal Microbicides Against HIV. First Edit. *Global HIV/AIDS Medicine.* Elsevier Inc.; 2008;595–601.

43. Mesquita L, Galante J, Nunes R, Sarmento B, Neves J Das. Pharmaceutical vehicles for vaginal and rectal administration of anti-hivmicrobicide nanosystems. *Pharmaceutics.* 2019;11(3).

44. Nandy B, Saurabh S, Sahoo AK, Dixit NM, Maiti PK. The SPL7013 dendrimer destabilizes the HIV-1 gp120–CD4 complex. *Nanoscale.* 2015;7(44):18628–41.

45. Mirani A, Kundaikar H, Velhal S, Patel V, Bandivdekar A, Degani M, et al. Tetrahydrocurcumin-loaded vaginal nanomicrobicide for prophylaxis of HIV/AIDS: in silico study, formulation development, and in vitro evaluation. *Drug Delivery and Translational Research.* 2019;9(4):828–47.

46. Mainardes RM, Diedrich C. The potential role of nanomedicine on COVID-19 therapeutics. *Therapeutic Delivery.* 2020 Jun 29;11(7):411–4.

47. Abd Ellah NH, Gad SF, Muhammad K, Batiha GE, Hetta HF. Nanomedicine as a promising approach for diagnosis, treatment and prophylaxis against COVID-19. *Nanomedicine.* 2020 Jul 29;15(21):2085–102.

48. Kerry RG, Malik S, Redda YT, Sahoo S, Patra JK, Majhi S. Nano-based approach to combat emerging viral (NIPAH virus) infection. *Nanomedicine.* 2019;18:196–220.

49. Huang X, Li M, Xu Y, Zhang J, Meng X, An X, et al. Novel gold nanorod-based HR1 peptide inhibitor for middle east respiratory syndrome Coronavirus. *ACS Applied Materials & Interfaces.* 2019 Jun 5;11(22):19799–807.

50. Han Y, Král P. Computational design of ACE2-based peptide inhibitors of SARS-CoV-2. *ACS Nano.* 2020 Apr 28;14(4):5143–7.

51. Pati R, Shevtsov M, Sonawane A. Nanoparticle vaccines against infectious diseases. *Front Immunol [Internet].* 2018 [cited 2020 Dec 9];9. Available from: www.frontiersin.org/articles/10.3389/fimmu.2018.02224/full

52. Rohovie MJ, Nagasawa M, Swartz JR. Virus-like particles: next-generation nanoparticles for targeted therapeutic delivery. *Bioengineering & Translational Medicine.* 2017;2(1):43–57.

53. Kato T, Takami Y, Kumar Deo V, Park EY. Preparation of virus-like particle mimetic nanovesicles displaying the S protein of Middle East respiratory syndrome coronavirus using insect cells. *Journal of Biotechnology.* 2019 Dec 20;306:177–84.

54. Zhao Z, Cui H, Song W, Ru X, Zhou W, Yu X. A simple magnetic nanoparticles-based viral RNA extraction method for efficient detection of SARS-CoV-2. *bioRxiv.* 2020 Feb 27;2020.02.22.961268.

55. Gong P, He X, Wang K, Tan W, Xie W, Wu P, et al. Combination of functionalized nanoparticles and polymerase chain reaction-based method for SARS-CoV gene detection. *Journal of Nanoscience and Nanotechnology.* 2008 Jan;8(1):293–300.

56. Kim H, Park M, Hwang J, Kim JH, Chung DR, Lee KS, et al. Development of label-free colorimetric assay for MERS-CoV using gold nanoparticles. *ACS Sensors.* 2019 May 24;4(5):1306–12.

57. Ahmed SR, Nagy É, Neethirajan S. Self-assembled star-shaped chiroplasmonic gold nanoparticles for an ultrasensitive chiro-immunosensor for viruses. RSC Advances. 2017 Aug 18;7(65):40849–40857.

58. Kupferschmidt K, Cohen J. Race to find COVID-19 treatments accelerates. *Science.* 2020 Mar 27;367(6485):1412–3.

59. Pison U, Welte T, Giersig M, Groneberg DA. Nanomedicine for respiratory diseases. *European Journal of Pharmacology.* 2006 Mar 8;533(1):341–50.

60. Li H, Liu SM, Yu XH, Tang SL, Tang CK. Coronavirus disease 2019 (COVID-19): current status and future perspectives. *International Journal of Antimicrobial Agents.* 2020 May;55(5):105951.

61. Mhatre S, Srivastava T, Naik S, Patravale V. Antiviral activity of green tea and black tea polyphenols in prophylaxis and treatment of COVID-19: a review. *Phytomedicine.* 2020 Jul 17;153286.

16 Chitosan Nanogel
Expanding Novel Phase in Drug Delivery System

Prashant Sahu, Varsha Kashaw, and Sushil K. Kashaw

ABBREVIATIONS

AFM	Atomic force microscopy
AIDS	Acquired immunodeficiency virus
APCs	Antigen presenting cell
ATRP	Atom transfer radical polymerization
BBB	Blood Brain Barriers
CNS	Central nervous system
CRP	controlled radical polymerization
DNA	Deoxyribonucleic acid
DSC	Differential scanning colorimetry
EGF	Epithelial growth factor
FT-IR	Fourier Transform Infra Red microscopy
GIT	Gastrointestinal tract
HPLC	High performance liquid chromatography
NIR	Near Infra red radiation.
NMR	Nuclear Magnetic Resonance
NSAIDs	Non-steroidal anti inflammatory drugs
O/W	Oil in water
PAAs	Poly acrylic acids
PCL	Polycaprolactone
PCRs	Polymerase chain reactions
PDMS	Polydimethylsiloxane
PEG	Poly ethylene glycol
PEI	Polyethylene amine
PHEMA	Polyhydroxyethyl methacrylate
PLGA	Polylactic-glycolic acid
PMMA	Polymethyl methacrylate
PVP	Polyvinyl pyrrolidone
SCC	Squamous cell carcinoma
siRNA	Small interfering Ribonucleic acid
SPF	Shirasu porous glass
SEM	Scanning electron microscopy
TEM	Transmission electron microscopy
UV	Ultraviolet
VEGF	Vascular endothelial growth factor
W/O	Water in oil

DOI: 10.1201/9781003130055-16

16.1 INTRODUCTION

In the last few decades nanotechnology has received significant interest for a wide range of applications. Nanotechnology and polymers have astounding interest in biomedical engineering, pharmaceutical industry and therapeutic innovation among others. Polymers in pharmaceutical technology constitute an indispensable class of excipients of constantly increasing significance; therefore, discovering their properties becomes vital [1]. Natural and synthetic polymers play an important role in formulating intelligent drug delivery systems, thus contributing to the improvement of achieved therapeutic effect. Aiming to overcome the drawbacks of oral route, immense attention has been paid in the field of mucoadhesive polymer system in formulations to prolong their residence time on mucosal membrane. Chitosan is an interesting polymer that has been used extensively for delivery of an active pharmaceutical ingredient owing to its biocompatible, biodegradable, and mucoadhesive properties [2]. Chitosan polymer has been used as drug excipients in the form of beads, films, nanoparticles, and nanogels etc. Recently, the development of Chitosan based nanogels have also been considerable attention because they can encapsulate various types of drugs, for instance poorly soluble drugs, and biotechnology based drugs etc., to minimize burst release, selectively release pattern inside or near a specific tissue or organ and enhance the efficiency [3]. Nanogels show promising as a suitable nanomedicine carrier in contrast to other nanoparticles especially in terms of drug loading, more residence time of drugs in specific tissue, protect drugs from degradation, and consequently enhance bioavailability of drugs. For example Lu *et al.* synthesized the hybrid nanogels for targeting effective positive folic acid, with three components i.e. hydrophilic polyacrylamide (PAm), the matrix of the nanogels and methotrexate (MTX) [4].

16.2 NANOGELS

Nanogels are nanosized aqueous dispersion of hydrogels formed by physical and chemical cross linked three dimensional (3D) polymers that can be used to facilitate the encapsulation of various classes of biological active molecules through self assembly involving salt bond, hydrogen bond, hydrophobic interactions between the drug and the polymer matrix [5]. Nanogels have received much interest for drug delivery because of their amendable chemical, three dimensional physical structures, high loading capacity, high stability, and biocompatibility [6].

The advantages of nanogels as a potential nanomedicines carrier system (Figure 16.1):

i. The Particle size of nanogels can be easily manipulated to achieve both passive and active drug targeting after intravenous administration because nanogels have tunable size from nanometers to micrometers.

ii. Nanogels have larger surface area; can be manipulated to avoid rapid clearance by phagocytic cells, which is significant for *in vivo* application.

iii. Controlled and sustained drug release at the target site, improving the therapeutic efficacy and reducing side effects because controlled release and degradation characteristic can be modulated by the choice of matrix constituents.

iv. Nanogels have considerable drug loading capacity, high aqueous dispersion stability and drug can be incorporated into the system without any chemical reaction; this is an important attribute for preserving the drug activity.

v. Nanogels are ideal candidate for intracellular drug delivery because they have ability to reach the smallest capillary vessels, due to their tiny volume, and to penetrate the tissue either through the Para cellular or the transcellular pathways.

vi. Nanogels are highly biocompatible and biodegradable drug delivery system.

vii. The nanogels based drug delivery system can be used for various route of administration including oral, parenteral, nasal, pulmonary, intra-ocular, topical, etc. [7–9].

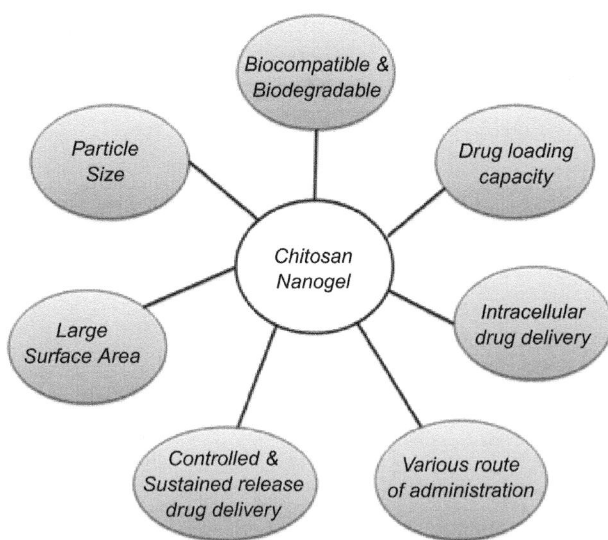

FIGURE 16.1   Advantages of chitosan nanogel system.

16.3   CHITOSAN

Chitosan *i.e.* poly [β-(1–4)—linked-2-amino-2-deoxy-D-glucose], is a natural, linear and cationic polyaminosaccharide obtained from the alkaline deacetylation of chitin. Together with chitin, Chitosan is considered the second most abundant polysaccharide after cellulose [10]. Chitosan is most widely used natural excipients in pharmaceutical formulations for novel drug delivery system. The reaction of Chitosan is significantly more versatile than cellulose due to presence of NH_2 group. When the degree of deacetylation of chitin reaches about 50% it becomes soluble by protonation of the $-NH_2$ on the C-2 position of the D-glucosamine repeat unit, wherewith the polysaccharide is converted to a polycationicin aqueous acidic medium and is called Chitosan [11]. The degree of deacetylation has a considerable effect on the solubility and rheological properties of the polymer. The NH_2 group of chitosan has a pKa in the range of 55 to 6.5, depending on the source of the polymer. At low pH, the polymer is soluble, with the sol-gel transition occurring at pH 7. The pH sensitivity, coupled with NH_2 group, make Chitosan an exceptional polymer for oral drug delivery applications [12]. A wide variety of pharmaceutical applications for Chitosan has been reported over the last few decades. Additionally to the good biocompatibility of chitosan and the abundance of natural sources of the material, Chitosan has a number of desirable properties that make its study more interesting. Being biocompatible, biodegradable, and muco-adhesive, Chitosan and its derivative have been used as drug vehicles in the forms of beads, films, nanoparticles, and nanogels, etc. [13].

16.3.1   CHEMICAL STRUCTURE OF CHITOSAN

Chitosanpoly [β-(1–4)—linked-2-amino-2-deoxy-D-glucose] is obtained by the alkaline deacetylation of chitin. Chitosan is a copolymer of N-acetyl-D-glucosamine and D-glucosamine. The sugar backbone consists of α-1, 4-linked D-glucosamine with high degree of N-acetylation [14]. It is structurally very similar to cellulose, but it has acetamide group ($-NHCOCH_3$) at the C-2 position (Figure 16.2).

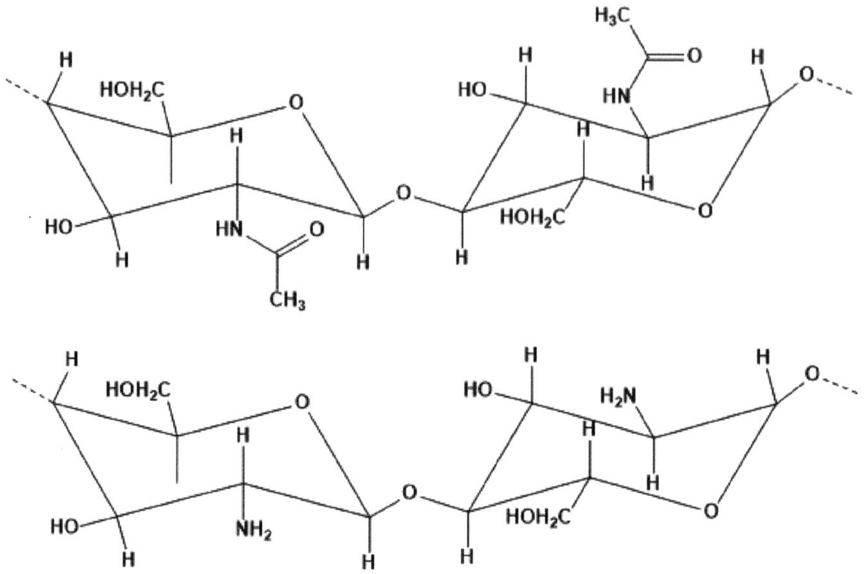

FIGURE 16.2   Structure of chitin and chitosan.

16.3.2   PROPERTIES OF CHITOSAN

Chitosan is distinct from other commonly available natural polysaccharides due to its glucosamine groups, cationicity, and capacity to form polyelectrolyte complexes, making it a versatile material with extensive application in drug delivery [15].

16.3.3   CHEMICAL PROPERTIES OF CHITOSAN

The chemical properties of Chitosan are as follow (Figure 16.3):
   i. Linear polyamine,
   ii. Reactive amino group,
   iii. Reactive hydroxyl group,
   iv. Highly basic polysaccharide,
   v. Solubility in various media, solutions, viscosity,
   vi. Polyelectrolyte behavior, polyoxysalt formation,
   vii. Chelates many transition metals [16–18]

16.3.4   BIOLOGICAL PROPERTIES OF CHITOSAN

The chemical properties of Chitosan are as follow (Figure 16.4):
   i. Biocompatible natural polymer
   ii. Biodegradable to body constituents
   iii. Mucoadhesion
   iv. Macrophage activation
   v. Adsorption enhancer
   vi. Analgesic action

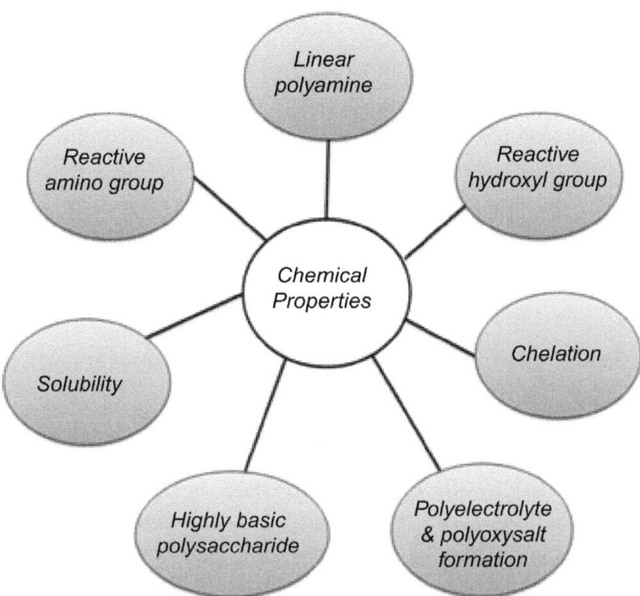

FIGURE 16.3   Chemical properties of chitosan nanogels.

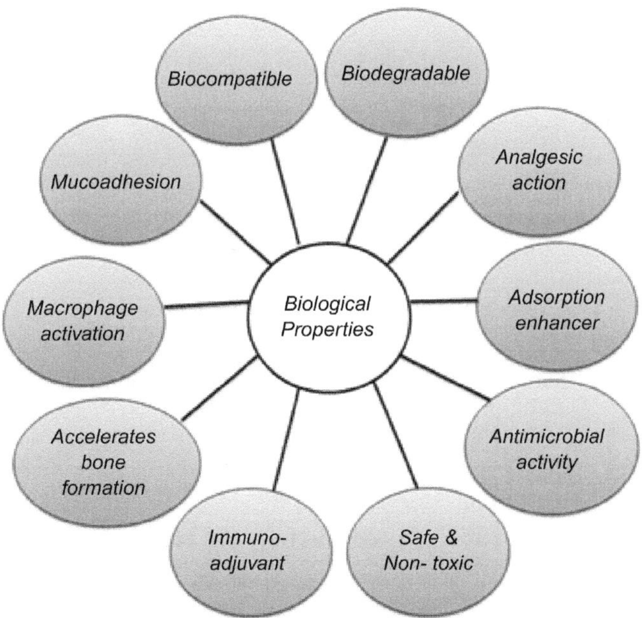

FIGURE 16.4   Biological properties of chitosan nanogels.

   vii. Antimicrobial activity

 viii. Immunoadjuvant

    ix. Accelerates bone formation

     x. Safe and non-toxic [19, 20]

16.4 CHITOSAN NANOGELS

In last few decades, nanogels based on Chitosan have received huge consideration because of its unique properties to encapsulate various types of drugs, peptides, proteins; to minimize burst release, improve selectivity, enhances the efficiency of the drug therapy [21]. Chitosan based Nanogels have advantages predominantly for the design and engineering of novel drug delivery due to their unique properties:

   i. Biodegradability
   ii. Biocompatible
   iii. Mucoadhesive
   iv. Hydrophilic character that facilitate administration of poorly absorbable drugs
   v. High aqueous dispersion stability [22, 23]

Nanogels are being explored drug delivery agents for site specific targeting due to their easy tailoring properties and ability to efficiently encapsulate therapeutics of diverse nature through simple mechanisms [24]. Nanogels are competently internalized by the target cells, avoid accumulation in non-target tissues thereby lower the therapeutic dosage and minimize harmful effects [25]. Chitosan nanogels have been prepared by several methodologies, for example, covalently cross-linked hybrid nanogels based on Chitosan chains provided a pH regulated release of the anticancer drug Temozolomide in the typical abnormal pH range of 5~7.4 found in a pathological zone and consequently enhanced the therapeutic efficiency. In particular, Chitosan based nanogels have been developed as a drug delivery platform for a wide range of active molecules [26].

16.4.1 Preparation of Chitosan Nanogels

Different methods have been used to prepare chitosan nanogel systems (Table 16.1, Figure 16.5). Various factors are responsible for selection such as thermal and chemical stability of the active constituent, reproducibility of the kinetic profiles of drug, particle size requirement and residual toxicity associated with the final product [27].

16.4.1.1 Emulsion Cross Linking

Chitosan solution is emulsified in oil (w/o emulsion) in this method. Use of appropriate surfactant stabilizes the aqueous droplets. Selection of suitable crosslinking agent such as glutaraldehyde,

TABLE 16.1

Commercial Methods Employed for the Production of Chitosan Nanogel

S. No.	Production Method	Matrix composition
1	Emulsification and crosslinking	Chitosan, glutaraldehyde
2	Reverse micellization	Chitosan, glutaraldehyde
3	Ionic gelation Chitosan,	Tripolyphosphate
4	Polyelectrolyte complexation	Chitosan, alginate, gum arabic, carboxymethyl cellulose, carrageenan, chondroitin sulfate, cyclodextrins, dextran sulfate, polyacrylic acid, poly-γ-glutamic acid, insulin, DNA
5	Modified ionic gelation with radical polymerization	Chitosan, acrylic acid, methacrylic acid, polyethylene glycol, polyether
6	Emulsion solvent diffusion	Chitosan

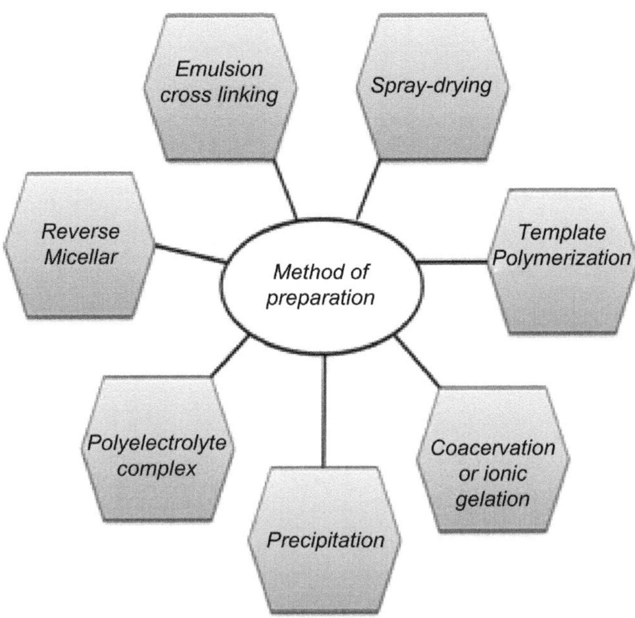

FIGURE 16.5   Method of preparations of chitosan nanogels.

stabilize the polysaccharide droplets of the gel (Figure 16.6). The nanogel prepared was then washed and dried. The utilization of the organic solvents and crosslinking agents are associated with major drawback that may harmfully affect the steadiness of proteins [28]. Furthermore, nanogel cross-linked with glutaraldehydes presents depressing effects on cell viability.

16.4.1.2 Spray-drying

This method is a fine practice to produce powders, granules or agglomerates from the combination of drug and excipient solutions as well as suspensions. A stream of hot air dries the atomized droplets is the basis of this method [29]. Firstly chitosan is dissolved or dispersed in this method then aqueous acetic acid solution, then drug is dissolved or dispersed in the solution and lastly an appropriate cross-linking agent is added [30]. This solution is then atomized in a flow of warm air. Formation of small droplets is result of atomization after which solvent evaporates immediately leading to the formation of free flowing particles. To achieved desired size of particles various process parameters are to be controlled. Inlet, size of nozzle, spray flow rate and atomization pressure results in different particle size [31].

16.4.1.3 Reverse Micellar Method

Firstly reverse micelles are produced by dissolving surfactant in organic solvent. To this, an aqueous solution of drug and chitosan are added with constant vortexing to avoid any turbidity (Figure 16.7). Microemulsion phase is obtained from the aqueous solution in such a way to keep the entire mixture optically transparent [32]. Nanogels of larger size are obtained by addition of water. To this solution, a crosslinking agent is added and the kept under continuous stirring overnight. To obtain the transparent dry mass the organic solvent is then evaporated. Then water is added, followed by the addition of suitable salt, will precipitate the surfactant out. Drug-loaded nanogels is obtained after centrifugation and decanting the supertant. Dialysis of aqueous dispersion through dialysis membrane immediately for 1 hr. and obtained solution is lyophilized to obtained dry powder [33].

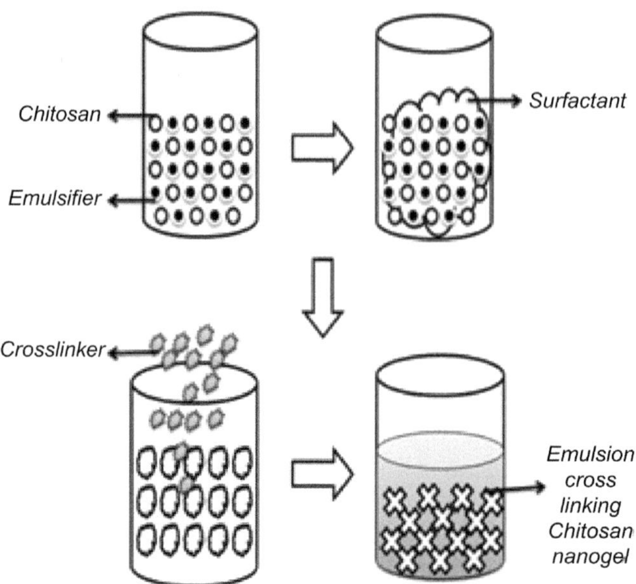

FIGURE 16.6   Emulsion crosslinking method.

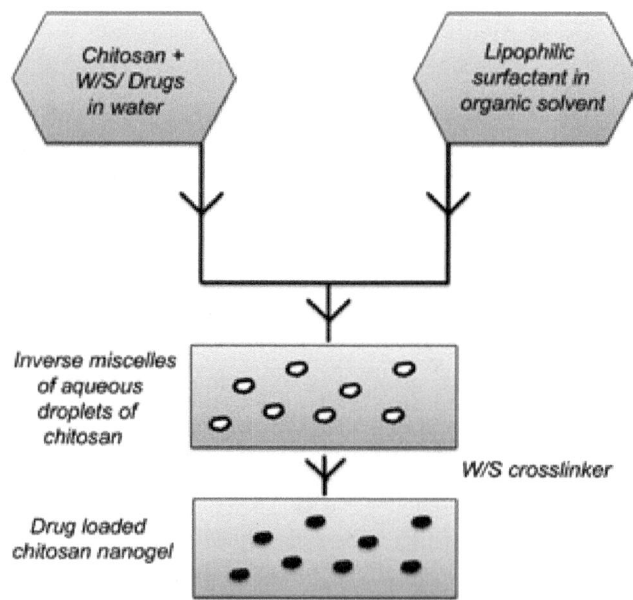

FIGURE 16.7   Reverse micellar method.

16.4.1.4   Template Polymerization Initiator

In this process, chitosan is dissolved in an acrylic monomer solution with continuous stirring. The negatively charged acrylic monomers line up along the chitosan molecules as a consequence of electrostatic interaction [34]. With the complete dissolution of chitosan, the polymerization is initiated by adding the $K_2S_2O_8$ under stirring at 70°C (**fig16.8**). Appearance of an opalescent solution which occurs after complete polymerization indicates the nanogels formation [35]. The residual monomers

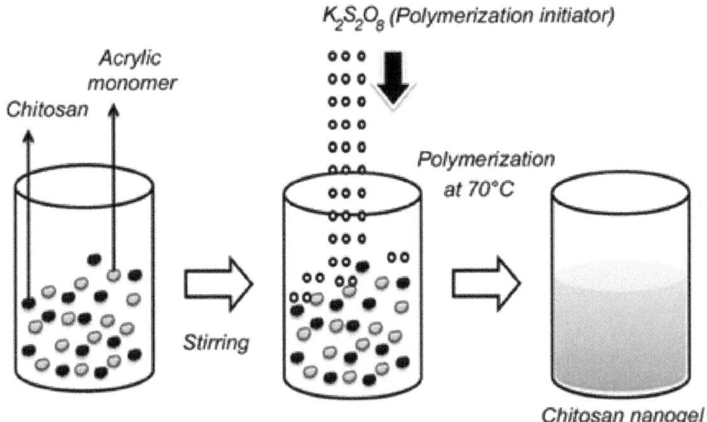

FIGURE 16.8   Template polymerization initiator.

and initiator are removed from the nanogels after filtration and dialysis. The size of the obtained nanogels is in the range of 50 to 400 nm and is positively charged. The complete polymerization leads to the emergence of an opalescent solution, indicating the Nanogels formation. The Nanogels solution are then filtered and dialyzed to remove the residual monomers and initiator. The obtained Nanogels are positively charged and present a size in the range of 50 to 400 nm [36].

16.4.1.5   Polyelectrolyte Complex (PEC)

Complexes formed or produced by self-assembly of the plasmid DNA and cationic charged polymer comes under self-assemble polyelectrolyte or polyelectrolyte complex. Usually, this procedure offers simple and mild preparation without involving ruthless conditions [37]. Mechanism of self-assembly polyelectrolyte involves charge neutralization between DNA and cationic polymer leading to subside in hydrophobicity as the constituent of self-assembly (Figure 16.9). Cationic polymers such as gelatin and polyethylenimine also have the same property [38]. Commonly, this method involves mild and simple preparation method without harsh conditions. Following the addition of DNA solution into Chitosan in acetic acid solution, nanogels are spontaneously formed with stirring under room temperature. The size of the formed complex is between 50nm to 700nm [39].

16.4.1.6   Precipitation

Formation of nanogels by precipitation occurs by two approaches. The first method is desolation, in which sodium sulfate (flocculants) is added to chitosan's water solution and solubility of Chitosan is decreased by the combination of water and sulfate, leading to the precipitation of managers due to hydrogen bonding between molecules. The second method is based on the diffusion of emulsified solvent [40]. The organic solvent is used in this method. Chitosan is dispersed in the organic phase under the action of emulsified solvent. Encapsulation occurs at the interface of the two phases where turbulence appears and then Chitosan is precipitated, resulting in the generation of nanogels. The size of nanogels obtained is large results in restriction of their application [41].

16.4.1.7   Coacervation or Ionic Gelation Method

Using biodegradable hydrophilic polymers such as gelation, sodium alginate and chitosan has been focused by many researchers for the preparation of nanogels [42]. The preparation of the nanogels for the development of chitosan nanogels is by ionic gelation (Figure 16.10). This method involves mixing of two aqueous phases of which one is the chitosan polymer, a di-block co-polymer propylene

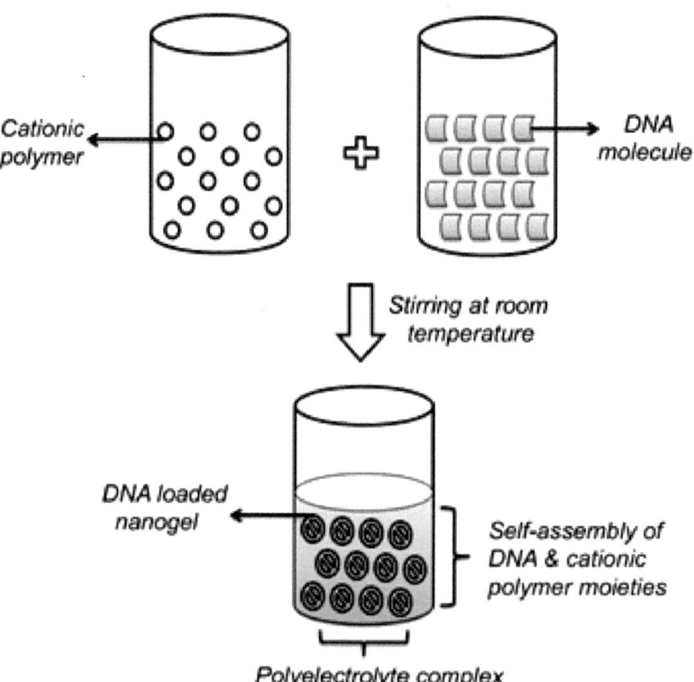

FIGURE 16.9   Polyelectrolyte complex (PEC).

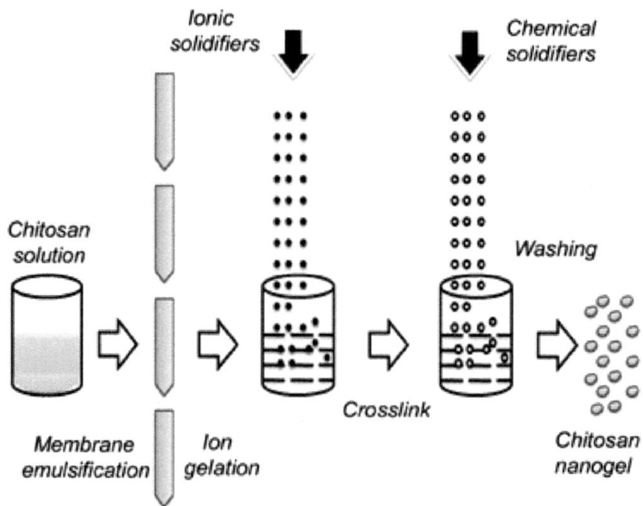

FIGURE 16.10   Coacervation or ionic gelation method.

oxide and the second one is a poly-anion sodium tri polyphosphate [43]. Positively charged amino group of chitosan interacts with negative charged anion TPP towards the formation of coacervates with size in the range of nanometer. As a result of electrostatic interaction between two aqueous phases coacervates are formed, whereas, in ionic gelation transition from liquid to gel occur due to ionic interaction conditions at room temperature [44].

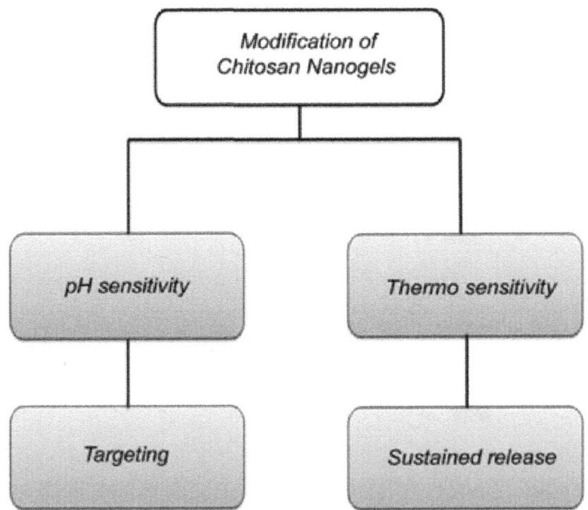

FIGURE 16.11 Modification of chitosan nanogels.

16.5 MODIFICATION OF CHITOSAN NANOGELS

Modifications of chitosan nanogels are focused on the increasing number of studies such as improve targeting, sustained or controlled release and bioavailability of chitosan (Figure 16.11). Thermosensitivity, pH sensitivity, and target accuracy are some important characteristics of nanogels [45].

16.5.1 MODIFICATION OF pH SENSITIVITY

Drug delivery system that increases drug release by changing carrier properties under acidic environment *in-vivo*, and targeting the abrasion tissue comes under pH-sensitive nanocarrier [46]. Polymer such as Poly(propylacrylic acid) (PPAA) is extremely sensitive to pH. High Membrane fragmentation of endosomal membrane occur at pH lower than 6.0 and let loose vesicular materials into cytochylema [47].

16.5.2 MODIFICATION OF THERMOSENSITIVITY

Structural alternation of thermosensitive drug carrier at dissimilar temperatures regulates release of drug. Extensively used thermoresponsive polymer as drug carriers is Poly (N-isopropyl acrylamide) [48]. At critical solution temperature of 38°C chitosan-poly-vinyl-caprolactane graft copolymer nanogels were sensitive to temperature. When 5-fluorouracil were used as a representative drug, release of drug occur at 38° C showing low toxicity to normal cells but high toxicity to tumor cells [49].

16.5.3 MODIFICATION OF TARGETING

Chitosan Nanogels with active targeting can be prepared through chemical modification, so as to make the drug identify the target precisely [50]. As a model drug, chitosan nanogels were prepared with resveratrol, using ligands of both avidin and biotin to modify the nanogels. Delivery system thus formed passively target the liver and positively target hepatoma cells. In this new drug delivery system two kinds of targeting mechanisms were combined to achieve targeting to specific cells in specific tissues, thus improving therapeutic effects, toxicity and side effects [51].

16.5.4 Modification of Sustained Release

Nanogels prepared with chitosan or lactic acid-chitosan were developed for increasing drug encapsulation, prolong drug release and increase chitosan solubility in solution of neutral pH, chitosan was modified by attaching L,D-lactic acid onto amino groups without using a catalyst [52]. Drug release rate were increased and drug encapsulation efficiency was decreased on increasing protein concentration. As chitosan is generally soluble only in acid solution, the chitosan grafted on lactic acid can be prepared from solutions of neutral pH, which will allow proteins or drugs to be uniformly incorporated in the matrix structure with minimal denaturation [53].

16.6 APPLICATION OF NANOGELS

Nanogels in a present scenario of medical era is progressed as an inspiring drug delivery system and creates varied structures like on site drug delivery system, sustained release formulation, high drug encapsulation properties, water solubility, biodegradability, low toxicity, tissue specificity, etc. (Figure 16.12) [54, 55]. Due to these intrinsic assets and individualities nanogel established extensively in many drug deliver streams. Mutual with polymers, metals, chelates and other active molecules nanogel emerged as extraordinary drug delivery system. The nanogel system commonly involved in many fields like pharmaceuticals, biotechnology, chemical technology, agriculture, medicine, diagnosing tool, food processing, etc. (Table 16.2) [56, 57].

The nanogel drug delivery system is commonly employed in following streams.

16.6.1 Nano Sized Drug Delivery System

Nanogel contains micro and nano molecules, drugs, and other therapeutic agents expressing small molecular weight in their organization competently [58]. This unlikely feature subsidizes nanogel system a very promising drug carrier for controlled and sustained release delivery of drugs and other therapeutic agents [59]. Merged with polymers these systems extensively used in the active delivery of bioactives, chemical and natural extracts. These nanogels are contrived typically with varied portion of polymers accounting synthetic and natural polymers [60].

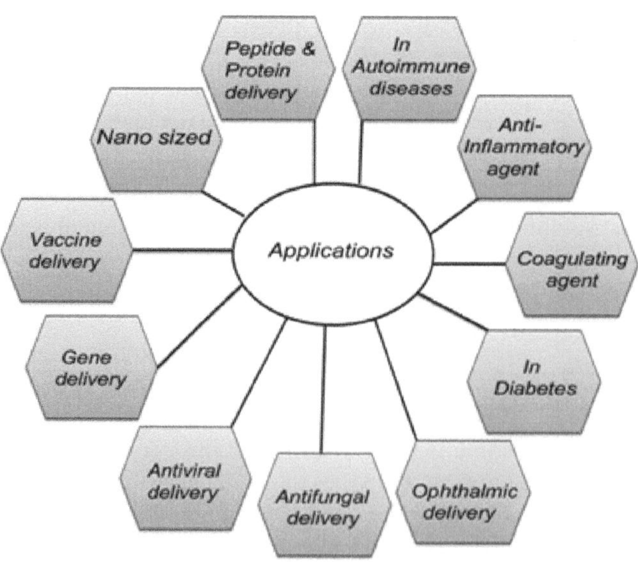

FIGURE 16.12 Application of chitosan nanogels.

TABLE 16.2

Commercial Applications of Chitosan Nanogel as Drug Delivery System

S. No.	Polymer	Type of nanogel	Remarks
1	Cross linked polyethylene mine & PEG/Pluronic	Biodegradable nanogel	5-triphosphorylated ribavirin reduced
2	Glycol chitosan grafted with 3-diethylaminopropyl group	pH responsive	Enhanced doxorubicin uptake
3	Polyethyleneimine nanogel	Size dependent nanogel	Enhanced gene hTERT-CD-TK delivered for lung cancer
4	Cholesterol bearing pullulan nanogel	Sustained release nanogel	Recombinant marineinterleukine-12 sustained tumor immunotherapy
5	Acetylated hyaluronic acid	Targeted nanogel	Doxorubicin loaded nanogel
6	Acrylate group modified cholesterol bearing pullulan	Cross-linked assembled nanogel	Fine interleukin-12 encapsulation & plasma level
7	Poly9(N-isopropylacrylamide) and chitosan	Thermosensitive magnetically active nanogel	Hyperthermia induced cancer treatment
8	PEo-b0PMA	Self-organizing nanogel	Enhance cisplatin or doxorubicin delivery
9	Carboxymethyl chitosan-linolenic acid	Biodegradable nanogel	Adryamycin siRNA anti-EGFR delivery

16.6.2 Peptide & Protein Delivery

Nanogel can be proficiently delivered via diverse routes like oral, parenteral, topical etc. Oral route is the most favored and the most suitable route of drug delivery but the main drawback of the oral route is the dilapidation of drug, poor bioavailability, low mucosal permeability, marginal stability, Gastrointestinal (GIT) irritation, etc. [61]. In case of sensitive drugs like proteins and peptides, the oral drug delivery turns out to be a lurid element. The nanogel drug delivery system opens new avenue in difficulty associated with the oral drug delivery [62]. Entrapment of drugs, peptides, proteins in nano formulation not only enhances drug therapeutic efficacy but also offers on-time and on-site drug delivery. The main benefit of nanogel deceived protein or peptides delivery is that, it requires very little amount of concentration of drugs and delivers directly to the desired site which eventually grasped into the systematic circulation without GIT degradation [63].

Introduction of polymers like chitosan, dextrin, PLGA (Poly-lactic glycolic acid) augmented the nanogel activity like sustained and controlled release, enzymatic cleavage etc. Polymeric nanogel offer decent therapeutic delivery of proteins which are very important in the medicinal era, since some of the supplies at its pinnacle level, for example Cytokines appears as noteworthy bioactive for vaccine and immunotherapy [64]. The nanogel containing growth hormones, cellular peptides, insulin emerge as new therapeutic drug delivery candidate to contest many life disturbing diseases like cancer, arthritis, diabetes, etc. [65]. PEGylation of polymeric nanogel is evolved as novel candidate in many diseases especially viral and bacterial diseases. For example, delivery of Bleomycin (an anticancer antibiotic drug) via PEGylated chitosan nanogel is appeared as effective drug system in the ailment of squamous cell carcinoma (SCC) transdermally.

Addition with intracellular delivery of Chitosan and PEG/heparin starts apoptosis in cancerous cell due to the stimulation of caspase proteins. Antihistamine activity of polymeric nanogel comprises of fluorescent heparin has been efficaciously estimated in rat mast cell. The *ex-vivo* trial proficiently established the inhibitory action of heparin nanogel in mast cell of rats [66].

16.6.3 Vaccine Delivery

Delivery of antigen or antibodies by mean of nano-formulation delivers the significant platform in the medical avenue. Conservative approach of drug delivery system containing the antigens or antibodies transact with the several tasks like integrity of antigen, deteriorations, stability, sterility, protection against infections, immune response, etc. [67]. Nanogel system not only offers the promise against the conventional tasks but guaranteed the delivery of both type of antigen i.e., humoral and cellular with the chief assertion of keeping actual immunity after the single delivery of vaccine. Vaccine nanogel system reproduces microbes or pathogens usually aware, phagocytosed and preceded by the dedicated antigen presenting cells (APCs) [68]. Generally most of the organism and pathogens are perceived and removed in very short time by the protection process, which are not antigen definite and does not need any extended period of induction. These contrivances are the imperious part of inborn immunity. Nanogel based cancer vaccines fetches the drug delivery system at its zenith innovative stature, articulating the improbable features like low adverse effects, stimuli specific, production of long term or life time immunity, etc. [69].

16.6.4 Gene Delivery

The appearance of Nucleic acids as biomedicines opens the mysteries of various fatal diseases treatment. Delivery of pDNA, oligonucleotides such as ODNs and siRNA displays their strong impression on variety of undying diseases counting cancer and HIVs [70]. Polymeric nanogel engulfed of active genes like siRNA and DNAs displays imperious tools in the cancer chemotherapy. Cancer currently scattering like a mushrooms globally, not only distressing the under developed countries but upsetting the super powers also [71]. Angiogenesis plays crucial role in the expansion and the initiation of cancer and tumor cells. PEG conjugated VEGF-siRNA/EGFR-siRNA complexes with PEI (polyethylenimine) displays extraordinary inhibition of VEGF/EGF appearance at tumor site, potently limiting tumor growth without creating the systemic side effects like inflammation of cells in tumor mice model [72].

The gene delivery via polymeric nanogel is demonstrating as commanding delivery carrier in competent anticipation of asthma, dropping the virus retention in lungs, prevention the inflammation in lungs and removing the hyper-infection related with asthma [73]. One of the key landmark has been attained by the gene therapy in the ailment of pulmonary asthma is the topical delivery of 5% Imiquimod gel composed with the siRNA targeting siNPRA (natri-uretic peptide receptor-A). The administration of polymeric siRNA fused with imiquimod cream effectively decline the airway hyper stimuli eosinophilia and pro-inflammatory cytokines IL-4 and IL-5 in lung homogenates when examined in asthmatic mice model [74].

16.6.5 Antiviral Nanogel Delivery

The drug delivery in the viral infection is always been the stimulating task. Research community discovering the trials related with the antiviral drug delivery system. After the efficaciously reconnoitering the antibacterial delivery of nanogel system, wide-ranging research has make the nanogel as a real dug carrier against the virus [75]. Viral diseases are most fatal and the life embellished diseases. Convention drug delivery against viruses comprises delivery of antiviral drug orally, parentally etc. which shows its own drawbacks like systemic toxicities, drug degradation, low therapeutic effects etc. With the appearance of nano-medicines the difficulties ascends due to the conventional drug delivery has been lessens to the great amount [76].

Polymeric silver nanogel has demonstrated the noteworthy antiviral activity against HIV-1 without persuading the toxicity and at very little concentration. In vitro research established the improved antiviral activity of silver nanogel against the HIV-1 viral strain. The silver nanogel shows the antiviral activity at an early phase of viral replication by hindering the cell division and striking the replication and translation progression. They also limit the binding, conjugation, fusion and infectivity of CD4 dependent virions [77]. They hold strong virus removing properties against the cell related and cell f0ree virus strains. Ligand anchored gold nanogel possess decent antiviral activity on variety of viruses. Amphiphilic sulphate tailored ligand conjugated Gold nanogel confers to the HIV envelope glycoprotein and hinders the HIV contagion of T-cells nano-concentration when evaluated and analyzed *invitro*.

Ligand conjugated nanogel particles augment the local concentration of bioactive particles at the targeted site which results in the better receptor binding of nanogel particles resulting in the good therapeutic effects at targeted site [78]. The polymeric gold nanogel are proficiently utilized against Herpes simplex virus Type-1 constituting MES showing strong antiviral activity targeting the virus through contrasting the binding to cellular heparin sulphate by its sulfonate end molecule. This blockage of the viral entrance into the cell results in removal of viral infection. The nanogel shows the ultra-fine action against the lethal Hepatitis-B virus. Research community professionally shows the silver nanogel delivery against the Hepatitis-B virus laterally with syncytial virus strain, HIV-1 virus and monkey-pox virus significantly [79].

16.6.6 Antifungal Nanogel Delivery

Fungal infection evolved as the big problem in present scenario of medicinal era subsidizing the higher risk and reason of impermanence and morbidity around the world [80]. Inadequate medicines and studies against the fungal infections results in more distressing condition. Polymeric silver nanogel estimated as potent fungi-static and fungicidal agent when examined against pathogen like yeasts. Silver nanogel also shows good antifungal activity against *Candida spp.*, at very low concentration of about 1–2 mg/ml of silver (Ag). The silver nanogel displays outstanding antifungal property against the species of *Candida* and *Trichophyton mentagrophytes* showing the IC80 value at very low concentration of 1–10µg/ml. The nanogel delivery suggestively exposes noteworthy action against the fungal pathogens as compare to the free drug like fluconazole or amphotericin B [81]. The chief phenomenon behind the antifungal activity of nanogel is to target the cell membrane and distracting the membrane potential, which results in the pores development in the cell membrane. Pores formation hints the leakage of cellular contents, eventually cause the cell death. Transmission electron microscopy (TEM) examination strongly reveals the disruption of cell membrane and pores in *Candida albicans* when the silver nanogel particles interact with the cell membrane of *C. albicans*. Antifungal metal nanogel also shows the subordinate actions like coating of particles, bio-stabilization of footwear materials, disinfectants of films against variety of fungal pathogens, etc. [82].

16.6.7 In Autoimmune Diseases

Nanogel demeanor liposomes entailed of MPA (mycophenolic acid) was effectively evaluated in treatment of autoimmune diseases [83]. The MPA liposomal nanogel solubilized by addition of cyclodextrin, Irgacure 2959 was presented as photo-initiator and PEG (Polyethylene glycol) was concluded with an acrylate end group. When the contact of UV radiation takes place, photopolymerization of PEG oligomer initiates. The nanogel system produces numerous intrinsic properties such as lodging of the MPA (drug) load at targeted site, active penetrating to the cell membrane for the effectual binding to the receptor cell triggers the rapid therapeutic response [84]. Polymeric nanogel delivery in the autoimmune conditions raises the therapeutic efficiency to the targeted site and evades the frequent dosing of drug, which leads to eradicate the risk of renal damage, liver injury and local tissue damages.

16.6.8 Ophthalmic Delivery

pH sensitive nanogel delivery discloses the usefulness of this nano-medicine in the arena of ophthalmology. Polymeric *pH* activated nanogel composed of polyvinyl pyrrolidone-poly acrylic acid (PVP/PAAc) which is contrived by the polymerization of PAAc in aqueous solution of PVP starts by gamma radiation. Pilocarpine compressed PVP/PAAc nanogel reveals enhance ophthalmic drug delivery of *pH* sensitive nanogel at the targeted site with negligible toxicity [85].

16.6.9 Diabetes

Glucose receptive insulin entrapped nanogel injection has been effectively evaluated and measured. The charge interaction plays crucial role between the nanogel particles and the glucose molecules [86]. Acidity of the nanogel particles rises by the accumulation of the dextran leads to fine interface of nanogel particles and evades the clearance from the body. Polymeric nanogel complexes with dextran entrapped insulin possess good antidiabetic activity when injected in the body with the benefit of less dose and better residing time. The elevated permeation of gel agreements the glucose molecules to enter and diffuse within the gel matrix [87]. At elevated glucose level, large amount of glucose molecules diffuses through the gel and release of insulin befalls due to the ionic interaction between the gel and glucose molecules. Conversion of glucose to glucuronic acid take place displays the noteworthy contribution of the nanogel delivery system in the condition of diabetes [88].

16.6.10 Coagulating Agent

Polymeric nanogel explored as a strong carrier unruffled of proteins molecules to restrict bleeding. The biodegradable chitosan anchored protein nanogel shows very strong and important coagulation response against wounds, rashes, bites, etc. [89].

16.6.11 Anti-Inflammatory Agent

Nanogels display very significant and effective anti-inflammatory action. Nanogel synthesized by PLGA/chitosan constitutes oleic acid as penetrator relish shows superfine anti-inflammatory activity [90]. Combined delivery of ketoprofen and spantide II via PLGA/chitosan nanogel displays good residing time and noteworthy anti-inflammatory action assessed *in-vivo*. The major benefit of PLGA/chitosan topical nanogel is the sustained release delivery with *pH* triggered release of ketoprofen and spantide II in allergic dermatitis and psoriatic plaque situations. The PLGA/chitosan topical nanogel elevates the percutaneous drug delivery of ketoprofen and spantide II and shows fine therapeutic action with low toxicities.

16.7 DISADVANTAGES OF NANOGEL

    i. Preparation of various nanogels is very tedious and expensive process for the removal of solvent, surfactants molecule after the complete synthesis of nanogel.

    ii. Toxicities problem can rise due to the residual of traces of surfactants or emulsifiers.

16.8 CONCLUSION

Chitosan nanogel delivery system emerges as a promising drugs carrier which plays imperative role in transport of abundant pharmaceuticals and therapeutics in fungal, bacterial and microbial ailments. Chitosan nanogels provide remarkable features and elude complications related with formulation like stability, absorption and compatibility. Nanogels offers a promising contestant in multiple directing like brain, lungs, colon, skin, GIT and heart with big advantage of numerous routes of administration. In future the limitations like site specificity, selectivity, adverse effects and therapeutic competence can be evades by controlling the detailed factors linked to formulation and delivery of nanogels which results in increasing vision of nanogel delivery system in drug delivery era. Further and widespread *in-vivo* and clinical research should be approved for the improved economic fabrication of nanogel at marketable stages.

REFERENCES

1. Agrawal, P., Strijkers, G.J., Nicolay, K., 2010. Chitosan-based systems for molecular imaging. Adv. Drug Deliv. Rev. 62, 42–58.
2. Ahad, A., Aqil, M., Kohli, K., Sultana, Y., Mujeeb, M., Ali, A., 2012. Formulation and optimization of nanotransfersomes using experimental design technique for accentuated transdermal delivery of valsartan. Nanomed.: Nanotechnol. 8, 237–249.
3. Ali, A.I., Jitender, M., Dinesh, K., Satish, S., Shankar, P.R., Asgar, A., 2011. Comparative study of transfersomes, liposomes, and niosomes for topical delivery of 5-fluorouracil to skin cancer cells: Preparation, characterization, in vitro release, and cytotoxicity analysis. Anti-cancer Drugs. 22, 774–782.
4. Andrade, F., Antunes, F., Nascimento, A.V., da Silva, S.B., das Neves, J., Ferreira, D., Sarmento, B., 2011. Chitosan formulations as carriers for therapeutic proteins. Curr. Drug Discov. Technol. 8, 157–172.
5. Anto, S.M., Kannan, C., Kumar, K.S., Kumar, S.V., Suganeshwari, M., 2011. Formulation of 5 fluorouracil loaded chitosan nanoparticles by emulsion droplet coalescence method for cancer therapy. Int J. Pharm. Biol. Arch. 2, 926–931.
6. Araujo, L.M.P.C., Thomazine, J.A., Lopez, R.F.V., 2010. Development of microemulsions to topically deliver 5-aminolevulinic acid in photodynamic therapy. Eur. J. Pharm. Biopharm. 75, 48–55.
7. Atyabi, F., Talaie, F., Dinarvand, R., 2009. Thiolated chitosan nanoparticles as an oral delivery system for amikacin: In vitro and ex vivo evaluations. J. Nanosci. Nanotechnol. 9, 4593–4603.
8. Avadi, M.R., Sadeghi, A.M.M., Mohammadpour, N., Abedin, S., Atyabi. F., Dinarvand, R., Rafiee-Tehrani, M., 2010. Preparation and characterization of insulin nanoparticles using chitosan and arabic gum with ionic gelation method. Nanomed. Nanotechnol. Biol. Med. 6, 58–63.
9. Azarbayjani, A.F., Venugopal, J.R., Ramakrishna, S., Lim, P.F.C., Chan, Y.W., Chan, S.Y., 2010. Smart polymeric nanofibers for topical delivery of Levothyroxine. J. Pharm. Pharm. Sci. 13, 400–410.
10. Azizi, E., Namazi, A., Haririan, I., Fouladdel, S., Khoshayand, M.R., Shotorbani, P.Y., 2010. Release profile and stability evaluation of optimized chitosan/alginate nanoparticles as EGFR antisense vector. Int. J. Nanomed. 5, 455–461.
11. Bahia, A.P., Azevedo, E.G., Ferreira, L.A., Frezard, F., 2010. New insights into the mode of action of ultradeformable vesicles using calcein as hydrophilic fluorescent marker. Eur. J. Pharm. Sci. 39, 90–96.
12. Baldrick, P., 2010. The safety of chitosan as pharmaceutical excipient. Regul. Toxicol. Pharmacol. 56, 290–299.
13. Bhattarai, N., Gunn, J., Zhang, M., 2010. Chitosan-based hydrogels for controlled, localized drug delivery. Adv. Drug. Deliv. Rev. 62, 83–99.
14. Bisht, S., Maitra, A., 2009. Dextran-doxorubicin/chitosan nanoparticles for solid tumor therapy. Wiley Interdiscip. Rev. Nanomed. Nanobiotechnol. 1, 415–25.
15. Biswas, S., Dodwadkar, N.S., Deshpande, P.P., Torchilin, V.P., 2012. Liposomes loaded with paclitaxel and modified with novel triphenylphosphonium-PEG-PE conjugate possess low toxicity, target mitochondria and demonstrate enhanced antitumor effects in vitro and in vivo. J. Control. Release. 159, 393–402.
16. Bouwstra, J.A., Gooris, G.S., 2010. The lipid organization in human stratum corneum model systems. Open. Derm. J. 4, 10–13.
17. Cai, S., Thati, S., Bagby, T.R., Diabw Mustafa, H., Davies, N.M., Cohen, M.S., Forrest, M.L., 2010. Localized doxorubicin chemotherapy with a biopolymeric nanocarrier improves survival and reduces toxicity in xenografts of human breast cancer. J. Control. Release. 146, 212–218.
18. Chakravarthi, S.S., De, S., Miller, D.W., Robbinson, D.H., 2010. Comparison of antitumor efficacy of paclitaxel delivered in nano- and microparticles. Int. J. Pharm. 383, 37–44.
19. Chan, H.K., Kwok, P.C.L., 2011. Production methods for nanodrug particles using the bottom-up approach. Adv. Drug Deliv. Rev. 63, 406–416.
20. Chang, R.S., Kim, J., Lee, H.Y., Han, S.-E., Na, J., Kim, K., Kwon, I.C., Kim, Y.B., Oh, Y.-K., 2010. Reduced dose-limiting toxicity of intraperitoneal mitoxantrone chemotherapy using cardiolipin-based anionic liposomes. Nanomed.: Nanotechnol. 6, 769–776.

21. Chaudury, A., Das, S., 2011. Recent advancement of chitosan-based nanoparticles for oral controlled delivery of insulin and other therapeutic agents. AAPS Pharm. Sci. Tech. 12, 10–20.

22. Cochran, M.C., Eisenbrey, J., Ouma, R.O., Soulen, M., Wheatley, M.A., 2011. Doxorubicin and paclitaxel loaded microbubbles for ultrasound triggered drug delivery. Int. J. Pharm. 414, 161–170.

23. Das, N.J., Bahia, M., Amiji, M.M., Sarmento, B., 2011. Mucoadhesive nanomedicines: Characterization and modulation of mucoadhesion at the nanoscale. Expert Opin. Drug Deliv. 8, 1085–1104.

24. Duceppe, N., Tabrizian, M., 2010. Advances in using chitosan-based nanoparticles for in vitro and in vivo drug and gene delivery. Expert Opin. Drug Deliv. 7, 1191–1207.

25. El Meshad, A.N., Tadros, M.I., 2011. Transdermal delivery of an anti-cancer drug via w/o emulsions based on alkyl polyglycosides and lecithin: Design, characterization, and in vivo evaluation of the possible irritation potential in rats. AAPS. Pharm. Sci. Tech. 12, 1–9.

26. Elsayed, A., Al-Remawi, M., Qinna, N., Farouk, A., Al-sou'od, K., Badwan, A., 2011. Chitosan-sodium lauryl sulfate nanoparticles as a carrier system for the in vivo delivery of oral insulin. AAPS Pharm. Sci. Tech. 12, 958–964.

27. Fan, W., Yan, W., Xu, Z., Ni, H., 2012. Formation mechanism of mono-disperse, low molecular weight chitosan nanoparticles by ionic gelation technique. Colloid Surf. B. Biointerfaces. 90, 21–27.

28. Ferlay, J., Shin, H.R., Bray, F., Forman, D., Mathers, C., Parkin, D.M., 2010. Estimates of worldwide burden of cancer in 2008: GLOBOCAN 2008. Int. J. Cancer. 127, 2893–2917.

29. Fernandez, C.B., Font, A.F., Merino, V., Diaz, D.C., Barroeta, M.E., Castellano, A.L., Diaz, M.C., 2011. Elastic vesicles of sumatriptan succinate for transdermal administration: Characterization and in vitro permeation studies. J. Liposome Res. 21, 55–59.

30. Gelfuso, G.M., Gratieri, T., Souza, J.G., Thomazine, J.A., Lopez, R.F.V., 2011. The influence of positive or negative charges in the passive and iontophoretic skin penetration of porphyrins used in photodynamic therapy. Eur. J. Pharm. Biopharm. 77, 249–256.

31. Gill, KK., Nazzal, S., Kaddoumi, A., 2011. Paclitaxel loaded PEG (5000)-DSPE micelles as pulmonary delivery platform: Formulation characterization, tissue distribution, plasma pharmacokinetics, and toxicological evaluation. Eur. J. Pharm. Biopharm. 79(2), 276–284.

32. Grabnar, P., Kristl, J., 2010. Physicochemical characterization of protein-loaded pectin-chitosan nanoparticles prepared by polyelectrolyte complexation. Pharmazie. 65, 851–852.

33. Grenha, A., Al-Qadi, S., Seijo, B., Remuñán-Lopez, C., 2010. The potential of chitosan for pulmonary drug delivery. J. Drug. Deliv. Sci. Technol. 20, 33–43.

34. Grenha, A., Gomes, M.E., Rodrigues, M., Santo, V.E., Mano, J.F., Neves, N.M., Reis, R.L., 2010. Development of new chitosan/carrageenan nanoparticles for drug delivery applications. J. Biomed. Mater. Res. 92A, 1265–1272.

35. Heney, M., Alipour, M., Vergidis, D., Omri, A., Mugabe, C., Thng, J., Suntres, Z., 2010. Effectiveness of liposomal paclitaxel against MCF-7 breast cancer cells. Can. J. Physiol. Pharmacol. 88, 1172–1180.

36. Hureaux, J., Lagarce, F., Gagnadoux, F., Marie-Christine, R., Moal, V., Urban, T., Benoit, J.P., 2010. Toxicological study and efficacy of blank and paclitaxelloaded lipid nanocapsules after i.v. administration in mice. Pharm. Res. 27, 421–430.

37. Jain, A., Agarwal, A., Majumder, S., Lariya, N., Khaya, A., Himanshu, A., Majumdar, S., Agrawal, G.P., 2010. Mannosylated solid lipid nanoparticles as vectors for sitespecific delivery of an anti-cancer drug. J. Control. Release. 148, 359–367.

38. Jemal, A., Siegel, R., Xu, J., Ward, E., 2010. Cancer statistics, CA. Cancer J. Clin. 60, 277–300.

39. Kaihara, S., Suzuki, Y., Fujimoto, K., 2011. In situ synthesis of polysaccharide nanoparticles via polyion complex of carboxymethyl cellulose and chitosan. Colloid Surf. B – Biointerfaces. 85, 343–348.

40. Kaminskas, L.M., Kelly, B.D., McLeod, V.M., Sberna, G., Owen, D.J., Boyd, B.J., Porter, C.J., 2011. Characterization and tumour targeting of PEGylated polylysine dendrimers bearing doxorubicin via a pH labile linker. J. Control. Release. 152, 241–248.

41. Kaur, N., Puri R, Jain S., 2010. Drug-cyclodextrin-vesicles dual carrier approach for skin targeting of anti-acne agent. APPS PharmSci. Tech. 11, 528–537.

42. Kean, T., Thanou, M., 2010. Biodegradation, biodistribution and toxicity of chitosan. Adv. Drug Deliv. Rev. 62, 3–11.

43. Keawchaoon, L., Yoksan, R., 2011. Preparation, characterization and in vitro release study of carvacrol-loaded chitosan nanoparticles. Colloid Surf. B – Biointerfaces. 84, 163–171.

44. Kievit, F.M., Wang, F.Y., Fang, C., Mok, H., Wang, K., Silber, J.R., Ellenbogen, R.G., Zhang, M., 2011. Doxorubicin loaded iron oxide nanoparticles overcome multidrug resistance in cancer in vitro. J. Control. Release. 152, 76–83.

45. Kilicay, E., Demirbilek, M., Turk, M., Guven, E., Hazer, H., Denkbas, E.B., 2011. Preparation and characterization of poly(3-hydroxybutyrate-co-3 hydroxyhexanoate) (PHBHHX) based nanoparticles for targeted cancer therapy. Eur. J. Pharma. Sci. 44, 310–320.
46. Kim, J.H., Bae, S.M., Na, M.H., Shin, H., Yang, Y.J., Min, K.H., Choi, K.Y., Kim, K., Park, R.W., Kwon, I.C., Lee, B.H., Hoffman, A.S., Kim, I.S., 2012. Facilitated intracellular delivery of peptide-guided nanoparticles in tumor tissues. J. Control. Release. 157, 493–499.
47. Kulkarni, S.S., Aloorkar, N.H., 2010. Smart polymers in drug delivery: An overview. J. Pharm. Res. 3, 100–108.
48. Lee, S., Yun, M.H., Jeong, S.W., Hoon, C., Kim, J.Y., Seo, M.H., Pai, C.M., Kim, S.O., 2011. Development of docetaxel-loaded intravenous formulation, Nanoxel-PM™ using polymer-based delivery system. J. Control. Release. 155, 262–271.
49. Li, X., Kong, X., Zhang, J., Wang, Y., Shi, S., Guo, G., Luo, F., Zhao, X., Wei, Y., Qian, Z., 2011. A novel composite hydrogel based on chitosan and inorganic phosphate for local delivery of camptothecin nano-colloids. J. Pharm. Sci. 100, 232–241.
50. Li, X.Y., Kong, X.Y., Wang, X.H., Shi, S., Guo, G., Luo, F., Zhao, X., Wei, Y., Qian, Z., 2010. Gel-sol-gel thermo-gelation behavior study of chitosan-inorganic phosphate solutions. Eur. J. Pharm. Biopharm. 75, 388–392.
51. Liang, Y., Qiao, Y., Guo, S., Wang, L., Zhai, Y., Xie, C., Hu, R., Deng, L., Dong, A., 2012. Investigation on injectable, thermally and physically gelable poly(ethylene glycol)/poly(octadecanedioic anhydride) amphiphilic triblock co-polymer nanoparticles. J. Biomater. Sci. Polym. Ed. 23, 465–482.
52. Lin, X., Deng, L., Xu, Y., Dong, A., 2012. Thermosensitive in situ hydrogel of paclitaxel conjugated poly (ε-caprolactone)-poly(ethylene-glycol)-poly(ε-caprolactone). Soft Matter. 12, 3470–3477.
53. Liu, X., Sun, J., Chen, X., Wang, S., Scot, H., Zhan, X., Zhan, Q., 2012. Pharmacokinetics, tissue distribution and anti-tumour efficacy of paclitaxel delivered by polyvinylpyrrolidone solid dispersion. J. Pharm. Pharmacol. 7, 757–782.
54. Luo, X., Xie, C., Wang, H., Liu, C., Yan, S., Li, X., 2012. Antitumor activities of emulsion electrospun fibers with core loading of hydroxyl camptothecin via intratumoral implantation. Int. J. Pharm. 425, 19–28.
55. Mackay, H.J., Provencheur, D., Heywood, M., Tu, D., Eisenhauer, E.A., Oza, A.M., Meyer, R., 2011. Phase II/III study of intraperitoneal chemotherapy after neoadjuvant chemotherapy for ovarian cancer. Curr. Oncol. 18, 84–90.
56. Macewan, S.R., Callahan, D.J., Chilkoti, A., 2010. Stimulus-responsive macromulecules and nanoparti-cules for cancer drug delivery. Nanomedicine UK. 5, 793–806.
57. Maestrelli, F., González-Rodríguez, M.L., Rabasco, A.M., Ghelardini, C., Mura, P., 2010. New "drug-in cyclodextrin-in deformable liposomes" formulations to improve the therapeutic efficacy of local anaes-thetics. Int. J. Pharm. 395, 222–231.
58. Mahdi, E.S., Sakeena, M.H.F., Abdulkarim, M.F., Abdullah, G.Z., Sattar, M.A., Noor, A.M., 2011. Effect of surfactant and surfactant blends on pseudo ternary phase diagram behavior of newly synthe-sized palm kernel oil esters. Drug Des. Devel. Ther. 5, 311–323.
59. Mahajan, A., Aggarwal, G., 2011. Smart polymers: Innovations in novel drug delivery. Int. J. Drug Dev. & Res. 3, 16–30.
60. Malam, Y., Lim, E.J., Seifalian, A.M., 2011. Current trends in the application of nanoparticles in drug delivery. Current Med. Chem. 18, 1067–1078.
61. Manchanda, R., Nimesh, R., 2010. Controlled size chitosan nanoparticles as an efficient, biocompatible oligonucleotides delivery system. J. Appl. Polym. Sci. 118, 2071–2077.
62. Maurya, S.K., Pathak, K., Bali, V., 2010. Therapeutic potential of mucoadhesive drug delivery systems – An updated patent review. Recent Patents Drug Deliv. Formul. 4, 256–265.
63. Naha, P., Bhattacharya, K., Tenuta, T., Dawson, K., Lynch, I., Gracia, A., Lyng, F., Byrne, H., 2010 Intracellular localisation, geno- and cytotoxic response of poly N-isopropylacrylamide (PNIPAM) nanoparticles to human keratinocyte (HaCaT) and colon cells (SW 480). Toxi. Lett. 198, 134–143.
64. Naik, S., Patel, D., Chuttani, K., Mishra, A.K., Misra, A., 2012. In vitro mechanistic study of cell death and in vivo performance evaluation of RGD grafted PEGgylated docetaxel liposomes in breast cancer. Nanomed.: Nanotechnol. 8, 951–962.
65. Nassier, O.A., 2010. Protein undernutrition in tumor-bearing mice, response and toxicity to paclitaxel. Int. J. Pharm. 6, 296–300.
66. Nava, G., Pinon, E., Mendoza, L., Mendoza, N., Quintanar, D., Ganem, A., 2011. Formulation and in vitro, ex vivo and in vivo evaluation of elastic liposomes for transdermal delivery of Ketorolac Tromethamine. Pharmaceutics. 3, 954–970.

67. Nepal, O., Rao, J.P., 2011. Haemolytic effects of hypo-osmotic salt solutions on human erythrocytes. Kathmandu. Univ. Med. J. 34, 35–39.

68. Paolino, D., Celia, C., Trapasso, E., Cilurzo, F., Fresta, M., 2012. Paclitaxel-loaded ethosomes: Potential treatment of squamous cell carcinoma, a malignant transformation of actinic keratoses. Eur. J. Pharm. Biopharm. 81, 102–112.

69. Park, J.H., Chi, S.C., Lee, W.S., Lee, W.M., Koo, Y.B., Yong, C.S., Choi, H.G., Woo, J.S., 2009. Toxicity studies of Cremophor-free paclitaxel solid dispersion formulated by a supercritical anti solvent process. Arch. Pharm. Res. 32, 139–148.

70. Ravichandiran, V., Masilamani, K., Senthilnathan, B., 2011. Liposome-A versatile drug delivery system. Der Pharmacia Sinica. 2, 19–30.

71. Shakeel, F., Ramadan, W., 2010. Transdermal delivery of anticancer drug caffeine from water-in-oil nanoemulsions. Colloids and Surfaces B: Biointerfaces. 75, 356–362.

72. Shaikh, R.P., Pillay, V., Choonara, Y.E., Toit, L.C., Ndesendo, V.M.K., Bawa, P., Cooppan, S., 2010. A review of multi-responsive membranous systems for rate-modulated drug delivery. AAPS Pharm. Sci. Tech. 2, 441–459.

73. Shapira, A., Livney, Y.D., Broxterman, H.J., Assaraf, Y.G., 2011. Nanomedicine for targeted cancer therapy: Towards the overcoming of drug resistsnce. Drug Resist. Updat. 14, 150–163.

74. Sheihet, L., Garbuzenko, O.B., Bushman, J., Gounder, M.K., Minko, T., Kohn, J., 2012. Paclitaxel in tyrosine-derived nanospheres as a potential anti-cancer agent: In vivo evaluation of toxicity and efficacy in comparison with paclitaxel in Cremophor. Eur. J. Pharm. Sci. 45, 320–329.

75. Stuart, M.A.C., Huck, W.T.S., Genzer, J., Muiller, M., Ober, C., Stamm, M., Sukhorukov, G.B., Szleifer, I., Tsukruk, V.V., Urban, M., Winnik, F., Zauscher, S., Luzinov, I., Minko, S., 2010. Emerging applications of stimuli-responsive polymer materials. Nat. Mater. 9(2), 101–113.

76. Su, M., Zhao, M., Luo, Y., Lin, X., Xu, L., He, H., Xu, H., Tang, X., 2011. Evaluation of the efficacy, toxicity and safety of vinorelbine incorporated in a lipid emulsion. Int. J. Pharm. 411, 188–196.

77. Teskac, K., Kristi, J., 2010. The evidence for solid lipid nanoparticles mediated cell uptake of Resveratrol. Int. J. Pharm. 390, 61–69.

78. Tsallas, A., Jackson, J., Burt, H., 2011. The uptake of paclitaxel and docetaxel into ex vivo porcine bladder tissue from polymeric micelle formulations. Cancer Chemother. Pharmacol. 68, 431–444.

79. Urbinati, G., Marsaud, V., Plassat, V., Fattal, E., Lesieur, S., Michel, J., 2010.Renoir liposomes loaded with histone deacetylase inhibitors for breast cancer therapy. Int. J. Pharm. 397, 184–193.

80. Utreja, P., Jain, S., Tiwary, A.K., 2011. Localized delivery of paclitaxel using elastic liposomes: Formulation development and evaluation. Drug Deliv. 18, 367–376.

81. Wang, C., Wang, Y.J., Fan, M., Luo, F., Qian, Z., 2011a. Characterization, pharmacokinetic and disposition of novel nanoscale preparations of paclitaxel. Int. J. Pharm. 414, 251–259.

82. Wang, S., Shanga, D., Lia, X., Jianga, T., 2009. Preparations and properties of hydroxycamptothecin emulsion and its tissue distribution in mice. Asian J. Pharm. Sci. 4, 299–307.

83. Wang, Y., Wu, K.C., Zhao, B.X., Zhao, X., Wang, X., Chen, S., Nie, S.F., Pan, W.F., Zhang, X., Zhang, Q., 2011b. Novel paclitaxel microemulsion containing a reduced amount of Cremophor EL: Pharmacokinetics, biodistribution, and in vivo antitumor efficacy and safety. J. Biomed. Biotechnol. 8, 352–360.

84. Wolinsky, J.B., Colson, Y.L., Grinstaff, M.W., 2012. Local drug delivery strategies for cancer treatment: Gels, nanoparticles, polymeric films, rods, and wafers. J. Control. Release. 159, 14–16.

85. Xiao, W., Luo, J Jain, T., Riggs, J.W., Teseng, H.P., Henderson, P.T., Cherry, S.R., Rowland, D., Lam, K.S., 2012. Biodistribution and pharmacokinetics of telodendrimer micellar paclitaxel nanoformulation in a mouse xenografts model of ovarian cancer. Int. J. Nanomedicine. 7, 1585–1597.

86. Yoshizawa, Y., Kono, Y., Ogawara, K.I., Kimura, T., Higaki, K., 2011. PEG liposomalization of paclitaxel improved its in vivo disposition and anti-tumor efficacy. Int. J. Pharm. 412, 132–141.

87. You, J., Almeda, D., Ye, G.J.C., Auguste, D.T., 2010. Bio responsive matrices in drug delivery. J. Biol. Eng. 4(15), 1–12.

88. Zaafarany, G.M., Awad, G.A., Holayel, S.M., Mortada, N.D., 2010. Role of edge activators and surface charge in developing ultradeformable vesicles with enhanced skin delivery. Int. J. Pharm. 397, 164–172.

89. Zhang, H., Wang, Z.Y., Gong, W., Li, Z.P., Mei, X.G., Lv, W.L., 2011. Development and characteristics of temperature-sensitive liposomes for vinorelbine bitartrate. Int. J. Pharm. 414, 56–62.

90. Zhao, Q.H., Zhang, Y., Liu, Y., Li, H., Shen, W.Y., Yang, W.J., Wen, L.P., 2010. Anticancer effect of realgar nanoparticles on mouse melanoma skin cancer in vivo via transdermal drug delivery. Med. Oncol. 27, 203–212.

17 Theranostic Nanocarriers for Cancer Applications

Pritish Kumar Panda, Amit Verma, Ankit Jain,
Sarjana Raikwar, and Sanjay K. Jain

17.1 INTRODUCTION

Theranostics is an important term in the diagnosis and treatment of any disease, including cancer [1]. Theranostic nanomedicine is used for cancer diagnosis, treatment, drug administration, and gene delivery. Understanding the molecular mechanisms, diagnostic techniques, therapeutic effectiveness, and toxicity connected with nanocarrier(s) is made possible by theranostics [2, 3]. Magnetic resonance imaging (MRI) is the most-used imaging method. It is used for early detection of cancers and also in cancer theranostics. Iron oxide, gold, silver, and other metal nanoparticles (NPs) are used in both cancer diagnosis and treatment. When contrasted to healthy tissues or cells, these NPs and MRI have been utilized to highlight sick tissues and cells. Theranostic research has been concentrated on this field because cancer is currently one of the most serious diseases [4, 5]. A cancer cell can affect any type of cell or tissue in the human body. It is caused by uncontrolled cell division, where normal cells accumulate with abnormal cells, forming a tumor that can be either benign or malignant [6]. Several factors are involved in cancer, such as unhealthy diet, genetic mutations, ultraviolet radiation (UV), drugs, occupational exposure, and consumption of tobacco and alcohol. There are various types of cancer, such as cancer of the colon, prostate, pancreas, lungs, brain, breast, and skin [7–9]. Today, cancer has become one of the leading causes of mortality worldwide despite advanced medical technologies. Currently, cancer treatment is limited to chemotherapy, surgery, and radiotherapy. However, all these treatment strategies are associated with the risk of affecting normal cells, which can cause undesirable effects. Therefore, new technology development is required for the secure and efficient treatment of cancer. A promising delivery system for the detection and treatment of cancer is nanoparticles containing therapeutic chemicals. Theranostic treatment for cancer mostly focuses on drug delivery and diagnosis. Theranostic systems, which are based on the use of many diagnostic and therapeutic mechanisms in a single moiety, are currently on the cusp of innovation [10].

An emerging field called nanotechnology may entail creating and using nanocarriers to improve the efficacy of current therapeutics [11]. These nanocarrier(s) are designed to deliver therapeutic agents to cancer cells. It may involve targeted drug delivery, stimuli-sensitive drug delivery, and controlled delivery of the drug. In cancer research, nanotechnology has wide potential to overcome the limitations associated with current chemotherapy. These nanocarrier(s) have unique characteristics such as small size (in nanometers), desirable drug release profile, and ability to recognize normal cells and cancer cells [12]. Thus, nanomedicine provides a great understanding of the development of nanocarriers varying in size to enhance the effectiveness of the entrapped drug and achieve safety via precise targeting of cancer cells [13]. Nanomedicines have also stimulated the creation of more sophisticated nanosystems, which can simultaneously assess therapy efficacy and provide anticancer medications with more specificity. They can be developed to a more advanced form with the applications of theranostic science in the treatment of cancer. Theranostic methods for the administration of anticancer drugs and diagnosis are covered in this chapter. It also covers theranostic nanocarriers used in the detection and treatment of cancer, including nanoparticles, liposomes, carbon nanotubes, nanofibers, nanoshells, dendrimers, and micelles. [14, 15]. Various

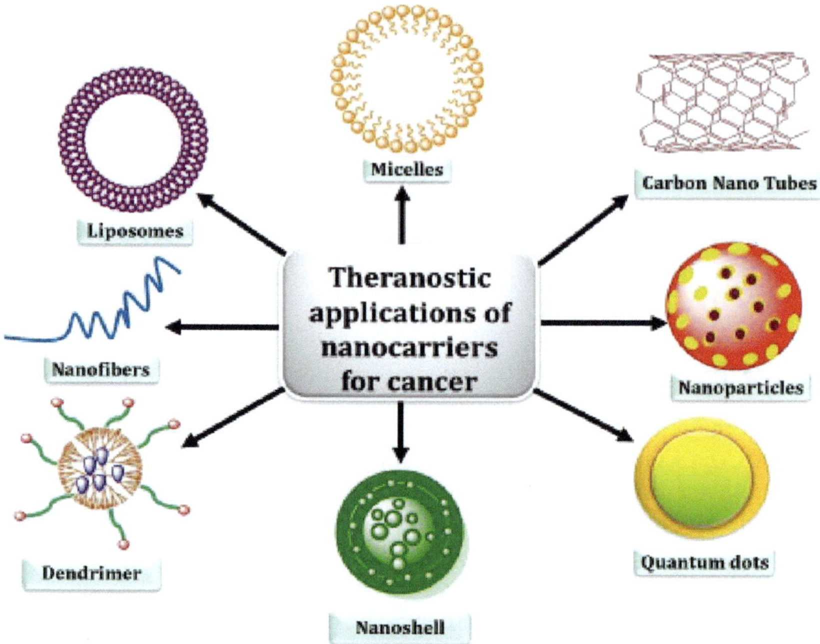

FIGURE 17.1 Various theranostic nanocarriers for cancer application.

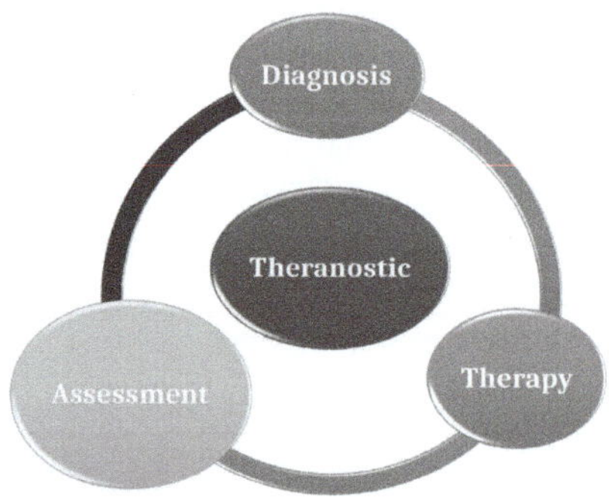

FIGURE 17.2 Action of theranostic agents.

theranostic nanocarriers for cancer application are depicted in Figure 17.1, and Figure 17.2 depicts the action of theranostic agents.

17.2 THERANOSTIC NANOCARRIERS FOR CANCER APPLICATIONS

Recently, nanocarriers have arisen to a great extent as one of the most important and promising implements for theranostic purposes. They have potential in a variety of areas, including imaging, diagnostics, and drug delivery, due to their inherent characteristics of being able to take an image of cancer cells/tissues, diagnose disease conditions, and/or detect cancer cells at an earlier stage. Moreover, nanocarriers can treat the diseases like cancer simultaneously. This method, also referred to as theranostic nanocarriers, is cleverly able to simultaneously identify and cure. These are distinctive in that they are easily biodegradable and compact, with a large surface area, and effectively functionalized by means of surface altering characteristics. They are quickly expanding as an intriguing and useful drug delivery technology for cancer treatment. Table 17.1 shows different theranostic nanocarriers utilized in cancer treatment delivery systems.

17.2.1 Nanoparticles in Cancer Theranostics

Theranostic nanoparticles can be developed in various ways. Most therapeutic substances, such as anticancer drugs, biomolecules, active chemicals in products, and photosensitizers, have been found to be conjugated to or loaded onto formerly existing imaging nanoparticles like gold nanocages, quantum dots, and iron oxide nanoparticles (IONPs). Additionally, they are formed by attaching a variety of radioisotopes, optical or magnetic nanoparticles, fluorescent dyes, and other imaging contrast agents to already-existing therapeutic nanoparticles [27]. Moreover, the encapsulation of both imaging and therapeutic agents is done together in a biocompatible nanocarrier (polymeric nanoparticles and porous silica nanoparticles). The surface of theranostic NPs is further changed using polyethylene glycol and other targeting ligands to give them an advanced form that is effective in targeting tumors [28]. These alterations help them improve blood circulation half-life and help in cancer therapy. Yang *et al.* developed multifunctional nanoparticles that illustrate theranostic applications. Because poly (aspartic acid) is biodegradable, it is used as a drug delivery vehicle. Iron oxide nanoparticles were produced using the thermal decomposition method. Then, using the emulsion process, they were loaded onto poly (aspartic acid) nanoparticles. The solvent diffusion approach was used to insert the anticancer drug doxorubicin (DOX) into the multifunctional nanoparticles. For imaging, IONPs were employed, and DOX was put to use as a cancer therapeutic. This has shown that DOX was released effectively from nanoparticles.

TABLE 17.1
Theranostic Nanocarriers for Cancer Drug Delivery

Type of Nanocarrier	Drugs/ Biomolecules	Theranostic Agent	Technique	Type of Cancer	References
Nanoparticles	Gemcitabine	Octabutoxyphthalocyanine palladium (II)	Photothermal	Pancreatic cancer	[16]
Gold nanoparticles	Paclitaxel	Rhodamine B-linked beta-cyclodextrin	Photothermal	Cancer	[17]
Nanoparticles	Paclitaxel	Glutathion	Chemo-photothermal/ photoacoustic	Cancer	[18]
Nanoparticles	Doxorubicin	Superparamagnetic iron oxide (SPIO)	Redox-responsive	Liver and other cancers	[19]
Nanoparticles	Doxorubicin	SPIO and Fe^{3+}	Photothermal	Liver cancer	[20]
Quantum-dot–based theranostic micelles	Amentoflavone	Indium phosphate/zinc sulfide	Photothermal	Breast cancer	[21]
Micelles	Paclitaxel	SPIO	Magnetic resonance imaging (MRI)	Breast and skin cancer	[22]
SPION	Doxorubicin	Iron oxide	MRI	Liver cancer	[23]
Liposomes	Sorafenib	Gadolinium	MRI	Liver cancer	[24]
Liposomes	Tirapazamine	Chlorin e6	Photodynamic therapy	Cancer	[25]
Liposomes	Doxorubicin	Gadolinium	Photothermal	Solid tumors	[26]

Additionally, IONPs conducted a magnetic resonance imaging study using a contrast agent to diagnose malignancy [29]. Xu *et al.* prepared nanocomposites with a block copolymer using DOX and IONPs. They demonstrated *in vitro* and *in vivo* imaging as well as drug delivery applications of prepared nanocomposites for cancer [30]. Yang *et al.* reported remarkable results in order to prepare theranostic agents and observed both *in vivo* and *in vitro* theranostic uses. They synthesized a nanocomposite using graphene oxide and iron oxide together for imaging as well as cancer-targeting drug delivery. A biocompatible polymer, like PEG, was used to produce the nanocomposites and functionalize them. It was done to reduce the toxicity raised by graphene oxide. It was able to create a photothermal study for the treatment of cancer, and the outcomes were successful for the efficient ablation of the tumor. Different doses were also prepared and tested to obtain no side effects using *in vivo* or *in vitro* toxicity study [31]. IONPs have received abundant attention from researchers as an important contrast agent due to their multidimensional action like superparamagnetic activity, biocompatibility, and very low cost. They are generally used in magnetite or hematite forms. To enable theranostic uses, they were surface modified and functionalized with various inorganic compounds, ligands, and polymeric and non-polymeric stabilizers. Magnetic NPs have also been used to deliver drugs to target different cancer cells using systemic injection so that a high magnetic field is created over the tumor. It enhances the accumulation of NPs by immobilizing the circulating particles for cargo release. SPIOs have been prepared for successful gene delivery to the Wistar rat gut. Labhasetwar *et al.* developed IONPs in which they loaded paclitaxel and doxorubicin for direct delivery to cancer cells, and the novel nanocarrier system showed concurrent MRI activity. A novel nanocarrier system was prepared for both diagnosis and therapeutic use in which DOX, an anthracycline derivative, was incorporated into INOPs to target lung cancer. Huh *et al.* developed IONPs coupled with trastuzumab, a monoclonal antibody that is known to interfere with cell membrane receptors and hence is used for both diagnosis and treatment of cancer [32]. They also reported the theranostic application of magnetic nanoparticles for both imaging and siRNA delivery. With the aid of a pH-labile hydrazone bond, SPIONs were formed by loading DOX. It assisted in overcoming tumors' *in vitro* multidrug resistance. The chemotherapeutics' effectiveness was also increased using PEG-coating [33]. In another study, PTX was shown to conjugate with IONPs and gold NPs and evaluated for *in vitro* study [34]. It revealed the dual docetaxel/SPION-loaded NPs for targeting prostate cancer cells and ultrasensitive MRI for theranostic uses [35]. However, many theranostic NPs consisting of IONPs and other magnetic NPs have new trends to offer multi-diagnostic opportunities. A theranostic nanocarrier system (FA-SPIONs) comprising an anti-cancer drug (DOX) for concurrent imaging (MR) and drug delivery into cancer cells is shown in Figure 17.3.

17.2.2 Quantum Dots in Cancer Theranostics

Nanocrystals called quantum dots (QDs) are fluorescent semiconductors used as nanocarriers for the targeting of many diseases like cancer. They have special characteristics like extraordinary brightness and photostability which make them more attractive for fluorescent labelling of biomolecules. They also have the ability to perform optical encoding of various cell membranes and tissues [36]. These have unique uses in areas like imaging and drug delivery. They are less useful in research because of their toxic behavior, but toxicity can be lessened by synthesizing QDs with silicon and carbon used for cancer therapeutics [37]. Gao *et al.* revealed the successful use of QD-based conjugates in mice cancer cells [38]. A novel QD conjugate was prepared combining the use of an aptamer and DOX for cancer targeting, imaging, and sensing. The main goal was to deliver DOX selectively to prostate cancer (PCa) cells [39]. Theranostic application of QDs is also investigated in PCa. In another study, an aptamer-based QD was prepared by conjugation with a specific DNA aptamer for the treatment of ovarian cancer.

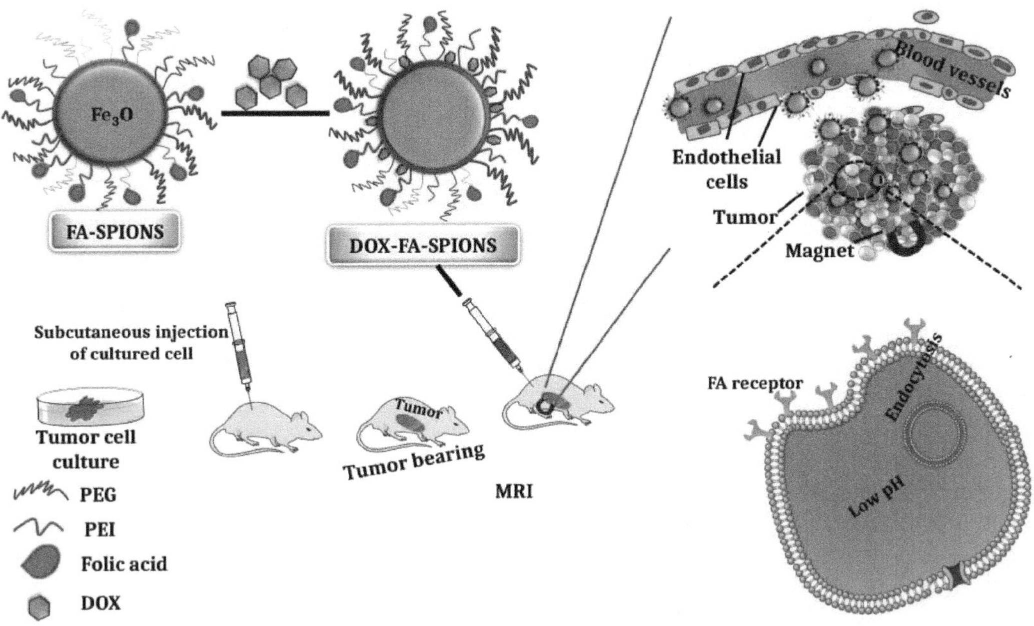

FIGURE 17.3 Theranostic nanocarrier system comprising DOX for concurrent imaging (MR) and drug delivery into cancer cells.

17.2.3 CARBON NANOTUBES IN CANCER THERANOSTICS

One of the newer nanocarrier systems being employed for theranostic purposes is carbon nanotubes (CNTs). These are allotropes of carbon. CNTs are single- or multi-layered cylindrical structures. They have inherent mechanical as well as electronic properties valuable in the field of nanotechnology. Recently, CNTs have been widely used for imaging and drug delivery. It has been noticed that the uptake of CNTs is increased by cells; nonetheless, the precise mechanism is still unknown. This increases the demand for CNTs. They are also used in drug delivery applications due to the efficient loading of active agents/biomolecules [40]. Due to their enormous surface area, CNTs have many advantages over current delivery vectors. This is because they allow for numerous drug attachment sites. CNTs have been functionalized by conjugating with several anticancer agents like doxorubicin, paclitaxel, cisplatin, methotrexate, and quercetin and were found effective in *in vivo* and *in vitro* testing [41]. Pal *et al.* developed CNTs coated with zirconium oxide that provide efficient loading of active materials and these nanoparticles demonstrated photothermal ablation therapy because of significant near-infrared optical absorption [42]. Sitharaman *et al.* synthesized CNTs coupled with paramagnetic gadolinium nanoparticles to offer high-performance MRI. They were prepared by an electric arc discharge process using Y/Ni as catalyst and then underwent pyrolysis at 1000°C, followed by fluorination in an inert environment. The CNTs were then loaded with gadolinium by soaking and sonicating using high performance liquid chromatography (HPLC)-grade DI water containing aqueous $GdCl_3$ [43].

17.2.4 LIPOSOMES FOR CANCER THERANOSTICS

Liposomes are important and successful nanocarrier systems for drug delivery that contain lipid bilayers enclosing an aqueous core. These are spherical vesicles. They can be used as a developing nanocarrier system for theranostic applications and can contain a variety of diagnostic and therapeutic chemicals. They have a special structure that allows them to trap hydrophobic substances inside the lipid bilayers [44]. Furthermore, they also encapsulate hydrophilic agents in the center of the aqueous compartment, which supports agents that do not degrade. Good biocompatibility, excellent agent-loading efficiency, stability in biological settings, and predictable release kinetics are liposomes' distinctive traits. Additionally, in clinical tests, they offer better pharmacokinetics and bio-distribution of theranostic drugs than other nanocarriers [45].

Theranostic liposomes are intended to expedite simultaneous diagnosis as well as being a treatment approach for cancer therapy [46]. Various nanosized imaging agents like gold NPs, INOPs, and QDTs should be bound covalently to the surface of theranostic liposomes or trapped within the hydrophobic core for the purpose of diagnosis. Additionally, anti-cancer medicines may be either embedded in the lipophilic bilayers or encapsulated in the core. These kinds of nanocarriers are called liposome-nanoparticle hybrids [47]. These kinds of theranostic liposomes can further be modified by conjugation with a molecular probe for effective targeting to cancer cells. These nanosized theranostic liposomes have additional advantages and can circulate for prolonged periods in the systemic circulation. These are also able to evade host defenses and target the tumor site for successful drug release and enabling *in vivo* or *in vitro* imaging concurrently [48]. These types of liposomes were developed by Yang *et al.* by loading of QDTs and targeting folate receptors and intended for cellular imaging for cancer theranostic applications [49]. In another study, liposomal formulations were prepared by loading with QDTs and the drug apomorphine for brain targeting [50]. Lu and his team prepared a liposomal formulation using phosphatidylethanolamine (PE) lipids as one of the lipid components and tried to bind it firmly with Hg^{2+} ions. The liposomal formulation was transformed into a theranostic nanocarrier system using a Hg^{2+} chelator, meso-2,3-dimercaptosuccinic acid (meso-DMSA), and a fluorescent dye [51]. Ostrowski and coworkers developed a phosphocholine-based liposomal system comprising a photochemical nitric oxide (NO) donor, mac-CrONO. As the mac-CrONO complex is fluorescent, it helps in imaging and makes the liposomes theranostic [52]. It has been investigated for the simultaneous incorporation of both the drugs and imaging agents into liposomes for cancer therapy. Another multifunctional liposomal system was investigated by Li *et al.*, in which liposomes were prepared using distearoyl phosphatidylcholine (DSPC) and loaded with DOX. Additionally, the liposome was coupled with radioactive ions like (99mTc) or (64Cu) for single-photon emission computed tomography imaging (SPECT) or position emission tomography (PET), as well as a near-infrared fluorescent dye (IR dye) and an MRI contrast agent (Gd-DOTA). Then, the formulations were tested in a mouse xenograft model of head and neck cancer. The result displayed effective theranostic use in cancer therapy [53].

17.2.5 Nanofibers for Cancer Theranostics

Recently, nanofibers/electrospun nanofibers are more in demand due to their exceptional features such as good flexibility, high drug loading capacity, high surface to volume area, and ease of production and operation. They are widely used in tissue engineering as well as in drug delivery approaches. Many studies have been done regarding the theranostic use of nanofibers for cancer. Nanofibers have the ability to contain different anticancer agents and target cancer cells. Surprisingly, it has been shown that these nanocarriers are found to deliver different combinations of drugs along with contrast agents to provide theranostic uses for cancer [54, 55]. Badrinath *et al.* prepared a CVV-PLGA nanofiber for theranostic use in cancer. PLGA, also known as poly (lactic-co-glycolic acid), is a biodegradable polymer that is used to create nanocarriers such as nanoparticles and nanofibers. CVV is a cancer-promoting oncolytic vaccinia virus (CVV). In this study, a PLGA nanofiber membrane with CVV implanted on it was used for theranostic applications. Further, it was assembled with a green fluorescent protein (GFP) to offer dual purposes of precise targeting as well as early imaging [56]. Darwesh *et al.* prepared nanofibers by the coaxial electrospinning method. They used Eudragit S100 (ES 100), gadodiamide (GDD), polyvinylpyrrolidone K90 (PVP K90), and hydroxypropyl-beta-cyclodextrin (HP-β-CyD) for the preparation of nanofibers. GDD is an MRI contrast agent. Coaxial nanofibers containing PVP K90, HP-CyD, and ES 100 as the shell and GDD as the core were stable. This could be used to make a dosage form which is proficient for the oral imaging of intestine and theranostic potential [57].

17.2.6 Nanoshells for Cancer Theranostics

A form of spherical nanoparticle known as a nanoshell (NSs) or nanoshell plasmon is made up of a metallic shell-like layer of gold over a dielectric core. It contains a plasmon, a quasiparticle capable of either the quantum plasma oscillation or the collective excitation. Due to this phenomenon, the electrons oscillate simultaneously among all the ions [58]. Gold nanoshells (AuNSs) displayed tunable surface plasmon resonance. Due to this inherent feature, they can be used to tune the near-infrared region for tissue penetration purposes. Using AuNSs and a laser, this very effective light-to-heat conversion causes thermal injury to cancer cells. Additionally, AuNSs function as a versatile nanocarrier system for the delivery of both therapeutic and diagnostic substances [59]. Yin *et al.* prepared AuNSs for theranostic purposes for cancer. They put together IONPs (inner cores) modified by polyethyleneimine (PEI) and used epigallocatechin gallate (EGCG) as a reducing agent to make NSs. The prepared nanocarrier system was further modified with PEG. A large amount of bio-stability, rapid cellular uptake, and outstanding *in vitro* and *in vivo* anti-tumor effectiveness have all been demonstrated by this highly integrated nanocarrier system. Additionally, the prepared AuNSs can be utilized as an MRI and X-ray imaging agent [60].

17.2.7 Dendrimers for Cancer Theranostics

A dendrimer is a structural macromolecule that has a low-density interior created by repeating branching units in the middle of the molecule. Additionally, it has a high-density exterior with surface functional groups. These are symmetrically shaped nanosized nanocarriers and can be reproduced on a large scale. Due to these inherent qualities, dendrimers are in high demand for drug delivery and other biomedical applications. Also, dendrimers have potential theranostic use for cancer therapy [61]. Mrówczyński and co-workers synthesized a multifunctional nanocarrier system based on generation (G) 4.0, 5.0, and 6.0 polyamidoamine (PAMAM) dendrimers. They were then added to magnetite nanoparticles (Fe_3O_4) coated in polydopamine (PDA). These dendrimers were used to treat liver cancer cells using a combination of chemo and photothermal therapy [62]. Siegwart and co-workers prepared a novel theranostic dendrimer (DLNPs) based on a lipid nanoparticle (LNP) system composed of PEGylated BODIPY dyes (PBD) for both *in vitro* and *in vivo* near-infrared (NIR) imaging as well as mRNA administration. To improve mRNA distribution, a pH-responsive PBD-lipid was used in the formulation. It showed greater potency *in vivo* even at a low dose. Moreover, it also illuminated tumors using pH-responsive NIR imaging. This novel theranostic dendrimer system is promising to simultaneously detect and treat cancer [63]. Also, a new phosphorus dendrimer/Cu(II) complex was investigated for nano-theranostic purposes using ultrasound-enhanced MR imaging-guided cancer therapy [64].

17.2.8 Micelles for Cancer Theranostics

Amphiphilic block copolymers work to create the core-shell structures known as polymeric micelles. Several block copolymers such as poly(L-amino acids), poly(esters), and poly(propylene oxides) are used for the development of micelles. In comparison to other nanocarriers, these nanocarriers are smaller (10–100 nm), which is suitable for efficient extravasation into cancer cells. These micelles are applicable for poorly soluble drugs and enhance the drug entrapment and targetability of cancer cells. They are used as solubilizing agents, leading to improve solubility and reduced toxicity associated with anticancer drugs like paclitaxel and doxorubicin [65]. Elzoghby and co-workers developed zein-chondroitin sulfate (ChS) micelles for theranostic use in cancer. The goal of this work was to combine celastrol's (CST) ability to inhibit NF-B with sulfasalazine's (SFZ) ability to inhibit glutathione, which inhibits CST inactivation and enhances CST's anti-tumor actions. The CD44-receptor-mediated uptake of developed micelles was observed in cancer cells. These micelles combine hydrophilic ChS with hydrophobic SFZ to form a micellar system. Furthermore, physical incorporation of oleic acid-capped SPIONs into the hydrophobic core of micelles promoted MRI along with magnetic tumor targeting. In MCF-7 and MDA-MB-231 breast cancer cells, increased cellular internalization of micelles was attained when magnetic targeting was combined with the active targeting activities of ChS. They concluded that the developed magnetically targeted micelles have promising potential in cancer theranostics [66].

17.3 CONCLUSION AND FUTURE PERSPECTIVES

In this chapter, a few theranostic nanocarriers that were looked into for cancer applications have been mentioned. These nanocarriers can possess many inherent theranostic properties that can be used for cancer treatment. Some nanocarriers could be loaded with advanced imaging/contrast agents with appropriate therapeutics for cancer theranostic applications. Although research on the use of nanocarriers for the effective treatment and diagnosis of the cancer is fast progressing, so far, no theranostic nanocarriers have been developed to meet the clinical standards. The theranostic nanocarriers so far developed are having promise and advantages and disadvantages. The cost of gold nanoparticles, intrinsically low sensitivity of IONPs as MRI contrast probes, toxicity of QDs, and non-biodegradability of CNTs are the main limitations that need to be solved. Each of these issues is being worked on, and future studies should continue to concentrate on them. Additionally, as drug carriers, site or specifictargeting is a subject that is never sufficiently discussed. Despite the promise, the related pieces of evidence are so far insufficient and require more focus for subsequent research.

REFERENCES

1. Ahmed, N., H. Fessi, and A. Elaissari, Theranostic applications of nanoparticles in cancer. *Drug Discovery Today*, 2012. **17**(17–18): p. 928–934.
2. Sumer, B. and J. Gao, Theranostic nanomedicine for cancer. *Nanomedicine*, 2008. **3**(2): p. 137–140.
3. Jain, A., et al., Nanocarrier based advances in drug delivery to tumor: an overview. *Current Drug Targets*, 2018. **19**(13): p. 1498–1518.
4. Souza, K., et al., Mesoporous silica–magnetite nanocomposite synthesized by using a neutral surfactant. *Nanotechnology*, 2008. **19**(18): p. 185603.
5. Saraf, S., et al., Targeting approaches for the diagnosis and treatment of cancer. *Frontiers in Anti-Cancer Drug Discovery*, 2020. **11**: p. 105.
6. Aljabali, A.A.A., et al., Albumin nano-encapsulation of piceatannol enhances its anticancer potential in colon cancer via downregulation of nuclear p65 and HIF-1α. *Cancers*, 2020. **12**(1): p. 113.
7. Tiwari, A., et al., Novel targeting approaches and signaling pathways of colorectal cancer: an insight. *World Journal of Gastroenterology*, 2018. **24**(39): p. 4428.
8. Panda, P.K., et al., Novel strategies for targeting prostate cancer. *Current Drug Delivery*, 2019. **16**(8): p. 712–727.
9. Subudhi, M.B., et al., Eudragit S100 coated citrus pectin nanoparticles for colon targeting of 5-fluorouracil. *Materials (Basel)*, 2015. **8**(3): p. 832–849.
10. Tran, S., et al., Cancer nanomedicine: a review of recent success in drug delivery. *Clinical and Translational Medicine*, 2017. **6**(1): p. 44.
11. Chellappan, D.K., et al., Targeting neutrophils using novel drug delivery systems in chronic respiratory diseases. *Drug Development Research*, 2020. **81**(4): p. 419–436.
12. Wang, J., et al., Precise design of nanomedicines: perspectives for cancer treatment. *National Science Review*, 2019. **6**(6): p. 1107–1110.
13. Arruebo, M., et al., Assessment of the evolution of cancer treatment therapies. *Cancers*, 2011. **3**(3): p. 3279–3330.

14. Jain, A. and S.K. Jain, Advances in tumor targeted liposomes. *Current Molecular Medicine*, 2018. **18**(1): p. 44–57.

15. Dangi, R., et al., Targeting liver cancer via ASGP receptor using 5-FU-loaded surface-modified PLGA nanoparticles. *Journal of Microencapsulation*, 2014. **31**(5): p. 479–487.

16. Wang, Q., et al., Theranostic nanoparticles enabling the release of phosphorylated gemcitabine for advanced pancreatic cancer therapy. *Journal of Materials Chemistry B*, 2020. **8**(12): p. 2410–2417.

17. Heo, D.N., et al., Gold nanoparticles surface-functionalized with paclitaxel drug and biotin receptor as theranostic agents for cancer therapy. *Biomaterials*, 2012. **33**(3): p. 856–866.

18. Li, Y., et al., A simple glutathione-responsive turn-on theranostic nanoparticle for dual-modal imaging and chemo-photothermal combination therapy. *Nano Letters*, 2019. **19**(8): p. 5806–5817.

19. Yang, H., et al., Redox-responsive nanoparticles from disulfide bond-linked poly-(N-ε-carbobenzyloxy-l-lysine)-grafted hyaluronan copolymers as theranostic nanoparticles for tumor-targeted MRI and chemotherapy. *International Journal of Biological Macromolecules*, 2020. **148**: p. 483–492.

20. Shu, G., et al., Sialic acid-engineered mesoporous polydopamine nanoparticles loaded with SPIO and Fe3+ as a novel theranostic agent for T1/T2 dual-mode MRI-guided combined chemo-photothermal treatment of hepatic cancer. *Bioactive Materials*, 2020. **6**(5): p. 1423–1435.

21. Wang, Y., et al., Quantum-dot-based theranostic micelles conjugated with an anti-EGFR nanobody for triple-negative breast cancer therapy. *ACS Applied Materials & Interfaces*, 2017. **9**(36): p. 30297–30305.

22. Upponi, J.R., et al., Polymeric micelles: theranostic co-delivery system for poorly water-soluble drugs and contrast agents. *Biomaterials*, 2018. **170**: p. 26–36.

23. Mouli, S.K., et al., Image-guided local delivery strategies enhance therapeutic nanoparticle uptake in solid tumors. *ACS Nano*, 2013. **7**(9): p. 7724–7733.

24. Xiao, Y., et al., Sorafenib and gadolinium co-loaded liposomes for drug delivery and MRI-guided HCC treatment. *Colloids and Surfaces B: Biointerfaces*, 2016. **141**: p. 83–92.

25. Zhang, K., et al., Light-triggered theranostic liposomes for tumor diagnosis and combined photodynamic and hypoxia-activated prodrug therapy. *Biomaterials*, 2018. **185**: p. 301–309.

26. Pitchaimani, A., et al., Design and characterization of gadolinium infused theranostic liposomes. *RSC Advances*, 2016. **6**(43): p. 36898–36905.

27. Xie, J., S. Lee, and X. Chen, Nanoparticle-based theranostic agents. *Advanced Drug Delivery Reviews*, 2010. **62**(11): p. 1064–1079.

28. Panda, P.K. and S.K. Jain, Doxorubicin bearing peptide anchored PEGylated PLGA nanoparticles for the effective delivery to prostate cancer cells. *Journal of Drug Delivery Science Technology*, 2023: p. 104667.

29. Yang, H.-M., et al., Multifunctional poly (aspartic acid) nanoparticles containing iron oxide nanocrystals and doxorubicin for simultaneous cancer diagnosis and therapy. *Colloids and Surfaces A: Physicochemical and Engineering Aspects*, 2011. **391**(1–3): p. 208–215.

30. Xu, H., et al., Polymer encapsulated upconversion nanoparticle/iron oxide nanocomposites for multimodal imaging and magnetic targeted drug delivery. *Biomaterials*, 2011. **32**(35): p. 9364–9373.

31. Yang, K., et al., Multimodal imaging guided photothermal therapy using functionalized graphene nanosheets anchored with magnetic nanoparticles. *Advanced Materials*, 2012. **24**(14): p. 1868–1872.

32. Huh, Y.-M., et al., In vivo magnetic resonance detection of cancer by using multifunctional magnetic nanocrystals. *Journal of the American Chemical Society*, 2005. **127**(35): p. 12387–12391.

33. Kievit, F.M., et al., Doxorubicin loaded iron oxide nanoparticles overcome multidrug resistance in cancer in vitro. *Journal of Controlled Release*, 2011. **152**(1): p. 76–83.

34. Hwu, J.R., et al., Targeted paclitaxel by conjugation to iron oxide and gold nanoparticles. *Journal of the American Chemical Society*, 2009. **131**(1): p. 66–68.

35. Ling, Y., et al., Dual docetaxel/superparamagnetic iron oxide loaded nanoparticles for both targeting magnetic resonance imaging and cancer therapy. *Biomaterials*, 2011. **32**(29): p. 7139–7150.

36. Ma, Y., et al., Quantum dots (QDs) for tumor targeting theranostics, in *Nanomaterials for Tumor Targeting Theranostics: A Proactive Clinical Perspective*. 2016, World Scientific. p. 85–141.

37. Tade, R.S. and P.O. Patil, Theranostic prospects of graphene quantum dots in breast cancer. *ACS Biomaterials Science & Engineering*, 2020. **6**(11): p. 5987–6008.

38. Gao, X., et al., In vivo cancer targeting and imaging with semiconductor quantum dots. *Nature Biotechnology*, 2004. **22**(8): p. 969–976.

39. Bagalkot, V., et al., Quantum dot– aptamer conjugates for synchronous cancer imaging, therapy, and sensing of drug delivery based on bi-fluorescence resonance energy transfer. *Nano Letters*, 2007. **7**(10): p. 3065–3070.

40. Ji, S.-R., et al., Carbon nanotubes in cancer diagnosis and therapy. *Biochimica et Biophysica Acta (BBA)-Reviews on Cancer*, 2010. **1806**(1): p. 29–35.

41. He, H., et al., Carbon nanotubes: applications in pharmacy and medicine. *BioMed Research International*, 2013. **2013**.

42. Pal, K., D.J. Kang, and J.K. Kim, Microstructural investigations of zirconium oxide—on core–shell structure of carbon nanotubes. *Journal of Nanoparticle Research*, 2011. **13**(6): p. 2597–2607.

43. Sitharaman, B., et al., Superparamagnetic gadonanotubes are high-performance MRI contrast agents. *Chemical Communications*, 2005. (31): p. 3915–3917.

44. Verma, A., et al., Folate conjugated double liposomes bearing prednisolone and methotrexate for targeting rheumatoid arthritis. *Pharmaceutical Research*, 2019. **36**(8): p. 123.

45. Verma, A., et al., Systematic optimization of cationic surface engineered mucoadhesive vesicles employing design of experiment (DoE): a preclinical investigation. *International Journal of Biological Macromolecules*, 2019. **133**: p. 1142–1155.

46. Choi, K.Y., et al., Theranostic nanoplatforms for simultaneous cancer imaging and therapy: current approaches and future perspectives. *Nanoscale*, 2012. **4**(2): p. 330–342.

47. Jain, A. and S.K. Jain, Stimuli-responsive smart liposomes in cancer targeting. *Current Drug Targets*, 2018. **19**(3): p. 259–270.

48. Al-Jamal, W.T. and K. Kostarelos, Liposomes: from a clinically established drug delivery system to a nanoparticle platform for theranostic nanomedicine. *Accounts of Chemical Research*, 2011. **44**(10): p. 1094–1104.

49. Yang, C., et al., Folate receptor–targeted quantum dot liposomes as fluorescence probes. *Journal of Drug Targeting*, 2009. **17**(7): p. 502–511.

50. Wen, C.-J., et al., Theranostic liposomes loaded with quantum dots and apomorphine for brain targeting and bioimaging. *International Journal of Nanomedicine*, 2012. **7**: p. 1599.

51. Yigit, M.V., et al., Inorganic mercury detection and controlled release of chelating agents from ion-responsive liposomes. *Chemistry & Biology*, 2009. **16**(9): p. 937–942.

52. Ostrowski, A.D., et al., Liposome encapsulation of a photochemical NO precursor for controlled nitric oxide release and simultaneous fluorescence imaging. *Molecular Pharmaceutics*, 2012. **9**(10): p. 2950–2955.

53. Li, S., et al., Novel multifunctional theranostic liposome drug delivery system: construction, characterization, and multimodality MR, near-infrared fluorescent, and nuclear imaging. *Bioconjugate Chemistry*, 2012. **23**(6): p. 1322–1332.

54. Doostmohammadi, M., H. Forootanfar, and S. Ramakrishna, New strategies for safe cancer therapy using electrospun nanofibers: a short review. *Mini Reviews in Medicinal Chemistry*, 2020. **20**(13): p. 1272–1286.

55. Purohit, A. and P.K. Panda, Thread of hope: weaving a comprehensive review on electrospun nanofibers for cancer therapy. *Journal of Drug Delivery Science and Technology*, 2023. **89**: p. 105100.

56. Badrinath, N., et al., Local delivery of a cancer-favoring oncolytic vaccinia virus via poly (lactic-co-glycolic acid) nanofiber for theranostic purposes. *International Journal of Pharmaceutics*, 2018. **552**(1–2): p. 437–442.

57. Darwesh, A.Y., M.S. El-Dahhan, and M.M. Meshali, New oral coaxial nanofibers for gadodiamide-prospective intestinal magnetic resonance imaging and theranostic. *International Journal of Nanomedicine*, 2020. **15**: p. 8933.

58. Loo, C., et al., Nanoshell-enabled photonics-based imaging and therapy of cancer. *Technology in Cancer Research & Treatment*, 2004. **3**(1): p. 33–40.

59. Zhao, J., M. Wallace, and M.P. Melancon, Cancer theranostics with gold nanoshells. *Nanomedicine*, 2014. **9**(13): p. 2041–2057.

60. Yin, Y., et al., Epigallocatechin gallate based magnetic gold nanoshells nanoplatform for cancer theranostic applications. *Journal of Materials Chemistry B*, 2017. **5**(3): p. 454–463.

61. Sk, U.H. and C. Kojima, Dendrimers for theranostic applications. *Biomolecular Concepts*, 2015. **6**(3): p. 205–217.

62. Jędrzak, A., et al., Dendrimer based theranostic nanostructures for combined chemo-and photothermal therapy of liver cancer cells in vitro. *Colloids and Surfaces B: Biointerfaces*, 2019. **173**: p. 698–708.

63. Xiong, H., et al., Theranostic dendrimer-based lipid nanoparticles containing PEGylated BODIPY dyes for tumor imaging and systemic mRNA delivery in vivo. *Journal of Controlled Release*, 2020. **325**: p. 198–205.

64. Fan, Y., et al., Phosphorus dendrimer-based copper (II) complexes enable ultrasound-enhanced tumor theranostics. *Nano Today*, 2020. **33**: p. 100899.

65. Verma, A., et al., Liposomes for advanced drug delivery, in *Advanced Biopolymeric Systems for Drug Delivery*. 2020, Springer. p. 317–338.

66. Elhasany, K.A., et al., Combination of magnetic targeting with synergistic inhibition of NF-κB and glutathione via micellar drug nanomedicine enhances its anti-tumor efficacy. *European Journal of Pharmaceutics and Biopharmaceutics*, 2020. **155**: p. 162–176.

18 Nanoparticulate Vaccines
Mechanistic Insight and Recent Advances

Kantrol Kumar Sahu, Krishna Yadav, Monika Kaurav, Madhulika Pradhan, and Sunita Minz

18.1 INTRODUCTION

As a complex biological network, our immune system plays a significant role in almost all disease pathogenesis. The advent of nanotechnology facilitates disease prevention and therapeutic measures based on the development of multifunctional nanoparticles [1, 2]. These nanoparticles attack dendritic cells (DCs) and exert strong immunotherapeutic effects in infectious diseases, including cancer [3]. Various types of nanoparticles (NPs) have been developed and designed for such delivery systems. These NPs, depending on their size (1–1000 nm), constitute a heterogeneous category and include lipid nanoparticles (LNPs), liposomes, virus-like particles (VLPs), and cationic polymers [4]. A simple production process and high immunogenicity are the two main factors for which NPs have become attractive for the delivery of antigens and adjuvants.

The vaccine against the hepatitis B virus (HBV) was the first nanoparticulate vaccine (1981) licensed for human use, and it is a virus-like particle (VLP)–based vaccine [5]. Currently, researchers all over the world are making great efforts to modulate and understand the immunity raised by NPs.

However, vaccine design is not an easy task; several studies are involved regarding the discovery of safe, economic, and effective vaccine systems [6]. The perfect blend of polymers along with loading of suitable antigens and adjuvants was a first step towards production of antigen-loaded polymeric nanoparticles. This new era of vaccination also includes phospholipid bilayer formulations such as liposomes to encapsulate or conjugate antigens. Nanovaccine design also includes gold-like inorganic materials [7]. These NPs contain both antigen and adjuvant and are capable of enhancing both arms (innate and adaptive) of the immune system [8].

This chapter deals with various types and preparation methods of nanoparticulate vaccines. The uptake, processing, and immunology behind them, along with recent advances, are also discussed in this chapter.

18.2 VARIOUS FORMS AND THEIR PREPARATION METHODS

18.2.1 VIRUS-LIKE PARTICLES

Virus-like particles are the most attractive and interesting of all the NP delivery systems studied due to their ease of production and ability to produce firm immune responses. VLPs usually have a size of 20–150 nm and are made from a single protein to construct a multimeric complex with a strong epitope density [9–11]. VLPs integrate without capturing any viral RNA; therefore, unlike viruses, they do not replicate and infect. In order to avoid the addition of the enfolded genome into the host cell and/or to prevent recombination with live or altered viruses in infected humans, viral integrase coding genes are often eliminated prior to transmission.

DOI: 10.1201/9781003130055-18

VLPs may be fabricated either by fusing the particles with proteins or by introducing several antigens to express additional proteins. VLPs that offer safeguards against the original virus as well as against heterologous antigens can be generated using that approach. In addition, the viral surface can be chemically bound to the VLP's biocouple with non-protein antigens such as small organic molecules or polysaccharides [12, 13]. The system of expression of the baculovirus has a good safety profile and is most widely used for generating VLPs because baculoviruses do not naturally infect people. The most widely researched VLP portion is the *Autographa california* multiple nuclear polyhedrosis virus (ACMNPV) [14].

The development of "humanized" cell cultures has been a significant approach for the synthesis of galactosylated glycoprotein and sialylated glycoproteins, those regulated and expressed by β-1, 4-galactosyltransferase, and α-2,6-sialyltransferase [15–17]. The subsequent cell degradation and insect cell lysis within a few days of baculovirus infection is another concern associated with the baculovirus expression mechanism. This can be troublesome for proteins that are chosen for isolation or vulnerable to deterioration. Subsequent struggles to alleviate that major issue have been made in the form of random mutagenesis and non-lytic baculoviruses, with the effect that cell lysis has fallen by almost ten times, and the degradation of the expressed protein is reduced.

18.2.2 Liposomes

Liposomes are self-assembled as VLPs, but they constitute a bilayer phospholipid membrane and aqueous core. They can be formed as a single bilayer phospholipid or multilamellar vesicle comprising many concentric phospholipid membranes stratified by aqueous layers and as a mono-laminate vesicle [18, 19]. This enables liposomes to incorporate hydrophilic substances into the aqueous center or/and hydrophobic substances into the phospholipid bilayer. Many published methodologies for the preparation of liposomes are beyond the scope of this observation. However, all of these usually exhibit reverse-phase evaporation mechanism by solubilizing phospholipids such as phosphatidylcholine and monophosphoryl lipid A in organic solvents (such as chloroform, methanol) and subsequent evaporation of the solvent followed by the addition of antigen and aqueous phases, leading to the formation of large unilamellar vesicles [18, 20]. Conversely, a high energy input which including sonication or high-pressure nitrogen gas may develop liposomes in water. This initially creates large vesicles, but a continuous energy input provides relatively small unilamellar vesicles. Lipid dissolution in a surfactant that contains a high amount of critical micelle concentrations such as octyl glucoside is a different technique for the preparation and is utilized for unilamellar vesicles with high-energy antigens, which can often be destructive. The solution is further dialyzed against the antigen buffer, which causes liposome development. Cholesterol can be (and sometimes is) applied to the lipid bilayer in one of these systems to ensure structural support. Other techniques for liposome encapsulation include a pH gradient, freeze-thaw cycles, or an antigen encapsulation process using ammonium sulfate at concentrations of 25–72% [18–20].

18.2.3 Immune-Stimulating Complexes

Immune-stimulating complexes (ISCOMs) are colloidal saponin micelles of ~45 nm, and self-adjuvanted conveyance structures for immunizations and are prevalently perceived as ISCOMs. There are two main kinds of ISCOMs, phospholipid (PL), most commonly phosphatidylethanolamine or phosphatidylcholine, and cholesterol (Chl) and saponin (Sap) [21, 22]. Proteins from microscopic organisms and parasites, which incorporate *E. coli*, *Brucella aborus*, and *P. falciparum*, are presently being utilized to develop ISCOMs. Virus without protein structures is also frequently utilized and is insinuated as ISCOM grids. ISCOMs self-amass at an ideal ratio (PL: Chl: Sap::1:1:5) for fabrication of ISCOMs under the influence of a non-ionic surfactant, which would then be able to be dissolve out [21–23].

18.2.4 Polymeric Nanoparticles

Polymeric nanoparticles have been extremely effective for their relevance to conveyance of therapeutics and their biodegradability. Furthermore, compositional alterations to the copolymer likewise offer controlled discharge of drugs from polymeric NPs. NPs can be fabricated with different polymers, such as poly(lactic acid)(PLA), poly(amino acids), poly(ɯ-hydroxy acids) or polysaccharides, poly(5-α-hydroxy-acids) and poly(lactic-co-glycolic acid)(PLGA). These polymers can hold as well as display antigens. These polymers are regularly utilized for production of nanoparticles through double emulsion technique followed by solvent evaporation. First, a synthetic polymer is solubilized with solvents like methylene chloride, ethyl acetic acid derivatives, and methyl acetate, and then the antigen is accumulated by vortexing to make the primary emulsion. Further, a W/O/W emulsion would form with the addition of an emulsifier (for example, polyvinyl pyrrolidine or polyvinyl alcohol). This brings about the precipitation of the polymer on the antigen. The solution is then evaporated and dried to prevent erosion of the polymer by water-catalyzed ester hydrolysis [21].

Usually, saline solution containing antigen is added to the selected polymer which is previously dissolved in DMSO. The mixture is then centrifuged to cast protein-loaded polymer NPs. The resultant embodiment in general has efficiency of between 30 and 60% and is consistent over in an acidic pH range [22]. Hydrophilic polysaccharide polymeric materials likewise may convey both dextran and chitosan based vaccines through the NPs. Much intrigue has been paid to chitosan NPs because of the biocompatibility, biodegradability, and its capacity to open adamant convergences between epithelial cells [23].

18.3 UPTAKE, *IMMUNE MODULATION AND FACTORS AFFECTING*

Vaccination is one of the most well-known traditional methods for disease prevention by training the body against specific antigens found on it [24]. Development of antigen containing NPs has attracted interest in treatment and prevention of various diseases including cancer. Nanoparticulate vaccines have ability to affect the function of immune cells (innate and adaptive) that results in induction, amplification, attenuation and prevention of immune response (**Figure 18.1**).

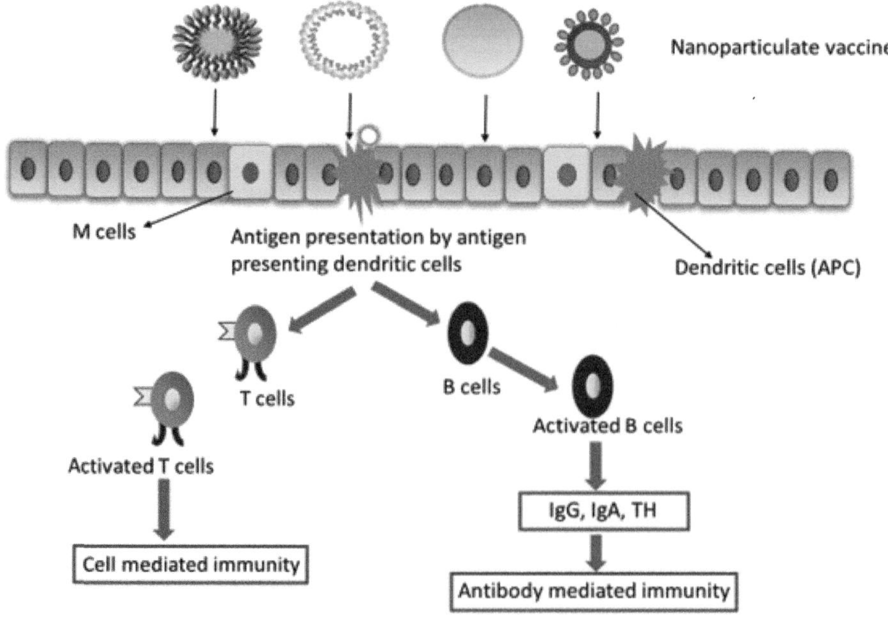

FIGURE 18.1 Mechanism of immunity induction by nanoparticulate vaccine.

This is called immune modulation by NPs which is useful in achieving therapeutic goals [25]. Such modulation and prevention extends from simple seasonal flus to many potential deadly infections. This can be well explained by successful eradication story of smallpox which have high mortality rate and even it has been defeated by vaccination [26].

Polymeric nanoparticles are effective immunogen. Various polymers appeared to be promising adjuvant and activator of immune responses in the host. Amphiphilic NPs activates DCs by mimicking natural pathogens similar to lipopolysaccharide (LPS). Whereas, DCs were activated by poly (methylvinyl ether-co-maleic anhydride) NPs through TLR stimulation in innate immune system. Thus various polymeric NPs activate immune system differently. Complement activation for improved immunity has also been done by chemical modification of NPs surface. This has been experimentally proved in murine model to facilitate vaccination purposes, where poly-hydroxylated NPs showed better result as compared to non-hydroxylated polymeric NPs. It has been found that, NPs containing pluronic-stabilized polypropylene sulfide (PPS) showed improved deposition and fixation of the C3b component. This leads to dendritic cells (DCs) activation and maturation more strongly as compared to non-hydroxylated nanospheres [35].

Another method of modulating immunity is use of an appropriate adjuvant. It helps in designing better nanoparticulate vaccine in many regards as it performs many functions. These are as follows:

TABLE 18.1

Factors Affecting Immunomodulation of NPs

Factors	Comments	References
Nanoparticle size	The immunogenicity of nanoparticles is strongly dependent on size as well as their aggregation. For example, antigen-specific polyfunctional CD4(+) T cells is profoundly influenced by 200 nm NPs as compared to 30 nm NPs in case of intranasal immunization.	[27]
Nanoparticle shape	It has been reported that shape determines the cellular uptake of NPs for further immunomodulation. Rod, elliptical or disk-shaped nanoparticles are less efficiently taken by the cell as compared to spherical nanoparticles.	[28]
Surface property	Surface property of NPs plays a vital role in the interactions between NPs and immune system. Surface curvature, charge and reactivity affect the aggregation, stability, and receptor binding. Cationic NPs strongly attracted towards negatively charged cell membrane and easily uptaken by macrophage and DCs. Moreover, surface displayed immunoactive surface ligands, can facilitate pathogen-mimetic immune cell activation.	[29–31]
Composition of NPs	It affects the functional outcome of NPs expression and different core composition gave different immune effect. Presence or absence of adjuvant determines the immunogenicity. Adjuvant generally increases the magnitude, induction, or durability of immune responses specially innate immunity.	[32]
Route of administration	Generally, intradermal or intramuscular administered NPs stimulate tissue residential cells, such as dermal DCs, Langerhans's cells and adipose tissue macrophages. Parenteral NPs interact with circulating immune cells and the complement system by plasma protein binding.	[33]
Plasma protein binding	NPs bind with plasma proteins such as immunoglobulins, apolipoproteins and other complement system proteins. This leads to conformational changes in the structure of adsorbed proteins and signal transduction. Thus the amount of protein present in plasma affects NPs interaction with immune cells.	[34]

1. Engaging immune cells for profound result
2. Increased antigen uptake and presentation to antigen-presenting cells (APC)
3. Up-regulation of immune messengers such as cytokines and chemokines.
4. Promoting lymph migration of immune cells
5. Sustained release of antigens providing long lasting immunity

Thus, it enhances the immunostimulatory activity of vaccine formulation which is required to induce higher antigen-specific immune response [36–38].

But, it is very tough to be accepted as vaccine adjuvant as it must be compatible with antigen molecules and non-toxic in nature. One such web-based central database study, suggests that only few have received licenses out of about hundred tested for human use [39]. One of the most widely used and accepted vaccine adjuvant is Monophosphoryl lipid A (MPLA). It is first approved adjuvant which is TLR agonist, frequently used for mass vaccination in human and compatible with large number of antigens [40]. Similarly, aluminum is one such powerful adjuvant for increased antibody production and has wide compatibility [41].

18.4 ROUTES OF ADMINISTRATION OF NANO-VACCINES

For administration of nanovaccines different routes of administration are employed, in which most commonly used routes are oral, parenteral, intradermal, subcutaneous, ocular, nasal and pulmonary [42]. Table 18.2 lists various routes of administration of vaccines and their features.

TABLE 18.2

Various Routes of Vaccine Administration Along with Their Advantages and Disadvantages

Route of administration	advantages	disadvantages
Oral	• Low cost vaccine production • Low delivery risk • Mucosal and systemic immunization • Securest route	• Instability in GI tract • High dose and potent adjuvant required • Small animal models available for viral and bacterial diseases
Intranasal	• Provide mucosal, lung and systemic antibody • Low delivery risk • Many animal models available for viral and bacterial diseases • High permeability and rapid absorption	• Mucociliary clearance • Need of potent adjuvant • Safety risk in humans
Pulmonary	• Provide lung and mucosal antibody mediated immunity • Delivery via inhalers/nebulizers/sprays	• Safety risk in humans
Topical	• Reduced systemic toxicity • Improved patient compliance • Self-applicability	• Patent adjuvant needs • Skin toxicity studies required
Vaginal	• Local and systemic vaccine delivery • High permeability and surface area • Avoid first pass metabolism	• Need special mucoadhesive delivery system
Ocular	• Provide mucosal immunity for infectious diseases	• Enzymatic degradation • Poor corneal permeability • Enzymatic degradation
Parenteral	• Provide humoral and cell mediated immunity • Low antigen dose needs • Clinical tested • Many clinical trials data available	• Sterile needle required • Trained personnel required • Potent adjuvant required

18.4.1 Oral Route

Majority of the contagious diseases are caused by colonization and invading of pathogens at host's mucosal surfaces. For example, number of bacterial, viral and parasites causes infection at the gastrointestinal tract (GIT) mucosal surfaces. In that cases, to stop personnel contact-based pathogen transmission and to further limit their proliferation at mucosal sites, stimulation of mucosal immunity is an essential necessity. The oral route is the one of the most commonly accessible and prevalent route of vaccination, which offers absorption of vaccines as of buccal via the rectal mucosa which provide improved local mucosal immune response protection to patients [42]. But the major disadvantage associated with oral route of administration is requirement of higher vaccination dose for effective working due to several hurdles such as strict gastric environment, low permeability of biological membranes, hepatic first pass metabolism and chemical instability of vaccines. Several number of nano vaccines delivery-based approaches have been employed to enhance immunogenicity and stability of oral vaccines [43–47].

18.4.2 Nasal Route

The nasal route of administration has been predominantly utilized for delivering nearby activity of the vaccines on the nasal mucosa surface. Although, nasal route provides several advantages such as great permeability of nasal epithelium for higher molecular weight vaccine candidates (≤1000 Da) and rapid absorption rate across nasal mucosa, but the accuracy and effectiveness of vaccine administered depends on mucociliary clearance, presence of enzymes in mucus secretions of nasal membrane, mucus secretion turnover and deposition and uptake of vaccine formulation in nasal mucosa. Novel nanocarrier mediated vaccine formulations efficiently enhance vaccine facilitation in nasal mucosa as well as provide stability and protection from enzymes [48–51].

18.4.3 Ocular Route

The ocular mucosal surface lining, due the exposure to environment, is an most prominent entry point as well as susceptible to many mucosal infection causing pathogenic substances and antigens. Thus, eye mucosa also has the huge possibility to deliver mucosal peptide/protein-based vaccines for ophthalmic infectious conditions [52]. However certain disadvantages also associated with vaccine delivery via this route such as poor corneal permeability, enzymatic degradation, low transport capacity, poor tear turnover and systemic absorption. In many ocular vaccination studies, it has been observed that nanocarrier mediated vaccination provide better results and surmounted the problems associated with this vaccination route [53, 54].

18.4.4 Vaginal Route

Vaginal mucosal surface is a threshold entry point for many infectious pathogens particularly virus and bacteria. Vaccine administration via vaginal site offers many benefits for local and systemic delivery of drugs, hormones, antigens and vaccines, due to high vaginal mucosal permeability, rich blood supply and large surface area and avoid first pass metabolism [55, 56]. Vaginal delivery of mucoadhesive vaccine system of recombinant human papilloma virus to enhance antibodies production against papilloma virus [57].

18.4.5 Topical Route

Vaccine delivery via topical route provides non-invasive delivery method for genetic DNA and naked plasmid DNA and also offers several benefits such as improved patient compliance, reduce toxicity, potential for multiple targets and needle free administration [58]. In recent era several practices such as electroporation, sonophoresis, iontophoresis and chemical induced diffusion are used, to produce antigen specific cell mediated and humoral immune response along with delivery systems approaches (liposomes, niosomes) [59].

18.5 RECENT ADVANCEMENT AND FUTURE PROSPECTS

In recent years, the discovery of vaccine adjuvants has progressed plenty of advancement, especially in understanding their modes of action in cells and molecules and how they'd be modified. NPs could be used to deliver multiple antigens to different parts of the body, offering biodegradable and biocompatible mechanisms with reduced toxicity and an important alternative to conventional vaccines. The thorough understanding of nanoparticles in the delivery of vaccines has made a significant contribution to nanoparticles being advanced in multiple immunotherapy approaches. It is now used to implement various therapeutic aspects in many important immune dysfunctions, including cancer and other immune conditions.

18.5.1 VACCINE DELIVERY IN CANCER IMMUNOTHERAPY

Nanoparticles could indeed directly influence vaccine delivery. The most studied nanostructures vaccines are antigens (e.g. peptides and proteins)-TLR agonist hybrid vaccines [60]. The blend of TLR agonists and antigen causes the antigen and adjuvant to be co-delivered to the very same immune cell. Descriptive research on anchored TLR7/8 agonists to polymer nanostructures asserted that minimal agonist-density polymer-TLR7/8 agonists would self-assemble to particles of 10–20 nm in diameter. The development of cytokines in lymph nodes was greater in non-formulated TLR7/8 agonists [61].

Numerous different inhibitory signals in the tumor microenvironment are aimed to provide by nanoparticles. A nanoparticles based approach for suppressing immune control points and the metabolism of tryptophan was created. Nanoparticles for therapeutic peptide assembly were manufactured together with NLG919 (indoleamine inhibitor 2, 3-dioxygenase 1, IdO-1) and were antagonistic to the programmed cell death ligand 1 (DPPA-1) [62]. The nanoparticles showed a spherical form and continued drug release that was encouraged in the presence of acidic pH and enzymes. Nanoparticle swelled and consequently collapsed and local releases of DPPA1 and NLG919 were found in the tumor stroma, which is useful for cytotoxic T Lymphocytes (CTL) activation and endurance. The fraction of CD8 + T cells in the tumor enhanced, and a strong anti-tumor immunity in the tumor was expended, thereby limiting the formation of melanoma. Summarizing this study, nanoparticles have shown a potential ability to cancer immunotherapy by attacking several tumor micro-environmental inhibitory signals.

Fe3O4 nanoparticles can also be targeted specifically to the immune checkpoint for the delivery of modulators in TME modulation. Ge et al. [63] have developed and tested a novel Fe3 O4 nanoparticle-based multipurpose therapeutic carrier. The carrier was produced with (1) mPEG-PLGA for spherical superparticles (sPs) encapsulation (2) imiquimod (R837), a non-immune adjuvant that could facilitate DCs and tumor-associated phagocytosis, and (3) Fe3O4 nanoparticles. The carrier was then referred to as Fe3O4-R837 SPs. The graphical representation of photothermic Fe3O4-R837 SPs with PD-L1 cancer immunotherapy blockage is shown in **Figure 18.2**. Tumors with near-infrared irradiation could be killed and powerful immune responses could be triggered by the messenger. The PD-L1 blocking approach has been shown to remove primary tumors, avoid metastases, and hinder the development of tumor-cell formation. The findings also revealed that the cancer immunotherapy of Fe3O4 nanoparticles can be aimed at the modulate tumor microenvironment modulation immune control stage [64].

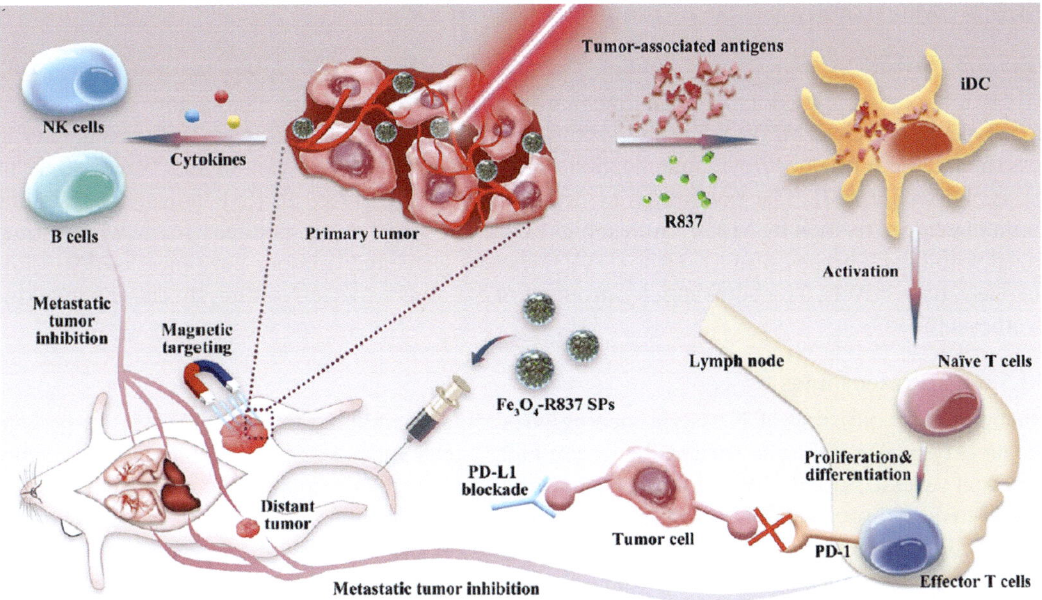

FIGURE 18.2 Graphical representation of Fe3O4-R837 SP photothermal therapy with PD-L1 checkpoint inhibitors for cancer immunotherapy; Adopted from [63].

18.5.2 Vaccine Delivery in COVID-19

The COVID-19 infected millions of people without a strong indication of infection and continued to spread due to lack of drugs or vaccines. In such situation modifying a viral strains is by far the most promising approach. The 2019-novel coronavirus (nCoV or SARS-CoV-2) genome pattern and associated proteins have been provided in record time, which enables the creation of inactively and/or mitigated viral vaccines alongside prophylactic and treatment sub-unit vaccines [65]. Nanotechnology has the advantage of modern vaccinating design because antigen-adjuvant nanomaterial and viral structure imitating are perfect for antigen delivery. In reality, an mRNA vaccine administered by lipid nanoparticles would be the first vaccine applicant to be initiated in clinical trials.

Advances in bio/nanotechnology and modern nano/production along with accessible information and data exchange provide the basis for the accelerated advancement of novel vaccine strategies in order to have an impact on the pandemic of COVID-19. Within 40 days following initial reporting of SARS-CoV-2 structure and genomics, the very first vaccine applicant has attempted to enter the therapeutic development pipeline and, from 1 June 2020, 16 vaccine applicant applicants already are present in a clinical study, many of them in phase II and even one in phase III. A multitude of nanotechnology systems are pivoting toward SARS-CoV-2; although highly encouraging, all of them may have an influence on the SARS-CoV-2 pandemic a couple of years from their implementation. It does, however, act as an instinct for research, funding organizations, and partners to work on the advancement of technological platforms to better brace for potential pandemics, as catastrophic as it is as COVID-19 [65]. Several nanomaterials have a technology platform that can be made flexible, stable, compact, distributed, and self-administered. Vaccinated applicants for SARS and MERS did not make it to the market, since the low levels of infections did not have financial rewards and the possibility of a major new virus pandemic was widely overlooked.

18.5.3 Miscellaneous

18.5.3.1 MF59

MF59, a human-approved nano-sized adjuvant is a commercial vaccine that is now being used as a therapeutic vaccine. MF59 is an o/w type of emulsion made up of droplets with a diameter of less than 250 nm produced by emulsification of Squalene along with Span 85 and Tween 80 in the citrate buffer [66, 67]. The preclinical evidence recorded by Ott et al. [68] indicates substantial immunogenic activation by MF59. Guinea pigs exhibit a 34-fold rise in antibody titers, when immunized with type 2 herpes simplex virus (HSV) whereas goats and baboons have increased 9–5-fold increase, respectively. The adjuvanticity protocol of MF59 is expected to directly cause a cytokine synthesis [67–69].

18.5.3.2 Proteosomes

Nanoparticles consisting of Neisseria meningitides' outer membrane proteins (OMPs) are perhaps the most typical proteosome variants being used for vaccine purposes. In a commercialized meningococcal vaccine since the 19th century, OMPs are being effectively implemented and are referred to as non-toxic and very well tolerated [70, 71]. This immunogenic supply mechanism is ideal to provide polar and/or amphiphilic antigen because of the hydrophobic structure of the OMPs and typically utilizes a noncovalent proteosome-antigen association to construct the related complexes [72].

18.6 CONCLUSION

Numerous varieties of particulate delivery systems for vaccines have been described, and each particulate vaccine have advantages over traditional methods of vaccines delivery. Instead of conventional vaccines these new generation vaccines enhance an immune response in better way. Naïve antigen has poor antigenic property on their own, in order to boost the immune response adjuvant is required. So these particulate system shows multiple benefits as adjuvant and carrier systems. It also has a significant role in antigen delivery too and simultaneously it will activate numerous cells of immune systems. Thus delivery of antigens using advance techniques has an intense effect on immune response.

18.7 ACKNOWLEDGMENT

The authors want to acknowledge Guru Ghasidas Vishwavidyalaya, Bilaspur, C.G., University Institute of Pharmacy, Pt Ravishankar Shukla University, Raipur, C.G., KIET Institute of Pharmacy, KIET Institute, Gaziabad, U.P., Rungta College of Pharmaceutical Sciences and Research, Bhilai, C.G., Department of Pharmacy, Indira Gandhi National Tribal University, Amarkantak, M.P. for providing necessary literature and infrastructural facilities required for compilation of work.

REFERENCES

1. A. Gokarna, L.H. Jin, J.S. Hwang, Y.H. Cho, Y.T. Lim, B.H. Chung, et al., Quantum dot-based protein micro-and nanoarrays for detection of prostate cancer biomarkers, *Proteomics* 8(9) (2008) 1809e-18. https://doi.org/10.1002/pmic.200701072
2. J. Yang, C.H. Lee, H.J. Ko, J.S. Suh, H.G. Yoon, K. Lee, et al., Multifunctional magnetopolymeric nanohybrids for targeted detection and synergistic therapeutic effects on breast cancer, *Angew. Chem. Int. Ed.* 46(46) (2007) 8836e-9. https://doi.org/10.1002/anie.200703554
3. C. Primard, N. Rochereau, E. Luciani, C. Genin, T. Delair, S. Paul, et al., Traffic of poly (lactic acid) nanoparticulate vaccine vehicle from intestinal mucus to subepithelial immune competent cells, *Biomaterials* 31(23) (2010) 6060e-8. https://doi.org/10.1016/j.biomaterials.2010.04.021
4. S.C. Semple, B.L. Mui, C.K. Cho, D.W.Y. Sah, D. Stebbing, E.J. Crosley, E. Yaworski, I.M. Hafez, J.R. Dorkin, J. Qin, et al., Rational design of cationic lipids for siRNA delivery. *Nat. Biotechnol.* 28 (2010) 172–76. https://doi.org/10.1038/nbt.1602

5. K.M. Saul, The newly licensed hepatitis B vaccine characteristics and indications for use, *J. Am. Med. Assoc.* 247 (1982) 2012–15. https://doi:10.1001/jama.1982.03320390074052

6. S. Li, H.I. Nakaya, D.A. Kazmin, J.Z. Oh, B. Pulendran, Systems biological approaches to measure and understand vaccine immunity in humans, *Semin. Immunol.* 25(3) (2013) 209–18. https://doi.org/10.1016/j.smim.2013.05.003

7. M. Luo, L.Z. Samandi, Z. Wang, Z.J. Chen, J. Gao, Synthetic nanovaccines for immunotherapy, *J. Contr. Release* 263 (2017) 200–10. https://doi.org/10.1016/j.jconrel.2017.03.033

8. F. Fontana, D. Liu, J. Hirvonen, H.A. Santos, Delivery of therapeutics with nanoparticles: what's new in cancer immunotherapy? *Wiley Interdiscip. Rev. Nanosci. Nanotechnol.* 9(1) (2017) 1–26. https://doi.org/10.1002/wnan.1421

9. A. Roldão, M.C.M. Mellado, L.R. Castilho, M.J.T. Carrondo, P.M. Alves, Virus-like particles in vaccine development, *Expert Rev. Vaccines* 9 (2010) 1149–76. https://doi.org/10.1586/erv.10.115.

10. S.M. Kingsman, A.J. Kingsman, Polyvalent recombinant antigens: a new vaccine strategy, *Vaccine* 6 (1988) 304–306. https://doi.org/10.1016/0264-410x(88)90174-0.

11. A. Zeltins, Construction and characterization of virus-like particles: a review, *Mol. Biotechnol.* 53 (2013) 92–107. https://doi.org/10.1007/s12033-012-9598-4.

12. K. Young, S. Mcburney, L. Karkhanis, T. Ross, Virus-like particles: designing an effective AIDS vaccine, *Methods* 40 (2006) 98–117. https://doi.org/10.1016/j.ymeth.2006.05.024.

13. K.G. Patel, J.R. Swartz, Surface functionalization of virus-like particles by direct conjugation using azide-alkyne click chemistry, *Bioconjug. Chem.* 22 (2011) 376–87. https://doi.org/10.1021/bc100367u.

14. Y. Hu, Baculovirus as a highly efficient expression vector in insect and mammalian cells, *Acta Pharmacol. Sin.* 26 (2005) 405–16. https://doi.org/10.1111/j.1745-7254.2005.00078.x.

15. R.L. Harrison, D.L. Jarvis, Protein N-glycosylation in the baculovirus-insect cell expression system and engineering of insect cells to produce "mammalianized" recombinant glycoproteins, *Adv. Virus Res.* 68 (2006) 159–91. https://doi.org/10.1016/S0065-3527(06)68005-6.

16. J.J. Aumiller, J.R. Hollister, D.L. Jarvis, A transgenic insect cell line engineered to produce CMP-sialic acid and sialylated glycoproteins, *Glycobiology.* 13 (2003) 497–507. https://doi.org/10.1093/glycob/cwg051.

17. D.L. Jarvis, D. Howe, J.J. Aumiller, Novel baculovirus expression vectors that provide sialylation of recombinant glycoproteins in lepidopteran insect cells, *J. Virol.* 75 (2001) 6223–7. https://doi.org/10.1128/JVI.75.13.6223-6227.2001.

18. N. Marasini, K.A. Ghaffar, M. Skwarczynski, I. Toth, Chapter twelve—liposomes as a vaccine delivery system, in: M. Skwarczynski, I.B.T.-M. and N.V.D. Toth (Eds.), *Micro Nano Technol*, William Andrew Publishing, 2017: pp. 221–39. https://doi.org/10.1016/B978-0-323-39981-4.00012-9.

19. R. Nisini, N. Poerio, S. Mariotti, F. De Santis, M. Fraziano, The multirole of liposomes in therapy and prevention of infectious diseases, *Front. Immunol.* 9 (2018) 155. https://doi.org/10.3389/fimmu.2018.00155.

20. R.A. Schwendener, Liposomes as vaccine delivery systems: a review of the recent advances, *Ther. Adv. Vaccines* 2 (2014) 159–82. https://doi.org/10.1177/2051013614541440.

21. T. Liu, Vaccine adjuvant delivery systems constructed using biocompatible nanoparticles formed through self-assembly of small molecules, in: R. Qian (Ed.), IntechOpen, 2018: Ch. 2. https://doi.org/10.5772/intechopen.79905.

22. M. Sanders, L. Brown, G. Deliyannis, ISCOM™-based vaccines: the second decade, *Immunol. Cell Biol.* 83 (2005) 119–28. https://doi.org/10.1111/j.1440-1711.2005.01319.x.

23. A.E. Gregory, R. Titball, D. Williamson, Vaccine delivery using nanoparticles, *Front. Cell. Infect. Microbiol.* 4 (2013) 13. https://doi.org/10.3389/fcimb.2013.00013.

24. Riedel, S. Edward Jenner and the history of smallpox and vaccination. *Bayl. Univ. Med. Cent. Proc.* 18 (2005) 21–5. https://doi.org/10.1080/08998280.2005.11928028

25. Gomes, A.C., Mohsen, M., Bachmann, M.F. Harnessing nanoparticles for immunomodulation and vaccines. *Vaccines* 5 (2017) 1–15. https://doi.org/10.3390/vaccines5010006

26. F. Fenner, Smallpox: emergence, global spread, and eradication. *Hist. Philos. Life Sci.* 15 (1993) 397–420. https://pubmed.ncbi.nlm.nih.gov/7529932/

27. A. Stano, C. Nembrini, M.A. Swartz, J.A. Hubbell, E. Simeoni, Nanoparticle size influences the magnitude and quality of mucosal immune responses after intranasal immunization, *Vaccine* 30(52) (2012) 7541–46. https://doi.org/10.1016/j.vaccine.2012.10.050

28. K.K. Sahu, R.S. Pandey, Immunological evaluation of colonic delivered hepatitis B surface antigen loaded TLR-4 agonist modified solid fat nanoparticles, *Int. Immunopharmacol.* 39 (2016) 343–52. https://doi.org/10.1016/j.intimp.2016.08.007

29. S.A.A. Rizvi, A.M. Saleh, Applications of nanoparticle systems in drug delivery technology, *Saudi Pharm. J.* 26(1) (2017) 64–70. https://doi.org/10.1016/j.jsps.2017.10.012

30. J.A. Rosenthal, L. Chen, J.L. Baker, D. Putnam, M.P. DeLisa, Pathogen-like particles: biomimetic vaccine carriers engineered at the nanoscale, *Curr. Opin. Biotechnol.* 28 (2014) 51–8. https://doi.org/10.1016/j.copbio.2013.11.005

31. K. Fytianos, S. Chortarea, L. Rodriguez-Lorenzo, F. Blank, C. Von Garnier, A. Petri-Fink, B. Rothen-Rutishauser, Aerosol delivery of functionalized gold nanoparticles target and activate dendritic cells in a 3D lung cellular model, *ACS Nano.* 11 (2017) 375–83. https://doi.org/10.1021/acsnano.6b06061

32. J.E. Crowe, Prevention of fetal and early life infections through maternal-neonatal immunization, in: *Section V Diagnosis and Management*, Elsevier, 2011: 1212–30.

33. L. Yuanchang, J. Hardie, X. Zhang, V.M. Rotello, Effects of engineered nanoparticles on the innate immune system, *Semin. Immunol.* 34 (2017) 25–32. https://doi.org/10.1016/j.smim.2017.09.011

34. M. Lundqvist, J. Stigler, G. Elia, I. Lynch, T. Cedervall, K.A. Dawson, Nanoparticle size and surface properties determine the protein corona with possible implications for biological impacts. *Proc. Natl. Acad. Sci. USA.* 105 (2008) 14265–70. https://doi.org/10.1073/pnas.0805135105

35. S.T. Reddy, A.J. Van der Vlies, E. Simeoni, V. Angeli, G.J. Randolph, C.P. O'Neil, L.K. Lee, M.A. Swartz, J.A. Hubbell, Exploiting lymphatic transport and complement activation in nanoparticle vaccines. *Eur. Cells Mater.* 25 (2007) 1159–64. https://doi.org/10.1038/nbt1332

36. J.C. Cox, A.R. Coulter, Adjuvants-A classification and review of their modes of action, *Vaccine* 15 (1997) 248–56. https://doi.org/10.1016/S0264-410X(96)00183-1

37. K. Hoebe, E. Janssen, B. Beutler, The interface between innate and adaptive immunity, *Nat. Immunol.* 5 (2004) 971–4. https://doi.org/10.1038/ni1004-971

38. C.K. Fraser, K.R. Diener, M.P. Brown, J.D. Hayball, Improving vaccines by incorporating immunological coadjuvants, *Expert Rev. Vaccines* 6 (2007) 559–78. https://doi.org/10.1586/14760584.6.4.559

39. B. Sun, T. Xia, Nanomaterial-based vaccine adjuvants. *J. Mater. Chem. B* 4 (2016) 5496–509. https://doi.org/10.1039/C6TB01131D

40. K.K. Sahu, M. Kaurav, R.S. Pandey, Chylomicron mimicking solid lipid nanoemulsions encapsulated enteric minicapsules targeted to colon for immunization against hepatitis B. *Int. Immunopharmacol.* 66 (2019) 317–29. https://doi.org/10.1016/j.intimp.2018.11.041

41. A.T. Glenny, C.G. Pope, H. Waddington, U. Wallace, Immunological notes. XVII–XXIV. *J. Pathol. Bacteriol.* 29 (1926) 31–40. https://doi.org/10.1002/path.1700290106

42. V.A. Erdmann, J. Barciszewski (Eds.), DNA and RNA nanobiotechnologies in medicine: diagnosis and treatment of diseases, *Springer Sci. Bus. Media* 20 (2013) 104–14.

43. M.D. Bhavsar, M.M. Amiji, Polymeric nano- and microparticle technologies for oral gene delivery, *Expert Opin. Drug Deliv.* 4 (2007) 197–213. https://doi.org/10.1517/17425247.4.3.197

44. C.R. Oliveira, C.M. Rezende, M.R. Silva, et al., Oral vaccination based on DNA-chitosan nanoparticles against Schistosoma mansoni infection. *Sci. World J.* (2012) 938457. https://doi.org/10.1100/2012/938457

45. R. Kumar. V.P. Ishaq Ahmed, V. Parameswaran, et al., Potential use of chitosan nanoparticles for oral delivery of DNA vaccine in Asian sea bass (Lates calcarifer) to protect from Vibrio (Listonella) anguillarum. *Fish Shellfish Immunol.* 25 (2008) 47–56. https://doi.org/10.1016/j.fsi.2007.12.004

46. T. Naito, Y. Kaneko, D. Kozbor, Oral vaccination with modified vaccinia virus Ankara attached covalently to TMPEG-modified cationic liposomes overcomes pre-existing poxvirus immunity from recombinant vaccinia immunization, *J. Gen. Virol.* 88 (2007) 61–70. https://doi.org/10.1099/vir.0.82216-0

47. S. Jain, P. Singh, V. Mishra, et al., Mannosylated niosomes as adjuvant-carrier system for oral genetic immunization against hepatitis B, *Immunol. Lett.* 101 (2005) 41–9. https://doi.org/10.1016/j.imlet.2005.04.002

48. D. Raghuwanshi, V. Mishra, D. Das, et al., Dendritic cell targeted chitosan nanoparticles for nasal DNA immunization against SARS CoV nucleocapsid protein, *Mol. Pharm.* 9 (2012) 946–56. https://doi.org/10.1021/mp200553x

49. J. Xu, W. Dai, Z. Wang, et al., Intranasal vaccination with chitosan-DNA nanoparticles expressing pneumococcal surface antigen a protects mice against nasopharyngeal colonization by Streptococcus pneumoniae, *Clin. Vaccine Immunol.* 18 (2011) 75–81. http://doi.org/10.1128/CVI.00263-10

50. B. Slutter, N. Hagenaars, W. Jiskoot, Rational design of nasal vaccines. *J. Drug Target.* 16 (2008) 1–17. https://doi.org/10.1080/10611860701637966

51. H.K.S.Yadav, M. Dibi, A. Mohammad, A.E. Srouji, Nanovaccines formulation and applications-a review, *J. Drug Deliv. Sci. Technol.* 44 (2018) 380–7. https://doi.org/10.1016/j.jddst.2018.01.015

52. J.W. Streilein, B.R. Ksander, A.W. Taylor, Immune deviation in relation to ocular immune privilege. *J. Immunol.* 158 (1997) 3557–60. www.jimmunol.org/content/158/8/3557.long

53. A.B. Nesburn, T.V. Ramos, X. Zhu, et al., Local and systemic B cell and Th1 responses induced following ocular mucosal delivery of multiple epitopes of herpes simplex virus type 1 glycoprotein D together with cytosine-phosphate-guanine adjuvant, *Vaccine* 23 (2005) 873–83. https://doi.org/10.1016/j.vaccine.2004.08.019

54. K. Hu, J. Dou, F. Yu, et al., An ocular mucosal administration of nanoparticles containing DNA vaccine pRSC-gD-IL-21 confers protection against mucosal challenge with herpes simplex virus type 1 in mice, *Vaccine* 29 (2011) 1455–62. https://doi.org/10.1016/j.vaccine.2010.12.031

55. A. Hussain, F. Ahsan, The vagina as a route for systemic drug delivery. *J. Control. Release* 103 (2005) 301–13. https://doi.org/10.1016/j.jconrel.2004.11.034

56. S. Gupta, R. Gabrani, J. Ali, et al., Exploring novel approaches to vaginal drug delivery. *Recent. Pat. Drug Deliv. Formul.* 5 (2011) 82–94. https://doi.org/10.2174/187221111795471418

57. J.S. Park, Y.K. Oh, M.J. Kang, et al., Enhanced mucosal and systemic immune responses following intravaginal immunization with human papillomavirus 16 L1 virus-like particle vaccine in thermosensitive mucoadhesive delivery systems. *J. Med. Virol.* 70 (2003) 633–41. https://doi.org/10.1002/jmv.10442

58. A. Nasir, Nanotechnology in vaccine development: a step forward, *J. Invest. Dermatol.* 129 (2009) 1055–9. https://doi.org/10.1038/jid.2009.63

59. S. Mehier-Humbert, R.H. Guy, Physical methods for gene transfer: improving the kinetics of gene delivery into cells. *Adv. Drug. Deliv. Rev.* 57 (2005) 733–53. https://doi.org/10.1016/j.addr.2004.12.007

60. B.J. Ignacio, T.J. Albin, A.P. Esser-Kahn, M. Verdoes, Toll-like receptor agonist conjugation: a chemical perspective, *Bioconjug. Chem.* 29 (2018) 587–603. https://doi.org/10.1021/acs.bioconjchem.7b00808.

61. G.M. Lynn, R. Laga, P.A. Darrah, A.S. Ishizuka, A.J. Balaci, A.E. Dulcey, M. Pechar, R. Pola, M.Y. Gerner, A. Yamamoto, C.R. Buechler, K.M. Quinn, M.G. Smelkinson, O. Vanek, R. Cawood, T. Hills, O. Vasalatiy, K. Kastenmüller, J.R. Francica, L. Stutts, J.K. Tom, K.A. Ryu, A.P. Esser-Kahn, T. Etrych, K.D. Fisher, L.W. Seymour, R.A. Seder, In vivo characterization of the physicochemical properties of polymer-linked TLR agonists that enhance vaccine immunogenicity, *Nat. Biotechnol.* 33 (2015) 1201–10. https://doi.org/10.1038/nbt.3371.

62. K. Cheng, Y. Ding, Y. Zhao, S. Ye, X. Zhao, Y. Zhang, T. Ji, H. Wu, B. Wang, G.J. Anderson, L. Ren, G. Nie, Sequentially responsive therapeutic peptide assembling nanoparticles for dual-targeted cancer immunotherapy, *Nano Lett.* 18 (2018) 3250–8. https://doi.org/10.1021/acs.nanolett.8b01071.

63. R. Ge, C. Liu, X. Zhang, W. Wang, B. Li, J. Liu, Y. Liu, H. Sun, D. Zhang, Y. Hou, H. Zhang, B. Yang, Photothermal-activatable Fe(3)O(4) superparticle nanodrug carriers with PD-L1 immune checkpoint blockade for anti-metastatic cancer immunotherapy, *ACS Appl. Mater. Interfaces* 10 (2018) 20342–55. https://doi.org/10.1021/acsami.8b05876.

64. Y. Huang, J. Zeng, Recent development and applications of nanomaterials for cancer immunotherapy, *Nanotechnol. Rev.* 9 (2020) 382–99. https://doi.org/10.1515/ntrev-2020-0027.

65. M.D. Shin, S. Shukla, Y.H. Chung, V. Beiss, S.K. Chan, O.A. Ortega-Rivera, D.M. Wirth, A. Chen, M. Sack, J.K. Pokorski, N.F. Steinmetz, COVID-19 vaccine development and a potential nanomaterial path forward, *Nat. Nanotechnol.* 15 (2020) 646–55. https://doi.org/10.1038/s41565-020-0737-y.

66. S. Calabro, E. Tritto, A. Pezzotti, M. Taccone, A. Muzzi, S. Bertholet, E. Gregorio, D. O'Hagan, B. Baudner, A. Seubert, The adjuvant effect of MF59 is due to the oil-in-water emulsion formulation, none of the individual components induce a comparable adjuvant effect. *Vaccine* 31 (2013). https://doi.org/10.1016/j.vaccine.2013.05.007.

67. D.T. O'Hagan, MF59 is a safe and potent vaccine adjuvant that enhances protection against influenza virus infection, *Expert Rev. Vaccines* 6 (2007) 699–710. https://doi.org/10.1586/14760584.6.5.699.

68. G. Ott, G.L. Barchfeld, D. Chernoff, R. Radhakrishnan, P. van Hoogevest, G. Van Nest, MF59. Design and evaluation of a safe and potent adjuvant for human vaccines, *Pharm. Biotechnol.* 6 (1995) 277–96. https://doi.org/10.1007/978-1-4615-1823-5_10.

69. M. Dupuis, T.J. Murphy, D. Higgins, M. Ugozzoli, G. van Nest, G. Ott, D.M. McDonald, Dendritic cells internalize vaccine adjuvant after intramuscular injection, *Cell. Immunol.* 186 (1998) 18–27. https://doi.org/10.1006/cimm.1998.1283.

70. R. Glück, Immunopotentiating reconstituted influenza virosomes (IRIVs) and other adjuvants for improved presentation of small antigens, *Vaccine* 10 (1992) 915–9. https://doi.org/10.1016/0264-410x(92)90325-e.

71. O.O. Bilukha, N. Rosenstein, Prevention and control of meningococcal disease. Recommendations of the advisory committee on immunization practices (ACIP), *MMWR. Recomm. Reports Morb. Mortal. Wkly. Report. Recomm. Reports* 54 (2005) 1–21.

72. J. Aucouturier, L. Dupuis, S. Deville, S. Ascarateil, V. Ganne, Montanide ISA 720 and 51: a new generation of water in oil emulsions as adjuvants for human vaccines, *Expert Rev. Vaccines* 1 (2002) 111–8. https://doi.org/10.1586/14760584.1.1.111.

19 Role of Nanobiotechnology in Cell-Based Nanomedicines

Yachana Mishra, and Vijay Mishra

19.1 INTRODUCTION

The creation and utilization of materials, devices, and systems by controlling matter at the nanoscale is known as nanotechnology. DNA has a width of around 2.5 nm. The protein molecule has a size of 1–20 nm. It was just a matter of time until nanotechnology was combined with biotechnology to create nanobiotechnology, given living cells already contain functioning nanoscale elements. Nanomedicine is the practice of using nanobiotechnologies in medicine [1].

Nanobiotechnology is already influencing the medical sector. Early nanotechnology ideas have evolved into various innovations over the last 50 years, and a few nanotechnology-based medicines are now on the market. The word "nanobiopharmaceuticals" can be applied to multiple pharmaceutical applications, including drug development and distribution. Nanotechnologies have the ability to change the world and show a significant impact on surgery and medicine. This is due to the fact that pathological and physiological cellular activities take place on a nanoscale. Nanomedicine is a refinement in molecular medicine that combines genomics and proteomics to produce personalized drugs. Figure 19.1 depicts the relationship between nanobiotechnology, nanomedicine, and other technologies. It illustrates how nanobiotechnology can influence nanomedicine growth directly and indirectly by developing other disciplines like molecular diagnostics and nanopharmaceutical delivery. Parallel to nanomedicine, nanotechnology assists personalized medicine development. Essential uses for drug delivery and molecular diagnostics will be briefly highlighted prior to exploring the function of nanotechnology in different disorders [2].

19.2 NANOBIOTECHNOLOGY AND NANOMEDICINES

Nanomedicine is a relatively new area of research. Only since the 1990s has there been research into how nanotechnology can be used in biology, medical science, and pharmacology [3]. Three pillars underpin the potential applications of nanotechnology in medicine:

1. Nanoinstruments and nanomaterials used as biosensors, treatment aids, and active substance delivery systems [4];
2. Understanding of genetics, artificially created or altered microbes, and proteomics in the context of molecular medicine;
3. Nanotechnology used for quick diagnosis and treatment, genetic material repair and cell surgery, and enhancing natural physiological functions, among other things [5].

Nanobiotechnology is a field in which nanotechnology techniques are created and used to investigate biological phenomena [6]. Nanoparticles, for example, may be used as sensors, probes, or vehicles for the transmission of biomolecules in cellular systems [7]. Biological therapies such as monoclonal antibodies (MAbs), gene therapy, cell therapy, recombinant human proteins, vaccinations, RNA interference (RNAi), and antisense techniques are becoming increasingly common in modern medicine [8].

DOI: 10.1201/9781003130055-19

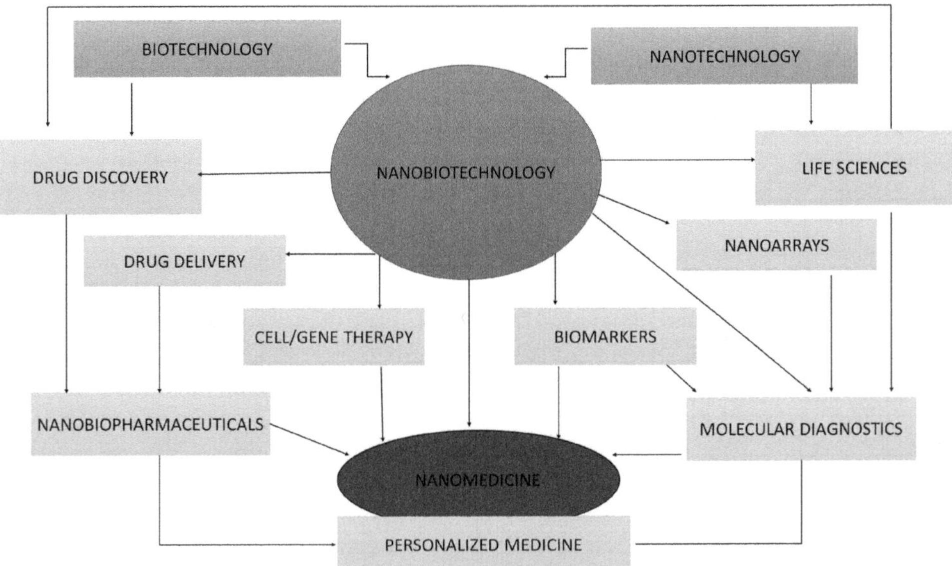

FIGURE 19.1 Inter-relationship between nanomedicine, nanobiotechnology, and other techniques.

19.3 NANOBIOTECHNOLOGY IN BIOLOGICAL THERAPIES

Biological therapies like vaccines and gene and cell therapy involve the use of molecular biology in therapeutics. The applications of nanobiotechnology may improve biological therapies, especially their delivery, which are discussed as follows [9].

19.3.1 VACCINATION

DNA vaccines can be new vaccines for essential pathogens like HIV, tuberculosis, and malaria, but existing delivery methods are inadequate. Nanoparticles (NPs) show promise as DNA vaccine delivery systems. The production of nanoemulsions or NP aerosol vaccines is also underway. Particles are recognized by immune system components more effectively than soluble proteins [10]. Due to similar size range of NPs and many pathogenic organisms including viruses, NP-based vaccines, also known as nanovaccines, improve both innate and adaptive immunity. Nanovaccines have been developed using non-infectious viruses without genetic material, that is, virus-like particles (VLPs) and polymeric NPs [11, 12].

19.3.2 CELL THERAPY

In order to treat or prevent human illness, cells that have been chosen, multiplied, and pharmacologically changed are administered through cell therapy. This therapy can be expanded to cover both pharmacological and nonpharmacological methods of influencing intrinsic functions of body cells for therapeutic objectives. The purpose of cell therapy is to substitute, restore, or improve the functionality of injured tissues or organs. The cells used may come from the patient, a donor, or a different species to produce cancer vaccines, cell lines, and cells from patients' tumors [11].

Recent developments in bone marrow–mesenchymal stem cell (BM-MSC) research offered an innovative method for treating chronic pulmonary diseases (COPD). MSCs have been shown to differentiate type I and type II alveolar epithelial cells in LPS and CS-induced lung injury rat models [13].

19.3.3 Gene Therapy

Gene therapy is characterized as transferring predetermined genetic material to a patient's specific target cells to prevent or alter a disease state. Viruses are commonly used as vectors, but nonviral methods are also used. DNA and gene are inserted into cells without vectors, and different approaches have been used to alter in vivo gene function without gene transfer [14].

Glioblastoma, the most prevalent adult brain cancer, nearly invariably returns after radiation therapy. The goal of recent studies is to pinpoint the clinically significant processes behind this recurrence. The same individuals' matched pre- and post-radiation therapy glioblastoma samples were used for microRNA (miRNA) profiling. The wild-type isocitrate dehydrogenase promoters (wtIDH) and O-methylguanine-DNA methyltransferase (umMGMT) were present in all samples. The bulk of miRNAs remained unchanged after treatment, with miR-603 being the most notable exception. Only a few particular miRNAs showed reduced levels in post-treatment specimens. The release of miR-603 from extracellular vesicles (EVs) was triggered by ionizing radiation (IR), enabling the de-repression of IGF1 and IGF1R. Additionally, miR-603 export depressed MGMT, a DNA repair protein in charge of cleansing agents that cause DNA alkylation, enabling cross-resistance to these agents. The expression of Ectopic miR-603 was more abundant than the cell's capacity to export it. This is combined with IR and DNA alkylating chemicals to exert a tumor-killing effect. Profiling of matched glioblastoma samples from before and after therapy revealed that radiation-induced disruption of many miRNAs' homeostasis. The CSC state was enhanced by radiation-induced EV export of miR-603, which also increased DNA repair to sustain acquired resistance. The expression of exogenous miR-603 reversed the results, suggesting its therapeutic use [15].

Colorectal cancer (CRC) patients are often administered 5-fluorouracil (5-FU), yet 5-FU resistance is the leading cause of CRC treatment failure. Due to their ability to regulate the signaling pathways associated with the start and progress, miRNAs have lately been recognized as a potential solution. The safe and effective distribution of miRNAs to the target cells is challenging. Engineered exosomes were employed to transport a miR-21 inhibitor oligonucleotide (miR-21i) and the anticancer drug 5-FU to cancer cells expressing the Her2 gene. Exosomes from donor cells that have been purified and modified to contain miR-21i and 5-FU are electroporated before being injected into the 5-FU-resistant CRC cell line HCT-1165FR. Additionally, animals with tumors were routinely administered exosomes laden with 5-FU and miR-21i. These exosomes had a strong anti-tumor impact. A miR-21i and 5-FU co-delivery system based on modified exosomes successfully boosted cellular absorption while drastically reducing miR-21 expression in 5-FU resistant HCT-1165FR cells. Because PTEN and hMSH2 are miR-21 regulatory targets, miR-21 downregulation resulted in the arrest of the cell cycle, diminished tumor growth, enhanced apoptosis, and restored hMSH2 and PTEN expression. Particularly interesting was the significant slowing of tumor development caused by the systematic injection of the miR-21i target in a mouse model of colon cancer. More intriguingly, drug resistance was successfully overcome when 5-FU and miR-21i were administered in combination with modified exosomes, and cytotoxicity was dramatically enhanced in 5-FU-resistant colon cancer cells compared to 5-FU or miR-21i alone. Exosome-based co-delivery of a miRNA and an anticancer drug foreshadows a possible strategy for reversing drug resistance in CRC and improving cancer treatment efficacy [16].

Exosomes can carry biological molecules between cells as endogenous nanocarriers in various ways. The exosome is limited in focusing on certain receiver cells. The authors developed a technique to identify exosome with elevated integrin v3 binding. An improved version of integrin and metalloproteinase 15 (A15) generated on exosomal membranes (A15-Exo) allowed for the simultaneous in vivo and in vitro delivery of cholesterol-modified miRNA 159 (Cho-miR159) and doxorubicin (DOX) to triple-negative breast cancer (TNBC) cells. The targeted A15-Exo was produced by persistent protein kinase C activation in macrophages generated from monocytes.

Cell-produced exosomes demonstrated better-targeting characteristics with a 2.97-fold greater yield. A15-Exo loaded with Cho-miR159 and DOX produced synergistic therapeutic effects in MDA-MB-231 cells. DOX and Cho-miR159 were delivered in vivo through vesicles, successfully silencing the TCF-7 gene and enhancing anticancer benefits without any negative side effects. The results demonstrated a synergistic impact of co-delivering DOX and miR159 through targeted exosomes for TNBC treatment [17].

Polymer-based gene/drug delivery holds promise for the treatment of inherited or acquired disorders due to the structural stability of the polymer, more impressive therapeutic agent ability, less host immunogenicity, and cheaper cost. Antisense treatment uses antisense oligonucleotides (AOs) to treat hereditary illnesses or infections. Unfortunately, naked AOs demonstrated poor therapeutic effects in vivo and in clinical trials because of their sluggish cellular uptake and quick circulation discharge. Specific triazine-cored amphiphilic polymers (TAPs) might enhance the transport of AOs, phosphorodiamidate morpholino oligomer (PMO), and 2'-O-methyl phosphorothioate RNA (2'-OMePS) in vivo and in vitro. TAPs markedly improved AO-induced exon-skipping in a GFP reporter-based myotube culture and myoblast system, and their observed cytotoxicity was lower than PEI 25K, Lipofectamine 2000, or Endoporter. In dystrophic mdx mice, the administration of optimized TAPs formulations with AO targeted to dystrophin exon 23 resulted in a marked improvement in exon-skipping performance. The strongest ones for PMO and 2'-OMePS administration in mdx mice were 11- and 15-fold stronger than the AO alone, respectively. The hydrophilic-lipophilic balance (HLB), content, and molecular size of the polymers, as well as the structure of the AO, all affect the carrier's efficiency. TAP polymers have demonstrated better exon-skipping efficacy of AOs in vitro and in mdx mice, as well as reduced cytotoxicity, suggesting they might be employed as a secure and effective delivery system for genes and drugs [18].

Over the past ten years, exosomes have developed as an innovative endogenous delivery system. It indicates that MicroRNA-210 (miR-2110) has a lot of potential to enhance angiogenesis for the recovery of damaged brain tissue following cerebral ischemia. However, it is still difficult to effectively and securely administer miR-210 intravenously. Exosomes contain cholesterol-modified miR-210 after being conjugated to the c(RGDyK) peptide (RGD-exo:miR-210). The RGD-exo:miR-210 targeted the damaged portion of the ischemic brain following intravenous injection in an animal model of temporary middle cerebral artery occlusion (MCAO), increasing miR-210 at the location. Vascular endothelial growth factor (VEGF), CD34, and integrin 3 are also noticeably elevated following 14 days of RGD-exo:miR-210 treatment. Additionally, the animal has a greater chance of surviving. The data provide an approach for delivering angiogenic agents and miR-210 to ischemic brain cells to treat ischemic stroke [19].

19.4 RELATIONSHIP OF NANOBIOTECHNOLOGY TO NANOMEDICINE

New opportunities are made possible by nanobiotechnology, particularly in regenerative medicine. Nanomaterials might artificially repair or create missing or damaged tissue, including muscle, organ, and nerve cells, by controlling and promoting cell development [8]. Nanoporous carrier materials are currently employed as matrices to track cell development in wound healing and plastic surgery. If targeted nerve cell development is effective, new therapies for neurological diseases like Alzheimer's that were hitherto incurable may be created [3].

19.5 NANOBIOTECHNOLOGY FOR PERSONALIZED TREATMENT

A variety of nanotechnologies and nanodevices (nanobiochips and nanobiosensors) are used to speed up drug discovery and growth. Although some widely used medicines are customized, some new medicines have been designed from the start with personalization in mind (Figure 19.2). Nanobiotechnology is now substantially influencing the pharmaceutical industry [20].

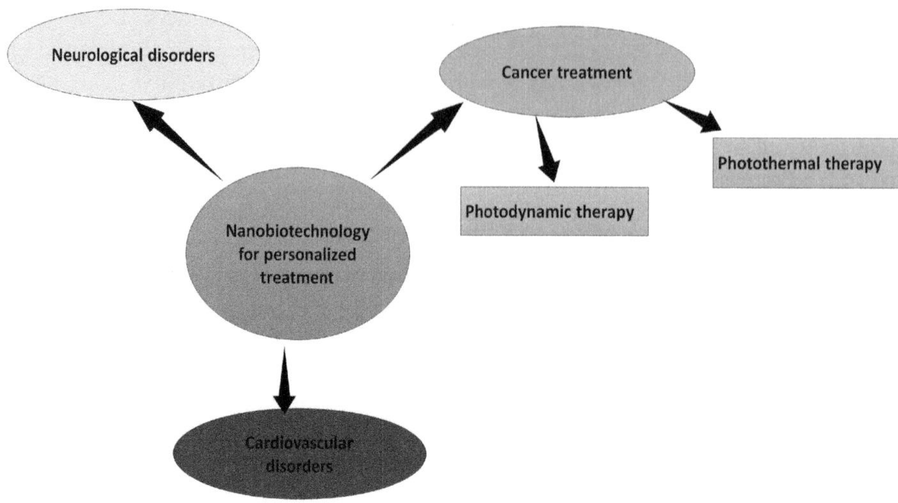

FIGURE 19.2 Nanobiotechnology for personalized treatment.

19.5.1 Cancer Treatment

Nanobiotechnology is vital for the advancement of personalized cancer treatment methods. Nanobiotechnologies will also aid in discovering cancer biomarkers, which will form the foundation for developing diagnostics and therapeutics. Here are a few examples of how nanobiotechnology is being used to help cancer patients. Using v3-targeted paramagnetic NPs, non-invasive identification of minor regions of angiogenesis associated with embryonic melanoma tumors was achieved. Metal atoms augment contrast in traditional MRI scans. Each particle has a material on its surface that sticks to newly created blood arteries in tumor areas. This allows molecular MRI to detect sparse biomarkers in vivo, while conventional MRI still misses the growths. Early detection, particularly in melanoma, can improve treatment effectiveness [21].

Hepatocellular carcinoma (HCC) is lethal cancer that affects the liver. The majority of HCC cases occur in cirrhotic/fibrotic livers. Desmoplastic tumors include substantial intercellular interaction between cancer cells and activated, cancer-associated fibroblasts. According to this research, EVs can store and distribute miR to desmoplastic tumors in vivo. It is unclear how exactly activated liver fibroblasts and stellate cells contribute to the development of HCC. Signals produced by activated fibroblasts are conveyed by EVs and aid in developing HCC. Researchers showed that messenger RNA (mRNA) targets for miR-335 were down-regulated following treatment with EV-miR-335–5p. This research informed future HCC therapeutic strategies, such as loading therapeutic nucleic acids into stellate cell-derived EVs and delivering them in vivo [22].

The time between relapse and death is short for TNBC, a rapidly progressing cancer form. A tumor's enhanced aggressiveness, medication resistance, illness recurrence, and metastasis are all associated with stem cells inside the tumor. The roles of several stem cell markers, such as CD133, CD44, CD24, ABCG2, and ALDH1, in the carcinogenesis of breast cancer, remain uncertain. Anti-microRNA (anti-miRNA) has been administered via RNA nanotechnology for the treatment of TNBC. An RNA aptamer that coupled to the CD133 receptor and a locked nucleic acid (LNA) sequence that inhibited miRNA21 were both held in place by the three-way junction (3WJ) motif. The NPs were specifically taken up by TNBC cells and breast cancer stem cells (BCSCs), according to binding experiments. Functional experiments revealed that cancer cell movement was slowed down. The expression of miR21 was suppressed, while PTEN and PDCD4—two downstream tumor suppressors—were expressed more. Neither in vivo nor in vitro cytokine production was induced by these therapeutic RNA NPs. Systemic injection of these RNA NPs demonstrated great specificity in targeting TNBC tumors and effectiveness in inhibiting tumor development in an animal investigation. These results demonstrated the RNA NPs' therapeutic translation efficacy for TNBC treatment [23].

19.5.1.1 Photothermal Therapy

Novel nanophotosensitizers are still being sought for photothermal treatment (PTT). As potential nanophotosensitizers in PTT, Depciuch et al. created PtAu nanoraspberries (PtAu NRs) with a fancy form and non-agglomerated core/shell. Two colon cancer cell lines (SW620 and SW480) were exposed to laser irradiation in conjunction with PtAu NRs. Light microscopy images revealed observable alterations in the cell morphology. Raman and FTIR spectroscopies revealed that laser irradiation in the presence of PtAu NRs changed the chemical composition of the DNA, phospholipids, lipids, and protein structures. In the MTS experiment, PtAu NRs in the cell culture caused a 25% reduction in the viability of cancer cells. In contrast, 650 and 808 nm lasers caused 65% and 60% death of cancer cells, respectively, when paired with laser irradiation and NPs. The 650 and 808 nm lasers' observed photothermal conversion efficiency was 62% and 51%, respectively. PtAu NRs might be effective light absorbers in PTT anticancer therapy [24].

19.5.1.2 Photodynamic Therapy

In photodynamic therapy (PDT), hydrophobic photosensitizers must become more water soluble and aggregate more in tumor tissue in vivo. Designing novel drugs with non-toxic structures would be a successful strategy to accomplish these aims in terms of future commercialization or clinical use. By joining many chlorin e6 (Ce6) molecules into gelatin polymer, Son et al. developed two gelatin-Ce6 conjugates with various quantities of Ce6: gelatin-Ce6–2 and gelatin-Ce6–8. Compared to hydrophobic Ce6, the conjugates produced were more soluble in aqueous solutions. When exposed to laser radiation, the conjugates might generate singlet oxygen and kill tumor cells. After being intravenously injected into mice with the SCC-7 tumor, gelatin-Ce6–2 showed prolonged blood circulation and greatly enhanced accumulation in tumor tissue, as revealed in real-time imaging in vivo. Gelatin-Ce6–2 completely reduced tumor development and improved PDT following laser irradiation in contrast to free Ce6 and gelatin-Ce6–8. This work demonstrated that the stability and solubility of water might be significantly enhanced by a straightforward construction built of photosensitizer and gelatin. Gelatin-Ce6 demonstrated more significant tumor tissue aggregation and enhanced therapeutic effectiveness during in vivo PDT, demonstrating its significant clinical potential [25].

NP-based gene delivery methods offer a lot of promise. A lot of research has been done on superparamagnetic iron oxide nanoparticles (SPIONPs), which are theranostic due to their great biocompatibility and diagnostic capacity. The widespread usage of cationic coatings results in significant toxicity and prevents the technique from being applied in the clinic. Highly biocompatible, portable, and non-cationic SPION-based theranostic NPs were introduced by Unal et al. as innovative gene therapy agents. Developed for an autophagy inhibitory microRNA, MIR376B, Argonaute 2 (AGO2) protein-conjugated, anti-HER2 antibody-linked, and fluorophore-tagged SPIONPs (SP-AH NPs) were used. By selectively delivering sufficient amounts of microRNA into HER2-positive breast cancer cell lines in vitro and in a xenograft nude mouse model of breast cancer in vivo, these functionalized NPs efficiently prevented autophagy [26].

19.5.2 Neurological Disorders

By applying nanobiotechnologies to the nervous system, researchers can develop and administer drugs for CNS illnesses and better understand neurological problems. Nanobiotechnology will improve molecular detection of neurological diseases, making combining diagnostics and treatments into personalized medicine easier. The creation of logical therapeutics centered on the pathomechanisms of neurological illnesses is another approach that nanotechnologies will support customized neurology. NPs are now being used to deliver targeted drugs to the brain, which is vital in creating personalized treatments for neurological disorders [27].

The most frequent pediatric brain cancers are atypical teratoid/rhabdoid tumors (AT/RT) and medulloblastoma (MB). The present treatment, radiation, carries a significant danger to a child's growth before the age of three. Consequently, more effective therapeutic approaches are required. Although cancer gene therapy is a potential medical alternative, administering viruses to young kids carries risks. Choi et al. created a library of poly(beta-amino ester) (PBAE) NPs and employed herpes simplex virus type I thymidine kinase (HSVtk), which allowed transfected cells to undergo regulated apoptosis for administering a suicide gene therapy to pediatric brain cancer models through plasmid delivery. AT/RT and MB-implanted mice demonstrated greater median overall survival rates in the PBAE-HSVtk treated groups ($P = 0.0083$ vs. control and $P = 0.0001$ vs. control, respectively). The information demonstrated the viability of employing biodegradable PBAE NPs as a secure and efficient nanomedicine for treating pediatric CNS tumors [28].

19.5.3 Cardiovascular Disorders

Nanosystems that can diagnose a condition and treat it with specialized delivery systems will influence cardiovascular diagnostics in the future. Cardiovascular disease may be seen and drugs can be delivered to the target field simultaneously when perfluorocarbon NPs are used for controlled drug delivery and molecular imaging. Site-selective drugs and image-based therapies can assist in guaranteeing that medicine is acting on its intended target and having a molecular impact, both of which are necessary for individualized treatment [29].

Many people throughout the world suffer from cardiovascular diseases (CVDs), which are fatal. Innovative treatment strategies for treating various disorders have been made possible by nanotechnology-based drug delivery. However, in order to properly understand the causes and/ or mechanisms that affect care and create better therapies to battle CVD, a mix of diagnostic and therapeutic skills is still required. Biodegradable photoluminescent polylactones (BPLPLs), which have good cytocompatibility, strong, long-lasting intrinsic fluorescence, and biodegradability, potentially fill this gap. Kuriakose et al. developed three different BPLPL-based NPs, BPLP-co-poly (lactic-co-glycolic acid) copolymers with lactic acid and glycolic acid ratios of 50:50 (BPLPL-PLGA50:50), 75:25 (BPLPL-PLGA75:25), and BPLP-co-poly (L-lactic acid) (BPLPL-PLLA). The authors determined that both BPLPL-based NPs were acceptable since they were both 160 nm in size, exhibited photoluminescence properties, and had customizable encapsulated protein release kinetics based on polylactones copolymerized with BPLP materials. Over two days, BPLPL-PLGA NPs outperformed BPLPL-PLLA NPs in several formulations, including simulated bodily fluid, deionized water, serum, and saline. Human umbilical vein-derived endothelial cells exposed to BPLPL-based NPs accumulated in a dose-dependent manner in vitro. BPLPL-PLGA NPs showed higher viability compatibility with endothelial cells without impacting biological processes like nitric oxide production. All BPLPL NPs further demonstrated hemocompatibility with no impact on whole blood kinetic profiles and non-hemolytic platelet responses comparable to those of FDA-approved PLGA. According to research, BPLPL-PLGA-based NPs have better physical and biological features than BPLPL-PLLA-based NPs, suggesting they might be employed as functional nanocarriers for CVD treatment and diagnostics [30].

Cardiovascular and metabolic disease (CMD) is still the foremost cause of mortality worldwide. A lipid-lowering phytoconstituent with a wide range of metabolic-disorder-fighting properties, Berberine (BBR) is a hopeful candidate for treating CMD. Since BBR targets the liver, liver-site accumulation may be critical for the drug's therapeutic impact. For successful BBR liver deposition, an engineered micelle (CTA-Mic) containing α-tocopheryl hydrophobic core and polyethylene glycol (PEG)-thiol shell was developed. The biodistribution study showed that micelles increased BBR accumulation in the liver by 248.8%. Several energy-related genes are upregulated in HepG2 cells and in vivo experiments. The BBR-CTA-Mic intervention significantly enhanced metabolic profiles and decreased the development of aortic arch plaque in mice fed a high-fat diet. The findings demonstrated the feasibility of a liver-targeting strategy to treat CMD with natural drugs aided by nanotechnology [31].

19.6 CONCLUSION AND FUTURE PROSPECTS

Nanobiotechnology applications are starting to have an impact on traditional medicine. Compared to other high-tech items and considering the strict regulatory requirements of the medical business, new medical technology takes 10 to 15 years to reach the market. Many approved nanodrugs or nanodevices are predicted due to early 2000s expenditures in fundamental nanomedicine research. Drugs with increased effectiveness, tailored administration, and lower toxicity will be produced and administered thanks to nanotechnology. Despite significant advancements in understanding the molecules that make up the mitochondrial machinery, illnesses brought on by mitochondria malfunction still have no cure. The National Institutes of Health (NIH) financed nanomedicine research that made it simple to obtain cutting-edge nanodevices and nanosystems based on the logical design and exact integration of functional nanomaterials for clinical nanomedicine progress.

Applications of nanotechnology and nanobiotechnology will significantly impact medicine in the next decades. Possibilities include developing individualized medicines with no side effects and improving current and introducing new, minimally invasive treatment methods for previously incurable diseases. Early detection of diseases at the molecular level could be accomplished by inexpensive and simple rapid tests and highly accurate imaging techniques.

REFERENCES

1. Patil A, Mishra V, Thakur S, Riyaz B, Kaur A, Khursheed R, Patil K, Sathe B. Nanotechnology derived nanotools in biomedical perspectives: an update. *Current Nanoscience*. 2019;15(2):137–46.
2. Qi B, Wang C, Ding J, Tao W. Applications of nanobiotechnology in pharmacology. *Frontiers in Pharmacology*. 2019;10:1451.
3. Mappes T, Jahr N, Csaki A, Vogler N, Popp J, Fritzsche W. The invention of immersion ultramicroscopy in 1912—the birth of nanotechnology? *Angewandte Chemie International Edition*. 2012;51(45):11208–12.
4. Jain KK. Advances in the field of nanooncology. *BMC Medicine*. 2010;8(1):1.
5. Jain KK. *The hand book of nanomedicine*. 2008a. Humana Press, New York, NY.
6. Fatouros PP, Corwin FD, Chen ZJ, Broaddus WC, Tatum JL, Kettenmann B, Ge Z, Gibson HW, Russ JL, Leonard AP, Duchamp JC. In vitro and in vivo imaging studies of a new endohedral metallofullerene nanoparticle. *Radiology*. 2006;240(3):756–64.
7. Gao X, Yang L, Petros JA, Marshall FF, Simons JW, Nie S. In vivo molecular and cellular imaging with quantum dots. *Current Opinion in Biotechnology*. 2005;16(1):63–72.
8. Krukemeyer MG, Krenn V, Huebner F, Wagner W, Resch R. History and possible uses of nanomedicine based on nanoparticles and nanotechnological progress. *Journal of Nanomedicine and Nanotechnology*. 2015;6(6):336.
9. Jain KK. Nanomedicine: application of nanobiotechnology in medical practice. *Medical Principles and Practice*. 2008b;17(2):89–101.
10. Akin D, Sturgis J, Ragheb K, Sherman D, Burkholder K, Robinson JP, Bhunia AK, Mohammed S, Bashir R. Bacteria-mediated delivery of nanoparticles and cargo into cells. *Nature Nanotechnology*. 2007;2(7):441–9.
11. Jain KK. Role of nanobiotechnology in drug delivery. In *Drug delivery systems*. 2020 (pp. 55–73). Humana Press, New York, NY.
12. Seth A, Ritchie FK, Wibowo N, Lua LH, Middelberg AP. Non-carrier nanoparticles adjuvant modular protein vaccine in a particle-dependent manner. *PloS One*. 2015;10(3):e0117203.
13. Passi M, Shahid S, Chockalingam S, Sundar IK, Packirisamy G. Conventional and nanotechnology based approaches to combat chronic obstructive pulmonary disease: implications for chronic airway diseases. *International Journal of Nanomedicine*. 2020;15:3803.

14. Chowdhury EH. pH-sensitive nano-crystals of carbonate apatite for smart and cell-specific transgene delivery. *Expert Opinion on Drug Delivery*. 2007;4(3):193–6.

15. Ramakrishnan V, Xu B, Akers J, Nguyen T, Ma J, Dhawan S, Ning J, Mao Y, Hua W, Kokkoli E, Furnari F. Radiation-induced extracellular vesicle (EV) release of miR-603 promotes IGF1-mediated stem cell state in glioblastomas. *E Bio Medicine*. 2020;55:102736.

16. Liang G, Zhu Y, Ali DJ, Tian T, Xu H, Si K, Sun B, Chen B, Xiao Z. Engineered exosomes for targeted co-delivery of miR-21 inhibitor and chemotherapeutics to reverse drug resistance in colon cancer. *Journal of Nanobiotechnology*. 2020;18(1):1–5.

17. Gong C, Tian J, Wang Z, Gao Y, Wu X, Ding X, Qiang L, Li G, Han Z, Yuan Y, Gao S. Functional exosome-mediated co-delivery of doxorubicin and hydrophobically modified microRNA 159 for triple-negative breast cancer therapy. *Journal of Nanobiotechnology*. 2019;17(1):1–8.

18. Wang M, Wu B, Tucker JD, Shah SN, Lu P, Lu Q. Triazine-cored polymeric vectors for antisense oligonucleotide delivery in vitro and in vivo. *Journal of Nanobiotechnology*. 2020;18(1):1–4.

19. Zhang H, Wu J, Wu J, Fan Q, Zhou J, Wu J, Liu S, Zang J, Ye J, Xiao M, Tian T. Exosome-mediated targeted delivery of miR-210 for angiogenic therapy after cerebral ischemia in mice. *Journal of Nanobiotechnology*. 2019;17(1):1–3.

20. Odiba A, Ottah V, Ottah C, Anunobi O, Ukegbu C, Edeke A, Uroko R, Omeje K. Therapeutic nanomedicine surmounts the limitations of pharmacotherapy. *Open Medicine*. 2017;12(1):271–87.

21. Daniel MC, Astruc D. Gold nanoparticles: assembly, supramolecular chemistry, quantum-size-related properties, and applications toward biology, catalysis, and nanotechnology. *Chemical Reviews*. 2004;104(1):293–346.

22. Wang F, Li L, Piontek K, Sakaguchi M, Selaru FM. Exosome miR-335 as a novel therapeutic strategy in hepatocellular carcinoma. *Hepatology*. 2018;67(3):940–54.

23. Yin H, Xiong G, Guo S, Xu C, Xu R, Guo P, Shu D. Delivery of anti-miRNA for triple-negative breast cancer therapy using RNA nanoparticles targeting stem cell marker CD133. *Molecular Therapy*. 2019;27(7):1252–61.

24. Depciuch J, Stec M, Klebowski B, Baran J, Parlinska-Wojtan M. Platinum–gold nanoraspberries as effective photosensitizer in anticancer photothermal therapy. *Journal of Nanobiotechnology*. 2019;17(1):1–2.

25. Son J, Yi G, Kwak MH, Yang SM, Park JM, Lee BI, Choi MG, Koo H. Gelatin–chlorin e6 conjugate for in vivo photodynamic therapy. *Journal of Nnanobiotechnology*. 2019;17(1):50.

26. Unal O, Akkoc Y, Kocak M, Nalbat E, Dogan-Ekici AI, Yagci Acar H, Gozuacik D. Treatment of breast cancer with autophagy inhibitory microRNAs carried by AGO2- conjugated nanoparticles. *Journal of Nanobiotechnology*. 2020;18:1–8.

27. de Jong WH, Roszek B, Geertsma RE. Nanotechnology in medical applications: possible risks for human health. 2005.

28. Choi J, Rui Y, Kim J, Gorelick N, Wilson DR, Kozielski K, Mangraviti A, Sankey E, Brem H, Tyler B, Green JJ. Nonviral polymeric nanoparticles for gene therapy in pediatric CNS malignancies. *Nanomedicine: Nanotechnology, Biology and Medicine*. 2020;23:102115.

29. Engel E, Michiardi A, Navarro M, Lacroix D, Planell JA. Nanotechnology in regenerative medicine: the materials side. *Trends in Biotechnology*. 2008;26(1):39–47.

30. Kuriakose AE, Pandey N, Shan D, Banerjee S, Yang J, Nguyen KT. Characterization of photoluminescent polylactone-based nanoparticles for their applications in cardiovascular diseases. *Frontiers in Bioengineering and Biotechnology*. 2019;7:353.

31. Guo HH, Feng CL, Zhang WX, Luo ZG, Zhang HJ, Zhang TT, Ma C, Zhan Y, Li R, Wu S, Abliz Z. Liver-target nanotechnology facilitates berberine to ameliorate cardio-metabolic diseases. *Nature Communications*. 2019;10(1):1–6.

20 Gold Nanoparticles
Multifunctional Nanocarriers for Drug Delivery and Biomedical Application

Rajkumari Lodhi, Ekta Gurnany, Samir Bhargava, Rishi Paliwal, Chetan Ram, Gaurav Saraogi, and Satish Shilpi

20.1 INTRODUCTION

Gold nanoparticles (GNPs) are a new drug carrier composed of an inorganic gold core surrounded by an organic monomolecular layer. Gold (Au) nanoparticles have been studied as molecular imaging agents due to their bright NIR fluorescence emission in the 700–900 nm range and their low toxicity [1, 2]. These metallic nanoparticles emit size and composition based radiation of different wavelengths. Gold nanoparticles are non-corrosive and biocompatible so they are widely used for medical purposes in the fields of medicine and biology, and their applications [3, 4]. The variety of shape (spherical, rod like, star shape and others) of gold-based drug delivery carriers are used for drug delivery but spherical shaped GNPs is the most common. GNPs relatively have good stability and non-toxic [5–7]. In addition, GNP can be used in combination with a variety of drugs to detect most cancers and is widely used in treatment. These particles demonstrate versatility in clinical programs or applications.

Due to high stability and biocompatibility, GNPs have been in nanomedicines field. It was used to diagnosis and drug delivery. GNPs has several unique characteristics and used widely in biomedical fields such as cancer phototherapy, targeting of therapeutically active molecules, labeling, imaging and biosensing. The gold nanoparticles can be prepared in rod-shaped, shell and cage-like, star shaped and each has different physiochemical and optical properties. It is also available in the form of nanoclusters. It is also available in the form of a sphere with a cage called a gold nanocage and gold nanosphere also called gold nanoparticles (Figure 20.1). Table 20.1 lists remarkable features of GNPs in drug delivery.

GNP, also known as colloidal gold, which typically obtained with 1.0–100.0 in diameter range. The unique characters of gold nanoparticles which is useful in electronic devices, environmental monitoring, biomedical fields, electrochemical and immunological assays, biochemical sensors, food processing and security screening. Colloidal gold was recorded in the Middle Ages as a substance used in the treatment and diagnosis of illness. Gold compound, i. H. K [Au (CN)] was first studied as a bacteriostatic agent, after which the metal and its salts were eventually consumed in modern medicine. In recent decades, gold has been used to deliver medicine. It is used to induce hyperthermia through external application of near-infrared and laser light. BSPs are used in a variety of applications such as sensors, catalysis, decorative purposes and antibacterial activity. It is used as a catalyst for many organic chemical reactions.

DOI: 10.1201/9781003130055-20

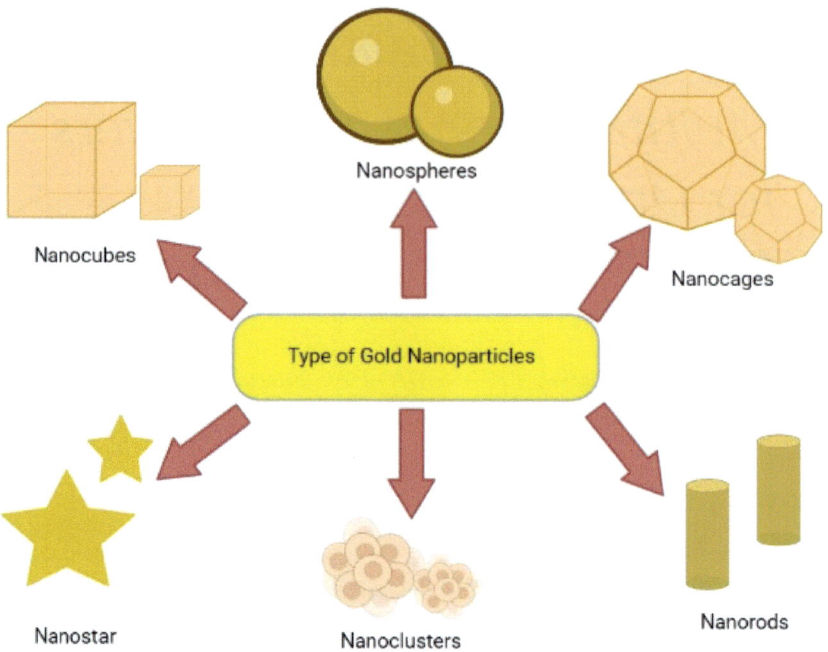

FIGURE 20.1 Types of different gold nanoparticles.

TABLE 20.1

GNPs Based Drug Delivery and Targeting.

Nanoparticles Type/ Modification	Therapeutic Molecules/ Active Drug	Purpose/Application	Reference
GNPs	DNAzyme	Dengue virus detection	Carter et al., 2013
GNPs	TNFα	Tumor targeting	Goel et al., 2009
GNPs	Doxorubicin	Target EphB4 receptors on tumor cell	You et al., 2013
Nitroreductase decorated GNPs	CB1954 prodrug	CB1954 anticancer pro-drug activity enhancement	Gwenin et al., 2011
Thiolated-PEG conjugated GNPs	Oxaliplatin, cisplatin, and carboplatin	Enhanced drug uptake in the lung and colon cancer cell lines	Brown et al., 2010
pH sensitive GNPs	Glycyrrhetinic acid	Tumor targeting	Tian et al., 2014
BSA conjugated GNPs	Methotrexate	Cancer cell targeting	Murawala et al., 2014

20.2 TYPES OF GOLD NANOPARTICLES

20.2.1 GOLD NANOROD

Gold nanorods shown anisotropic characters and it is because of the presence of vertical and horizontal Plasmon resonances excitation peaks. Longitudinal plasmon resonance can exhibit near-infrared absorption. It's often an essential consideration when utilizing for drug delivery. The gold nanorods showing short and log axis absorption band. As the rod length increases, then the vertical band due to the redshift is increase. This character of gold nano-rods is useful for cell imaging and photo thermal based cancer treatment [8].

20.2.2 Gold Nano Cage

Gold nanocage can be obtained with 45 nm of size that generates strong near-infrared which are beneficial for the tumor retardation [9]. It has porous sturdy walls structure with significant SPR near 810 nm [10]. It is a porous, and size of the pore can be control by varying the process and formulation variables or via a surrogate galvanic response between syncopated silver particles and aqueous solution of chloroauric acid (HAuCl4) (Grabtchak et al., 2015). It has maximum absorbance at 820 nm [11]. Its outer edge is about 50nm and inner boundary with 42 nm, wall consistency 4 nm when estimated with an electron microscope. The finite difference timeline system showed a substantial enhanced in the electromagnetic radiation of the multi version of GNCs when compared to monoversion of GNCs [12].

20.2.3 Gold Nanospheres and Microspheres

Gold particles are generally spherical and uniform in shape and size and can be used as a diagnostic agent and drug delivery as well as it make targetable by conjugating targeting ligands, antibodies or other targeting moiety. It can be obtained in the 2 to 250 nm diameter. Gold nanospheres are shown an absorption maximum in the visible range from 510 nm to 550 nm [13]. Due to the very high uniformity of shape and size, these nanospheres are scattered only once. Bright colors under a dark field microscope. The sharp light scattering character of gold particles makes suitable for tissue imaging.

20.2.4 Gold Nano Star

Gold Nanostars widely utilized in plasmonics, spectroscopy, medical field, and energy transformation [14]. They have unique features such as outstanding optical and physicochemical properties. Star-shaped GNP can be used for biosensing and bioimaging, photothermia, and targeted drug delivery. Due to their nontoxicity and high therapeutic load efficiency, they are utilized in the targeted drug delivery and imaging in the treatment of tumor-like diseases.

20.2.5 Gold Nanoclusters (AuNCs)

The NIR luminescence of BSA conjugated GNCs at 675 nm can be further increased by using cysteine and cupric ion (Cu2+). It increase the tissue imaging power of the gold nancarriers. BSA steadied gold nanoclusters supported cell and animal growth in comparison to plain BSA. Drug loaded gold nonocluster reported enhanced uptaken by tumor [9, 10]. Gold nanoclusters shown emission of fluorescent light make it appropriate for cell imaging and researchers focusing on this properties and utilized the same for diagnosis [15]. Ultra-small gold nanoclusters (AuNCs) are arising as implicit antibacterial agents and have drawn violent attention within the biomedical fields due to their excellent biocompatibility and weird physicochemical parcels. It was found in previous study that gold nanoclusters conjugated with glutathione bypass the RES uptake. It can be prepared for radiation therapy that shows the minimum tissue damage.

20.2.6 Synthesis of Gold Nanoparticles

20.2.6.1 Chemical Synthesis

Chemical Method: In this method the solution chemically reduced from gold ion to gold atom by using some suitable reducing agent and then followed by stabilization or capping process. The size can be controlled by different stabilizing agents and by some process variables such stirring/sonication speed and time. The method can provide <2 nm of spherical gold nanoparticles with controlled stabilizing process. Amino acid, sod. Citrate, ascorbic acid are used as a reducing agent to reduce the gold ions. This method is very simple and can produce gold nanoparticles in very short time.

Seeding Method: In this method the aqueous gold salt is transform and reduced to organic gold atom solution using tetraoctylammonium bromide and sodium borohydride. The stabilization of synthesized gold nanoparticles is carried out by alkanthiol. The brown color is indication of reaction and formation of nanoparticles. It provides spherical gold nanoparticles below 5nm in diameter. The ascorbic acid promotes the formation of gold nanoparticles and prevent the nucleation. This method can provide different sizes of rod shaped gold particles.

In this method seeding process is occur in which seeds particles is formed first by using a reducing agent to reduce the gold salt. Then the seed particles is then convert in gold salt in the presence of ascorbic acid.

Digestive Method: In this method the gold salt solution is heated at approx 140°C for two min and then reduce the temperature 110°C for five minutes in the presence of alkanthiol. It synthesized unidispersed nanoparticles.

20.2.6.2　Biological Synthesis

In this methods, the gold nanoparticles can be synthesized on living bacterial and fungal and plant cells. In the case of gold nanoparticles synthesis in bacterial cells, the ionic interaction between positive charge of gold ion and negative charge of cell wall of bacteria is occur which result in the formation gold nanoparticles. The intracellular and extracellular bacterial enzymes (NADPH-dependent enzymes) are responsible for the reduction of gold ion (Au^{3+}) to gold atom (Au^0). Similarly the biological synthesis of gold nanoparticles can be carried out using fungal cells. The variety of enzymes secreted and excreted intracellular and extracellular is responsible for the reduction of gold ion to atom for the formation of gold nanoparticles.

The gold nanoparticles can be synthesized using plant cells and its extract. It is very cost effective, fast and environment friendly. Phytonanotechnology has gained attention with time as it comprises an eco-friendly, cheap, and rapid process for the synthesis of nanoparticles. Every plant contain variety of active phytoconstituents such as alkaloids, flavonoids, glycosides, ascorbic acids, sterols etc. is responsible for reducing the gold ions into gold atom. The synthesis process of gold nanoparticles can be carried out within the plant and externally in the plant extract. Every part of the plant contain active constituent which can be used for the synthesis of gold nanoparticles. This method can provides different size of nanoparticles and it is depends upon the type of active constituent of different plants. It is found that from the literature this method can synthesized the gold nanoparticles in the range of 5–100nm in diamters in size range.

20.2.7　BIOMEDICAL APPLICATION OF GOLD NANOPARTICLES

GNPs are suitable for controlled and target drug delivery, anti-cancer, tissue imaging, diagnostics and many other reasons like excellent response to human being, low toxicity, adjustable stability, and ability to interact with a wide variety of substances. The nanotechnology are the result of formulation of delicate nanoparticles. Efficiently, metal nanoparticles are widely used under biomedical field.

20.2.8　GOLD NANOPARTICLES IN VIRUS DETECTION

It can utilize to detect the virus in living things. The best treatment for viral infections is the host's own immune system of the body. In other words, the first exclusion of viral infections is an alternative approach to treat infections.

Dengue virus detection: Dengue virus belongs to the flavivirus family and can affect more than one million population annually. Approximately 70% patient required special care in hospitals [15–17]. Most of peoples of tropical countries have risk for the dengue virus (DENV) infection. It is come under the category of world most dangerous viruses [17]. Carter et al., 2013 reported DNAzyme conjugated gold nanoparticles (AuNP) was efficiently utilized to identification of dengue virus [18].

Detection Human papillomavirus (HR-HPV): It is responsible to causes cervical cancer. It obtained in two different strain papilloma virus-16, and papilloma virus-18. DNA can be detect by Loop-mediated isothermal amplification (LAMP) [19]. It explore the utility of DNA attached GNPs for the detection of human papillomavirus (HPV-16, 18). AuNP mediated color change is the indication for the presence HPV16 and HPV18 strain of virus that was further compared with visual turbidity. The LAMP with the AuNP based colorimetric assay offers an easy and quick diagnostic tool for virus diagnosis.

20.2.9 GOLD NANOPARTICLES IN TREATMENT OF CANCER

Traditionally, surgery, chemotherapy, and radiation therapy are the main treatment approaches for the cancer that can precipitate with serious side effect. Some alternate approaches based on GNPs that can overcome the toxicity risk occur with conventional therapy. It includes the photothermia, photodynamic therapy and tumor targeting.

20.2.9.1 Photothermal Therapy

Photothermal therapy (PTT) is a potential treatment approach for the cancer treatment. After GNPs administration PTT need solar radiation to induce thermal energy that irradiate metastatic cancer cells. It also reduces the risk of metastatic. If this therapy is applied with chemotherapy, then it synergises the action of each other against cancer. Nam et al., 2008 prepared polydopamine-coated spiked gold nanoparticles shown enhanced physical stable that was applied against tumor which shown significant anti-tumor activity. It was reported that about 5,000 gold nanoshells per prostate adenocarcinoma cell required achieving killing. Khasid et al., 2015 developed PEGylated nanoshells shown NIR absorption peak that were administered via IV route in tumor bearing nude mice [20]. It was revealed significant tumor regression in comparison to without PEGylated nanoshells. Kashid et al. (2015) also reported that 93% tumor regression required 8.5 µL/g of nanoshells and below this concentration it retard the tumor progression [20, 21].

20.2.9.2 Photodynamic Therapy

Gold nanoparticles (GNPs) are being extensively examined in medical field due to its low toxicity and highly compatible with biological system. GNP is widely used in photodynamic therapy and provides a photosensitizer in the treatment of cancer [22]. Surface engineering of gold nanoparticles with photosensitizers and targeting ligands has been used to target receptors that are overexpressed in cancer cells. The initial use of GNP as a simple carrier of photosensitizers for PDT has evolved significantly to include the application of PEGylation modifications to impart stealth properties to the gold nanoparticles of the host body. Gold nanoparticles have been reported to induce oxygen-free radicals that can kill cancer cells. The functionalization of ligands that target gold nanoparticles allows them to target and target overexpressed receptors on cancer cells. In another study, gold nanoparticles bound to cannabidiol were used for photothermal treatment [23]. Radiation sensitization and effectiveness depends upon the quantity and retention time of gold nanomaterials in the biological system. In vivo biodistribution confirms that 12.1 and 27.3 nm PEG-coated gold nanoparticles (10 to 30nm in size range) were found uptaken by cancer cells and found [24].

20.2.10 TUMOR TARGETING BY GNPS

GNPs can be surface modify with targeting ligands for selective target to different part of tumor cells. This concept can minimize the toxicity and dose of chemotherapeutic agents. It can be used to transport drugs, nucleic acid materials, and other biomaterial or proteins. Peptide-bonded nanoparticles have been reported for the diagnosis and treatment of cancer. Here, a human-programmed Death Ligand 1 (PD-L1) peptide was used to surface-modify GNP and make GNP targetable. Multifunctional nanoparticles, i. H. Ce6-PD-L1 peptide-bonded gold nanoparticles using polyethylene glycol as the linker used for photothermal and photodynamic therapy imaging. In this study, the peptide PD-L1 was used as the targeting ligand. Both confocal imaging and flow cytometry experiments revealed an interesting affinity of the as-prepared nanoprobes GNPs @ PEG/Ce6-P for cancer cells (HCC827) showing high PD-L1 receptors expression. In vitro and in vivo studies have shown that the generated conjugates are useful tools for real-time visualization with PTT, PDT, and fluorescence and photoacoustic imaging [24, 25]. Gold nanoparticles as a drug delivery system are attracting more attention from researchers due to their high cellular uptake, biocompatibility, hydrophilicity, non-immunogenicity, and low toxicity [26, 27] Nanoparticles based drug targeting can beneficial with enhanced bioavailability and therapeutic effect and it can change the pharmacokinetic and pharmacodynamics parameters of targeted drug with less side effect [28–30].

20.2.11 GENE AND PROTEIN DELIVERY

Gold nanoparticles (GNPs) are non-toxic carriers and may be compatible with a variety of active pharmaceutical ingredients including monoclonal antibodies, genetic material and other protein and peptides for its administration to the body. Cellular delivery of recombinant genetic materials is come under the field of bioscience and *biotechnology*. There are so many techniques available for transfection of genetic material but still unmet need to develop a technique which can deliver gene efficiently to the target cells [31, 32]. DNA delivery is often mediated by viral and non-viral carriers. Viral carriers generally have excellent transfection properties. However, the difficulty of large-scale production of these agents and their immunogenicity has led to increased interest in the development of non-viral delivery systems [33]. Although various non-viral gene carriers have been developed, the basic understanding of the basic structure-activity relationships that determine the transfection efficiency of these systems is still limited [33, 34]. For example, in the case of PEI, some reports have shown that branched PEI is a less efficient carrier than linear PEI of the same molecular weight [35–37]. Sylvester et al., 2010 discussed different type urothelial and bladder cancer [38]. Intravesical therapy with adjuvant-decorated GNP is a selective adjuvant therapy that may be beneficial in the treatment of urothelial cancer. One study reports TNFα-inducible protein 8-like2 molecule used to sustain immune homeostasis which retard the growth of tumor. The over-expressed TIPE2 receptor on tumor cells was the target to block their functioning which revealed its role in TIPE2 in tumor progression. It was confirmed by retardation growth of 4T1 cancer [24]. They prepared a vector with small plasmid having TIPE2 receptor overexpression for targeting which inhibited the tumor growth significantly. In general, overexpression of TIPE2 enhanced the production of IFN-α and γ and CD8 + in T cells and NK cells while suppressing MDSC, and suppressed the metastasis of breast tumor.

20.2.12 DELIVERY OF THERAPEUTIC MOLECULES

The developments of therapeutically active genetic material have made significant progress for the treatment of canner and neurodegenerative disease. Drug delivery systems provide positive aspect for the delivery of free drug molecules by improving solubility, protection from biological environment, and its distribution in biological system. Other authors expected from delivery system include high encapsulation and an ideal release kinetic property for any active therapeutic molecule. They can also alter inauspicious pharmacokinetics of some "free" drugs. It can entrapped or large amount of therapeutic active molecules and can release it in controlled and sustained manner that maintain the therapeutic level in the body. Several studies have reported the use of GNPs as drug delivery vehicles because it has very high drug loading efficiency, for examples GNPs with

2.0 nm in size can coupled around 100 targeting. Farook et al., 2018 synthesized gold nanoparticles loaded with chemotherapeutic drugs doxorubicin and bleomycin [39]. The anticancer potential of this combinational therapy was carried out on HeLa cells. The passive tumor targeting is achieved by size depended EPR effect and it also uptaken actively due to its surface modification. This study reported that prepared bleomycin and doxorubicin capped gold nanoparticles blocked the cell cycle of the cancer cells. Kalimuthu et al., 2018 synthesized a peptide (P4) containing chlorambucil, melphalan or bendamustine which was further conjugate with gold nanoparticles with the help of PEG linker [40]. The prepared conjugate was revealed with significantly killed the A20 cancer cell invitro. It was also reported that the used peptide has only 10–15 min of biological half-life but when it conjugated on the gold nanoparticles then the half-life of the peptide increase to 22–24 hr and it worked actively in the biological system to 72 hr.

Huang et al., 2007 prepared tiopronin conjugated gold nanoparticles for effective targeting to breast tumor. In this study author examined the size depended penetration of prepared nanoparticles in the tumor environment and found that 2–6 nm of gold nanoparticles were found to penetrate efficiently whereas larger particles with average diameter of 15nm were found unable to penetrate deeply environment of the tumor cells [41]. Su et al., 2022 prepared M1 macrophage polarization specific polyaniline-glyco compound attached simultaneously with anti-apoptosis agent (PD-1) to the surface of gold nanoparticles and administered for the treatment of lung cancer and found that it induce the secretion of immunogenic cytokinin and create hot-cold tumor microenvironment responsible for T-cell activation which retard the growth of tumor significantly [42].

20.2.13 ENZYME IMMOBILIZATION AND DELIVERY

Nanoporous Gold (NPG) have potential to immobilize the enzymes. It bind or adsorbed the enzyme on its large surface in a very large amount [43]. GNP turned out to be a novel carrier suitable for enzyme immobilization. Doxorubicin-containing lysozyme-dextran nanogel loaded with biocompatible gold nanoparticles prepared using lysozyme-dextran nanogel as a reducing agent and stabilizer. GNPs with carboxyl-terminated thiol groups are functionalized by the binding of the enzyme glucose oxidase. NPGs prepared in various forms from alloys containing less than 50 atomic % gold by delegation [44]. The corresponding high surface area gold structure is manufactured using the template approach. Immobilization of the covalent enzyme is often achieved by forming a self-assembled monolayer on an NPG with terminal reactive functional groups, followed by binding to the enzyme via an amide bond to a lysine residue will be immobilized. The immobilized enzymes are not directly affected by environmental factors in comparison to free enzymes. The immobilized enzyme can be recover and reuse multiple times [45]. Table 20.2 lists immobilization techniques used with GNPs.

20.2.14 GOLD NANOPARTICLES IN IMAGING

Optical imaging is a foremost potential tools in biological research. Despite major advances, available biooptical imaging techniques are less sensitive or resolution power. Use of GNPs in conjuction with the available techniques can overcome the previous problem and improver the sensitivity in biological system [46–48]. Gold nanoparticles were shown better result to diagnose the ophthalmic associated issues. Although many ophthalmic diagnostic imaging methods are available, there are important unmet needs for ophthalmic molecular diagnostic imaging, especially for the first detection of disease before morphological changes become more apparent [48–52]. Gold nanoparticles (GNPs) have recently attracted attention as X-ray contrast agents due to their high X-ray attenuation, non-toxicity, simple in preparation, provide wide area to conjugate targeting ligands to make it site or cell specific drug delivery carrier and coating of some suitable protective agent such PEG and other polymer to make it non-immunogenic. It is a potential diagnostic agent because it can apply to moniterning the blood pumping and its flow pattern in the body. The active and passive targeting

TABLE 20.2

Application of Gold Nanoparticle in Enzyme Immobilization

Immobilization principle	Application	Reference
Adsorption on GNPs surface	Inversion of carbohydrates	Gomes-Ruffi et al., 2012
Enzyme bind covalently on GNPs	Enhanced activity of proteases, and oxidases	Huang et al., 2012 and Schuckel et al., 2011
Entrapped in liposomes	Enzyme-replacement	Rao et al., 2009
Immobilization of enzyme on polymeric nanoparticles	Control release for enzyme and replacement therapy	Soldatkin et al., 2010

TABLE 20.3

Gold Nanoparticles in Imaging

Biomarker/therapeutic molecules	Objectives	Imaging Methodology	Reference
Methylene blue	Analyze plasmon characters	Raman Spectroscopy	Laurent et al., 2005
Monoclonal antibody	Cells imaging	Raman Spectroscopy	Oyelere et al., 2000
Gadolinium chelates as in diethylene-triamine-penta-acetic-acid	Improvement in diagnosis and imaging property	MRI	Rajagopal et al., 2011
Antibodies conjugated Au-nanomaterials	Cells specific Imaging	CT Scan	Popovtzer et al., 2008
Di-thiolated-polyamino-carboxylate radiosubstances (99m)-Tc, (111)-In and gadolinium on gold particle surface.	bio-distribution behavior	MRI, X-Ray	Raghavender et al., 2011

of gold based nanomaterial can be monitored by using computer tomography. AuNP is also used as X-ray contrast agents within the critical structure-characteristics-functional relationship paradigm [46, 48, 53–62]. Perry et al., 2020 discussed the application of gadolinium chelates conjugated gold nanoparticles for MRI guided cell imaging [53]. Rajagopal et al., in 2011 prepared gadolinium chelates conjugated gold nanoparticle to improve MRI guided diagnosis [54]. The more specific cell imaging can be achieved by conjugating the monoclonal antibodies on the surface of gold nanomaterial. Popovtzer et al., 2008 conjugated monoclonal antibodies on the surface of the gold nanoparticles and the cell specific imaging was carried out by CT scan. It has theranostics properties. Theranostics is a character of a drug carrier system which has drug delivery as well as diagnostic properties simultaneously [55]. It can become targeted by attaching a ligand or targeting moiety in their surface. Silva et al., 2020 prepared such type of radiotheranostics targeted drug delivery carrier in which gold nanoparticles were loaded with bombesin. Bombesin has receptor specific activity it target the gastrin releasing peptide receptor (GRPr) which is generally overexpressed on the surface of cancer cells [56]. The carrier system is attached with ^{67}Ga/Gd radioactive substances that are responsible for imaging with MRI and Single Photon Emission Computed Tomography (SPECT) respectively. The prepared targeted radiotheranostics gold nanoparticles were revealed with good targeting, distribution and imaging properties simultaneously in tumor bearded mice model. It was found that prepared bombesin containing gold nanoparticles efficiently target the GRPr and have good diagnosing power. Significantly it target and block the GRPr in case of prostate cancer. Table 20.3 lists a few reports using GNPs in imaging applications.

20.2.15 CONSIDERATION OF TOXICITY OF GOLD NANOPARTICLES

Gold nanoparticles (GNPs) are biocompatible and more biologically active. Gold nanoparticles are known to be a safe material and have no toxic effects [56–58]. It was found that gold nanomaterials accumulated in many organs of rats [59–61]. The effectiveness and accumulation of gold nanomaterials depend upon size and duration of exposure [24, 63, 64].

20.2.16 CONCLUSION

Gold nanoparticles are biocompatible, non-toxic, multifunctional drug nanocarrier systems consisting of an inorganic gold core surrounded by an organic substances. It is utilized as molecular imaging agents and can emit radiation of different wavelengths depending on their size, shape and composition. The unique properties that colloidal gold depends on are widely used in the medical and biological fields such as cell and organ imaging, photothermal and photodynamic therapy for cancer, and antibacterial agents. They can come in a variety of shapes and sizes, including nanoclusters, spheres, stars, rods, and cubes, each with its own biomedical uses. They have high loading efficiency of therapeutic molecules and high surface engineering potential that can be used to target specific organs or cells in the body.

20.3 ACKNOWLEDGMENT

The authors would like to acknowledge the SERB-DST, New Delhi, and MP Council of Science and Technology, Bhopal, for providing research grant that promote the writing the chapter.

REFERENCES

1. Vosch, T., Antoku, Y., Hsiang, J. C., Richards, C. I., Gonzalez, J. I., Dickson, R. M. Strongly emissive individual DNA-encapsulated Ag nanoclusters as single-molecule fluorophores. *Proc Natl Acad Sci U S A* 2007, 104(31):12616–21.
2. Chithrani, B. D., Ghazani, A. A., Chan, W. C. Determining the size and shape ependence of gold nanoparticle uptake into mammalian cells. *Nano Lett* 2006, 6(4):662–8.
3. Martin, C. R. A membrane-based synthetic approach. *Science* 1994, 266(5193):1961–6.
4. Babak, N., El-Sayed, M. A. Preparation and growth mechanism of gold nanorods (NRs) using seed-mediated growth method. *Chem Matter* 2003, 15: 1957–62.
5. El-Sayed, I. H., Huang, X., El-Sayed, M. A. Selective laser photo-thermal therapy of epithelial carcinoma using anti-EGFR antibody conjugated gold nanoparticles. *Cancer Letters* 2006, 239(1):129–35.
6. Huisman, H. J., Fütterer, J. J., Van Lin, E. N. J. T. et al. Prostate cancer precision of integrating functional MR imaging with radiation therapy treatment by using fiducial gold markers. *Radiology* 2005, 236(1):311–7.
7. Ackerson, C. J., Sykes, M. T., Kornberg, R. D. Defined DNA/nanoparticle conjugates. 2005, 102(38):13383–5.
8. Stone, J., Stephen, J., David, W. Development of a biosensor for dengue virus using gold nanorods technology. *Wiley Interdiscip Rev Nanomed Nanobiotechnol* 2011, 3(1):100–9.
9. Chen, J., Chen, Q., Liang, C., Yang, Z., Zhang, L., Yi, X., Dong, Z., Chao, Y., Chen, Y., Liu, Z. Albumin-templated biomineralizing growth of composite nanoparticles as smart nano-theranostics for enhanced radiotherapy of tumors. *Nanoscale* 2017, 9:14826–35.
10. Chen, J., Saeki, F., Wiley, B. J., Cang, H., Cobb, M. J., Li, Z. Y., Au, L., Zhang, H., Kimmey, M. B., Li, X., Xia, Y. Gold nanocages bioconjugation and their potential use as optical imaging contrast agents. *Nano Lett* 2005, 5(3):473–7.

11. Song, K. H., Kim, C., Cobley, C. M., Xia, Y., Wang, L. V. Near-infrared gold nanocages as a new class of tracers for photoacoustic sentinel lymph node mapping on a rat model. *Nano Lett* 2009, 9(1):183–8.

12. Cai, W., Gao, T., Hong, H., Zun, J. Applications of gold nanoparticles in cancer nanotechnology. *Nanotechnol Sci Appl* 2008, 1:17–32.

13. Kao, H., Lin, Y., Chen, C. Evaluation of EGFR-targeted radioimmuno-gold-nanoparticles as a theranostic agent in a tumor animal model. *Bioorg Med Chem Letter* 2013, 23:3180–5.

14. Wenxin, N., Yi An Alvin, C., Weiqing, Z., Hejin, H., Xianmao Lu, J., Highly symmetric gold nanos tars crystallographic control and surface-enhanced raman scattering property. *Am Chem Soc* 2015 Aug 26, 137(33):10460–3.

15. Wu, X., He, X., Wang, K., Xie, C., Zhou, B., Qing, Z. Ultrasmall near-infrared gold nanoclusters for tumor fluorescence imaging in vivo. *Nanoscale* 2010, 2:2244–9.

16. Randolph, S. E., Rogers, D. J. The arrival, establishment and spread of exotic diseases: patterns and predictions. *Nat Rev Microbiol* 2010, 8:361–71.

17. Clyde, K., Kyle, J. L., Harris, E. Recent advances in deciphering viral and host determinants of dengue virus replication and pathogenesis. *J Virol* 2006, 80:11418–31.

18. Carter, J. R., Balaraman, V., Kucharski, C. A. et al. A novel dengue virus detection method that couples DNAzyme and gold nanoparticle approaches. *Virol J* 2013, 10:201.

19. Kumvongpin, R., Jearanaikool, P., Wilailuckana, C., Sae-Ung, N., Prasongdee, P., Daduang, S., Wongsena, M., Boonsiri, P., Kiatpathomchai, W., Swangvaree, S. S., Sandee, A., Daduang, J. High sensitivity, loop-mediated isothermal amplification combined with colorimetric gold-nanoparticle probes for visual detection of high risk human papillomavirus genotypes 16 and 18. *J Virol Methods* 2016, 234:90–5.

20. Kashid, S. B., Tak, R. D., Raut, R. W. Antibody tagged gold nanoparticles as scattering probes for the pico molar detection of the proteins in blood serum using nanoparticle tracking analyzer. *Colloids Surf B Biointerfaces* 2015, 133:208–13.

21. Grabtchak, S., Montgomery, L. G., Pang. B., Wang, Y., Zhang, C., Li, Z., Xia. Y., Whelan, W. M. Interstitial diffuse radiance spectroscopy of gold nanocages and nanorods in bulk muscle tissues. *Int J Nanomedicine* 2015, 10:1307–20.

22. Calavia, P. G., Bruce, G., Pérez-García, L., Russell, D. A. Photosensitiser-gold nanoparticle conjugates for photodynamic therapy of cancer. *Photochem Photobiol Sci* 2018, 17:1534–52.

23. Mokoena, D., George, B. P., Abrahamse, H. Conjugation of hypericin to gold nanoparticles for enhancement of photodynamic therapy in MCF-7 breast cancer cells. *Pharmaceutics* 2022 Oct 18, 14(10):2212.

24. Zhang, X. D., Wu, D., Shen, X., Chen, J., Sun, Y. M., Liu, P. X., Liang, X. J. Size-dependent radiosensitization of PEG-coated gold nanoparticles for cancer radiation therapy. *Biomaterials* 2012, 33(27):6408–19.

25. Liu, W. W., Li, P. C. Photoacoustic imaging of cells in a three-dimensional microenvironment. *J Biomed Sci* 2020, 27:3.

26. Astruc, D., Boisselier, E., Ornelas, C. Dendrimers designed for functions from physical photophysical and supramolecular properties to applications in sensing catalysis molecular electronics photonics and nanomedicine. *Chem Rev* 2010, 110(4):1857–959.

27. Davis, M. E., Chen, Z., Shin, D. M. Nanoparticle therapeutics: an emerging treatment modality for cancer. *Nat Rev Drug Discov* 2008, 7(9):771–82.

28. Xu, P., VanKirk, E. A., Zhan, Y., Murdoch, W. J., Radosz, M., Shen, Y. Targeted charge-reversal nanoparticles for nuclear drug delivery. *Angew Chem Int* 2007, 46(26):4999–5002.

29. Langer, R., Tirrell, D. A. Designing materials for biology and medicine. *Nature* 2004, 428(6982):487–92.

30. Allen, T. M., Cullis, P. R. Drug delivery systems entering the mainstream. *Science* 2004, 303(5665):1818–22.

31. Neumann, E., Schaefer-Ridder, M., Wang, Y., Hofschneider, P. H. Gene transfer into mouse lyoma cells by electroporation in high electric fields. *EMBO J* 1982, 1(7):841–5.

32. Kaczmarczyk, S. J., Sitaraman, K., Young, H. A., Hughes, S. H., Chatterjee, D. K. Protein delivery using engineered virus-like particles. *Proc Natl Acad Sci USA* 2011, 108(41):16998–7003.

33. Pack, D. W., Hoffman, A. S., Pun, S., Stayton, P. S. Design and development of poly-mers for gene delivery. *Nat Rev Drug Discov* 2005, 4:581–93.

34. Wong, S. Y., Sood, N., Putnam, D. Combinatorial evaluation of cations, pH-sensitive and hydrophobic moieties for polymeric vector design. *Mol Ther* 2009, 17:480–90.

35. Jeong, G. J., Byun, H. M., Kim, J. M., Yoon, H., Choi, H. G. Bio distribution and tissue expression kinetics of plasmid DNA complexed with polyethylenimines of different molecular weight and structure. *Control Release* 2007, 118:118–25.

36. Bragonzi, A., Boletta, A., Biffi, A. et al. Comparison between cationic polymers and lipids in mediating systemic gene delivery to the lungs. *Gene Ther* 1999, 6:1995–2004.

37. Wightman, L., Kircheis, R., Rössler, V. et al. Different behavior of branched and linear polyethylenimine for gene delivery in vitro and in vivo. *Gene Med* 2001, 3:362–72.

38. Sylvester, R. J., Brausi, M. A., Kirkels, W. J. Long-term efficacy results of EORTC genito-urinary group randomized phase 3 study 30911 comparing intravesical instillations of epirubicin, bacillus Calmette-Guerin, and bacillus Calmette-Guerin plus isoniazid in patients with intermediate- and high-risk stage Ta T1 urothelial carcinoma of the bladder. *Eur Urol* 2010, 57(5):766–73.

39. Farooq, M. U., Novosad, V., Rozhkova, E. A. et al. Retracted article: gold nanoparticles-enabled efficient dual delivery of anticancer therapeutics to HeLa cells. *Sci Rep* 2018, 8:2907.

40. Kalimuthu, K., Lubin, B. C., Bazylevich, A. et al. Gold nanoparticles stabilize peptide-drug-conjugates for sustained targeted drug delivery to cancer cells. *J Nanobiotechnol* 2018, 16:34.

41. Huang, X., Jain, P. K., El-Sayed, I. H., El-Sayed, M. A. Gold nanoparticles: interesting optical properties and recent applications in cancer diagnostics and therapy. *Nanomedicine (Lond)* 2007, 2(5):681–93.

42. Su, W. P., Chang, L. C., Song, W. H., Yang, L. X., Wang, L. C., Chia, Z. C., Chin, Y. C., Shan, Y. S., Huang, C. C., Yeh, C. S. Polyaniline-based glyco-condensation on Au nanoparticles enhances immunotherapy in lung cancer. *ACS Appl Mater Interfaces* 2022, 14(21):24144–59.

43. Stine, K. J., Jefferson, K., Shulga, O. V. Nanoporous gold for enzyme immobilization. *Methods Mol Biol* 2017, 1504:37–60.

44. Cai, W., Gao, T., Hong, H., Sun, J. Applications of gold nanoparticles in cancer nanotechnology. *Nanotechnol Sci Appl* 2008, 1:17–32.

45. Homaei, A. A., Sariri, R., Vianello, F., Stevanato, R. Enzyme immobilization: an update. *J Chem Biol* 2013, 6(4):185–205.

46. Wu, H. L., Tsai, H. R., Hung, Y. T. et al. A comparative study of gold nanocubes, octahedra, and rhombic dodecahedra as highly sensitive SERS substrates. *Inorg Chem* 2011, 50(17):8106–11.

47. Shilpi, S., Khatri, K. Gold nanoparticles as carrier (s) for drug targeting and imaging. *Pharm Nanotechnol* 2015, 3(3):154–70.

48. Shilpi, S., Jain, A., Gupta, Y., Jain, S. K. Colloidosomes: an emerging vesicular system in drug delivery. *Crit Rev™ Ther Drug Carr Syst* 2007, 24(4):361–91.

49. Schcukel, J., Matura, A., Van Pee, K. H. One-copper laccase-related enzyme from Marasmius sp. purification, characterization and bleaching of textile dyes. *Enzyme Microb Technol* 2011, 48(3):278–84.

50. Murawala, P., Tirmale, A., Shiras, A., Prasad, B. L. V. In situ synthesized BSA capped gold nanoparticles Effective carrier of anticancer drug Methotrexate to MCF-7 breast cancer cells. *Mater Sci Eng* 2014, 34:158–67.

51. Onaciu, A., Braicu, C., Zimta, A.-A. et al. Gold nanorods from anisotropy to opportunity an evolution update. *Nanomed (Lond)* 2019, 14(9):1203–26.

52. Bin, L., Guanglei, Q., Yu, H. E. et al. Targeted theranostics of lung cancer: PD-L1-guided delivery of gold nanoprisms with chlorin for enhanced imaging and photothermal/photodynamic therapy. *Acta Biomater* 2020, 117:361–73.

53. Perry, H. L., Botnar, R. M., Wilton-Ely, J. D. E. T. Gold nanomaterials functionalised with gadolinium chelates and their application in multimodal imaging and therapy. *Chem Commun (Camb)* 2020, 56(29):4037–46.

54. Rajagopal, A., Aravinda, S., Raghothama, S., Shamala, N., Balaram, P. Chain length effects on helix-hairpin distribution in short peptides with Aid-DAla and Aib-Aib segments. *Biopolymers (Pept Sci)* 2011, 96:744–56.

55. Popovtzer, R., Agrawal, A., Kotov, N. A., Popovtzer, A., Balter, J., Carey, T. E., Kopelman, R. Targeted gold nanoparticles enable molecular CT imaging of cancer. *Nano Lett* 2008, 8(12):4593–6.

56. Silva, F., Paulo, A., Pallier, A. et al., Dual imaging gold nanoplatforms for targeted radiotheranostics. *Materials (Basel)* 2020, 13(3):513.

57. Abdelhalim, M. A. K., Moussa, S. A. A. The gold nanoparticle size and exposure duration effect on the liver and kidney function of rats in vivo. *Saudi J Biol Sci* 2013, 20:177–81.

58. Pourali, P., Badiee, S. H., Manafi, S., Noorani, T., Rezaei, A., Yahyaei, B. Biosynthesis of gold nanoparticles by two bacterial and fungal strains, Bacillus cereus and Fusarium oxysporum, and assessment and comparison of their nanotoxicity in vitro by direct and indirect assays. *Electron J Biotechnol* 2017, 29:86–93.

59. Abdelhalim, M. A. K., Jarrar, B. M. Gold nanoparticles administration induced prominent inflammatory, central vein intima disruption, fatty change and Kupffer cells hyperplasia. *Lipids Health Dis* 2011a, 10:133.

60. Abdelhalim, M. A. K., Jarrar, B. M. Gold nanoparticles induced cloudy swelling to hydropic degeneration, cytoplasmic hyaline vacuolation, polymorphism, binucleation, karyopyknosis, karyolysis, karyorrhexis and necrosis in the liver. *Lipids Health Dis* 2011b, 10:166.

61. Abdelhalim, M. A. K., Jarrar, B. M. Renal tissue alterations were size-dependent with smaller ones induced more effects and related with time exposure of gold nanoparticles. *Lipids Health Dis* 2011c, 10:163.

62. Mohamed Shehata, D., Hadi, S. Applications of gold nanoparticles in virus detection. *Theranostics* 2018 Feb 15, 8(7):1985–2017.

63. Darweesh, R. S., Ayoub, N. M., Nazzal, S. Gold nanoparticles and angiogenesis: molecular mechanisms and biomedical applications. *Int J Nanomedicine* 2019, 14:7643–63.

64. Kashid, S. B., Tak, R. D., Raut, R. W. Antibody tagged gold nanoparticles as scattering probes for the pico molar detection of the proteins in blood serum using nanoparticle tracking analyzer. *Colloids Surf B Biointerfaces* 2015, 133:208–13.

21 Nanoparticles for Controlled Delivery of Proteins and Peptides

Raghuraj Singh, Krishna Yadav, Eupa Ray,
Kalpesh Vaghasiya, and Rahul Kumar Verma

21.1 INTRODUCTION

The multidisciplinary field of engineered drug delivery systems, that combines materials engineering, biology and medicine, is a mounting research field dealing with the engineering of materials at different level for controlled and targeting based treatments. The final aim of Pharmaceutical formulator is to design successful cost effective dosage forms for safe and effective therapy, allowing for individual patient requirements and compliance[1]. With the recent development in biotechnology, a huge number of novel proteins and peptides produced are design protein delivery an important area of pharmaceutical research. In recent times, with the development of nanotechnology and polymer science, materials can be manipulated at an atomic level, and more sophisticated drug delivery systems can be developed to overcome the limitations associated with conventional delivery of proteins and peptides[2,3]. Proteins and peptides are most effective therapeutics that have been widely considered as efficient therapeutic agents for the treatment of different types diseases such as cancer, metabolic disorders (diabetes), autoimmune disorders like rheumatoid arthritis (RA), anemia, hemophilia, hepatitis C virus infection, Gaucher's disease and so on[4]. Protein and peptide have numerous advantages like higher specificity and affinity to target with low toxicity as compare to small chemical drugs molecule. On the other hand, both protein and peptide are unstable and easily degraded inside the body while administered, which leads to the low bioavailability[5].

The use of NPs as a delivery system facilitates transportation to exist accelerated to the site of action, decreased side effects and prolonged occurrence in the body. Due to multi-functionality, NPs protects the proteins and peptides from rapid breakdown or clearance, and enhanced the concentration at particular site, in that way lowering the dosage and frequency of the therapeutic agents. Therapeutic molecules such as protein and peptides might be located inside or sometimes attached on the surface of NPs. The use of NPs in proteins and peptides transportation allows the release of conjugate into specific site by active or passive transport mechanism. The release of the drug from the NPs depends on the physiochemical properties of polymeric materials and the mechanism used for the construction of NPs, because several polymers that have been used in the construction of NPs respond on the physiological changes in the local environment, such as pH, temperature, osmolality, and enzymatic level or reaction[6,7]. NPs used to improve both therapeutic as well as pharmacological properties of proteins and peptides. The use of NPs as the delivery system might improve the administration and effectiveness of therapeutic proteins and peptides because of their small in size, NPs are able to cross different biological barriers such as the blood-brain barrier (BBB) and act at the cellular level[8].

The various nanotechnology-based delivery systems that can protect the proteins and peptides from enzymatic degradation, improve permeation through the epithelial cells. The other challenge for the formulation scientists is designing and developing of NPs delivery systems that can attain three key objectives, viz. Multirate or pulsatile delivery, self-regulated mechanism and site specific controlled or targeted delivery proteins and peptides[9].

The different routes of administration for the delivery of proteins and peptides including oral, nasal, pulmonary, transdermal (TD), and intravenous (IV), subcutaneous (SC) are available, but still protein and peptides therapeutic delivery is an challenging due to their several hostile properties including large molecular weight, short biological half-life, sensitivity to enzymatic degradation, immunogenicity, propensity to undergo aggregation, adsorption, denaturation, reticuloendothelial system (RES) uptake, ion permeability, and accumulation in healthy organs and tissues[10,11]. In addition to this, both manufacturing as well as environmental factors may also lead to denaturation of protein and peptides, decrease their biological activity, render the proteins immunogenic, precipitation and induce aggregation of protein and peptides. Therefore, development effective engineered nano-formulations of therapeutic proteins and peptide are essential to overcome these problems and improving bioavailability as well as patient compliance[12,13.]

21.2 PROTEINS AND PEPTIDES

Protein and peptide are biopolymers of amino acids sequence, involve in broad range of biological activity. The peptide is a low molecular weight compound may have molecular weight less than 5000 whereas protein is a high molecular weight compound having molecular weight more than 10,000 and the categories between the proteins and peptides which have molecular weights between5,000 to 10,000 are known as polypeptides[14,15]. These are the important molecules for life and they are having fundamental roles in approximately all biochemical processes in the body16. Both Proteins as well as peptides having a broad range of functions including catalysis of reactions, signal transduction, regulation of gene expression, transportation, immune related functions and also involved in different pathological conditions such as hypertension, diabetes, and cancer and so on[17].

The molecular sizes of proteins and peptides therapeutics are larger than those in traditional therapeutic agents, and proteins have primary, secondary and tertiary structures, which make them extremely liable to physicochemical degradation. Molecular weight and size of proteins and peptides significantly influence the diffusion through the epithelial layer. Several research studies have investigated the effects of molecular weight and size upon the gastrointestinal absorption of various hydrophilic therapeutic compounds. Normally, therapeutic proteins are referred to as globular proteins because they are of almost spherical shape in solution. Proteins have different levels of structure which are generally referred as the primary, secondary, tertiary, and quaternary structures[18,19].

21.2.1 STRUCTURE OF PROTEINS AND PEPTIDES

The idea about proteins and peptides structure is most important in order to minimize the different problems arrived during development of novel controlled drug delivery system[15]. The molecules composed of 50 or more amino acids called protein and molecules contain less than 20 amino acids known as peptide[20]. Between the proteins and peptides, polypeptides are categories which contain about 20 to 50 amino acids. In the polymeric structure of proteins and peptides, amino acids connected together via amide linkages known as peptide bonds[21] (Figure 21.1).

21.2.1.1 Primary Structure

The primary structure of proteins denotes the specific sequence and number of amino acids which are covalently bonded in the protein structure. The primary structure of proteins started from the amino terminal to carboxyl terminal end. In DNA molecules, the primary structure of proteins is determined by sequence of nucleotides.

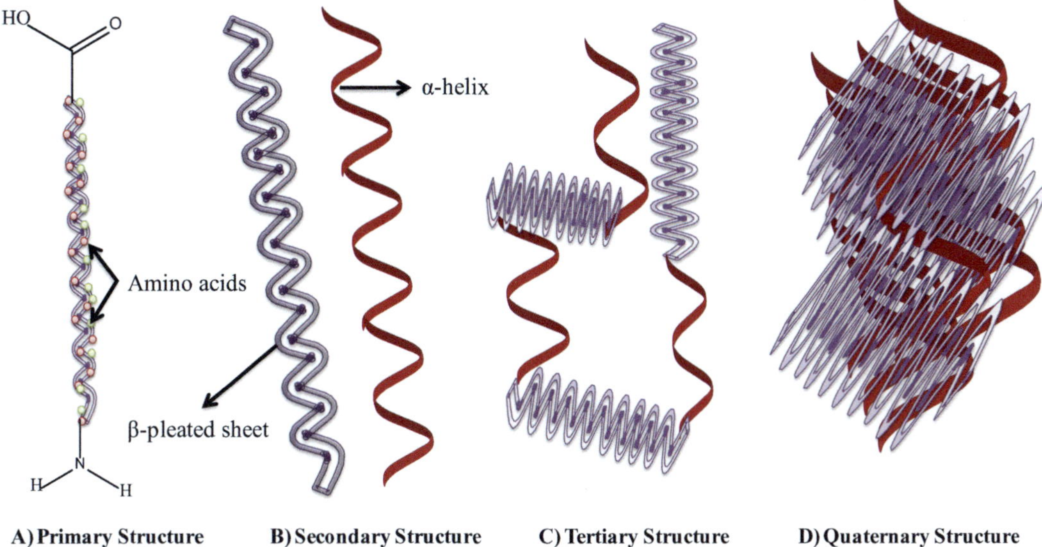

FIGURE 21.1 Structure of proteins and peptides.

21.2.1.2 Secondary Structure

The secondary structure denotes the arrangement of individual amino acids along with the polypeptide backbone in the protein structure. The α-helix and β-pleated sheet are most common types of secondary structures. The loops and turns of the polypeptide chain comprise the secondary structure. The alpha helices and beta sheets are the ordinary conformations of secondary structure, through the rest individual small loops, β-bends and random coils. The different bends such as hairpin bends, β-bends are connected anti-parallel β-strands which are important to maintain the globular shape of proteins. In the secondary structure of proteins these elements help to neutralize its polar atoms through hydrogen bonding.

21.2.1.3 Tertiary Structure

The tertiary structure denotes the three dimensional arrangement of a single protein molecule in the structure and quaternary structure denotes the proteins that contain two or more than two polypeptide chains linked by non-covalent bonds. Disulfide bonds one of the special types of covalent bond which contribute into the tertiary structure of proteins. These covalent linkages are much stronger as compare to other types of linkages between the sulfur containing side chains of cysteines which contribute to tertiary structure of proteins[22–24].

21.2.1.4 Quaternary Structure

Numerous proteins are composed of a single polypeptide chain and having only three different levels of structure. On the other hand, some proteins are composed of several polypeptide chains known as subunits. While these subunits join together, they provide the protein structure called quaternary structure. One of the best examples of a protein quaternary structure is hemoglobin that has quaternary structure.

21.2.2 THERAPEUTIC APPLICATION OF PROTEINS AND PEPTIDES

Peptide and protein therapeutics classified as bio-pharmaceuticals or bio-drugs, encompass an growing share of pharmaceutical market. Both proteins as well as peptides have an important and rapidly increasing role as therapeutic medicines, due to their specificity, high affinity and low toxicity[25]. Proteins and peptides are biological therapeutic agent that has been used for the treatment of a wide range of diseases such as cancer, metabolic disorders (diabetes), autoimmune disorders (RA), anemia, hemophilia, Gaucher's disease etc., but numerous others under in clinical development[26]. The most commonly marketed protein and peptide based pharmaceuticals comprises different monoclonal antibody products for the treatment and/or managements of different types of autoimmune diseases and cancer, therapeutic vaccines for hepatitis A and B treatments, insulin for the treatment of diabetes, growth hormone for hormone deficiency, and interferon for hepatitis B and C treatment (Figure 21.2).

21.2.3 Issues Related with the Delivery Proteins and Peptides

In this decades proteins and peptides emerges out as versatile medicine with low potency and low toxicity because these are endogenous compound which regulate many physiological process in the body. The proteins and peptides such as insulin, growth hormones, monoclonal antibodies and oligopeptides have wide market application for different ailments. But still shortcoming are associated in terms of delivery and disposition, henceforth protein and peptides are available in parenteral injection delivery due to their GI instability, poor permeability (hydrophilicity and high molecular mass) and extensive biotransformation subsequently leads to low oral bioavailability[27]. The physicochemical properties of protein and peptides such as large size, surface charge and susceptibility

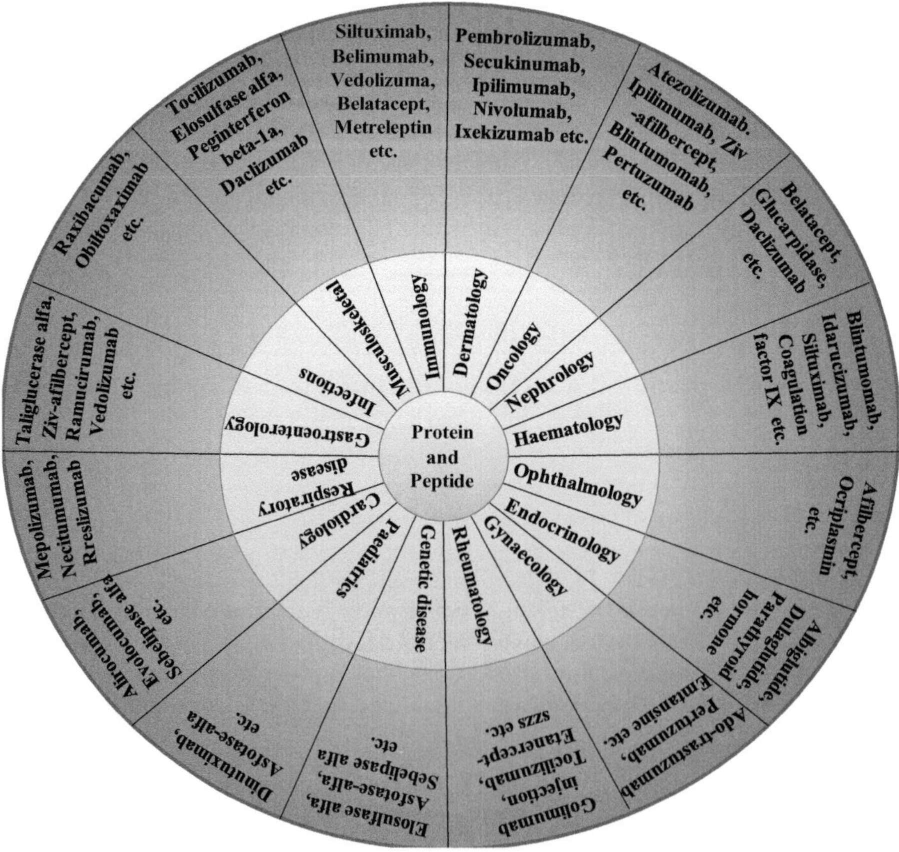

FIGURE 21.2 Therapeutic application of FDA approved bio-pharmaceuticals.

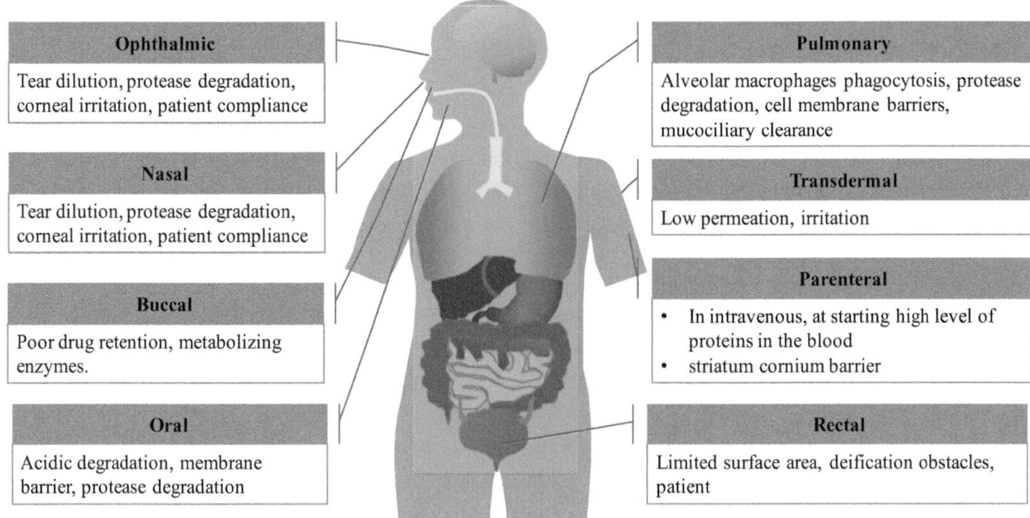

FIGURE 21.3 Barriers for delivery of protein and peptides.

to enzymatic degradation have wide impact on selection of key delivery vehicle for administration. Generally molecular mass less than 500 Da are easily accessible for GI absorption and skin by passive diffusion. Owing to large size needed active diffusion using carrier mediated transport or endocytosis through transmembrane. Hydrophilicity is another features affecting cellular entry of protein and peptides. Surface charge formed by isomerization, deamination, post-translation modification and surrounding pH may compromise absorption property28 (Figure 21.3).

This surface charge on protein leads to interaction with different molecule on membrane or tissue components, thus altering ADME of therapeutic proteins. Moreover, proteins are also prone to physicochemical and enzymatic degradation in the lifecycle of products. There are some biological barrier which are affecting stability and absorption particularly, different pH conditions, enzymatic barrier and mucosal barrier. Proteins are unstable in stomach acidic conditions and high pH condition in ileum or colon causes destabilization. Enzymatic barrier includes destabilization of protein in the gastrointestinal (GI) tract by pepsin and proteases are highly active in the intestine. The proteolytic effect in colon is relatively lower, hence this create opportunity to targeted delivery to colon. All Mucosal epithelia covered with mucus, which form protective layer which form physical barrier for diffusion of large molecules[29,30].

21.3 APPROACHES/METHODS TO ENHANCE PROTEINS AND PEPTIDES DELIVERY

There are numerous biological and bio-pharmaceutical obstructions including physical, chemical and enzymatic destabilization of proteins and peptides, which limits their effective delivery at the site of action. Accordingly, effective formulations of proteins and peptides are required to overcome these different physical, chemical and biological obstacles. The different strategies are reported by several researchers for improving the drug delivery and systemic bioavailability of protein and peptides includes enzymatic inhibition, chemical modification, surface modification, mucus adhesion systems, absorption enhancers, and NPs based approach. NPs based approaches are more effective because of small size, improved surface area, invasive and non-invasive delivery of protein and peptides NPs. In addition to this NPs help to overcome many of the barriers including enzymatic degradation, gastric destabilization and poor permeability through biological membrane.

21.3.1 Parenteral Delivery

Parenteral route is the invasive method for delivery of proteins and peptides therapeutics. NPs may protect bio-therapeutics from degradation, increase *in-vivo* half life and provide extended drug release. However, different researchers developed polymeric NPs for parenteral drug delivery of bio-therapeutics. A number of targeted and controlled release injectable NPs based delivery systems have been investigated for proteins and peptides delivery at particular site, optimum therapeutic concentration, at a desired rate which reduces side effects. These systems include SLN, liposomes, nanospheres, dendrimers and polymeric NPs are being widely estimated for their targeted and controlled delivery of proteins and peptides via parenteral route[31]. The development of nanotechnology based formulation for therapeutic proteins and peptides, depends on the biophysiochemical and physiological characteristics of proteins and peptides molecules, including their molecular weight, immunogenicity, biological half-life, stability, dose requirement, site, rate of administration, and pharmacokinetic as well as pharmacodynamic behavior. Most commonly used polymers for the development of parenteral NPs includes PLGA, PLA, poly(methyl methacrylates), polycaprolactone (PCL), albumin, alginate, and chitosan. The surface modification of NPs such as PEGylation was done by several researchers to achieve long-term systemic circulation, site-specific delivery and controlled release of proteins and peptides therapeutics[32]. Glowka and co-workers developed salmon calcitonin (sCT) loaded PLGA NPs and found sCT loaded PLGA NPs have high bioavailability and sustained drug release as compared to sCT solution[33].

21.3.2 Oral Delivery

Oral delivery is characteristically most preferred way of administration for proteins and peptides due to better patient compliance and cost effective as compared to parental delivery. The oral formulations development for proteins and peptides presents a complicated challenge due to numerous barriers such as enzymatic barriers, pH of biological fluids, mucosal barriers and many others including first pass metabolism and these challenges can overcome by nanotechnology based NPs approaches[34]. A variety of NPs have been investigated as potential nano-carriers for oral delivery of proteins and peptides due to non-immunogenic and biocompatible. Because of NPs improve the physical and chemical stability of peptides and proteins therapeutic in the gastrointestinal tract by incorporating peptides and proteins into the polymeric matrix structure of NPs. A variety of natural, synthetic and smart modified polymers such as poly (lactic-co-glycolic acid) (PLGA), poly (lactic acid) (PLA), poly-methyl-methacrylates, chitosan, and gelatin, are the most extensively used for the development of NPs. Chitosan is most widely used polymers due to high biocompatibility, enhances cellular uptake, mucoadhesion, and low toxicity which make it a most suitable candidate as proteins and peptides delivery polymeric carriers[35,36]. Mukhopadhyay and co-workers developed and evaluated the self-assembled insulin loaded chitosan NPs for successful oral delivery with spherical shapes, high encapsulation efficiency and average particle size range from 200–550 nm. After oral administration of insulin loaded chitosan NPs in diabetic mice, blood glucose level were significantly decreased and suggesting that chitosan NPs have enormous potential as oral carriers for proteins and peptides delivery[34].

21.3.3 Pulmonary Delivery

Pulmonary route is clinically accepted way to deliver protein and peptides bio-therapeutic compared with other routes due to large surface area (around 80–140 m^2), high blood supply and especially thin alveolar thickness (approximately 0.1–0.5 mm) of epithelium which allow fastest and higher absorption of bio-therapeutic. Pulmonary delivery of bio-therapeutic is beneficial because its bypass the hepatic first-pass metabolism, effective at lower doses, non-invasive and applicable for both local as well as systemic delivery. Generally proteins and peptides with 6000 to 50,000 D in molecular weights have excellent bioavailability and following inhalation. This route is easily targeted with 5 μm mean aerodynamic mass diameter through aerosol delivery or devices such as ultrasonic nebulizers, jet nebulizers, metered dose inhalers (MDI) and dry powder inhalers (DPI). Commonly, NPs appear to be assuring as a pulmonary drug delivery carrier of proteins and peptides due to their controlled release of bio-therapeutics and targeting capability. In addition to this, NPs below 200 nm in size might getaway the appreciation by alveolar macrophages, which results in more efficient drug uptake and therapeutic action[30]. The different polymeric, lipid and polymeric-lipid hybrid NPs are most widely used as a carrier for pulmonary delivery due to high biocompatibility biodegradation, biocompatibility, non-immunogenicity and the effortlessness of copolymerization and surface modification[37]. Alfagih and co-workers developed bovine serum albumin (BSA) loaded NPs by using a biodegradable biocompatible polymer, poly (glycerol adipate-co-ω-penta decalactone) (PGA-co-PDL), for pulmonary drug delivery. The effective uptake of NPs by targeted dendritic cells with more than 85% cell viability was observed and results indicate protein loaded PGA-co-PDL NPs suitable for inhalation[38].

21.3.4 TRANSDERMAL DELIVERY

Delivery of bio-therapeutics by the use of skin offers some advantages comprising decreased frequency dosing with sustained release, avoiding the hepatic first-pass effect, and better patient compliance[39]. In compression to oral delivery, transdermal delivery may avoid the chemical and enzymatic deterioration of proteins and peptides in the harsh environment of gastrointestinal tract. The different approaches have been developed to overcome the skin barriers (tight junctions of viable epidermis), includes chemical penetration enhancers such as polyethylene glycols (PEG), terpenes and penetration enhancement techniques such as sonophoresis, iontophoresis, electroporation, and microneedles[40]. Sadhasivam and co-workers developed insulin loaded chitosan NPs for transdermal delivery. These NPs exhibited a quasi-circular polymeric structure with the sizes ranging from 465 to 661 nm. Transdermal patches of chitosan NPs were developed using HPMC, PEG 400 and PVP K30, using tween 80 as a plasticizer[41].

21.3.5 OCULAR DELIVERY

The NPs based ocular delivery proteins and peptides have shown huge promise as a novel bio-therapeutics for the treatment of different ocular diseases, with several advantages including less toxicity, high potency, and improved chemical and biological diversity. The various NPs including liposomes, nanospheres, dendrimers and polymeric micelles are being widely estimated for their targeted and controlled delivery of proteins and peptides via this route30. Cho and co-workers developed thermo-sensitive hexanoyl glycol chitosan (HGC) nano-carrier for the ocular drug delivery, by means of modulating the extent of N-hexanoylation to control the thermogelling and achieved superior bioavailability and increased the duration of action as compared to marketed formulation[42].

21.3.6 DELIVERY BY OTHERS ROUTE

The several others non-invasive routes such as nasal and rectal also tried by different researchers for enhance delivery of proteins and peptides. The nasal delivery based mucoadhesive NPs are effective drug carriers for nasal delivery of proteins and peptides as they present higher residence time among improved permeation thereon the nasal membrane. Rectal delivery of NPs might increase the bioavailability of proteins and peptides which are very susceptible to physical, chemical and enzymatic deterioration. The rectal delivery of proteins and peptides helpful when patient are liable to nausea, vomiting and convulsion[30,39].

21.4 CONTROLLED DELIVERY OF PROTEINS AND PEPTIDES

The clinical application of the bio-therapeutics such as protein and peptides are still hindered by delivery associated issues. To compensate these issues, various novel approaches are explored to deliver protein and peptides to the site of action with functional conformation. The primary objective of controlled release formulations is to prolong the effect of drug for longer period by continuous releasing drug at predetermined rate, which results in reduction of dose and subsequently to reduced toxicity. The novel approaches including in situ gel, micro-particle and osmotic controlled system has proved their potential to deliver protein biologics and clinically available in market[43]. Controlled delivery of proteins and peptides therapeutic depends on the polymer concentration and types of polymer used and mechanism of polymer degradation. The most common mechanism of drug release are diffusion, dissolution and erosion. The control release of any bio-therapeutic from polymeric matrix depends on the local microenvironment (such as enzymes, pH, temperature and volume of dissolution media, etc.) where the delivery system is present[44].

21.4.1 POLYMERS FOR CONTROLLED DELIVERY OF PROTEINS AND PEPTIDES

The polymers play a key role in pharmaceutical field to develop controlled release formulation and continuous improvement in the polymers leading the drug delivery systems to new horizon. The proper combination of drug with polymers leads the sustained or controlled release of drug from delivery system and triggered by external environment which leads to reduction in dosing frequency. A variety of polymers tested for their controlled release behavior of small molecules as well as large molecules such as protein and peptides. This controlled release of bio-therapeutics from delivery systems mediated by different mechanism such as degradation controlled, diffusion controlled, chemically and solvent-mediated systems. The different type of classification is available for polymer which is based on sources, solubility, structure, origin and molecular sources (Table 21.1). This classification of polymer described in below table 21.2 [45].

The developments of polymer science, several co-polymers are generated from two different polymers with desirable hydrophilic and hydrophobic characteristics leads to formation of block copolymers. The resultant block copolymers may provide controlled release, microencapsulation or enzymes immobilization. Several research groups working on the preparation of novel polymers to advances the drug delivery systems. With several advances in single entity polymers, novel blend of polymers are also in the development for drug delivery application such as bends of hydrocolloids and carbohydrate. Combining two polymers always offer some drawbacks such as low mechanical strength, poor film formation, and lower gelling capacity since use in optimum ratio can manage this drawback easily. In future, polymer blend prepared from hot melt extrusion (HME) techniques may broad the application of polymers to the new level[46,47].

21.4.2 ADVANTAGES OF CONTROLLED DELIVERY OF PROTEINS AND PEPTIDES

Protein and peptides is complex framework of amino acid with integral structural and chemical properties. This structural framework poses functional conformation to this bio-therapeutics, which must be retaining throughout lifecycle to access the biological activity. This is commonly available in injectable due to poor in-vivo stability, large molecular size and concise half-life *in vivo* through oral or skin delivery. Henceforth require frequent dosing for therapeutic efficacy, which leads to patient discomfort and non-compliance[48]. In order to minimize frequent dosing, controlled delivery of protein and peptides proposes safeguard against in vivo degradation, reduced toxicity, improved patient compliance and efficient benefits of drug with small doses. Several efforts are made towards controlled delivery using chemical modification, micro- and nano-formulations[49,50].

TABLE 21.1

Various Polymers Used for Controlled Release of Proteins and Peptides

Mechanism of release	Polymers used	Model proteins and peptides
Bulk erosion polymers	PLGA	carbonic anhydrase, Interleukin-2, insulin
	Polycyanoacryalate	insulin, growth hormone-releasing factor, calcitonin
	Block polymers of PEG	BSA, bone morphogenetic Protein, immunoglobulin
Surface erosion polymers	Poly(anhydrides)	Insulin, myoglobin, lysozyme
	Poly(ortho esters)	cytochrome c, myoglobin, somatotropin
Hydrogel systems	Pluronic Polyols	BSA, Interleukin-2, urease
	Poly(Vinyl alcohol)	cytochrome c, myoglobin, somatotropin
	PVP	chymotrypsin, BSA
	Maleic anhydrides-Alkyl vinyl ether copolymers	IFNa, HSA
	Cellulose derivatives	TGF-Dl, aFGF
	Hyaluronic acid derivatives	insulin, NGF
	Alginates	albumin, TGF-Pl, bFGF
	Collagen	IL-2, NGF, insulin, EGF
	Gelatine	Interferon-α, Insulin, albumin
	Albumin	Insulin, gp120 peptide, growth hormone
	Starch and Dextran	Interferon-α, carbonic anhydrase
Composite systems	Combination (synthetic polymers with natural materials)	LHRH, insulin and vasopressin

21.5 NANOPARTICLES FOR CONTROLLED DELIVERY OF PROTEINS AND PEPTIDES

Nanoparticles (NPs) are nanoscale colloidal particles ranging from about 10 nm to 1000 nm in the dimension, made up of different biocompatible and biodegradable materials like natural, semi-synthetic, synthetic lipids, or phospholipids, polymers, and even organometallic compounds[25,51]. The most important goal in designing NPs for proteins and peptides delivery is to control the release of therapeutically active agents by surface modification, particle size, and surface properties in order to attain the site-specific drug delivery. The different types of NPs such as organic NPs (dendrimers, liposomes, SLN etc.), inorganic NPs (mesoporous silica NPs, gold NPs etc.) and hybrid NPs (lipid polymer hybrid NPs) have unique properties for the controlled and also targeted release of therapeutic agents due to their surface modification and nanoscale structures[8]. The a variety of novel carriers like liposomes, dendrimers, SLN, gold NPs hybrid NPs used as delivery system for different proteins and peptides therapeutic are listed in table (Table 21.3).

21.5.1 ORGANIC NANOPARTICLES

The organic NPs structured from a variety of materials such as polymers and lipids, have great consideration of researchers due to their different advantages over free drugs, including high encapsulation, better controlled or triggered drug release, targeting to specific sites and elevated versatile application in the field of drug delivery of various biological and nonbiological therapeutic agents[73]. The controlled drug release kinetics is an important issue in drug delivery because

TABLE 21.2

Summary of Featured Smart Stimuli-Responsive Drug Delivery System for Proteins and Peptides

Mechanism of release	Polymers used	Model proteins and peptides
Bulk erosion polymers	PLGA	carbonic anhydrase, Interleukin-2, insulin
	Polycyanoacryalate	insulin, growth hormone-releasing factor, calcitonin
	Block polymers of PEG	BSA, bone morphogenetic Protein, immunoglobulin
Surface erosion polymers	Poly(anhydrides)	Insulin, myoglobin, lysozyme
	Poly(ortho esters)	cytochrome c, myoglobin, somatotropin
Hydrogel systems	Pluronic Polyols	BSA, Interleukin-2, urease
	Poly(Vinyl alcohol)	cytochrome c, myoglobin, somatotropin
	PVP	chymotrypsin, BSA
	Maleic anhydrides-Alkyl vinyl ether copolymers	IFNa, HSA
	Cellulose derivatives	TGF-Dl, aFGF
	Hyaluronic acid derivatives	insulin, NGF
	Alginates	albumin, TGF-Pl, bFGF
	Collagen	IL-2, NGF, insulin, EGF
	Gelatine	Interferon-α, Insulin, albumin
	Albumin	Insulin, gp120 peptide, growth hormone
	Starch and Dextran	Interferon-α, carbonic anhydrase
Composite systems	Combination (synthetic polymers with natural materials)	LHRH, insulin and vasopressin

pharmacokinetics directly influences the therapeutic efficacy and toxicity. By selecting appropriate materials and design features for the NPs fabrication, therapeutic agent can be delivered in a controlled or triggered manner. Also in order to provide better controlled and targeted drug delivery, organic NPs are surface functionalized with various biomolecules or other polymeric materials[74] (Figure 21.4).

21.5.1.1 Dendrimer

Dendrimers also known as the "Polymers of 21st century" are novel three-dimensional spherical nano-polymeric structure having nano-scopic particle dimension range from 1 to 100 nm, characterized by highly branched 3Darrangement that provides a high degree of surface functionality as well as versatility. Generally, dendrimers consist of three different components a central core with at least two reactive functional groups, repeated branches, and surface functional groups[75,76]. Dendrimers assist in achieving improved bioavailability, controlled as well as targeted release of therapeutic agents and reduction in the systemic toxicity with increased therapeutic efficacy. The different types of dendrimers such as Poly(amidoamine) dendrimers (PAMAM), Polypropylene Imine dendrimer (PPI), Poly-l-lysine dendrimers, Fréchet's dendrimer, Chiral Dendrimers, Peptide dendrimers, Multiple antigen peptide dendrimers, Glyco-dendrimers, Hybrid dendrimers have been developed for delivery of biological therapeutic agent that has been used for the treatment of a wide range of diseases such as cancer, metabolic disorders, autoimmune disorders and so on. Surface modified PAMAM dendrimers are mainly used in target-specific controlled drug delivery of chemotherapeutical agents, peptides, and other therapeutic agents [77–79]. The different methods are used

TABLE 21.3

Different Types of NPs Developed for Controlled Drug Delivery of Proteins and Peptides

Protein/peptides	Therapeutic application	Types of NPs developed	Ref.
Insulin	Anti-diabetic	Polymeric NPs, Ceramic NPs, Dendrimers, Liposomes, SLN,	52–54
Etanercept	RA, Psoriatic arthritis, Plaque psoriasis, Ankylosing spondylitis	Gold NPs, SLN	55
Enalapril maleate	Anti-hypertensive	Magnetic-nanoparticles, Gold NPs	56
Salmon calcitonin	Symptomatic Paget's disease, Osteoporosis	PLGA-nanoparticles	57,58
Leuprolide	Prostate cancer, Central precocious puberty, Endometriosis	Liposomes	58,59
Octreotide	Tumors, Hypoglycemic neonates, Bleeding esophageal varices	Liposomes	60
Calcitonin	Hypercalcemia or osteoporosis	SLN	61
Thymopentin	Immuno-stimulant	SLN	62
Gonadotropin	Primary hypothalamic amenorrhea and hypogonadotropic hypogonadism	SLN	63
Tacrolimus and siRNA	Psoriasis	NLCs	64
Throtropin	CNS dysfunction	polymeric NPs	65
Cyclosporine A	Immunosuppressant	polymeric NPs	66
Human Growth Hormone	Deficiency of growth hormone	PLA-PEG-PLA and mPEG-PLA NPs	67
Cytochrome C	Anticancer	Mesoporous silica NPs	68
Cell-penetrating peptide (CPP)	Anticancer	Quantum dots	69
Pro-apoptotic protein caspase-3	Anticancer	Carbon nanotubes (CNTs)	70
Tocilizumab	Rheumatoid Arthritis	Gold nanoparticles	55
Growth factor Wnt3a	Stem cell proliferation	Magnetic Iron Oxide-Based NPs	71
Lysozyme	Delivery vehicle	Lipid polymer hybrid NPs	72

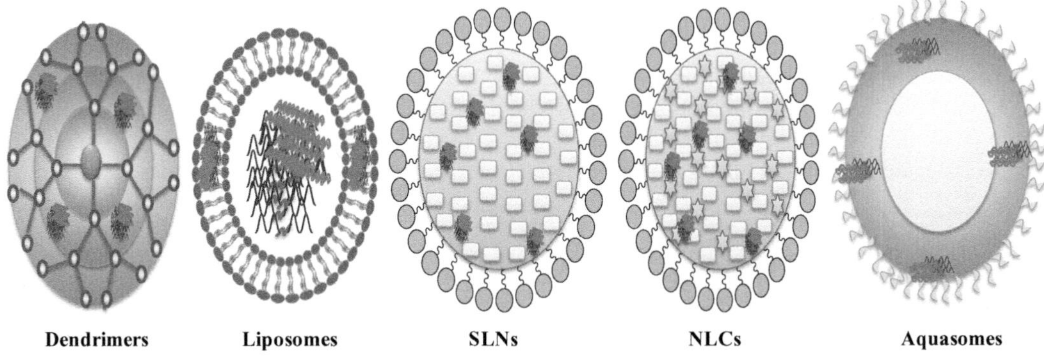

FIGURE 21.4 Organic nano-particles for controlled drug delivery of proteins and peptides.

for the synthesis of dendrimers includes divergent technique convergent technique hypercores and branched monomers technique, double exponential and mixed growth technique. The divergent and convergent are two most commonly complementary approaches, used in the synthesis of dendrimers. In the divergent approach, synthesis of dendrimers starts from "central core" and expand toward the surface. This technique completed by two steps, first activation of surface functional groups and second addition of monomers units to form branching. The advantages of this technique are successful production of large amount of dendrimers. In the convergent approach, synthesis of dendrimers starts from end groups and continuing inwards and finally attaches a suitable "central core" to complete the dendrimers structure. The easy purification of final products is the main advantage of this method[80,81]. Kojima and co-worker developed and evaluated the collagen attached dendrimers for controlled delivery. Developed dendrimers was characterized by the 1H NMR and circular dichroism (CD) spectrometry. The developed dendrimers form hydrogel which act as thermo-sensitive carrier and used as a cellular matrix for the controlled release of different therapeutic agents[82].

21.5.1.2 Liposomes

Liposomes exhibit large potential as a nano-lipid-carrier system for systemically administered peptide and protein therapeutics. Liposomes have two compartments; one is aqueous core that preserves the structure as well as conformation of the protein, other is lipid court that helps to improve absorption from biological membranes. If liposomes constructed by biodegradable and biocompatible materials, they cause very modest to no antigenic, pyrogenic, and toxic reactions inside human body[83,84]. The delivery of liposomes is possible by different routes such as oral, pulmonary, intranasal, parenteral, transdermal et cetera. Liposomes based depot formulations have been developed and characterized for controlled drug delivery of protein such as insulin and peptides such as octreotide and leuprolide[59].

The four basic steps involve in the preparation of liposomes are first drying down the lipids from organic solvent, secondly dispersing the lipid into aqueous phase third is purification of the resultant liposome and fourth analyzing final liposomal product. The methods used in the preparation and loading of therapeutic agents into the liposomes are passive loading and active loading techniques. Passive drug loading techniques comprise three different dispersion methods such as mechanical dispersion, solvent dispersion and detergent removal methods. The mechanical dispersion method includes sonication, micro-emulsification, film hydration by hand shaking or by freeze drying, freeze-thawed and extrusion by French pressure cell or by membrane[85]. Sonication is the most widely used for the preparation of small unilamellar vesicles (SUV) liposomes. The extrusion by the French pressure cell engages the extrusion of multilamellar vesicles (MLV) through a small orifice. French pressure extrusion method has numerous advantages as compare to sonication method and resulting liposomes are moderately larger than sonicated liposomes. In freeze-thawed method liposomes are rapidly frozen and then thawed slowly. The solvent dispersion method includes ether injection, ethanol injection and reverses phase vanishing method. The main advantage of this method is high encapsulation efficiency and used for encapsulating the small as well as large molecules. The detergent removal method involves the removal of non-encapsulated materials (detergent) by different techniques such as dialysis, gel-permeation chromatography and dilution[86]. Zhang et al. developed and evaluated insulin loaded lectin modified liposomes for oral delivery and investigated that liposomes are the potential carriers for proteins and peptides therapeutics delivery[53].

21.5.1.3 Solid Lipid Nanoparticles

Solid Lipid Nanoparticles (SLN) are submicron colloidal drug carriers with 50–1000 nmin diameter composed of lipids, which are solid at room temperatures as well as body temperature. SLN is a combination of both noisome and liposome which includes phospholipids along with surfactant as stabilizer. The reason behind using solid lipids instead of liquid lipids is an attractive approach towards achieve controlled release of therapeutic agent, because of the diffusion of drug from solid lipid should be significantly lower as compared to liquid lipids[87,88]. As compared to niosome and liposome, SLN have superior stability, better protection beside degradation of drugs and less production cost. Delivery of protein such as insulin, cyclosporine A, somatostatin and other biological therapeutics like peptides have been investigated through this lipid-based NPs. This lipid-based SLN NPs are also most suitable to load chemically synthetic lipophilic drugs such as Etomidate, Prednisolone and Etracaine for extended release at the particular site of action for specific period of time[89].

The different methods are used in the preparation of SLNs which includes high pressure homogenization (HPH), high speed homogenization with ultrasonication, double emulsion method, melting dispersion Technique, microemulsion method, solvent evaporation methods, super critical fluid technique, electro-spray technique and other. The high pressure homogenization with slight modification is most widely used method for SLNs and NLCs preparation. In this method formulation materials (drug, lipids and other excipients) are pushed through a narrow gap (few micron ranges) by means of high pressure (around 100–200 bars). Due to high shear stress and cavitation (by sudden reduction of pressure) forces, particle disrupt into submicron range. The SLN produce by HPH follow two basic techniques, one is hot and second is cold homogenization techniques. The basic difference in between hot and cold homogenization is that, in cold homogenization melted lipid containing drug is quickly cooled with dry ice or liquid nitrogen[90]. In solvent emulsification diffusion method, the lipid is dissolved in the organic solvents (water immiscible) followed by emulsification in the aqueous phase and results SLN dispersion formed by precipitation of lipid in aqueous phase after evaporation of solvents. The main advantage of this method is avoidance of heat during SLN preparation. The solvent evaporation is another method for SLN and NLC preparation in which lipophilic material dissolved in organic solvent (water immiscible) and then emulsified into the aqueous phase. After the evaporation of organic solvent, NPs dispersion is formed due to precipitation of lipid in the aqueous phase. In microemulsion method, first microemulsion are prepared by mixing the drug with melted lipid, surfactants and co-surfactants by keeping the temperature above melting points of lipids and then obtained microemulsion is disseminated in aqueous phase at temperature range between 2–10 °C. The electro-spray technique is recently developed novel technique for the preparation of lipid NPs like SLN, the electrodynamic atomization used to create narrow sized spherical dispersed SLN less than 1 μm in size. This method used to obtain SLN in powder form directly[91]. Muller et al. developed and evaluated SLN for oral delivery of cyclosporine A and identified that lipid matrix provide more flexible release of drug from SLN as compared to nano-crystals and in addition to this Reddy et al. developed tamoxifen citrate (TC) loaded SLN and mention that SLN is the potential carriers for proteins and peptides therapeutics delivery[92,93].

21.5.1.4 Nanostructured Lipid Carriers

Nanostructured lipid carriers (NLCs) are second generation, modified form of SLN that composed both solid as well as liquid lipids in the nanostructure, which results in a moderately crystallized or amorphous arrangement of lipids that imparts many advantages and overcome the limitations of SLN such as increased capacity of drug loading, improved entrapment of both lipophilic as well as hydrophilic drugs, extend drug release flexibility and better physical stability by preventing expulsion of drug during storage[94]. Excipients used in the fabrication of NLCs are biodegradable, biocompatible, non-irritating and the majority of them are GRAS listed. The surface modifications of NLCs by various polymeric and other materials are applied to achieve controlled drug delivery of protein and peptides. Depending on the composition of the solid and liquid lipid blends in the structure, NLCs are three types a) imperfect type b) amorphous type and c) multiple types. The different methods are available for NLCs preparation. The most widely used method is the high pressure homogenization (HPH) method, this method utilizes both high pressure and high temperature and another is high-pressure homogenization with low-temperature. The method used for the preparation of NLCs same as the method employing for the preparing SLN. These techniques include HPH,

HPH with ultrasonication, solvent dispersion, ultrasonic emulsion evaporation, supercritical fluid (SCF) method, electro-spray technique and other[95,96]. Viegas and co-worker successfully developed tacrolimus and siRNA loaded multifunctional NLCs and found that release of therapeutic agents from NLCs is controlled[64,97].

21.5.1.5 Aquasomes

Aquasomes are new class of solid drug nano-particulate carrier system having three-layered structures of core, coating, and drug which are self-assembled through ionic bonds, noncovalent bonds, and van der Wals forces. The solid phase nano-crystalline core decorated with the oligomeric film by which pharmacologically active drug molecules are adsorbed with and/or without modification. Aquasomes are spherical with particle size of 60–300 nm used for controlled delivery of protein and peptide therapeutics[98]. Aquasomes present a smart mode of delivery for therapeutic agents that belonging to the category of proteins and peptides, because they are capable to overcome various inherent problems related with these proteins and peptides therapeutics molecules. These problems include appropriate route of drug delivery, physiochemical instability, poor bioavailability, and immunogenicity[99].

The general procedure of aquasomes preparation is the formation inorganic core and this core coated with lactose structuring polyhydroxylated core that finally loaded by model therapeutic agents. Aquasomes are prepared by utilizing the principle of self-assembling, and follow three steps process, first preparation of ceramic core, second coating of core and third drug molecule immobilization. The ceramic core prepared by using colloidal precipitation with sonication, plasma condensation and inverted magnetron sputtering and coating of core by carbohydrate such as pyridoxal-5-phosphate, cellobiose, trehalose and sucrose, finally model drug immobilized with the help of partial adsorption electron microscopy[100].

Damera and co-worker successfully developed BSA loaded aquasomes and found that the aquasomes having multifunctional role in drug delivery and capable to deliver bioactive molecules such as proteins and peptides[101].

21.5.2 Inorganic Nanoparticles

The inorganic nanoparticles have acquired great attention of researchers due to their versatile application in the field of drug delivery system, diagnostic imaging and cell tracking. The therapeutic benefits of inorganic nanoparticles such as large surface area, better bioavailability, lower side effects, resistant towards organic solvents and controlled drug release proven potential for drug delivery vehicle. The various inorganic nanoparticles were explored such as gold nanoparticles, quantum dots, carbon nanotubes, mesoporous silica and magnetic nanoparticles[74]. The controlled delivery of cargo could be achieved by two probable mechanisms, passive actuation of cargo material's in which release of drug could be trigger by efflux or desorption from NP core or surface and active actuation in which "on demand" in response to an applied stimulus such as pH, enzyme, redox sensitive and so on102 (Figure 21.5).

21.5.2.1 Mesoporous Silica Nanoparticles

Mesoporous silica nanoparticles, an inorganic nanoparticles comprised of well-ordered range of honeycomb or hexagonal porous architecture, the robust structure provide large pore volume, well defined pore structure, surface multi-functionalization, adjustable pore size, superior biocompatibility, along with good physicochemical and thermal stability. This feature has proven MSN as a promising delivery platform for peptides and proteins to attain controlled release of cargoes. Also, the surface functionalization property of MSN have introduces new generation of nanoparticles that is stimuli responsive delivery system. Surface functionalization achieved by employing various external or internal stimuli such as pH, redox reaction, temperature, Enzymes etc. this type of multifunctional nanoparticles are widely investigated for targeted drug delivery and controlled

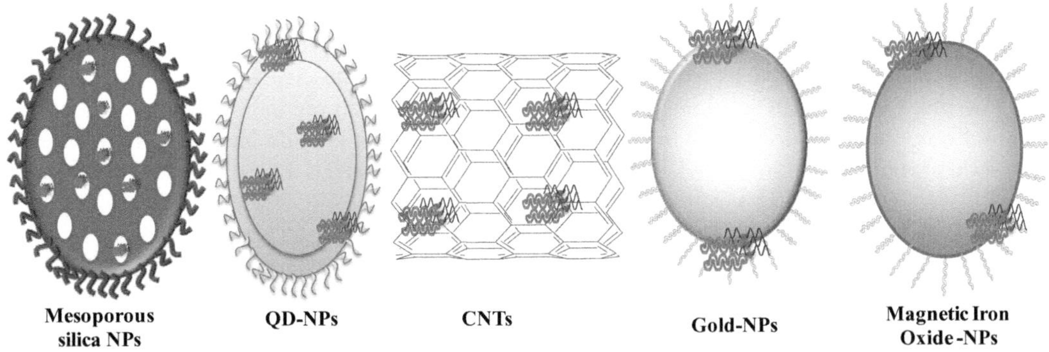

FIGURE 21.5   Inorganic nano-particles for controlled drug delivery of proteins and peptides.

release of payload[103,104]. Cytochrome-c is membrane impermeable protein delivered to tumour cells (HeLa cells) by using MSNPs. Different techniques employed to prepare MSNPs comprising sol-gel method, templating method, chemical etching method and microwave assisted techniques. In the sol-gel method, firstly colloidal suspension (sol) of hydrolyzed precursor formed to create initial framework. Subsequently, controlled aggregation or condensation of sol leads to form spherical or gel network depending reaction conditions105. Templating methods using surfactants and porous solid as a template to prepare mesoporous structure, on that basis they termed soft and hard templating method respectively. This method is widely explored and economical to process. Chemical etching techniques used to create hollow interior of mesoporous structure by structure modality based selective etching. Etching process take place at interior part while shell remain intact to create hollow structure. The Specific etching agents such as Na_2CO_3 solution and ammonia solution under hydrothermal treatment used for etching process. Microwave assisted techniques also used to create mesoporous silica structure but due rapid heating leads to decrease in the pore size[106,107]. Slowing and co-workers developed cytochrome-c entrapped MSNPs with large pore size (5.4 nm) serve as effective transmembrane delivery vehicle by avoiding endosomal entrapment into cytoplasm. The release profile and cell update studies revealed controlled release of cyt-c to tumour cell and induced apoptosis. The activity of cytochrome-c was retained after release from MSNPs and improvement in therapeutic effect[68].

21.5.2.2   QD-Based Nanostructures

Quantum dots (QDs) or semiconductor nanocrystals prepared from CdSe/ZnS core/shell, have emerged as excellent multifunctional vehicle for targeted and traceable delivery vehicle. The nanostructure holds preeminent optical and spectroscopic attributes that provide unique opportunity to treasure mechanism of targeted delivery vehicle. Besides responsive to various attachment and/or cargoes loading, additionally providing diagnosis imaging, drug tracking and controlled drug release[108]. The synthesis of quantum dots can be achieved by two approaches, One pot synthesis method in which preparation of QD depend on semiconductor source are rapidly injected into stirring and hot organic solvents containing molecules interact with different surface and precipitated on surface. The second approach for QD synthesis, lithography assisted technique blend of high-resolution electron beam lithography followed by etching. But this method deals with some drawbacks such as contamination, no uniform size, and expensive. Hence new refined method introduced termed epitaxial method. Epitaxial method of QDs preparation is widely used in techniques due to the detection of different biomolecules at a time[109,110].

Stimuli sensitive QDs was designed which exhibit "on demand" intracellular release of cell penetrating peptides (CPP), this peptide facilitate entry of conjugate into endocytic pathway. The peptide appended to QD that trigger controlled release of cargoes and modulation of drug efficacy. The controlled release of peptide inside cell is mediated by stimuli responsive linkage, ester, disulfide and hydrazine which is cleaved by internal stimuli such as enzymatic cleavage, reducing conditions and low pH. The QD-CPP conjugate creates self-assembly which regulate the ratio of peptide to QD and dose delivered to cells. This study showed uses of QD-peptide bioconjugate as versatile framework which enable improved cellular drug uptake with reduced toxicity[69].

21.5.2.3 Carbon Nanoparticles (Carbon Nanotubes)

Carbon nanotubes are hollow tubular assembly formed by carbon atom rolling of graphene enclosed into cylinder like framework with high aspect ratio. CNTs deliver notable unique structural, mechanical and electrical properties which render them as excellent application in biomedical field. CNTs, if formed by single sheet of carbon termed single wall CNTs (SWCNTs) and if prepared from co-axial multiple sheet of carbon termed multi wall CNTs (MWCNTs)[111]. Several novel biofunctionalization strategies such as nanotube-biomolecule conjugate for SWCNTs were employed for controlled release of cargoes from nanotube sidewall via biologically triggered bond cleavage of bioconjugate. CNTs employed as a carrier for several peptides and protein including protein A, bovine albumin serum, streptavidin and cytochrome C. The PLGA functionalized CNTs to enhance permeability and tumor penetration along with reduces toxicity issue, which provide attachment site for pro-apoptotic protein caspase-3 (CP3), with the controlled release of CP3 to bone cancer cell. The controlled release of protein manipulated by weight and ratio of PLGA conjugate, which allows release of CP3 to shows antitumor effect for a week without further dose. This study results demonstrated that functionalized CNTs are efficient nanocarrier for peptide and protein with controlled release profile[70].

21.5.2.4 Gold Nanostructures

Gold nanoparticles (AuNP) have demonstrated widespread application in the field of drug delivery, bio-sensing and vaccine delivery. These applications are attributable to unique optical properties, facile functionalization and tunable size and shapes. However, gold nanoparticle has potential applications, it has tendency to aggregate and toxicity associate, which inhibit their clinical application[112]. Various peptide and protein like Herceptin, bombesin are appended on gold nanoparticles to reduce the associated toxicity, also provide controlled release over period of time113. There are three commonly used methods for CNT preparations are reported. The arc discharge evaporation method using electric arc formed between two graphite placed following by creation of high temperature under vacuum condition. Subsequently evaporation of one of the carbon electrode from surface and condensation of other electrode to form rod shaped single or multi-walled CNTs based on catalyst used or not respectively. In the laser Ablation Method, vaporization of graphite achieved by pulsed and constant laser source under argon or helium gas. This method also uses high temperature as arc discharge method, with the aid of gas and catalyst mix. Another commonly used method is catalyzed chemical vapor sorption (CVP), in which carbon source (e.g. methane, ethane, etc.) are vaporized by heating and resultants nanostructure deposited on substrate such as silica, zeolite etc. the different heat sources are explored with CVD including thermal, photo-assisted and plasma enhanced to increased efficiency in processing[114]. For preparation of gold nanoparticles two approaches are used including top down approach and bottom-up approach. The top down approaches involve electron beam lithography and photolithography, wherein bottom-up approach includes chemical, sono-chemical, electrochemical templating, and thermal reduction techniques. Both type of approach provide gold nanoparticles in controlled size and shape. Chemical method involves reduction of Au by reducing agents such as borohydride, citric acid, oxalic acid, hydrazine etc. and to avoid aggregation stabilized using tri-sodium citrate, phosphorous ligands, oxygen based ligands or surfactants like cetyl-trimethyl-ammonium bromide (CTAB). Turkevich method and Brust method are commonly used method, where reduction of Au using reducing agent and stabilized. The electrochemical synthesis of gold nanostructure revealed size could be controlled electrochemically; nanostructure stabilized using tetra alkyl ammonium salts. This method is proved to be excellent for nanoparticle production, due to its modest equipment, low cost, lower processing temperature, high quality, and ease of controlling the yield. Another simple, fast and economic process reported for gold nanoparticle preparation i.e. seeding growth method. This method involves trisodium citrate as –OH source in seeding step and sodium borohydrate as a reducing agent[115]. Lee and co-workers successfully prepared hyaluronate-gold nanoparticle/Tocilizumab (HA-AuNP/TCZ) complex for the treatment of Rheumatoid arthritis (RA). TCZ is a monoclonal antibody used as an immunosuppressive drug by inhibiting interleukin-6 (IL-6) receptor in the pathogenesis of RA. HA was chemically conjugated to gold nanoparticles and tailored with TCZ. The HA-AuNP/TCZ complex was characterized and therapeutic effect was evaluated model mice[55].

21.5.2.5 Magnetic Iron Oxide-Based Nanostructures

Superparamagnetic iron oxide nanoparticles (SPIONs) is most exciting theranostic nanostructure prepared from synthetic Y-Fe_2O_3 (maghemite), Fe_3O_4 (magnetite) or α-Fe_2O_3 (hematite) core, usually occur in range 5–150 nm size. Due to inherent magnetic property, iron oxide nanoparticles can address maximum drug targeting, directed by external magnetic field applied to the desired site of action116. To realize controlled delivery of cargo, the nanoparticles can be functionalized with various moieties such as stimuli sensitive (pH, temperature etc.) and biomolecules (protein and peptides). Moreover peptide and protein functionalized iron oxide nanoparticles provide better biocompatibility, less side effects and targeted drug delivery[117,118]. Precisely, depends on required feature and application, different methods are employed to prepare Iron Oxide NPs (IONP). Co-precipitation is commonly used method for preparation IONPs in aqueous solution of ferrous and ferric salts under inert environment. This technique offer simple and economic process but results in non-uniform particle size and time consuming. In thermal decomposition method, commonly two approaches are followed. Firstly continuous heating of precursor constituent to the required temperature above which NPs start clustering. Second, injection of hot precursor into surfactant solution leads to nucleation to generate homogeneous IONPs. Microemulsion method based IONPs synthesis involves preparation of thermodynamic stable dispersion of two immiscible liquid with the aid of stabilizers. Another efficient method in terms of scalability is polyol method, in which metal oxide, acetate are dipped into diol solvents at low temperature[119]. Walker and co-worker developed super-paramagnetic iron oxide NPs (SPIONs) appended with a thermo-sensitive polymer, subsequently entrapped growth factor Wnt3a for stem cell proliferation. The loaded protein is in inactive state until magnetically responsive release to enhanced mesenchymal stem cell proliferation. The study results revealed that as triggered response of magnetic heating, which crumpled polymer shell around nanostructure core leads to controlled release the protein cargo at bulk solution[72].

21.5.3 HYBRID NANOPARTICLES

Lipid polymer hybrid nanoparticles (LPHNs) are hybrid nanostructure comprising positive edges of both lipidic and polymeric nanoparticles. The hybrid nanoparticles possess polymeric core shell entrapped payload, lipidic moiety appended onto surface of polymeric core and polyethylene glycol (PEG) layer facing aqueous milieu prolonging circulation time. These hybrid nanostructure exhibit unique advantages such as better biocompatibility, storage stability, high drug loading, controlled release profile and promising pharmacokinetic profile[120,121]. Many studies have performed to dip into the efficiency of hybrid nanoparticles in the delivery of peptide and protein cargo. The LPNs were prepared from Poly-ε-caprolactone (PCL) as a hydrophobic polymeric core and tailored with lipid layer prepared from lipid and lipid surfactant i.e. Glyceryl tripalmitate and L-α phosphatidylcholine (PC), the resultant nanostructure entrapped lysozyme as model protein. The in-vitro release study results of LNPs showed initial burst release of lysozyme from nanostructure due to lysozyme facile or entrapped on lipid layer of LNPs, but afterward controlled release of lysozyme ascribed to dispersed protein inside polymeric core. The essence of LPNs including high payload, high structure integrity, low cytotoxicity, higher cellular uptake and controlled release of lysozyme from nanostructure make it ideal delivery platform of peptide and protein[71,122]. Many studies have performed to dip into the efficiency of hybrid nanoparticles in the delivery of peptide and protein cargo. The LPNs were prepared from Poly-ε-caprolactone (PCL) as a hydrophobic polymeric core and tailored with lipid layer prepared from lipid and lipid surfactant i.e. Glyceryl tripalmitate and L-α phosphatidylcholine (PC), the resultant nanostructure entrapped lysozyme as model protein. The in-vitro release study results of LNPs showed initial burst release of lysozyme from nanostructure due to lysozyme facile or entrapped on lipid layer of LNPs, but afterward controlled release of lysozyme ascribed to dispersed protein inside polymeric core. The essence of LPNs including high payload, high structure integrity, low cytotoxicity, higher cellular uptake and controlled release of lysozyme from nanostructure make it ideal delivery platform of peptide and protein[71,122].

There are two common strategies employed to prepare LPNPs i.e. two step and one step process. Two step methods is typical approach, in which polymeric nanoparticles are mixed with dried lipid film followed by hydration or hydrated lipid vesicles. In both cases LPNPs assembled in response to external energy by simple vortexing, ultra-sonication or heating above phase transition temperature of lipid constituent. The efficient alternative technique developed i.e. one step method in which exclusively involves mixing of polymer and lipid lead to form self-assembled LPHNPs. The most common processes is nanoprecipitation which requires drug and polymer are dissolved in water miscible organic solvents (e.g. Ethanol, acetone) and lipid constituents dissolved in water above transition temperature to achieve homogeneous dispersion and then subsequent drop-wise addition of polymer solution into the lipid dispersion under constant stirring to create self-assembled hybrid NPs[123].

21.6 SPECIFIC TARGETING OF PROTEIN PEPTIDES

Traditional way of delivering molecules to its desired location leads to lower therapeutic effect and required high dose delivery to get desired therapeutic effects. This created opportunity for specific targeting method for guiding payload to the desired site to reduce drug dosage. Numerous nanoscale delivery systems are directed to targeted site such as polymeric nanocarriers, micelles, dendrimers, liposome, lipid NPs and inorganic NPs (e.g. silica NPs). The presence of functional group on surface of protein and peptides particularly -COOH and NH_3 group) offers functionalization site for different targeting ligand. The delivery system designed for anticancer drugs, mainly achieved by passive and active targeting (Figure 21.6).

In passive targeting, the attachment of PEG to protein or delivery system can prolong circulation time. In addition, reduction in non-immunogenicity and better accumulation into tumour cells due to enhanced permeation and retention effect (EPR effect). The long chain of PEG forms hydrophilic shell around delivery systems which could protect the cargo from interaction with serum proteins, subsequently reduction of reticuloendothelial system (RES) uptake. Another approach is nanocarriers with size less than 200 nm can be easily accessible to tumour cell due to disturbed vasculature and active targeting by attaching different targeting ligand to the nanocarrier for tumour accumulation[124]. In active targeting, diverse range of targeting ligand (carbohydrates, vitamins, antibodies, aptamers, proteins and peptides) were capped over nano-delivery system. Since last decades, varieties of ligands are attached to payload for targeting to specific receptors or cells like tumour cells. Amongst, proteins and peptides ligands retain better advantages such as higher specificity for specific receptor than other. Various protein and peptides are targeted for various receptors or cells like tumour cells, integrin receptor, thrombin receptors and pancreatic cells[125]. The facile functionalization of anti-human epidermal growth factor receptor 2 (Anti-HER2) antibodies such as trastuzumab (Herceptin) on different nanoparticles (PLGA, Gelatin, albumin, PLA NPs) was endeavored to target HER2 overexpressing cells in controlled manner. The internalization of antibodies capped NPs by receptor mediated endocytosis[126]. The facile functionalization of anti-human epidermal growth factor receptor 2 (Anti-HER2) antibodies such as trastuzumab (Herceptin) on different nanoparticles (PLGA, Gelatin, albumin, PLA NPs) was endeavored to target HER2 overexpressing cells

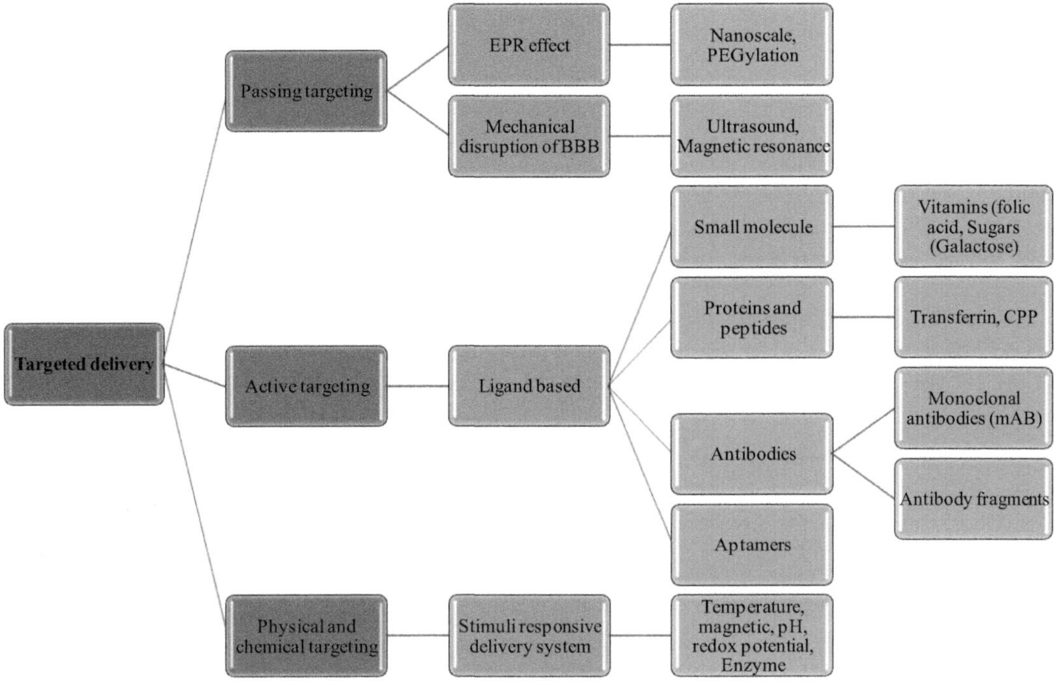

FIGURE 21.6 Targeted delivery of protein and peptides.

in controlled manner. The internalization of antibodies capped NPs by receptor mediated endocytosis126. The transferrin was anchored on albumin NPs to explore potential in brain delivery. The albumin nanoparticle prepared by ultra-emulsification method and incorporating azidothymidine (AZT) as model drug administered through intravenous route. The AZD loaded Tf anchored and non-anchored albumin nanoparticles evaluated for biodistribution after intravenous administration. The in-vivo biodistribution study evidently revealed that selective localization for Tf capped albumin NPs compared to non-capped NPs. The uptake of transferrin (Tf) modified NPs to the receptors associated with blood brain barrier (BBB) by absorptive endocytosis. In addition, net positive charge and co-ordination targeting achieved through uptake by monocyte make Tf anchored NPs potential candidate for localization in brain across BBB[127].

21.7 SMART DRUG DELIVERY SYSTEMS

The smart stimuli-responsive drug delivery system also known as intelligent delivery system is another approach to regulate drug release to the specific site by integrating different modalities compared with simple platform. The combination of targeting molecule with stimuli sensitivity can integrate into versatile system for selective localization and decrement in side effects. This can be achieved by selection of proper building block with endogenous trigger, which has inherent stimuli responsiveness to regulate release of molecules. In the recent years, stimuli responsive polymer garnered attention because of their responsiveness of physical and chemical properties towards external or internal stimuli such as temperature, pH, redox potential, etc. (Figure 21.7).

These stimuli responsive polymers are also termed "smart polymers" due to their different behavioral changes upon triggered by varieties of stimulus. Smart polymers also considered as "intelligent polymer" bears dramatic changes in structure or properties attributed to slight changes in their environment due to external or internal stimuli. This physical transition includes changes in

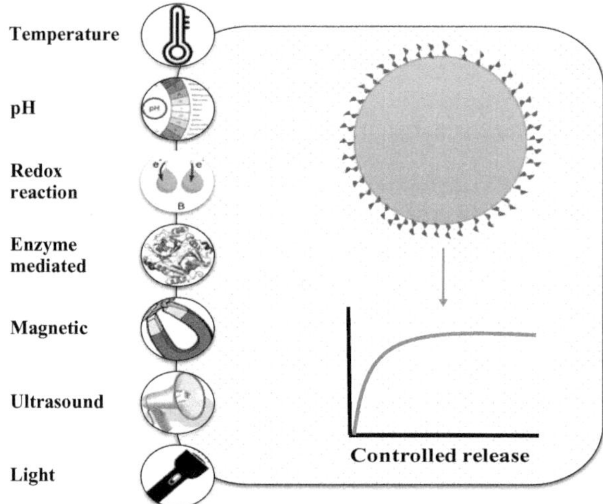

FIGURE 21.7   Stimuli responsive delivery of protein and peptides.

the solubility, physical form, conductivity, shape and solvent mediated swelling or shrinking[128,129]. The impelling cause behind this physical transition are disturbance in hydrogen bonding due to temperature shift, neutralization of charged polymer by variation in pH, drift in HLB value. The occurred physical transition in polymers paves the way to manipulate drug release of payload in controlled manner from drug delivery platform. This strategy unfolded versatile application of smart polymers for site specific delivery, shortened side effects improved stability and controlled release of protein and peptides[130].

REFERENCES

1. Yu M, Wu J, Shi J, Farokhzad OC. Nanotechnology for protein delivery: Overview and perspectives. *Journal of Controlled Release* 2016, 240:24–37.
2. Vaishya R, Khurana V, Patel S, Mitra AK. Long-term delivery of protein therapeutics. *Expert Opinion on Drug Delivery* 2015, 12(3):415–440.
3. Deb PK, Al-Attraqchi O, Chandrasekaran B, Paradkar A, Tekade RK. Protein/peptide drug delivery systems: Practical considerations in pharmaceutical product development. *Basic Fundamentals of Drug Delivery* 2019, 651–684.
4. Asfour MH. Advanced trends in protein and peptide drug delivery: A special emphasis on aquasomes and microneedles techniques. *Drug Delivery and Translational Research* 2021, 11(1):1–23.
5. Agnihotri SA, Mallikarjuna NN, Aminabhavi TM. Recent advances on chitosan-based micro-and nanoparticles in drug delivery. *Journal of Controlled Release* 2004, 100(1):5–28.
6. Suri SS, Fenniri H, Singh B. Nanotechnology-based drug delivery systems. *Journal of Occupational Medicine and Toxicology* 2007, 2(1):16.
7. Nevozhay D, Kańska U, Budzyńska R, Boratyński J. Current status of research on conjugates and related drug delivery systems in the treatment of cancer and other diseases. *Postepy higieny i medycyny doswiadczalnej* (Online) 2007, 61:350–360.
8. Pudlarz A, Szemraj J. Nanoparticles as carriers of proteins, peptides and other therapeutic molecules. *Open Life Sciences* 2018, 13(1):285–298.
9. Ratnaparkhi MP, Chaudhari SP, Pandya VA. Peptides and proteins in pharmaceuticals. *International Journal of Current Pharmaceutical Research* 2011, 3(2):1–9.
10. Keservani RK, Sharma AK, Jarouliya U. Protein and peptide in drug targeting and its therapeutic approach. *Ars Pharmaceutica* 2015, 56(3):165–177.
11. Indurkhya A, Patel M, Sharma P, Abed SN, Shnoudeh A, Maheshwari R, Deb PK, Tekade RK. Influence of drug properties and routes of drug administration on the design of controlled release system. *Dosage Form Design Considerations* 2018, 179–223.

12. Zhou XH, Po ALW. Peptide and protein drugs: I. Therapeutic applications, absorption and parenteral administration. *International Journal of Pharmaceutics* 1991, 75(2–3):97–115.
13. Choonara BF, Choonara YE, Kumar P, Bijukumar D, du Toit LC, Pillay V. A review of advanced oral drug delivery technologies facilitating the protection and absorption of protein and peptide molecules. *Biotechnology Advances* 2014, 32(7):1269–1282.
14. Mellstedt HK. Clinical considerations for biosimilar antibodies. *European Journal of Cancer Supplements* 2013, 11(3):1–11.
15. Tuncer Degim I, Çelebi N. Controlled delivery of peptides and proteins. *Current Pharmaceutical Design* 2007, 13(1):99–117.
16. Oh EJ, Park K, Kim KS, Kim J, Yang J-A, Kong J-H, Lee MY, Hoffman AS, Hahn SK. Target specific and long-acting delivery of protein, peptide, and nucleotide therapeutics using hyaluronic acid derivatives. *Journal of Controlled Release* 2010, 141(1):2–12.
17. Lin JH. Pharmacokinetics of biotech drugs: Peptides, proteins and monoclonal antibodies. *Current Drug Metabolism* 2009, 10(7):661–691.
18. Jacobs I, Petersel D, Shane LG, Ng C-K, Kirchhoff C, Finch G, Lula S. Monoclonal antibody and fusion protein biosimilars across therapeutic areas: A systematic review of published evidence. *BioDrugs* 2016 30(6):489–523.
19. Gupta H, Sharma A. Recent trends in protein and peptide drug delivery systems. *Asian Journal of Pharmaceutics* 2009, 3(2).
20. Jain A, Jain A, Gulbake A, Shilpi S, Hurkat P, Jain SK. Peptide and protein delivery using new drug delivery systems. *Critical Reviews in Therapeutic Drug Carrier Systems* 2013, 30(4).
21. Craik DJ, Fairlie DP, Liras S, Price D. The future of peptide-based drugs. *Chemical Biology & Drug Design* 2013, 81(1):136–147.
22. Pauling L, Corey RB, Branson HR. The structure of proteins; two hydrogen-bonded helical configurations of the polypeptide chain. *Proceedings of the National Academy of Sciences of the United States of America* 1951, 37:205.
23. Vhora I, Patil S, Bhatt P, Misra A. Protein- and peptide-drug conjugates: An emerging drug delivery technology. *Advances in Protein Chemistry and Structural Biology* 2015, 1–55.
24. Brown LR. Commercial challenges of protein drug delivery. *Expert Opinion on Drug Delivery* 2005, 2(1):29–42.
25. Buchanan A, Revell JD. Novel therapeutic proteins and peptides. *Novel Approaches and Strategies for Biologics, Vaccines and Cancer Therapies* 2014, 171–197.
26. Antosova Z, Mackova M, Kral V, Macek T. Therapeutic application of peptides and proteins: parenteral forever? *Trends in Biotechnology* 2009, 27(11):628–635.
27. Drucker DJ. Advances in oral peptide therapeutics. *Nature Reviews Drug Discovery* 2020, 1–13.
28. Muheem A, Shakeel F, Jahangir MA, Anwar M, Mallick N, Jain GK, Warsi MH, Ahmad FJ. A review on the strategies for oral delivery of proteins and peptides and their clinical perspectives. *Saudi Pharmaceutical Journal* 2016, 24(4):413–428.
29. Tibbitts J, Canter D, Graff R, Smith A, Khawli LA. Key factors influencing ADME properties of therapeutic proteins: A need for ADME characterization in drug discovery and development. *InMAbs* 2016, 8(2):229–245.
30. Bajracharya R, Song JG, Back SY, Han H-K. Recent advancements in non-invasive formulations for protein drug delivery. *Computational and Structural Biotechnology Journal* 2019, 17:1290–1308.
31. Patel A, Cholkar K, Mitra AK. Recent developments in protein and peptide parenteral delivery approaches. *Therapeutic Delivery* 2014, 5(3):337–365.
32. Zhang XG, Teng DY, Wu ZM, Wang X, Wang Z, Yu DM, Li CX. PEG-grafted chitosan nanoparticles as an injectable carrier for sustained protein release. *Journal of Materials Science: Materials in Medicine* 2008, 19(12):3525–3533.
33. Glowka E, Sapin-Minet A, Leroy P, Lulek J, Maincent P. Preparation and in vitro-in vivo evaluation of salmon calcitonin-loaded polymeric nanoparticles. *Journal of Microencapsulation* 2010, 27(1):25–36.
34. Mukhopadhyay P, Sarkar K, Chakraborty M, Bhattacharya S, Mishra R, Kundu PP. Oral insulin delivery by self-assembled chitosan nanoparticles: In vitro and in vivo studies in diabetic animal model. *Materials Science and Engineering: C* 2013, 33(1):376–382.
35. Luangtana-anan M, Nunthanid J, Limmatvapirat S. Potential of different salt forming agents on the formation of chitosan nanoparticles as carriers for protein drug delivery systems. *Journal of Pharmaceutical Investigation* 2019, 49(1):37–44.

36. Sandri G, Bonferoni MC, Rossi S, Ferrari F, Boselli C, Caramella C. Insulin-loaded nanoparticles based on N-trimethyl chitosan: In vitro (Caco-2 model) and ex vivo (excised rat jejunum, duodenum, and ileum) evaluation of penetration enhancement properties. *AAPS Pharmaceutical Science and Technology* 2010, 11(1):362–371.

37. Osman N, Kaneko K, Carini V, Saleem I. Carriers for the targeted delivery of aerosolized macromolecules for pulmonary pathologies. *Expert Opinion on Drug Delivery* 2018, 15(8):821–834.

38. Alfagih I, Kunda N, Alanazi F, Dennison SR, Somavarapu S, Hutcheon GA, Saleem IY. Pulmonary delivery of proteins using nanocomposite microcarriers. *Journal of Pharmaceutical Sciences* 2015, 104(12):4386–4398.

39. Jitendra PK, Bansal S, Banik A. Noninvasive routes of proteins and peptides drug delivery. *Indian Journal of Pharmaceutical Sciences* 2011, 73(4):367.

40. Zeb A, Arif ST, Malik M, Shah FA, Din FU, Qureshi OS, Lee E-S, Kim J-K. Potential of nanoparticulate carriers for improved drug delivery via skin. *Journal of Pharmaceutical Investigation* 2019, 49(5):485–517.

41. Sadhasivam L, Dey N, Francis AP, Devasena T. Transdermal patches of chitosan nanoparticles for insulin delivery. *International Journal of Pharmacy and Pharmaceutical Sciences* 2015, 7(5):84–88.

42. Cho IS, Park CG, Huh BK, Cho MO, Khatun Z, Li Z, Kang S-W, Choy YB, Huh KM. Thermosensitive hexanoyl glycol chitosan-based ocular delivery system for glaucoma therapy. *Acta Biomaterialia* 2016, 39:124–132.

43. Srinivas L, Manikanta V, Jaswitha M. Protein and peptide drug delivery-a brief review. *Research Journal of Pharmacy and Technology* 2019, 12(3):1369–1382.

44. Park K. Controlled drug delivery systems: Past forward and future back. *Journal of Controlled Release* 2014, 190:3–8.

45. Allen TM, Cullis PR. Liposomal drug delivery systems: From concept to clinical applications. *Advanced Drug Delivery Reviews* 2013, 65(1):36–48.

46. Tekade RK, Youngren-Ortiz SR, Yang H, Haware R, Chougule MB. Designing hybrid onconase nanocarriers for mesothelioma therapy: A Taguchi orthogonal array and multivariate component driven analysis. *Molecular Pharmaceutics* 2014, 11(10):3671–3683.

47. Mendes SC, Reis RL, Bovell YP, Cunha AM, van Blitterswijk CA, de Bruijn JD. Biocompatibility testing of novel starch-based materials with potential application in orthopaedic surgery: A preliminary study. *Biomaterials* 2001, 22(14):2057–2064.

48. Fu K, Klibanov AM, Langer R. Protein stability in controlled-release systems. *Nature Biotechnology* 2000, 18(1):24–25.

49. Elgersma AV, Zsom RLJ, Norde W, Lyklema J. The adsorption of bovine serum albumin on positively and negatively charged polystyrene latices. *Journal of Colloid and Interface Science* 1990, 138(1):145–156.

50. Ostuni E, Chapman RG, Holmlin RE, Takayama S, Whitesides GM. A survey of structure-property relationships of surfaces that resist the adsorption of protein. *Langmuir* 2001, 17(18):5605–5620.

51. Singh D, Dubey P, Pradhan M, Singh MR. Ceramic nanocarriers: Versatile nanosystem for protein and peptide delivery. *Expert Opinion on Drug Delivery* 2013, 10(2):241–259.

52. Pan Y, Li Y-J, Zhao H-Y, Zheng J-M, Xu H, Wei G, Hao J-S. Bioadhesive polysaccharide in protein delivery system: Chitosan nanoparticles improve the intestinal absorption of insulin in vivo. *International Journal of Pharmaceutics* 2002, 249(1–2):139–147.

53. Zhang N, Ping QN, Huang GH, Xu WF. Investigation of lectin-modified insulin liposomes as carriers for oral administration. *International Journal of Pharmaceutics* 2005, 294(1–2):247–259.

54. Goto T, Morishita M, Nishimura K, Nakanishi M, Kato A, Ehara J, Takayama K. Novel mucosal insulin delivery systems based on fusogenic liposomes. *Pharmaceutical Research* 2006, 23(2):384–391.

55. Lee H, Lee M-Y, Bhang SH, Kim B-S, Kim YS, Ju JH, Kim KS, Hahn SK. Hyaluronate-gold nanoparticle/tocilizumab complex for the treatment of rheumatoid arthritis. *ACS Nano* 2014, 8(5):4790–4798.

56. Shahverdi N, Heydarinasab A, Panahi HA, Moniri E. Synthesis and evaluation of enalapril-loaded PVA/PMC modified magnetic nanoparticles as a novel efficient nano-carrier. *ChemistrySelect* 2019, 4(18):5246–5250.

57. Yoo HS, Park TG. Biodegradable nanoparticles containing protein-fatty acid complexes for oral delivery of salmon calcitonin. *Journal of Pharmaceutical Sciences* 2004, 93(2):488–495.

58. Arulsudar N, Subramanian N, Mishra P, Chuttani K, Sharma RK, Murthy RSR. Preparation, characterization, and biodistribution study of technetium-99m-labeled leuprolide acetate-loaded liposomes in Ehrlich ascites tumor-bearing mice. *AAPS Pharmaceutical Science and Technology* 2004, 6(1):45–56.

59. Carafa M, Marianecci C, Annibaldi V, Di Stefano A, Sozio P, Santucci E. Novel O-palmitoylscleroglucan-coated liposomes as drug carriers: Development, characterization and interaction with leuprolide. *International Journal of Pharmaceutics* 2006, 325(1–2):155–162.

60. Ye Q, Asherman J, Stevenson M, Brownson E, Katre NV. DepoFoam(TM) technology: A vehicle for controlled delivery of protein and peptide drugs. *Journal of Controlled Release* 2000, 64(1–3):155–166.

61. Olbrich C, Gessner A, Kayser O, Müller RH. Lipid-drug-conjugate (LDC) nanoparticles as novel carrier system for the hydrophilic antitrypanosomal drug diminazenediaceturate. *Journal of Drug Targeting* 2002, 10(5):387–396.

62. Morel S, Ugazio E, Cavalli R, Gasco MR. Thymopentin in solid lipid nanoparticles. *International Journal of Pharmaceutics* 1996, 132(1–2):259–261.

63. Bajoria R, Sooranna SR. Liposome as a drug carrier system: Prospects for safer prescribing during pregnancy: A review. *Placenta* 1998, 19:265–287.

64. Viegas JSR, Praça FG, Caron AL, Suzuki I, Silvestrini AVP, Medina WSG, Del Ciampo JO, Kravicz M, Bentley MVRLB. Nanostructured lipid carrier co-delivering tacrolimus and TNF-α siRNA as an innovate approach to psoriasis. *Drug Delivery and Translational Research* 2020, 1–15.

65. Miyamoto S, Takaoka K, Okada T, Yoshikawa H, Hashimoto J, Suzuki S, Ono K. Polylactic acid-polyethylene glycol block copolymer: A new biodegradable synthetic carrier for bone morphogenetic protein. *Clinical Orthopaedics and Related Research* 1993, (294):333–343.

66. Sanchez A, Vila-Jato JL, Alonso MJ. Development of biodegradable microspheres and nano-spheres for the controlled release of cyclosporin A. *International Journal of Pharmaceutics* 1993, 99(2–3):263–273.

67. Ghasemi R, Abdollahi M, Zadeh EE, Khodabakhshi K, Badeli A, Bagheri H, Hosseinkhani S. mPEG-PLA and PLA-PEG-PLA nanoparticles as new carriers for delivery of recombinant human growth hormone (rhGH). *Scientific Reports* 2018, 8(1):1–13.

68. Slowing II, Trewyn BG, Lin VSY. Mesoporous silica nanoparticles for intracellular delivery of membrane-impermeable proteins. *Journal of the American Chemical Society* 2007, 129(28):8845–8849.

69. Sangtani A, Petryayeva E, Wu M, Susumu K, Oh E, Huston AL, Lasarte-Aragones G, Medintz IL, Algar WR, Delehanty JB. Intracellularly actuated quantum dot–peptide–doxorubicin nanobioconjugates for controlled drug delivery via the endocytic pathway. *Bioconjugate Chemistry* 2018, 29(1):136–148.

70. Cheng Q, Blais M-O, Harris G, Jabbarzadeh E. PLGA-carbon nanotube conjugates for intercellular delivery of caspase-3 into osteosarcoma cells. *PLOS One* 2013, 8(12):e81947.

71. Devrim B, Kara A, Vural İ, Bozkır A. Lysozyme-loaded lipid-polymer hybrid nanoparticles: Preparation, characterization and colloidal stability evaluation. *Drug Development and Industrial Pharmacy* 2016, 42(11):1865–1876.

72. Walker M, Will I, Pratt A, Chechik V, Genever P, Ungar D. Magnetically-triggered release of entrapped bioactive proteins from thermally responsive polymer-coated iron oxide nanoparticles for stem cell proliferation. *ACS Applied Nano Materials* 2020, 3(6):5008–5013.

73. Mitragotri S, Stayton P. Organic nanoparticles for drug delivery and imaging. *Mrs Bulletin* 2014, 39(3):219–223.

74. Gessner I, Neundorf I. Nanoparticles modified with cell-penetrating peptides: Conjugation mechanisms, physicochemical properties, and application in cancer diagnosis and therapy. *International Journal of Molecular Sciences* 2020, 21(7):2536.

75. Tripathy S, Das MK. Dendrimers and their applications as novel drug delivery carriers. *Journal of Applied Pharmaceutical Science* 2013, 3(9):142–149.

76. Liu J, Gray WD, Davis ME, Luo Y. Peptide-and saccharide-conjugated dendrimers for targeted drug delivery: A concise review. *Interface Focus* 2012, 2(3):307–324.

77. Srinageshwar B, Peruzzaro S, Andrews M, Johnson K, Hietpas A, Clark B, McGuire C, Petersen E, Kippe J, Stewart A. PAMAM dendrimers cross the blood-brain barrier when administered through the carotid artery in C57BL/6J mice. *International Journal of Molecular Sciences* 2017, 18(3):628.

78. Baig T, Nayak J, Dwivedi V, Singh A, Srivastava A, Tripathi PK. A review about dendrimers: Synthesis, types, characterization and applications. *International Journal of Advances in Pharmacy, Biology and Chemistry* 2015, 4:44–59.

79. Thanh VM, Nguyen TH, Tran TV, Ngoc U-TP, Ho MN, Nguyen TT, Chau YNT, Tran NQ, Nguyen CK, Nguyen DH. Low systemic toxicity nanocarriers fabricated from heparin-mPEG and PAMAM dendrimers for controlled drug release. *Materials Science and Engineering: C* 2018, 82:291–298.

80. Grayson SM, Frechet JMJ. Convergent dendrons and dendrimers: From synthesis to applications. *Chemical Reviews* 2001, 101(12):3819–3868.

81. Astruc D, Boisselier E, Ornelas C. Dendrimers designed for functions: From physical, photophysical, and supramolecular properties to applications in sensing, catalysis, molecular electronics, photonics, and nanomedicine. *Chemical Reviews* 2010, 110(4):1857–1959.

82. Kojima C, Tsumura S, Harada A, Kono K. A collagen-mimic dendrimer capable of controlled release. *Journal of the American Chemical Society* 2009, 131(17):6052–6053.

83. Park KH, Choi JM, Cho E, Jeong D, Shinde VV, Kim H, Choi Y, Jung S. Enhancement of solubility and bioavailability of quercetin by inclusion complexation with the cavity of mono-6-deoxy-6-aminoethylamino-β-cyclodextrin. *Bulletin of the Korean Chemical Society* 2017, 38(8):880–889.

84. Qiu M, Zhang Z, Wei Y, Sun H, Meng F, Deng C, Zhong Z. Small-sized and robust chimaeric lipopepsomes: A simple and functional platform with high protein loading for targeted intracellular delivery of protein toxin in vivo. *Chemistry of Materials* 2018, 30(19):6831–6838.

85. Eloy JO, de Souza MC, Petrilli R, Barcellos JPA, Lee RJ, Marchetti JM. Liposomes as carriers of hydrophilic small molecule drugs: Strategies to enhance encapsulation and delivery. *Colloids and Surfaces B: Biointerfaces* 2014, 123:345–363.

86. Akbarzadeh A, Rezaei-Sadabady R, Davaran S, Joo SW, Zarghami N, Hanifehpour Y, Samiei M, Kouhi M, Nejati-Koshki K. Liposome: Classification, preparation, and applications. *Nanoscale Research Letters* 2013, 8(1):102.

87. Müller RH, Mäder K, Gohla S. Solid lipid nanoparticles (SLN) for controlled drug delivery-a review of the state of the art. *European Journal of Pharmaceutics and Biopharmaceutics* 2000, 50(1):161–177.

88. zur Mühlen A, Schwarz C, Mehnert W. Solid lipid nanoparticles (SLN) for controlled drug delivery-drug release and release mechanism. *European Journal of Pharmaceutics and Biopharmaceutics* 1998, 45(2):149–155.

89. Almeida ANJ, Souto E. Solid lipid nanoparticles as a drug delivery system for peptides and proteins. *Advanced Drug Delivery Reviews* 2007, 59(6):478–490.

90. Duan Y, Dhar A, Patel C, Khimani M, Neogi S, Sharma P, Kumar NS, Vekariya RL. A brief review on solid lipid nanoparticles: Part and parcel of contemporary drug delivery systems. *RSC Advances* 2020, 10(45):26777–26791.

91. Siekmann B, Westesen K. Submicron-sized parenteral carrier systems based on solid lipids. *Pharmaceutical and Pharmacological Letters* 1992, 1(3):123–126.

92. Harivardhan Reddy L, Vivek K, Bakshi N, Murthy RSR. Tamoxifen citrate loaded solid lipid nanoparticles (SLN™): Preparation, characterization, in vitro drug release, and pharmacokinetic evaluation. *Pharmaceutical Development and Technology* 2006, 11(2):167–177.

93. Müller RH, Runge S, Ravelli V, Mehnert W, Thünemann AF, Souto EB. Oral bioavailability of cyclosporine: Solid lipid nanoparticles (SLNÂ®) versus drug nanocrystals. *International Journal of Pharmaceutics* 2006, 317(1):82–89.

94. Ketabat F, Pundir M, Mohabatpour F, Lobanova L, Koutsopoulos S, Hadjiiski L, Chen X, Papagerakis P, Papagerakis S. Controlled drug delivery systems for oral cancer Treatmentâ-current status and future perspectives. *Pharmaceutics* 2019, 11(7):302.

95. Khosa A, Reddi S, Saha RN. Nanostructured lipid carriers for site-specific drug delivery. *Biomedicine & Pharmacotherapy* 2018, 103:598–613.

96. Souto EB, Baldim I, Oliveira WP, Rao R, Yadav N, Gama FM, Mahant S. SLN and NLC for topical, dermal, and transdermal drug delivery. *Expert Opinion on Drug Delivery* 2020, 17(3):357–377.

97. Lee SG, Kim CH, Sung SW, Lee ES, Goh MS, Yoon HY, Kang MJ, Lee S, Choi YW. RIPL peptide-conjugated nanostructured lipid carriers for enhanced intracellular drug delivery to hepsin-expressing cancer cells. *International Journal of Nanomedicine* 2018, 13:3263.

98. Umashankar MS, Sachdeva RK, Gulati M. Aquasomes: A promising carrier for peptides and protein delivery. *Nanomedicine: Nanotechnology, Biology and Medicine* 2010, 6(3):419–426.

99. Andrade F, Videira M, Ferreira D, Sarmento B. Nanocarriers for pulmonary administration of peptides and therapeutic proteins. *Nanomedicine* 2011, 6(1):123–141.

100. Jain SS, Jagtap PS, Dand NM, Jadhav KR, Kadam VJ. Aquasomes: A novel drug carrier. *Journal of Applied Pharmaceutical Science* 2012, 2(1):184–192.

101. Damera DP, Kaja S, Janardhanam LSL, Alim S, Venuganti VVK, Nag A. Synthesis, detailed characterization, and dual drug delivery application of BSA loaded aquasomes. *ACS Applied Bio Materials* 2019, 2(10):4471–4484.

102. Dongying Q, Lan L, Qian D. Targeting of ovarian cancer cell through functionalized gold nanoparticles by novel glypican-3-binding peptide as a ultrasound contrast agents. *Process Biochemistry* 2020, 98:51–58.

103. Deodhar GV, Adams ML, Trewyn BG. Controlled release and intracellular protein delivery from mesoporous silica nanoparticles. *Biotechnology Journal* 2017, 12(1):1600408.

104. Scaletti F, Hardie J, Lee Y-W, Luther DC, Ray M, Rotello VM. Protein delivery into cells using inorganic nanoparticle-protein supramolecular assemblies. *Chemical Society Reviews* 2017, 47(10):3421–3432.

105. Díaz A, Katsarava R, Puiggalí J. Synthesis, properties and applications of biodegradable polymers derived from diols and dicarboxylic acids: From polyesters to poly(ester amide)s. *International Journal of Molecular Sciences* 2014, 15(5):7064–7123.

106. Kumar S, Malik MM, Purohit R. Synthesis methods of mesoporous silica materials. *Materials Today: Proceedings* 2017, 4(2):350–357.

107. Wu S-H, Mou C-Y, Lin H-P. Synthesis of mesoporous silica nanoparticles. *Chemical Society Reviews* 2013, 42(9):3862–3875.

108. Aladesuyi OA, Oluwafemi OS. Synthesis strategies and application of ternary quantum dots-in cancer therapy. *Nano-Structures & Nano-Objects* 2020, 24:100568.

109. Drbohlavova J, Adam V, Kizek R, Hubalek J. Quantum dots-characterization, preparation and usage in biological systems. *International Journal of Molecular Sciences* 2009, 10(2):656–673.

110. Blackburn NK, Schoub BD, O'Connell K. Reliability of the clinical surveillance criteria for measles diagnosis. *Bulletin of the World Health Organization* 2000, 78(6):861.

111. Saikia N. Functionalized carbon nanomaterials in drug delivery: Emergent perspectives from application. *Novel Nanomaterials-Synthesis and Applications*. IntechOpen. 2018.

112. Khoshnevisan K, Daneshpour M, Barkhi M, Gholami M, Samadian H, Maleki H. The promising potentials of capped gold nanoparticles for drug delivery systems. *Journal of Drug Targeting* 2018, 26(7):525–532.

113. Kumari Y, Singh SK, Kumar R, Kumar B, Kaur G, Gulati M, Tewari D, Gowthamarajan K, Karri VVSNR, Ayinkamiye C. Modified apple polysaccharide capped gold nanoparticles for oral delivery of insulin. *International Journal of Biological Macromolecules* 2020, 149:976–988.

114. Jagadeesan AK, Thangavelu K, Dhananjeyan V. Carbon nanotubes: Synthesis, properties and applications. *Surface Science*. IntechOpen. 2020.

115. Shah M, Badwaik V, Kherde Y, Waghwani HK, Modi T, Aguilar ZP, Rodgers H, Hamilton W, Marutharaj T, Webb C. Gold nanoparticles: Various methods of synthesis and antibacterial applications. *Frontiers in Bioscience* 2014, 19(8):1320–1344.

116. Vangijzegem T, Stanicki D, Laurent S. Magnetic iron oxide nanoparticles for drug delivery: Applications and characteristics. *Expert Opinion on Drug Delivery* 2019, 16(1):69–78.

117. Laurent S, Saei AA, Behzadi S, Panahifar A, Mahmoudi M. Superparamagnetic iron oxide nanoparticles for delivery of therapeutic agents: Opportunities and challenges. *Expert Opinion on Drug Delivery* 2014, 11(9):1449–1470.

118. Mohammed L, Gomaa HG, Ragab D, Zhu J. Magnetic nanoparticles for environmental and biomedical applications: A review. *Particuology* 2017, 30:1–14.

119. Ansari SAMK, Ficiarà E, Ruffinatti FA, Stura I, Argenziano M, Abollino O, Cavalli R, Guiot C, D'Agata F. Magnetic iron oxide nanoparticles: Synthesis, characterization and functionalization for biomedical applications in the central nervous system. *Materials* 2019, 12(3):465.

120. Date T, Nimbalkar V, Kamat J, Mittal A, Mahato RI, Chitkara D. Lipid-polymer hybrid nanocarriers for delivering cancer therapeutics. *Journal of Controlled Release* 2018, 271:60–73.

121. Wu C, Baldursdottir S, Yang M, Mu H. Lipid and PLGA hybrid microparticles as carriers for protein delivery. *Journal of Drug Delivery Science and Technology* 2018, 43:65–72.

122. Devrim B, Bozkır A. Preparation and characterization of protein-loaded lipid-polymer hybrid nanoparticles with polycaprolactone as polymeric core material. *Journal of Biomolecular Research & Therapeutics* 2014, 3(115):2.

123. Mukherjee A, Waters AK, Kalyan P, Achrol AS, Kesari S, Yenugonda VM. Lipid-polymer hybrid nanoparticles as a next-generation drug delivery platform: State of the art, emerging technologies, and perspectives. *International Journal of Nanomedicine* 2019, 14:1937.

124. Zhang X-X, Eden HS, Chen X. Peptides in cancer nanomedicine: Drug carriers, targeting ligands and protease substrates. *Journal of Controlled Release* 2012, 159(1):2–13.

125. Elzoghby AO, Elgohary MM, Kamel NM. Implications of protein-and peptide-based nanoparticles as potential vehicles for anticancer drugs. *Advances in Protein Chemistry and Structural Biology*. Elsevier. 2015, p 169–221.

126. Steinhauser I, Spänkuch B, Strebhardt K, Langer K. Trastuzumab-modified nanoparticles: Optimisation of preparation and uptake in cancer cells. *Biomaterials* 2006, 27(28):4975–4983.

127. Mishra V, Mahor S, Rawat A, Gupta PN, Dubey P, Khatri K, Vyas SP. Targeted brain delivery of AZT via transferrin anchored pegylated albumin nanoparticles. *Journal of Drug Targeting* 2006, 14(1):45–53.
128. James HP, John R, Alex A, Anoop KR. Smart polymers for the controlled delivery of drugs—a concise overview. *Acta Pharmaceutica Sinica B* 2014, 4(2):120–127.
129. Cardoso VF, Correia DM, Ribeiro C, Fernandes MM, Lanceros-Méndez S. Fluorinated polymers as smart materials for advanced biomedical applications. *Polymers* 2018, 10(2):161.
130. Al-Tahami K, Singh J. Smart polymer based delivery systems for peptides and proteins. *Recent Patents on Drug Delivery & Formulation* 2007, 1(1):65–71.

22 Nanotechnology and Regenerative Medicine

Taihaseen Momin, Anamika Sahu Gulbake,
Shivaji Kashte, Rahul Tiwari, and Arvind Gulbake

22.1 INTRODUCTION

The normal process of replacing or restoring damaged cells, tissues, organs and even whole-body parts to their original function is known as regeneration. Some tissue has high regeneration potential, such as the skin and liver, while other tissues have little or no capacity for regeneration. Today ongoing studies on regeneration focus on acquiring knowledge that will improve the range of regenerative medicine. The new interdisciplinary regenerative medicine area utilizes medical sciences, life science and engineering principles to encourage regeneration of injured tissues as well as whole organs. The potential for healing or replacing tissues and organs damaged by age, disease or trauma increases the importance of regenerative medicine. Until now, many preclinical and clinical studies have been carried out on regenerative medicine that have shown promising effects in the treatment of chronic and acute conditions such as wounds, cardiovascular diseases, traumas, certain types of cancer and many more [1–3]. The limited donor supply and other immune system–related complications are the main hurdle for using current transplant therapies, but the use of regenerative medicine could provide a better solution for this problem [4]. The use of nanomaterials and cells, or the combination of both, in regenerative medicine can be used as a structural and functional substitute for missing tissue or to contribute to tissue healing [5]. Apart from this, the innate healing response of the body can be utilized to enhance regeneration [6]. Stem cells have natural capacity to regenerate various therapeutically useful cells. These regenerated cells are useful for variety of disorders (i.e., diabetes; Parkinson's and Alzheimer's; aggressive and recurrent cancers and degenerative disorders such as osteoporosis, spine injuries, chronic liver injuries and arthritis; and muscular, skin, lung, eye and digestive disorders) [7]. For regenerative medicine, stem cells are widely used, as they have all the ideal raw material properties, such as the ability to produce a variety of cells and infinite development morphology. Recently, it has been successfully shown that in vitro regeneration can be performed for functional tissues. For this, the use of a natural or synthesized porous scaffold is developed on which stem cells are loaded for in-vitro and in-vivo cellular regeneration. Various biological molecules are used for functionalization of scaffolds depending on the targeted cell type. Bioreactors are useful for in-vitro tissue regeneration under controlled conditions. In industrial applications, these bioreactors can be combined with a variety of biomedical microelectromechanical systems (BioMEMS) to control specific operational conditions. Various biosensors and lab-on-a-chip approaches are combined with bioreactors for real-time observation and investigation of particular cellular processes [8].

Human tissues are made up of nanoscale structure. The progress in nanotechnology has provided the alternative ways to develop architectures, surfaces and materials with nanoscale properties which can simulate the cellular environment and promote functions i.e., cellular adhesion, mobility, and differentiation [9–10]. Nanoparticles are useful for the delivery of drugs and growth factors to the targeted site in regenerative medicine, whereas for preparation of scaffolds, nanofibers and biosensors are used for modification of surface-implantable materials. The chapter briefly covers the various aspects related to the application of nanotechnology for tissue regeneration and promising strategies in the field.

DOI: 10.1201/9781003130055-22

22.1.1 Nanoscaffolds for Tissue Regeneration

The repair or regeneration of various tissues can be achieved by standard approaches like autografts, allografts and xenografts. Autografts have achieved great success in the treatment of tissue deformity; however, donor site illness, prolonged recuperation, increased chance of serious infection and constrained availability are major limitations, whereas allografts may produce risks of transmissible diseases, viral infection and immunological rejections. Therefore, there is limited application of autografts, allografts or xenografts to treat bone [11], skin [12], nerve [13–14] and vascular tissue defects [15–16]. Presently there are no synthetic biological substitutes available with the same biological and mechanical properties compared to natural tissue. Therefore, there is a need to create a unique treatment as complementary or addition to traditional approaches used for tissue rejuvenation. The recent developments in nanotechnology and regenerative medicine can achieve biological substitutes which restore, maintain and improve tissue function to replace conventional grafts (Figure 22.1).

22.1.2 Bone Tissue Regeneration

The bone is a rigid tissue which protects the organs and provides support to the body. The repair and/or alteration of damaged bone with healthy (regenerated) bone is a critical issue in orthopedics worldwide. Tissue-engineered scaffolds have great possibility for bone tissue regeneration [11]. Overall, the performance and cytocompatibility of tissue-engineered scaffolds are significantly enhanced with the integration of nanoparticles and growth factors. Nanomaterials provide physiochemical signals that increase stem cell differentiation into bone-forming cells like osteoblasts and often improve the biocompatibility of inert scaffold materials [17–18].

Carbon nanofibers (CNFs) derived from electrospun polyacrylonitrile (PAN) nanofibers are used as the substrate for bone tissue healing showed good cytocompatibility *in vitro*. For example, CNFs seeded with MG-63 cells experienced direct current (DC) electrical stimulation that could have improved proliferation and activity of alkaline phosphatase (ALP) in bone cells [19]. A porous scaffold of polycaprolactone (PCL) coated with chitosan and an optimal amount of 45S bioactive glass (BG) nanoparticles bearing 7 wt% strontium (Sr) was found to be biodegradable, hydrophilic and biocompatible and improved both ALP expression and cell attachment *in vitro* [20]. An electrospun PCL-polyvinylidene fluoride (PCL-PVDF) hybrid nanofibrous scaffold embedded with

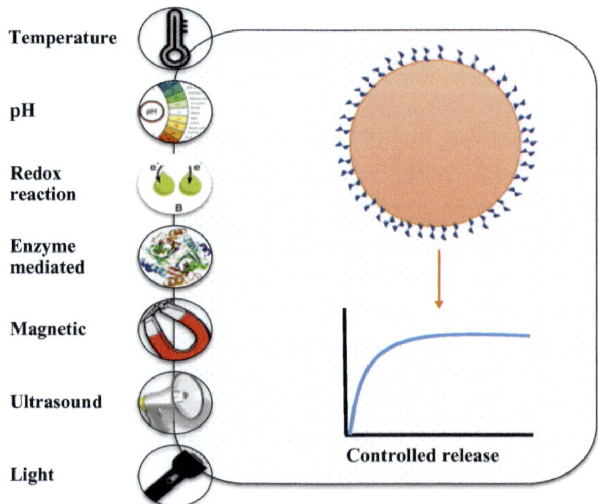

FIGURE 22.1 Nanoscaffolds and regenerative medicine.

basic fibroblast growth factor significantly increased osteogenic differentiation of human induced pluripotent stem cells (iPSCs) in contrast to a PCL-PVDF scaffold. There was the highest ALP expression and mineralization on the PCL-PVDF-bFGF scaffolds [21]. Super-paramagnetic iron oxide nanoparticles (IONPs) incorporated with calcium phosphate cement (IONP-CPC) and the effect of IONP inclusion with an exterior static magnetic field (SMF) on the accumulation, osteogenic distinction, and bone mineral creation of human dental pulp stem cells were investigated. It was observed that IONP-CPC enhanced cellular performance of hDPSCs, with increased ALP activity about threefold, and increased expressions of osteogenic marker genes than to CPC control and nonmagnetic IONP-CPC. In rat mandible defects, IONP-CPC caused vigorous osteogenesis as compared to a CPC control [22]. Calcium phosphate 2-D nanoflake (CaP)–decorated chitosan (CTs) functionalized with supermagnetic halloysite nanotubes (M-HNTs-CTs-CaP) scaffold has been synthesized with stepwise modification process. M-HNTs-CTs-CaP exhibited the highest osteogenesis and osteoconduction in comparison with HNTs, M-HNTs and M-HNTs-CTs owing to the improved CaP distribution on M-HNTs-CT surfaces and enhanced collaborative osteoconduction in human adipose-derived stem cells (hADMSCs) due to Fe_3O_4, chitosan and CaP [23]. Hydroxyapatite (HAP)-Tragacanth (GT) gum scaffolds showed the formation of apatite *in vitro* in simulated body fluid (SBF). These scaffolds were biocompatible with Vero cells [24]. Bio-composite scaffolds of chitosan (CS), nano-hydroxyapatite (nHAp) and nano zirconium dioxide ($nZrO_2$) along with miR-590–5p (microRNA) has been formulated using freeze drying method. In this case, the results showed that an amalgam of miR-590–5p along with a scaffold been increased osteoblast differentiation of mouse mesenchymal stem cells (C3H10T1/2) owing to trigger various signaling pathways in cells [25]. Bone morphogenic protein-2 (BMP-2) was conjugated with TiO_2 nanoparticles on a Zein-polydopamine (PDA) based nanofiber scaffold. It has been observed that significantly higher amount of mineralization lead the ALP activity in human fetal osteoblast (hFOB) cells cultured on nanofiber matrix than those cultured with only Zein, Zein-PDA and Zein-PDA-TiO_2 nanofiber scaffolds [26]. Polyethersulphone (PES) nanofibers coated with bioactive glass (BG) showed significantly enhanced biocompatibility and osteoconductivity in MG-63 cells and the highest reconstruction at the defect site *in-vivo* compared to the control group [27]. Layer by layer modified PCL-graphene oxide (GO)-*Cissus quandrangularis* (CQ) extract scaffolds showed improved osteoblastic differentiation of human umbilical cord–derived mesenchymal stem cells (hUCMSCs) along with osteoinduction and osteoconduction *in vitro* [28]. PCL-GO-CQ scaffolds planted with hUCMSCs scaffolds revealed the highest bone regeneration after 3 months of transplantation in a critical size rat model by assisting in complete healing of the defect site [29]. Although studies showed potential for bone regeneration and repair, more research is needed to develop biomimicking scaffolds to replace defective bone or cure bone defects and diseases via bone regeneration.

22.1.3 Skin Tissue Regeneration

In the human body, skin is the leading organ, providing protection from infectious agents, chemicals and mechanical and thermal stress and counteracting dehydration of the body. Though skin has the potential of self-healing without any external manipulation in most cases [30–32], cutaneous diseases, abrasions, burns and other traumatic events cause wounds which are critical to heal [33]. Generally, there are two types of wounds, acute and chronic. Within an expected time, acute wounds heal, but chronic wounds require a long time and are more prone to infection, are difficult to manage and require external interventions. A modern approach for the healing of chronic wounds is the fabrication of skin substitutes by tissue engineering to keep cell functional activity alive [34–35].

Adipose tissue-derived mesenchymal stem cells (ADMSCs) and keratinocytes seeded into gelatin/chitosan/β-glycerol phosphate (GCGP) nanoscaffold were transplanted in a rat model with an excisional wound (full thickness skin). A remarkable increase in wound closure rate in the keratinocyte-ADMSC-seeded GCGP nanoscaffolds was observed [36]. RL/RS 100 nanofibers carrying gentamicin sulphate (GS) and human epidermal growth factor (rhEGF) were electrospun to

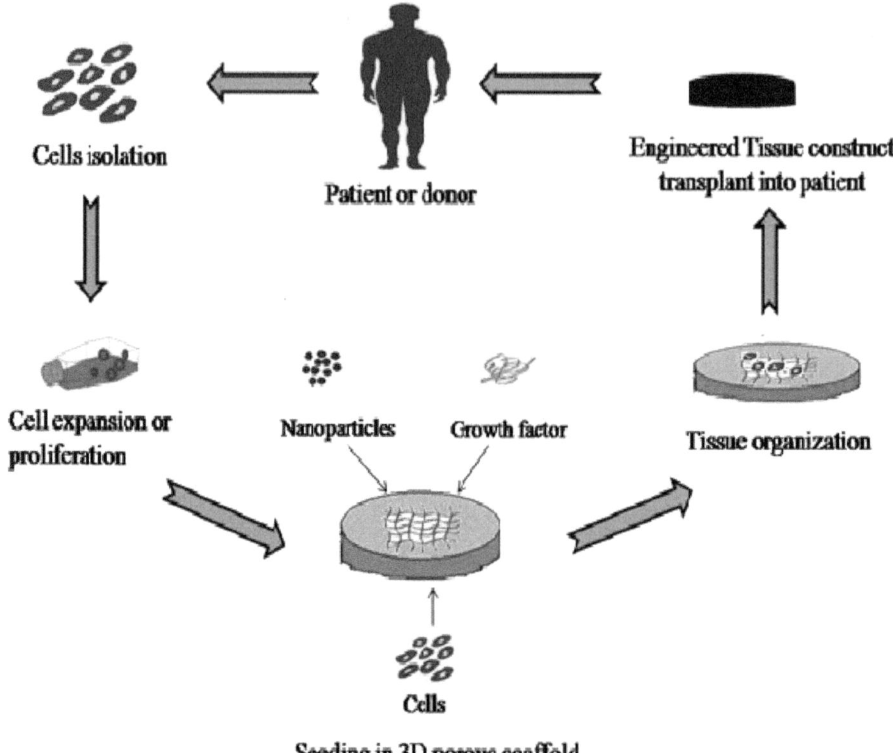

FIGURE 22.2 Tissue regeneration process.

yield nanofiber scaffolds. These nanoscaffolds showed antibacterial activity and encouraged quick wound-healing activity in dorsal wounds in mice [37]. A 3D hybrid nanoscaffold of polypropylene fumarate (PPF): diethyl fumarate (DEF) resin incorporated with gold nanoparticles (Au NPs) was prepared and when it was seeded with macrophages and mouse autologous adipose stem cells (ASCs), there was larger cell dispersion and cell adhesion than PPF scaffolds without Au NPs. In an experimental generated in-vivo wound model, an ASC-seeded 3D hybrid nanoscaffold stimulated tissue regeneration in muscle [38].

A tailored tri-layer PCL-gelatin scaffold showed mechanical firmness like skin layers, i.e., epidermis, dermis and hypodermis. An *in vitro* co-culture model accomplished by keratinocytes and human dermal fibroblast cells showed that multilayered scaffold encouraged proliferation and differentiation of various cells into organized tissue. *In-vivo* study suggested that the regenerated tissue showed comparable morphology to native skin [39]. A poloxamer (P407)-chitosan (CTS)-hyaluronic acid (HA)–based thermosensitive hydrogel was loaded with vitamins A, D and E (V-PCH3). This hydrogel was biocompatible, with optimum wettability, leakage and thermosensitive gelation properties. This hydrogel was antimicrobial and showed wound healing in mice [40]. To prepare a PVA/Chi/Cur patch, nano-curcumin was integrated into polyvinyl alcohol and chitosan. The PVA/Chi/Cur patch was biocompatible and showed increased cell proliferation of NIH3T3 cells. When these patches were studied in a rat model, there was an increased rate of wound rehabilitation [41]. Chitosan hydrogel was constructed by mixing the three different glycosaminoglycans such as HA, chondroitin sulfate (CS) and dermatan sulfate (DS) and collagen (CO). After hMSC encapsulation in these scaffolds, it provided a perfect microenvironment for viability and morphology of hMSCs up to 1 week. These scaffolds promoted healing and epidermal regeneration [42].

22.1.4 Nerve Tissue Regeneration

In the nervous system, the central nervous system (CNS) does not have the capacity to regenerate, but the peripheral nervous system (PNS) has the specific ability to regenerate after injury [43–44]. Peripheral nerve injury generally occurs due to physical damage such as trauma or accidents. The severity of the damage may directly affect the patient's quality of life [13–14]. Tissue engineering with nanomaterials is showing great possibilities for neural tissue regeneration. Nanoscaffolds have a greater surface-to-volume ratio that is suitable for cellular growth and adhesion. The permeability of nanoscaffolds can control the release of bioactive and growth factors which significantly stimulate peripheral nerve tissue regeneration [45–46].

Silk fibroin–reinforced gold nanorod (SF/GNR) nanocomposites showed improved cellular adherence, growth, proliferation and overexpression of nestin and neuron-specific enolase (NSE) in comparison to bulk SF scaffolds without any toxicity. GNRs considerably enhanced the insulation property of the bulk silk fibroin scaffold [47]. There was a significant amount of myelin formation, and it was firmly enclosed over the axons of the neurons. Electrospun SF nanofibers can offer an increased positive charge as well as purely topographical clues that can simulate the cellular micro-environment and can provide faster formation and maintenance of myelin [48].

22.1.5 Vascular Tissue Regeneration

Vascular tissues like arteries, blood vessels injury or other impairments causes cardiovascular diseases such as atherosclerosis and coronary arterial restenosis leading to mortality and morbidity. Myocardial infarction is often caused due to plaque formation in coronary arteries. Tissue engineering provides the potential to construct blood vessels. From the secretion of the extracellular matrix (ECM) to the formation of new tissues, the interaction of cells and scaffolds plays a vital role. The administration of a nanofiber template may direct the structural cells deportment to further grow as a new tissue [15–16].

Graphene oxide nanoscaffolds embedded in hydrogel were engrafted instantly in later spinal cord transection. These scaffolds were biocompatible and showed inward growth of connective tissue, blood vessels, neurofilaments and Schwann cells in the vicinity of nanoscaffolds [49]. The electrical, mechanical and biochemical properties of single-walled carbon nanotubes (SWNTs) blended with electrospun polyurethane nanofibers showed enhanced adsorption and retention of the culture media's protein. In vitro assessment showed that SWNTs exhibit exceptional physiochemical properties that might enhance cellular proliferation. These observations suggest that the polyurethane nanofibers containing SWNTs simulate the biological characteristics of blood vessels and ECM in vascular tissue engineering [15]. The matrix of poly (lactic acid) (PLA) and poly (butylene succinate) (PBS) was strengthened by cellulose nano fibrils developing a composite scaffold. CNF (cellulose nano fibrils) composite scaffolds made up of a poly (lactic acid) (PLA) and poly (butylene succinate) (PBS) matrix supports the connection and propagation of human fibroblast cells more than PLA, PBS or their mixture alone. This study showed that the formulated composite scaffolds proved their strength for vascular tissue engineering applications [50].

22.1.6 Cardiac Tissue Regeneration

Cardiovascular illnesses, heart failure and myocardial infarction are leading causes of morbidness and fatality in developed nations [51]. The cardiovascular breakdown is because the heart fails to siphon blood, and the grown-up heart muscle is unequipped for recovering harmed myocardial tissue. Right now, complete heart transplantation is a standard clinical system to reestablish the harmed myocardium and a few medications that slender blood, making it simpler to siphon by a faltering heart. Consequently, there is a need to grow new strategies to fix harmed heart tissue. Late cardiovascular tissue designing advanced as a promising way to heart unites, either entire heart substitutes or tissues that can be proficiently embedded in an organic entity. Tissue designing gives profoundly controllable three-dimensional conditions to intercede cell separation and advance useful gathering for use as high-devotion models to consider the cardiovascular turn of events and Cardiovascular illnesses [52].

Buckytubes (CNTs) introduced into poly(octamethylene maleate (anhydride) 1,2,4-butanetricarboxylate) (124 polymer), and built up an elastomeric scaffold for cardiovascular tissue designing. These 124 polymer-CNT materials showed the better conductance of scaffolds and expanded electrical signaling between cardiomyocytes (CMs) considering more rapid tissue association and development [53]. Bioactive glass nanoparticles fused hydrogel platforms boosted the differentiation of human endometrial stromal cells (EnSCs) into the endothelial lineage and expanded the degree of vascular endothelial growth factor (VEGF) expression. These endothelial lineage cells separated into cardiomyocytes and can be utilized for myocardial tissue engineering [54]. Cardiomyocytes cultivated onto Gold nanorod (GNR)-fused gelatin methacrylate (GelMA) hybrid hydrogels showed superb cell retention, feasibility, and metabolic movement. The improved operational and purposeful properties of the tissue were obtained due to the nanoengineered architecture of the matrix developed in advanced cell-matrix interface and cell-cell coupling [55]. Cardiovascular progenitor cells (CPCs) were cultivated onto nanofibrous poly(l-lactic acid) (PLLA) scaffolds differentiated into cardiomyocytes, smooth muscle cells, and endothelial cells. The frameworks empowered cell attachment, extension, and separation. At a point when these frameworks alongside CPCs were relocated subcutaneously in a bare mouse model there was endurance of the joined cells and their obligation to the three desired cell lineages. These permeable nanofibrous platforms and CPCs derived from patient iPSCs can be utilized for patient-specific cardiac fix [56].

22.2   NANODEVICES IN REGENERATIVE MEDICINE

Late advancement in nanotechnology has promoted the creation of nanodevices that can act or identify at the nanoscale. This innovative development has been made conceivable through advances in microfabrication innovation. The manufacture of biomicro-electromechanical systems (BioMEMS) has empowered the application of nanodevices in biomedicine [10]. These nanodevices incorporate biocapsules, bioreactors, biosensors, and laboratory-on-chip. Biocapsules basically contains the nanodevices used to transport or store the bioactives to be conveyed or gathered in a controlled manner. Development of biocapsules can be completed for specifically segregating explicit particles within device. Smart capsules can be produced that convey nanodevices for examining captured particles, and in this way can go about as neighborhood, touchy, and ongoing symptomatic instrument

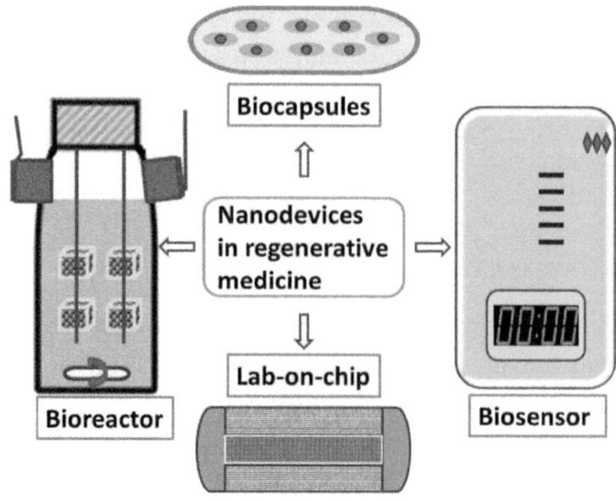

FIGURE 22.3   Nanodevices.

in illness identification. Bioreactors give controlled environment for cell and tissue recovery for in vitro systems like temperature, pH, pressure, supplement supply, and waste control. Biosensors are utilized to notice the progressions happening inside the bioreactor [57].

22.2.1 BIOREACTORS

The bioreactors provide the microenvironment for cell and tissue regeneration. Various sorts of bioreactors like spinner jars or rotating wall systems, a perfusion framework having possible applications in tissue designing for example, high efficiency cell seeding, enhanced functionality, extended cell viability and greater cell to cell contact [58].

Utilization of stirred suspension bioreactors (SSBs) for the extension of incited pluripotent stem cells (iPSCs) were researched and set up porcine iPSC (piPSCs) line and a recently produced cell line can fill in static and SSB culture. They announced that porcine iPSCs which grown in SSB keeps up attributes of pluripotency and karyotypic stability like cells grown in customary two-dimensional static culture. Investigation demonstrated that, SSBs are the reasonable for scale up of piPSCs in vitro [59]. Various bioreactors have been developed and reported for heart valve scaffold designs but most of them have faced serious regulatory challenges. Converse et al. reported the design for development of full scale, functional prototypes for tissue engineered heart valve (TEHV) and assessed the viability. The framework has set up efficacious in cultivating and mechanical molding of decellularized, aortic valves. Confinement of human mesenchymal stem cells (hMSCs) to the leaflet of the decellularized valve was accomplished via a utilization of mechanical molding utilizing the bioreactor, devoid of undesirable effects on cell phenotype or leaflet performance [60]. Bar et al. proposed a flow bioreactor for in vitro assessment of osteochondral defect (OCD) microenvironment, intended to support cell enrollment from the modeled bone marrow section within alginate hydrogel. The bioreactor permitted to check cell infiltration and hydrogel disintegration though live imaging, while it was additionally available for biochemical examinations for the assessment of chondrogenic separation of hMSCs inside the bioreactor. The bioreactor effectively showed its capacity to enroll cells to the deserted region by convectional stream alone and furthermore equipped for recognizing diverse cell infiltration profiles, contingent upon the matrix composition [61]. Buildup a 3D-culture stem cell bioprocess to make and approve a platform fit for creating mesodermal starting point tissue, for example, cardiomyogenic and skeletal tissue-like builds from embryonic stem cells (ESCs) in large scale production. Through underlying management of HepG2-CM, the 3D-ESCs embodied inside alginate/gelatin hydrogel effectively arrived at the initial enrichment of mesodermal differentiation throughout the successive embryonic body development period. By setting off terminal separation at different time focuses, enormous quantities of cardiomyogenic or osteogenic cell could be produced, with altogether enhanced contributor tissue properties [62]. The proper development of bioreactor who can provides a biomimetic physiological program is vital for the evolution of engineered tissue and for transforming tissue engineering approaches into clinical functions.

22.2.2 LABORATORY ON CHIP

In conventional 2D culture, frameworks are not equipped for cell separation and tissue association, but 3D cell culture model promotes level of cell differentiation and tissue organization. 3D-designed tissues entrapped into microfluidic gadgets can imitate in vivo construction, capacity, and responses to drugs in human tissues even more precisely prompting better in vitro viability and wellbeing screening before human preliminaries. The inadequacies of existing 2D and 3D culture framework are generally the aftereffect of long term and expensive in vivo experiments. The organ on chip is one of the dynamic in vitro models which provide investigation of human physiology in an organ-explicit setting, empower advancement of novel in vitro infection models, and may conceivably fill in as substitutes for creatures utilized in drug improvement, poison testing and evaluating for bio threat and chemical warfare agents [58]. Awaja et al. ascertain a time-cost effective lab-on-chip device via autohesion of polyether ether ketone (middle core) and two polystyrene outer layers by oxygen and methane plasma treatments at temperature near Tg (115 °C) without adhesive. The main advantage of the technology is to produce the chips with clear and specific precise sealing free from the toxic adhesives [63]. Alexander et al. developed a noninvasive technique to evaluate cells cultured in 2D and 3D on porous membranes. The transepithelial electrical resistance (TEER) values showed that skin simulate would be evaluated in culture up to 24 h and hold up the cellular lysis when brought to SDS medium. They give idea with a proof to ascertain the potential of IMOLA-IVD tool for developing noninvasive cellular assays with automation on complex 3D tissue [64]. Manufacture of nanoscaffolds by electrospinning PCL and three nanocarbons i.e., carbon nanotubes, graphene, and fullerene. The cell viability assay studied by Almar Blue showed that the PCL-nanomaterial nanofibers was not poisonous to the refined astrocytes. The development and morphology of astrocytes on nanofiber scaffolds studied by immunolabeling. This investigation revealed that PCL nanofibers comprising materials are biocompatible and would be suitable for biomolecules transport to the nervous system [65]. Grown new microfluidic model of glioblastoma that copies the elements of pseudo palisade arrangement by using SU-8 innovation. This framework showed that supplement and oxygen starvation trigger a solid transient interaction prompting pseudo palisade generation in vitro [66]. The lab-on-chip based detection devices are more pertinent with the present COVID-19 pandemic situation, exclusively for quick, robust, specific, sensitive, cost effective and may provide results instantly [67–68].

22.2.3 BIOSENSORS

The biosensor is a device used to detect biochemical changes based on blends of biological factor along with a physicochemical sensor. The first biosensor was developed in 1960s for glucose detection through electrochemical electrode [69]. Biosensors convert any changes into conductive signals received through an immobilized enzymes/biological receptor-based probe which are highly selective or specific for target moiety. Biosensors are having two basic features selective/specific binding and response to biological moiety [70]. Zhu et al. evaluated the release of pre-entrapped norepinephrine on MEMS device through the G protein coupled receptors for living cell-based biosensor [71]. Son et al. developed fluorescent microbead-based biosensor for the detection of transforming growth factor-β and hepatocyte growth factor from the hydrogel barrier to abutting sensor [72]. Biosensor also contribute a suitable technique to observe several signals from cells, expressing that biosensor-based systems exhibit great use for diagnosis of diseases. The cell-based biosensors have proven to be significant in neurological research and the MEA technique is useful to determine neuronal circuits, physiology, and abnormalities [73]. The biosensors are basically divided into two types, label-based and flexible biosensor. The tissue engineering in microfluidic technique with biosensor. The exploitation of a dual-transduction-incorporated biosensor evaluates electrical resistance combined with imaging facility while studying 3D based cell culture. To simulate the lively deposition of extracellular matrix (ECM) in 3D culture models and perceive osteogenesis through various quantities of bone–ECM elements (collagen, hydroxyapatite [HAp], and HA) within hydrogels (alginate-based). Electrical impedance spectroscopy (EIS) results depict that the impedances raised in a line with collagen and HA but complexly altered in case of HAp. They also produced two models comprised of primary osteoblast cells (OBs), to enhanced green fluorescent protein (EGFP), and 4T1 cells, secreted the EGFP-HA, in the hydrogel. They observed that the capacitance raised with initial embedded OBs and EGFP signal was observed by fluorescent picturing to confirm the cell proliferation over 3 days. Further, they transfect (through adenovirus) the primary OBs in rats with EGFP and cells were encapsulated in scaffolds (alginate). They demonstrated that a developed biosensing system could analyze the dynamic process of 3D culture in a non-invasive and real-time manner [74].

22.2.4 NANOMATERIALS FOR CELL IMAGING AND MOLECULAR IMAGING

Magnetic nanoparticles (MNPs) help to isolate and sort the stem cells. Superparamagnetic property of magnetic nanoparticles is extensively explored for numerous potentials use such as hyperthermia therapy, magnetic resonance imaging (MRI), repairing of injured tissues, immunoassay, drug/gene delivery, cell separation etc. [75–76]. Multifunctional carrier made up of PEG-PCL (polyethylene glycol-co-polycaprolactone) micelles were developed through O/W emulsion-solvent evaporation technique and encapsulating busulphan for drug delivery, VivoTag 680XL for optical imaging (fluorescence) and SPIONs for MR imaging. The SPION-bearing PEG-PCL micelles show a high contrast under MRI. There was superior drug loading and gradual drug release through PEG-PCL nanocarriers. There was no cytotoxicity of PEG-PCL micelles with HL60 cells. The biodistribution study of fluorescent probe labeled-PEG-PCL micelles suggests that multifunctional PEG-PCL micelles can be suitable for *in vivo* imaging and controlled drug delivery [77]. The imaging behavior of ME (magneto-endosymbionts) contrast agents were studied *in vitro* in MDA-MB-231BR and *in vivo* in foxn1 Nu/nu. A small number of 100 ME-labeled 231BR cells were visible *in vivo* through normal MRI (7T) protocol. MEs showed good contrast like conventional contrast agents (iron oxide nanoparticles) [78]. The viability of BMSCs (bone mesenchymal stromal cells) tagged with the Fluc (firefly luciferase), CyI dye and USPIO (ultra-small super-paramagnetic iron oxide) particles investigated *in vitro* and *in vivo* via bioluminescence, fluorescence, and MRI. Transplanted Fluc-USPIO BMSCs can be vigorously analyzed by using bioluminescence. It was found that the results are comparable to MRI and histology [79]. The magnetic nanoparticles were coated with P127 and T908 and analyzed for MRI cell tracking with MSCs and a multipotent neural progenitor cell. These cells were tagged with MNPs by a simple co-incubation of MNP cell uptake. It was found that P-MNPs and T-MNPs could be useful as MRI agent for tracking of stem cell, due to their higher sensitivity for *in-vivo* cell detection efficiency for labeling of cell [80]. Melanin-based gadolinium3+-chelate NPS (MNP-Gd3+) as a contrast agent was used to chase BMSCs *in-vivo*. These MNP-Gd3+ found good stability and sensitivity, great cell tracking efficiency with good biocompatibility as compared with commercial products [81]. When USPIO, and glucosamine-functionalized IONPs (GlcN) were evaluated in MSCs, they showed promising results for cell tracking, revealing better biocompatibility, increased uptake by MSCs both *in-vitro* and *in-vivo* [82]. The viability of ADSCs were tracked *in vivo* using USPIO revealed that it can efficiently label cells, self-renewal, and good proliferation capacity [83]. Lanthanide ions, Eu3þ and Gd3þ, same at a time doped into the mesoporous silica nanoparticles (MSN) for dual-imaging functions (EuGd-MSNs), this linkage facilitated the controlled release of CPT and improved therapeutic effect. The theranostic MSNs (EuGd-SS-CPT-FA-MSNs) could be used to target folate receptor-rich cancer cells via same time photoluminescence and MR imaging [84]. Fluorophore doped siloxane core nano emulsions showed potential to track NPSCs (neural progenitor/stem cells) using PDMS-based dual modality (MRI/fluorescence), dual functional (contrast/oximetry) nanoprobes [85]. When neural stem (NS) cells labeled with SPION transplanted into mouse striatum they showed normal cell proliferation, migration, differentiation and neurosphere formation [86]. Dextran coated SPIONs were synthesized by co-precipitation method with colloidal stable surface potential ranging from −1.5 mV to +18.2 mV. The change in the surface charge can affect the stem cell uptake behavior and the highly positive charged SPIONs showed greater uptake through MSCs with respect to neutral dextran [87]. When human muscle precursor cells (hMPCs) were labeled with SPIO nanoparticles, it revealed consistent detection of hMPCs by MRI *in vivo*. It can be safely used to track muscle regeneration [88].

22.3 CONCLUSION

Presently, in case of organ failure or damage, transplantation therapy is the only option, but the major problem associated with this is rejection. To overcome this problem new field is emerging like tissue engineering which helps to develop tissue construct and replaced with damaged tissue i.e., bone, heart, nerve, vascular and skin. The ECM mimicking structure are formed with the help of scaffold and nanomaterials. The potential of scaffold improved by combining nanomaterials such as nanofibers, nanoparticles with scaffold. The nanodevices such as bioreactor, biosensor and lab-on-chip provides a controlled and real time tissue regeneration. Magnetic nanoparticles used for cell sorting, cell tracking and imaging. Thus, for tissue regeneration, combination of tissue engineering with nanotechnology having great future.

22.4 ACKNOWLEDGMENT

Dr. Gulbake would like to thank SERB, New Delhi, for extending facilities to write this chapter (EEQ/2016/000789).

REFERENCES

1. Rubino CM, Bradley JS. Optimizing therapy with antibacterial agents: use of pharmacokinetic-pharmacodynamic principles in pediatrics. *Pediatric Drugs.* 2007 Nov;9:361–9.
2. Lopez-Cabezas C, Muner DS, Massa MR, Mensa Pueyo JM. Antibiotics in endophthalmitis: microbiological and pharmacokinetic considerations. *Current Clinical Pharmacology.* 2010 Feb 1;5(1):47–54.
3. Dasgupta A. Advances in antibiotic measurement. *Advances in Clinical Chemistry.* 2012 Jan 1;56:75.
4. Miller-Kasprzak E, Jagodziński PP. Endothelial progenitor cells as a new agent contributing to vascular repair. *Archivum Immunologiae et Therapiae Experimentalis.* 2007 Aug;55:247–59.
5. Chen WH, Wang HM. Experimental research progress of warming yang and reinforcing kidney of Chinese medicine to promote the differentiation of bone marrow stromal cells. *Zhongguo gu Shang= China Journal of Orthopaedics and Traumatology.* 2011 Apr 1;24(4):352–6.
6. Petit-Zeman S. Regenerative medicine. *Nature Biotechnology.* 2001 Mar;19(3):201–6.
7. Leterrier C, Potier J, Caillol G, Debarnot C, Boroni FR, Dargent B. Nanoscale architecture of the axon initial segment reveals an organized and robust scaffold. *Cell Reports.* 2015 Dec 29;13(12):2781–93.
8. Wegst UG, Bai H, Saiz E, Tomsia AP, Ritchie RO. Bioinspired structural materials. *Nature Materials.* 2015 Jan;14(1):23–36.
9. Alarçin E, Guan X, Kashaf SS, Elbaradie K, Yang H, Jang HL, Khademhosseini A. Recreating composition, structure, functionalities of tissues at nanoscale for regenerative medicine. *Regenerative Medicine.* 2016 Dec;11(8):849–58.
10. Engel E, Michiardi A, Navarro M, Lacroix D, Planell JA. Nanotechnology in regenerative medicine: the materials side. *Trends in Biotechnology.* 2008 Jan 1;26(1):39–47.
11. Kashte S, Jaiswal AK, Kadam S. Artificial bone via bone tissue engineering: current scenario and challenges. *Tissue Engineering and Regenerative Medicine.* 2017 Feb;14:1–4.
12. Vig K, Chaudhari A, Tripathi S, Dixit S, Sahu R, Pillai S, Dennis VA, Singh SR. Advances in skin regeneration using tissue engineering. *International Journal of Molecular Sciences.* 2017 Apr 7;18(4):789.
13. Marinescu SA, Zărnescu O, Mihai IR, Giuglea C, Sinescu RD. An animal model of peripheral nerve regeneration after the application of a collagen-polyvinyl alcohol scaffold and mesenchymal stem cells. *Romanian Journal of Morphology and Embryology.* 2014 Jan 1;55(3):891–903.
14. Mackinnon SE, Hudson AR. Clinical application of peripheral nerve transplantation. *Plastic and Reconstructive Surgery.* 1992 Oct 1;90(4):695–9.
15. Tondnevis F, Keshvari H, Mohandesi JA. Physico-mechanical and in vitro characterization of electrically conductive electrospun nanofibers of poly urethane/single walled carbon nano tube by great endothelial cells adhesion for vascular tissue engineering. *Journal of Polymer Research.* 2019 Nov;26:1–6.
16. Ezhilarasu H, Sadiq A, Ratheesh G, Sridhar S, Ramakrishna S, Ab Rahim MH, Yusoff MM, Jose R, Reddy VJ. Functionalized core/shell nanofibers for the differentiation of mesenchymal stem cells for vascular tissue engineering. *Nanomedicine.* 2019 Jan;14(2):201–14.
17. Nowicki M, Castro NJ, Rao R, Plesniak M, Zhang LG. Integrating three-dimensional printing and nanotechnology for musculoskeletal regeneration. *Nanotechnology.* 2017 Aug 24;28(38):382001.
18. Cui H, Nowicki M, Fisher JP, Zhang LG. 3D bioprinting for organ regeneration. *Advanced Healthcare Materials.* 2017 Jan;6(1):1601118.
19. Samadian H, Mobasheri H, Hasanpour S, Ai J, Azamie M, Faridi-Majidi R. Electro-conductive carbon nanofibers as the promising interfacial biomaterials for bone tissue engineering. *Journal of Molecular Liquids.* 2020 Jan 15;298:112021.

20. Shaltooki M, Dini G, Mehdikhani MJ. Fabrication of chitosan-coated porous polycaprolactone/strontium-substituted bioactive glass nanocomposite scaffold for bone tissue engineering. *Materials Science and Engineering: C.* 2019 Dec 1;105:110138.

21. Abazari MF, Soleimanifar F, Enderami SE, Nematzadeh M, Nasiri N, Nejati F, Saburi E, Khodashenas S, Darbasizadeh B, Khani MM, Ghoraeian P. Incorporated-bFGF polycaprolactone/polyvinylidene fluoride nanocomposite scaffold promotes human induced pluripotent stem cells osteogenic differentiation. *Journal of Cellular Biochemistry.* 2019 Oct;120(10):16750–9.

22. Xia Y, Chen H, Zhao Y, Zhang F, Li X, Wang L, Weir MD, Ma J, Reynolds MA, Gu N, Xu HH. Novel magnetic calcium phosphate-stem cell construct with magnetic field enhances osteogenic differentiation and bone tissue engineering. *Materials Science and Engineering: C.* 2019 May 1;98:30–41.

23. Lee YJ, Lee SC, Jee SC, Sung JS, Kadam AA. Surface functionalization of halloysite nanotubes with supermagnetic iron oxide, chitosan and 2-D calcium-phosphate nanoflakes for synergistic osteoconduction enhancement of human adipose tissue-derived mesenchymal stem cells. *Colloids and Surfaces B: Biointerfaces.* 2019 Jan 1;173:18–26.

24. Lett JA, Sundareswari M, Ravichandran K, Latha B, Sagadevan S. Fabrication and characterization of porous scaffolds for bone replacements using gum tragacanth. *Materials Science and Engineering: C.* 2019 Mar 1;96:487–95.

25. Balagangadharan K, Chandran SV, Arumugam B, Saravanan S, Venkatasubbu GD, Selvamurugan N. Chitosan/nano-hydroxyapatite/nano-zirconium dioxide scaffolds with miR-590-5p for bone regeneration. *International Journal of Biological Macromolecules.* 2018 May 1;111:953–8.

26. Babitha S, Annamalai M, Dykas MM, Saha S, Poddar K, Venugopal JR, Ramakrishna S, Venkatesan T, Korrapati PS. Fabrication of a biomimetic ZeinPDA nanofibrous scaffold impregnated with BMP-2 peptide conjugated TiO2 nanoparticle for bone tissue engineering. *Journal of Tissue Engineering and Regenerative Medicine.* 2018 Apr;12(4):991–1001.

27. Ardeshirylajimi A, Farhadian S, Jamshidi Adegani F, Mirzaei S, Soufi Zomorrod M, Langroudi L, Doostmohammadi A, Seyedjafari E, Soleimani M. Enhanced osteoconductivity of polyethersulphone nanofibres loaded with bioactive glass nanoparticles in in vitro and in vivo models. *Cell Proliferation.* 2015 Aug;48(4):455–64.

28. Kashte S, Sharma RK, Kadam S. Layer-by-layer decorated herbal cell compatible scaffolds for bone tissue engineering: a synergistic effect of graphene oxide and Cissus quadrangularis. *Journal of Bioactive and Compatible Polymers.* 2020 Jan;35(1):57–73.

29. Kashte S, Dhumal R, Chaudhary P, Sharma RK, Dighe V, Kadam S. Bone regeneration in critical-size calvarial defect using functional biocompatible osteoinductive herbal scaffolds and human umbilical cord Wharton's Jelly-derived mesenchymal stem cells. *Materials Today Communications.* 2021 Mar 1;26:102049.

30. Levengood SL, Erickson AE, Chang FC, Zhang M. Chitosan-poly (caprolactone) nanofibers for skin repair. *Journal of Materials Chemistry B.* 2017;5(9):1822–33.

31. Ahmadi-Aghkand F, Gholizadeh-Ghaleh Aziz S, Panahi Y, Daraee H, Gorjikhah F, Gholizadeh-Ghaleh Aziz S, Hsanzadeh A, Akbarzadeh A. Recent prospective of nanofiber scaffolds fabrication approaches for skin regeneration. *Artificial Cells, Nanomedicine, and Biotechnology.* 2016 Oct 2;44(7):1635–41.

32. Clark RA, Ghosh K, Tonnesen MG. Tissue engineering for cutaneous wounds. *Journal of Investigative Dermatology.* 2007 May 1;127(5):1018–29.

33. Bonvallet P, Culpepper B, Bain J, Schultz M, Thomas S, Bellis S. Microporous dermal-like electrospun scaffolds promote accelerated skin regeneration. *Tissue Engineering Part A.* 2014;20(17–18): 2434–45.

34. Olson JL, Atala A, Yoo JJ. Tissue engineering: current strategies and future directions. *Chonnam Medical Journal.* 2011 Apr 1;47(1):1–3.

35. Mohammadzadeh L, Rahbarghazi R, Salehi R, Mahkam M. A novel egg-shell membrane based hybrid nanofibrous scaffold for cutaneous tissue engineering. *Journal of Biological Engineering.* 2019 Dec;13:1–5.

36. Lotfi M, Naderi-Meshkin H, Mahdipour E, Mafinezhad A, Bagherzadeh R, Sadeghnia HR, Esmaily H, Maleki M, Hasssanzadeh H, Ghayaour-Mobarhan M, Bidkhori HR. Adipose tissue-derived mesenchymal stem cells and keratinocytes co-culture on gelatin/chitosan/β-glycerol phosphate nanoscaffold in skin regeneration. *Cell Biology International.* 2019 Dec;43(12):1365–78.

37. Dwivedi C, Pandey I, Pandey H, Patil S, Mishra SB, Pandey AC, Zamboni P, Ramteke PW, Singh AV. In vivo diabetic wound healing with nanofibrous scaffolds modified with gentamicin and recombinant human epidermal growth factor. *Journal of Biomedical Materials Research Part A.* 2018 Mar;106(3):641–51.

38. Zsedenyi A, Farkas B, Abdelrasoul GN, Romano I, Gyukity-Sebestyen E, Nagy K, Harmati M, Dobra G, Kormondi S, Decsi G, Nemeth IB. Gold nanoparticle-filled biodegradable photopolymer scaffolds induced muscle remodeling: in vitro and in vivo findings. *Materials Science and Engineering: C.* 2017 Mar 1;72:625–30.

39. Haldar S, Sharma A, Gupta S, Chauhan S, Roy P, Lahiri D. Bioengineered smart trilayer skin tissue substitute for efficient deep wound healing. *Materials Science and Engineering: C.* 2019 Dec 1;105:110140.

40. Soriano-Ruiz JL, Calpena-Campmany AC, Silva-Abreu M, Halbout-Bellowa L, Bozal-de Febrer N, Rodriguez-Lagunas MJ, Clares-Naveros B. Design and evaluation of a multifunctional thermosensitive poloxamer-chitosan-hyaluronic acid gel for the treatment of skin burns. *International Journal of Biological Macromolecules.* 2020 Jan 1;142:412–22.

41. Niranjan R, Kaushik M, Prakash J, Venkataprasanna KS, Arpana C, Balashanmugam P, Venkatasubbu GD. Enhanced wound healing by PVA/Chitosan/Curcumin patches: in vitro and in vivo study. *Colloids and Surfaces B: Biointerfaces.* 2019 Oct 1;182:110339.

42. Soriano-Ruiz JL, Gálvez-Martín P, López-Ruiz E, Suñer-Carbó J, Calpena-Campmany AC, Marchal JA, Clares-Naveros B. Design and evaluation of mesenchymal stem cells seeded chitosan/glycosaminoglycans quaternary hydrogel scaffolds for wound healing applications. *International Journal of Pharmaceutics.* 2019 Oct 30;570:118632.

43. Gu X, Ding F, Williams DF. Neural tissue engineering options for peripheral nerve regeneration. *Biomaterials.* 2014 Aug 1;35(24):6143–56.

44. Gu X, Ding F, Yang Y, Liu J. Construction of tissue engineered nerve grafts and their application in peripheral nerve regeneration. *Progress in Neurobiology.* 2011 Feb 1;93(2):204–30.

45. Aijie C, Xuan L, Huimin L, Yanli Z, Yiyuan K, Yuqing L, Longquan S. Nanoscaffolds in promoting regeneration of the peripheral nervous system. *Nanomedicine.* 2018 May;13(9):1067–85.

46. Shah S, Solanki A, Lee KB. Nanotechnology-based approaches for guiding neural regeneration. *Accounts of Chemical Research.* 2016 Jan 19;49(1):17–26.

47. Afjeh-Dana E, Naserzadeh P, Nazari H, Mottaghitalab F, Shabani R, Aminii N, Mehravi B, Rostami FT, Joghataei MT, Mousavizadeh K, Ashtari K. Gold nanorods reinforced silk fibroin nanocomposite for peripheral nerve tissue engineering applications. *International Journal of Biological Macromolecules.* 2019 May 15;129:1034–9.

48. Liu S, Niu C, Xu Z, Wang Y, Liang Y, Zhao Y, Zhao Y, Yang Y. Modulation of myelin formation by combined high affinity with extracellular matrix structure of electrospun silk fibroin nanoscaffolds. *Journal of Biomaterials Science, Polymer Edition.* 2019 May 30;30(12):1068–1082.

49. Palejwala AH, Fridley JS, Mata JA, Samuel EL, Luerssen TG, Perlaky L, Kent TA, Tour JM, Jea A. Biocompatibility of reduced graphene oxide nanoscaffolds following acute spinal cord injury in rats. *Surgical Neurology International.* 2016;7.

50. Abudula T, Saeed U, Memic A, Gauthaman K, Hussain MA, Al-Turaif H. Electrospun cellulose nano fibril reinforced PLA/PBS composite scaffold for vascular tissue engineering. *Journal of Polymer Research.* 2019 May;26:1–5.

51. Kashte S, Kadam S. Stem cell therapy: a hope business or a magic wand? *British Biomedical Bulletin.* 2013. hal-03710934.

52. Mohammadi Nasr S, Rabiee N, Hajebi S, Ahmadi S, Fatahi Y, Hosseini M, Bagherzadeh M, Ghadiri AM, Rabiee M, Jajarmi V, Webster TJ. Biodegradable nanopolymers in cardiac tissue engineering: from concept towards nanomedicine. *International Journal of Nanomedicine.* 2020 Jun 18;15:4205–24.

53. Ahadian S, Huyer LD, Estili M, Yee B, Smith N, Xu Z, Sun Y, Radisic M. Moldable elastomeric polyester-carbon nanotube scaffolds for cardiac tissue engineering. *Acta Biomaterialia.* 2017 Apr 1;52:81–91.

54. Barabadi Z, Azami M, Sharifi E, Karimi R, Lotfibakhshaiesh N, Roozafzoon R, Joghataei MT, Ai J. Fabrication of hydrogel based nanocomposite scaffold containing bioactive glass nanoparticles for myocardial tissue engineering. *Materials Science and Engineering: C.* 2016 Dec 1;69:1137–46.

55. Navaei A, Saini H, Christenson W, Sullivan RT, Ros R, Nikkhah M. Gold nanorod-incorporated gelatin-based conductive hydrogels for engineering cardiac tissue constructs. *Acta Biomaterialia.* 2016 Sep 1;41:133–46.

56. Liu Q, Tian S, Zhao C, Chen X, Lei I, Wang Z, Ma PX. Porous nanofibrous poly (L-lactic acid) scaffolds supporting cardiovascular progenitor cells for cardiac tissue engineering. *Acta Biomaterialia.* 2015 Oct 15;26:105–14.

57. Arora P, Sindhu A, Dilbaghi N, Chaudhury A, Rajakumar G, Rahuman AA. Nano-regenerative medicine towards clinical outcome of stem cell and tissue engineering in humans. *Journal of Cellular and Molecular Medicine.* 2012 Sep;16(9):1991–2000.

58. Kashte S, Maras JS, Kadam S. Bioinspired engineering for liver tissue regeneration and development of bioartificial liver: a review. *Critical Reviews™ in Biomedical Engineering.* 2018;46(5):413–27.

59. Burrell K, Dardari R, Goldsmith T, Toms D, Villagomez DA, King WA, Ungrin M, West FD, Dobrinski I. Stirred suspension bioreactor culture of porcine induced pluripotent stem cells. *Stem Cells and Development.* 2019 Sep 15;28(18):1264–75.

60. Converse GL, Buse EE, Neill KR, McFall CR, Lewis HN, VeDepo MC, Quinn RW, Hopkins RA. Design and efficacy of a single-use bioreactor for heart valve tissue engineering. *Journal of Biomedical Materials Research Part B: Applied Biomaterials.* 2017 Feb;105(2):249–59.

61. Bar A, Ruvinov E, Cohen S. Live imaging flow bioreactor for the simulation of articular cartilage regeneration after treatment with bioactive hydrogel. *Biotechnology and Bioengineering.* 2018 Sep;115(9):2205–16.

62. Cha JM, Mantalaris A, Jung S, Ji Y, Bang OY, Bae H. Mesoderm lineage 3D tissue constructs are produced at large-scale in a 3D stem cell bioprocess. *Biotechnology Journal.* 2017 Sep;12(9):1600748.

63. Awaja F, Wong TT, Arhatari B. Lab-on-a-chip device made by autohesion-bonded polymers. *Biomedical Microdevices.* 2018 Mar;20:1–9.

64. Alexander Jr FA, Eggert S, Wiest J. Skin-on-a-chip: transepithelial electrical resistance and extracellular acidification measurements through an automated air-liquid interface. *Genes.* 2018 Feb 21;9(2):114.

65. Srikanth M, Asmatulu R, Cluff K, Yao L. Material characterization and bioanalysis of hybrid scaffolds of carbon nanomaterial and polymer nanofibers. *ACS Omega.* 2019 Mar 8;4(3):5044–51.

66. Ayuso JM, Monge R, Martínez-González A, Virumbrales-Muñoz M, Llamazares GA, Berganzo J, Hernández-Laín A, Santolaria J, Doblaré M, Hubert C, Rich JN. Glioblastoma on a microfluidic chip: generating pseudopalisades and enhancing aggressiveness through blood vessel obstruction events. *Neuro-oncology.* 2017 Apr 6;19(4):503–13.

67. Burklund A, Tadimety A, Nie Y, Hao N, Zhang JX. Advances in diagnostic microfluidics. *Advances in Clinical Chemistry.* 2020 Jan 1;95:1–72.

68. Tadimety A, Zhang Y, Kready KM, Palinski TJ, Tsongalis GJ, Zhang JX. Design of peptide nucleic acid probes on plasmonic gold nanorods for detection of circulating tumor DNA point mutations. *Biosensors and Bioelectronics.* 2019 Apr 1;130:236–44.

69. Li YC, Lee IC. The current trends of biosensors in tissue engineering. *Biosensors.* 2020 Aug 3;10(8):88.

70. Fathi F, Rahbarghazi R, Rashidi MR. Label-free biosensors in the field of stem cell biology. *Biosensors and Bioelectronics.* 2018 Mar 15;101:188–98.

71. Zhu H, Stybayeva G, Macal M, Ramanculov E, George MD, Dandekar S, Revzin A. A microdevice for multiplexed detection of T-cell-secreted cytokines. *Lab on a Chip.* 2008;8(12):2197–205.

72. Son KJ, Gheibi P, Stybayeva G, Rahimian A, Revzin A. Detecting cell-secreted growth factors in microfluidic devices using bead-based biosensors. *Microsystems & Nanoengineering.* 2017 Jul 3;3(1):1–9.

73. Seymour JP, Wu F, Wise KD, Yoon E. State-of-the-art MEMS and microsystem tools for brain research. *Microsystems & Nanoengineering.* 2017 Jan 2;3(1):1–6.

74. Kozhevnikov E, Qiao S, Han F, Yan W, Zhao Y, Hou X, Acharya A, Shen Y, Tian H, Zhang H, Chen X. A dual-transduction-integrated biosensing system to examine the 3D cell-culture for bone regeneration. *Biosensors and Bioelectronics.* 2019 Sep 15;141:111481.

75. Solanki A, Kim JD, Lee KB. Nanotechnology for regenerative medicine: nanomaterials for stem cell imaging. *Nanomedicine.* 2008;3(4): 567–78.

76. Yi DK, Nanda SS, Kim K, Selvan ST. Recent progress in nanotechnology for stem cell differentiation, labeling, tracking and therapy. *Journal of Materials Chemistry B.* 2017;5(48):9429–51.

77. Asem H, Zhao Y, Ye F, Barrefelt Å, Abedi-Valugerdi M, El-Sayed R, El-Serafi I, Abu-Salah KM, Hamm J, Muhammed M, Hassan M. Biodistribution of biodegradable polymeric nano-carriers loaded with busulphan and designed for multimodal imaging. *Journal of Nanobiotechnology.* 2016;14(82):1–16.

78. Brewer KD, Spitler R, Lee KR, Chan AC, Barrozo JC, Wakeel A, Foote CS, Machtaler S, Rioux J, Willmann JK, Chakraborty P. Characterization of magneto-endosymbionts as MRI cell labeling and tracking agents. *Molecular Imaging and Biology.* 2018 Feb;20:65–73.

79. Cao J, Li X, Chang N, Wang Y, Lei J, Zhao D, Gao K, Jin Z. Dual-modular molecular imaging to trace transplanted bone mesenchymal stromal cells in an acute myocardial infarction model. *Cytotherapy.* 2015 Oct 1;17(10):1365–73.

80. Argibay B, Trekker J, Himmelreich U, Beiras A, Topete A, Taboada P, Pérez-Mato M, Iglesias-Rey R, Sobrino T, Rivas J, Campos F. Easy and efficient cell tagging with block copolymer-based contrast agents for sensitive MRI detection in vivo. *Cell Transplantation.* 2016 Oct;25(10):1787–800.

81. Cai WW, Wang LJ, Li SJ, Zhang XP, Li TT, Wang YH, Yang X, Xie J, Li JD, Liu SJ, Xu W. Effective tracking of bone mesenchymal stem cells in vivo by magnetic resonance imaging using melanin-based gadolinium3+ nanoparticles. *Journal of Biomedical Materials Research Part A*. 2017 Jan;105(1):131–7.

82. Guldris N, Argibay B, Gallo J, Iglesias-Rey R, Carbó-Argibay E, Kolen'ko YV, Campos F, Sobrino T, Salonen LM, Bañobre-López M, Castillo J. Magnetite nanoparticles for stem cell labeling with high efficiency and long-term in vivo tracking. *Bioconjugate Chemistry*. 2017 Feb 15;28(2):362–70.

83. Zhou S, Yin T, Zou Q, Zhang K, Gao G, Shapter JG, Huang P, Fu Q. Labeling adipose derived stem cell sheet by ultrasmall super-paramagnetic Fe3O4 nanoparticles and magnetic resonance tracking in vivo. *Scientific Reports*. 2017 Feb 21;7(1):42793.

84. Chan MH, Lin HM. Preparation and identification of multifunctional mesoporous silica nanoparticles for in vitro and in vivo dual-mode imaging, theranostics, and targeted tracking. *Biomaterials*. 2015 Apr 1;46:149–58.

85. Addington CP, Cusick A, Shankar RV, Agarwal S, Stabenfeldt SE, Kodibagkar VD. Siloxane nanoprobes for labeling and dual modality functional imaging of neural stem cells. *Annals of Biomedical Engineering*. 2016 Mar;44:816–27.

86. Azevedo-Pereira RL, Rangel B, Tovar-Moll F, Gasparetto EL, Attias M, Zaverucha-do-Valle C, Jasmin, Mendez-Otero R. Superparamagnetic iron oxide nanoparticles as a tool to track mouse neural stem cells in vivo. *Molecular Biology Reports*. 2019 Feb 1;46:191–8.

87. Barrow M, Taylor A, Nieves DJ, Bogart LK, Mandal P, Collins CM, Moore LR, Chalmers JJ, Lévy R, Williams SR, Murray P. Tailoring the surface charge of dextran-based polymer coated SPIONs for modulated stem cell uptake and MRI contrast. *Biomaterials Science*. 2015;3(4):608–16.

88. Azzabi F, Rottmar M, Jovaisaite V, Rudin M, Sulser T, Boss A, Eberli D. Viability, differentiation capacity, and detectability of super-paramagnetic iron oxide-labeled muscle precursor cells for magnetic-resonance imaging. *Tissue Engineering Part C: Methods*. 2015 Feb 1;21(2):182–91.

23 Nanomedicine for Cancer Immunotherapy

Renuka Khatik, Monika Dwivedi, Bhattarai Prapanna, and Sushesh Srivatsa Palakurthi

23.1 INTRODUCTION

Cancer is accretion of events involving genetic alterations in normal cells that grades in severe abnormalities in cell functioning. At cellular level, series of cascade induce immune response in human body to combat cancer cells. In tumorigenesis, neoantigens are discharged by tumor cells and then restricted by dendritic cells (DCs) [1]. Altogether, in this immuno-cascade, various multiple signals are delivered in the form of pro-inflammatory cytokines and biological factors to T cells. These signals activate effector T-lymphocyte, which trigger the T-lymphocyte response to cancer-specific antigens [2]. Subsequently, the actuated T-lymphocyte including CD8+ effector T-lymphocyte accommodate and invade the tumor after recognizing it and finally, terminating the targeted cancer cells. Following the cell death, several other biomarkers like tumor-associated antigens provide to the succeeding anti-tumor immune responses [3]. Contrary to normal conditions, the cell apoptosis mechanism exhibits an abnormal pattern in cancer patients. However, DCs and T-cells may not be able to detect heterologous tumor antigens, resulting in a regulatory T-cell response against tumor cells. Varied mechanisms play protagonist for conserved or acquired somatic mutations that can relate to the T-cell exhaustions that further indications to the abnormal T-cell functioning and limited intrusion in the tumors [4].

Current treatment practices for cancer rely on major surgical resection, hormonal therapy, chemotherapy, radiotherapy and immunotherapy. However, bio therapeutics such as MicroRNA replacement therapy, exosome, also conjoined the cancer therapy area as an emerging novel mode to address in cancer and cancer metastasis [5–7]. Immunotherapy can efficiently work for targeting the tumor microenvironment (TME). Thus, offering a minimal side effect and toxicity based individualized treatment for patients [8, 9]. Altogether, immunotherapy unveils imperative aspects of tumor associated immune-regulatory pathways directing an effective response of patient's body to cancer immunotherapy [10]. Therefore, cancer immunotherapy has triggered a widespread collection of molecular and cellular tools to limit the growth of cancer cells by arming the immune system, thus promoting anti-cancer immunity as a biological intervention.

Nanomedicine emerged as revolutionary intervention technology for cancer therapy. Owing to small size of nanomedicine, they are in high demand for modulation of pharmacokinetic, biodistribution profile of bio-actives, target site specificity. Nanomedicines demonstrated extreme efficiency in explicating maximum bioactivity of the chemotherapeutics drugs with reducing the toxic effect of drugs by cutting down the effective dose of anti-cancer treatment. With advent of biological agents in chemotherapy, nanomedicines serve as excellent delivery agents for these biological agents. The clinical success of biological agents in the form of immunotherapy suppression, T cell therapy, cancer vaccines, cytokines and other biological therapies depends on the act of the nano-drug delivery system.

Altogether, nanomedicines come up as platform for delivery immunotherapy agents simultaneously adding desired functionality in delivery system for intended delivery for preferred site, dose reduction, stability, enhanced bioeffect and reducing toxicity burden. Conversely, nanomedicine-based immunotherapy results in effective response, escalated survival rate and favored

DOI: 10.1201/9781003130055-23

immunological response through anti memory. To express this response, various strategies are under progress such as combination therapy of immunotherapy with other immunotherapies, biotherapeutics, chemotherapy and radiotherapy [11].

However, although the efficacy enhancement of these strategies has only modest, they have shown an improve in the frequency of serious side effects. Therefore, there is still a need for safe and potential alternative methods that can synergistically play the role of cancer immunotherapeutic effect to fully realize the effective of immunotherapy [12, 13].

With advancement of nanomedicine in immunotherapy field, two modes emerged for delivering biotherapeutics including localized delivery through injectable nanocarriers for localized effect at tumor site, systemic immunity modulation for tumors and bio potentiation of anti-cancer immune effect. Therefore, based on the route of administration, nanomedicine is designed to reaching the specific target site, direct its interaction with specific bio-molecules, which endorsing the attribution of specific cell populations, target its payloads to sub-cellular sections and temporarily control immunity signal [14]. Amongst the various causes of cancer, viral infection through HPV, PBV, bacterial infections like helicobacter pylori, ultraviolet radiation, carcinogen exposure and genetic mutations exists as major risks. As human immune-system rescues our human body from foreign molecules like viruses, bacteria and pre-cancerous cells for protection and differentiation of uncomplimentary foreign bodies, for instance, B- and T-lymphocytes deficient Rag2-/- mice have tendency to develop aggressive malignancies that spread in multiple organs. Henceforth, the immune system work through identifying cancerous and pre-cancerous stages of cells using -specific antigens articulated on surface of cells. This process of prevention and eradication of growth and development of malignant tumor is known as immune-surveillance. Numerous immune-cells, as well as B and T-cells, Natural killer cells, dendritic cells (DC), macrophages, and polymorphonuclear leukocytes (PMNs), are enlisted for recognition of cancerous cells; however, the cancerous cells can still avoid the immune surveillance [14].

23.2 APPROACHES TO CANCER IMMUNOTHERAPY

Innate immune activation and immune response against tumor are the two approaches of cancer immunotherapy created on immune editing [15]. Both non-specific and specific approaches work for eliminating tumor cells in two ways a) by improving cancer antigen performance and prompting a specific cytotoxic T lymphocyte (CTL). activity b) Down regulating tumor T-reg cells by guiding T-cells to the active site.

Various studies involving non-specific immune activation for treating different cancers were published to date [16]. Treatments with cytokines, interferons, or toll-like receptor (TLR) agonists

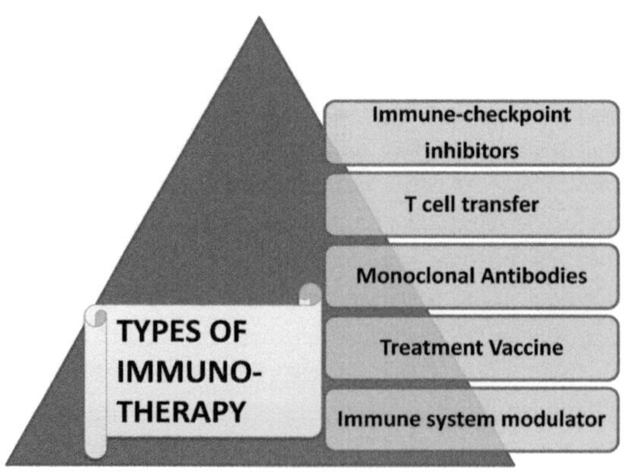

FIGURE 23.1 Illustration for types of immunotherapy.

are included in the innate immune stimulation approach. The different type of immune therapies as shown in Figure 23.1.

23.2.1 IMMUNE CHECKPOINT INHIBITORS (ICI)

ICI are specially functionalized anti-bodies that reduce the cells capacity to detriment immune-system. Checkpoint and respective partner proteins interaction leads to shutdown signal to the T-lymphocytes of immune-system resulting in subduing the immune signal preventing cancer cell destruction. Anti-cytotoxic T-lymphocyte antigen 4 (CTLA-4) antibody is the current U.S. Food and Drug Administration (FDA) approved ICI that has ability to release T-lymphocytes to stimulate T-cell responses against cancer. Some other checkpoint inhibitors interrupt the tumor cells signals for immune response suppression. Pro-grammid cell death protein 1 (PD-1) is such ICI that interact with T lymphocytes besides ligand (PD-L1) on cell surface and augment T-cell response inducing anti activity inside body [17].

23.2.2 T CELL TRANSFER

As T-cells are important counterparts of immunotherapy that stimulate immune cells to strengthen self-immune system [18]. Recent advances in immunotherapy through T cells involves: T cell therapy using infiltrating lymphocytes and CAR T-cell based therapy. These therapies include collection self-immune cells and *in vitro* culture of cells and replenishment of own immune cells in patient's body via vein. TIL infiltrating therapy utilized infiltrating lymphocytes whereas CAR T cell therapy utilized specific protein CAR and supplement it to patient's body. Thus, this therapy is known as T cell transferor immunological transfer therapy [19].

23.2.3 TUMOR TARGETING ANTIBODIES

Tumor targeting antibodies are advance biologically derived monoclonal antibodies designed for target specific binding on tumor cells. Monoclonal antibodies exhibit role of a bio-marker for tumor cells, thus, promoting better recognition along with demolition of targeted cancer cells by immune system as displayed in Figure 23.2. Monoclonal antibodies are FDA approved cancer anti-metastasis therapies for aggressive cancers. Targeting antibodies served via various mechanisms to combat cancer cells including antibody-dependent cellular cytotoxic effect (ADCC), induction of T-cell immunity and complement-dependent cytotoxic effect (CDC). For instance mAb-based immunotherapy for cancer contain (1) alemtuzumab (Campath), it is an anti-CD52 monoclonal antibody

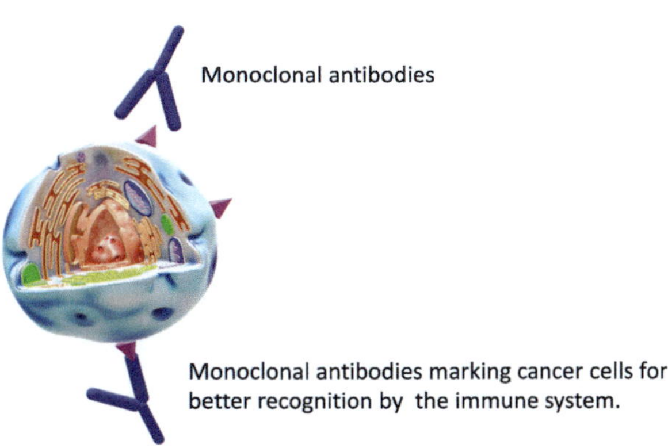

FIGURE 23.2 Image detailing binding of monoclonal antibody with antigen on cancer cell surface.

designed for eradicating leukemia cells for management of B cell chronic lymphocytic leukemia, second is rituximab (Rituxan), this is anti-CD20 monoclonal antibody to eradicate s; and third is trastuzumab (Herceptin), an anti-HER2 antibody serve to manage HER2-+ve metastatic breast cancer by inhibiting proliferation [20, 21].

23.2.4 Cancer Treatment Vaccine

The vaccines used for prevent cancer are also major protagonist of tumor immunotherapy, they explicit response through strengthening the innate immune response to cancer. Cancer vaccines are used for pre-existing cancer conditions. Because there are a huge figure of related antigens in tumor cells other than normal-cells, it can train components of the immune system to identify and terminate cancer cells related to these antigens [17]. Cancer vaccines follow three underline strategies:

(i) They can be designed as custom made exploiting patient's own cells. In such, they explicit the specificity and can express strong response through immune system against the recognizable features of cancer of the patients.

(ii) Cancer treatment vaccines derived from antigens communicated on the surface of specific cancer cells. These particular cancer vaccines explicit responses only for that specific antigen in patients.

(iii) Cancer treatment vaccines derived from self-dendritic cells (which are specific immune cells). DCs vaccines trigger innate immune system that response to reaction interaction with an antigen associated with cells. Sepultura-T is an approved DCs vaccine that specifically targets progressive prostate cancer [17].

Another therapy involves oncolytic virus treatment for chemotherapy, which uses an oncolytic virus to abolish cancerous cells that leave normal cells. Talimogene laherparepvec (T-VEC) or (Imlygic) is the main FDA approved oncolytic virus treatment designed for herpes simplex virus type 1 [22].

23.2.5 Immune System Modulators

Immune system modulators improve the innate immune response against melanoma through immunomodulators. Types of immunomodulators include as follow:

23.2.5.1 Treatment with Cytokines

Cytokine signaling molecule IL-2 improves cytotoxicity by proliferating the effector immune cell [23]. To counteract the enhanced immune activity, IL-2 activates a negative regulator like programmed death-1 (PD-1)[24]. It was also described that cytokine-induced killer (CIKs) cells possessing anti-tumor activity are liberated by IL-2 [25]. CIK is a minor histo-compatibility complex MHC controlled cytotoxic lymphocyte [26, 27]. It was found that route of administration of IL-2 was originated to suppress the tumor growth factor and exhibited clinical ability in treating melanoma and liver carcinoma. IL-2 was also found efficacious in vaccine therapy and adoptive immune therapy [28].

Besides its therapeutic benefits, IL-2 is an up-regulator for Treg-cells, which aggravates the tumor [29]. T-reg cells collected at the ovarian tumor site during the treatment with IL-2 and significantly dropped after cessation of the treatment. Dose dependent morbidity also occurs due to IL-2 toxicity, which occurs in many organs such as heart, kidneys, liver, central nervous system, and lungs [30].

Effector cells are stimulated but not the Treg cells in treatment approaches with additional cytokines like IL-21 and IL-18. IL-21 suppresses Treg cells besides activating NK-cells, CD4+ T-cells,

CD8+ T-cells and B-cells [31]. Activation of T-cells causes improved invention of TNF-α, INF-γ, IL-6, IL-1β and granulocyte-macrophage colony stimulating factor (GM-CSF)[32]. Combined treatment of IL-21 with anti-DR-5 antibody treatment promotes the tumor specific CTL motion and improved memory responses to tumor metastases besides suppressing TRAIL-sensitive tumor metastases [31]. Phase-I clinical trial clearly depicted that IL-21 solely exhibits anti-tumor activity in renal carcinoma and metastatic melanoma patients [33].

Alongside IL-21, IL-18 also exhibits effective anti-tumor activity by inducing INF-γ, GM-CSF, IL-2, TNF-α, IL-1α and increasing T-cell activity and NK-cell cytotoxicity [34]. In mice the protection against tumor challenges was observed with IL-18 [35]. In vivo studies discovered that IL-18 combined with doxorubicin found to significantly suppress ID8 ovarian tumor growth than compared with monotherapy of IL-18 [36].

23.2.5.2 Treatment with NK-cells

NK-cells are an acute factor of natural immunity that retain the power to identify and extinguish transformed cells by liberating cytotoxic granules [37]. NK-cells are mandatory for prime anti-tumorCD8+ T cell immune reaction by manufacturing chemo attractants including CCL5, XCL1that leads to the buildup of Conventional type 1 dendritic cells (c-DC1s) in tumors [38]. Emerging indication displays that the prognosis of patients with epithelial cell lung cancer, gastric tumor, colorectal tumor, and melanoma is significantly better than that of NK-cell infiltration [39]. Chimeric antigen receptors (CARs) endorse the anti-cancer response of immune effector cells and two independent studies have observed antitumor control activity of CD19-CAR engineered human NK cells against murine

Chimeric antigen receptors (CARs) promote the anti-cancer stimulate of immune effector cells. Two autonomous publications have noticed the anti-cancer regulator activity of person NK cells modified by CD19-CAR on mice [14] or humanCD19+ leukemia in animal and humanized mice settings [40]. A modern record has used prompted pluripotent somatic cells (iPSC) as an effective ready source for expanding NK-cells to adjust the NK-CAR engineering process [41].

23.3 NANOMEDICINES BASED CANCER IMMUNOTHERAPY

23.3.1 Liposomes

Liposomes are self-assembled closed structures completed of non-toxic lipids that self-assemble into more than one bilayer. They can bring hydrophilic components (in the aqueous core) or hydrophobic components (in the lipid bilayer) or both. This property of liposomes along with their biocompatibility and ease of functionalization makes them one of the commonly used nano-carriers [42]. Launched in 1995 in the US, Doxil, practiced for ovarian cancer and AIDS-related Kaposi's malignancy, is the initial ever liposome to be used clinically in cancer therapy. Other products like DaunoXome, Depocyte, Myocet, Amphotec, Ambisome, etc. have been permitted for clinical use in diseases including cancer and fungal infection [43].

However, we do not have any immune liposomes for cancer therapy in the market as of now, although, numerous pre-clinical successes have been achieved. A melanoma targeting TRP2 peptide was delivered to dendritic cells (DC) using liposomes coated with cytosine-guanine (CpG) adjuvant and DC affecting mannose by Lai et al. This led to increase in DC activation which further improved T-cell activation and proliferation of CD8+ T-cells and interferon-gamma fabricating cells. These liposomes have also been shown to prevent tumor growth and extend survival in B16 melanoma mice [44].

Similarly, Li et al. showed their liposomes can be used to distribute 6-carbon prodrug of an impermeable chemo- and immunotherapeutic agent, ceramide, in a hepatocellular carcinoma model. The formulation was able to slow the tumor growth, increase cancer cell apoptosis, and reduce cancer-related macrophages [45].

Targeting STAT3 signaling by Liao et al., novel-tumor targeting STAT3 inhibitor loaded liposomes has been another successful strategy in returning cancer immunity. STAT3 transcription factor suppresses antigen demonstration and costimulatory molecules. It also increases proliferation of regulatory T cells, responsible for cytotoxic CD8+ T cell inhibition. Systemic management of these liposomes displayed higher proliferation of activated T cells, M1-like macrophages, and DC in the tumor microenvironment [46].

23.3.2 DENDRIMERS

Dendrimers (DC) are a new session of polymers which are nano-sized, radially symmetric molecules with distinct, homogeneous and mono-disperse assembly. They entrap drugs in three major sites with different mechanisms: a) interior void spaces (by molecular entrapment); b) interior branching (by hydrogen bonding); and c) external sets (charge-charge interactions).

As the generations increase, the diameter of the DC increases linearly and the shape becomes more spherical [47]. Each generation has accurately binary the amount of external molecules, therefore the size and binding positions can be accurately controlled. One of the most common DC is polyamidoamine (PAMAM) because of its biocompatibility, external functionalizabilty, and ease of synthesis. Garcia-Vallejo et al. were able to demonstrate important induction of CD4+ and CD8+ T-cells through antigen presentation when 16–32 glycan units carrying dendrimers were conjugated with Lewis[b] glycopeptides to object dendritic cell-specific ICAM-3-grabbing nonintegrin (DC-SIGN). (4) In additional study, Daftarian et al. delivered DNA based vaccines into APCs, *in vivo*, by PAMAM dendrimers conjugated with MHC II targeting peptides. These dendrimers when administered subcutaneously, selectively transfected DCs in the draining lymph nodes, increased expansion of antigen-specific T-cells, and prove that recognized tumors are rejected [48].

23.3.3 CARBON NANOTUBES

Carbon nanotubes (CNTs) are the affiliate of fullerene family of carbon allotropes. They are long cylindrical molecules having either single (single-walled CNTs) or multiple walls (multiple-walled CNTs) made by rolling of graphene pieces which are capped at both ends by fullerene hemispheres. CNTs can be chemically functionalized or shortened chemically or physically to serve as drug carriers [49]. Hassan et al. OVA antigen and CpG and CD40 agonists were integrated on CNTs to display OVA-specific cellular immune responses and delayed tumor progress in a cancer animal model. These CNTs can come into cells via energy-dependent and passive an pathway, which is the opposite of PLGA encapsulation, which is only through energy-dependent mechanisms. In addition, compared with the free mixture of OVA and CpG, the chemical conjugate that integrates CpG and OVA can produce more anti-OVA IgG and IgG2c antibodies [50].

23.3.4 VIRUS-LIKE PARTICLES

Virus-like particles (VLPs) are made of viral basic proteins are self-accumulate into the shape resembling that of the parental virus. The proteins can be organized in 1–3 layers to yield VLPs in the range of 20–200 nm in size [51]. Devoid of viral genomic material, VLPs are not capable of replicating, but can present antigens to APCs thus activating B-cell and subsequently both CD4+ and CD8+ T-cells. They can be designed to immunogenic ligands, target immune cells, or enhance vaccine effectiveness through site-directed mutagenesis or bio-conjugation. Nowadays, VLPs in the clinical stage are directed against viral pathogens, but VLPs for cancer immunotherapy are also emerging [50]. A VLPs (AX09–0M6) by Bolli et al., targeted cystine-glutamate anti-porter protein, xCT, which protects breast tumor stem cells against oxidative and chemical stress. The VLPs was found to show strong antibody response against xCT and increase the level of NK cells in metastatic tissue of lung in mice. When tumors derived from Her2+ TUBO injected into mice, the VLPs significantly prevented the development of pulmonary nodules. They were also displayed to strongly hamper the growth and development of pulmonary metastases [52]. Similarly, Lizotte et al. Inhaled VLP derived from cowpea mosaic virus (CPMV) was used to demonstrate the reduction of established B16F10 melanoma lung metastasis and the generation of general anti-cancer immunity against comparatively non-immunogenic B16F10 in the skin. The VLPs inhalation resulted in potentially enhance in the tumor-infiltrating neutrophil (TIN) and $CD11b^+Ly6G^+$ activated neutrophils as well as a decrease in $CD11b^-Ly6G^+$ quiescent neutrophils. The TIN and $CD11b^+Ly6G^+$ activated neutrophils indicated potential antigen exhibition and T-cell priming ability by expressing MHC-II as well as high levels of co-stimulatory marker CD86 by TIN specifically [53]

23.3.5 Gold Nanoparticles

Gold nanoparticles (GNPs) are colloidal gold particles in submicron size range having oxidation state. GNPs, as carriers of therapeutic agents, have advantages over conventional systems in that they have huge area to volume ratio, efficient functionalization and cellular uptake, higher biocompatibility, and lesser non-specific toxicity [54, 55]. They have been used in various studies in cancer immunotherapy, some of which are summarized in table 23.1.

23.3.6 Hybrid/Organic Particle

In the last several decades, Nano Targeted Drug Delivery System (TDDS) has proven its potential to revolutionize therapeutic diagnosis and cancer immune-therapy. Inorganic nanoparticles are broadly used, gold, Silicon dioxide, Iron oxide are broadly used for medical diagnostics and therapies. although they have few advantages and disadvantage such as unstable, cytotoxicity, and free radical formation in certain genetic environments, while they are extremely biological compatible, chemically inactive, surface chemistry-tunable properties making them useful as adjustable nanocarriers [61, 62]. However, one of the main significant issues associated with metal nanocarrier is the assembly of reactive oxygen species (ROS) from the inorganic shells, which turns as a catalyst for adverse reactions, the inability of metallic nanoparticles to be biodegraded, or direct cytotoxicity leads to not only tumor cells but also normal tissues apoptosis. Dendritic cells (DCs) are well known potentially inhibited by factors existing in the tumor microenvironment (TME), and that changes the performance of DCs [63].

Fogli et al. prepared gold-functionalized silica nanoparticles and observed that different NPs bind to different biomolecule libraries in the cell lysate, and therefore have a significant impact on the maturation of DC via an up-regulation of CD80 and CD83 [64].

Although NPs offers a technology to encapsulate particles in the interior or surface conjugates by combining different particles to form hybrid nano-formulations. Xiao et al. The CpGoligodeoxynucleotide delivery system that has been prepared significantly promotes the expression of CD80 in macrophages, representing that the CpGoligodeoxynucleotide delivery can effectively regulate the polarity of macrophages to the anticancer M1 phenotype. The multifunctional hybrid delivery system displays high potential in the delivery of targeted nanoparticles in cancer immune-therapy [65].

23.3.7 Polymeric Micelles

Polymer micelles (PM) are self-collected bodies of amphiphilic copolymers with spherical shell-like structures and have been used as beneficial carriers for drug-delivery [50]. Because of their many excellent properties, including the capability to effectively dissolve various poorly soluble drugs, biocompatibility, excellent *in vitro/in vivo* stability, and the ability to assemble in the pathological range. In addition, these micelles can be given other functions by modifying their surfaces with several ligands and contrasting agent that cell penetrating parts to achieve exact drug targeting

TABLE 23.1

Gold Nanoparticles in Cancer Immunotherapy

Gold NPs	Immunogenic/Targeting Ligand	Mechanism	Function of GNPs	Results	Reference
Gold nanorods (GNR) **Aspect ratio (length divided by width)=3.9**	anti-EGFR mAbs	Anti-EGFR mAbs target malignant oral epithelial cells (HOC 313 clone 8 and HSC 3) resulting in concentration of GNR. Exposure to NIR laser at 800 nm results in heat generation by GNR killing tumor cells	Absorb laser light and convert it to heat	HOC 313 and HSC 3 cells were destroyed with smaller than half the laser energy needed to destroy normal cells	[56]
GNPs **15–30 nm** **3 designs:** **i) CpG-SH** **ii) CpG-T11-SH** **iii) CpG-TEG-T11-SH**	CpGoligodeoxynucleotide (CpG ODN)	CpG ODN binds to TLR9 of APCs which increase the expression of co-stimulatory molecules, secretion of inflammatory cytokines and activate CD8+ T cells	Enhance the effect of CpG by acting as effective carrier and reducing need for higher dose	Triethylene glycol (TEG) modified CpG-GNP significantly reduced tumor formation and endorsed survival in animal compared with free CpG	[57]
GNPs **30 nm**	Ovalbumin (OVA) peptide antigen	GNP-OVA induce significantly higher release of IL-6 when presented to Bone marrow resulting dendritic cells (BMDC). This works like vaccine and leads to antibody production.	GNP act as both carrier of OVA and adjuvant	GNP-OVA elicit higher immune reaction and subsequently higher anti-tumor effect and longer survival in mice compared to free OVA or another adjuvant like GNP-CpG	[58]
Gold nanorods **Length=50 nm** **Width=13 nm**	Macrolides (azithromycin, clarithromycin)	Macrolides accumulate preferentially in macrophages. Tumor associated macrophages (TAM) infiltrate into solid tumors, making up to 50% of breast carcinoma. Macrolide conjugated GNR are delivered to breast tumor cells via TAMs. Exposure to NIR laser at 806 nm induces phototoxicity in tumor cells.	Absorb laser light and convert to heat	NIR laser exposure resulted in substantial cytotoxicity in breast adenocarcinoma co-culture (MCF 7) containing macrolide-GNR treated TAMs compared to only NIR treated and PEG-GNR treated TAMs	[59]
GNPs		GNPs act as radio-enhancer during radiotherapy which enhance the expression of carcinoembryonic antigen (CEA) expression in human epithelial lung carcinoma cell line A549. Immunoadjuvants can be combined which activate APCs and present overexpressed CEA to T-cells	Radio-enhancer	Presence of GNP before irradiation in A549 cells showed increased overexpression of CEA compared to absence of GNP.	[60]

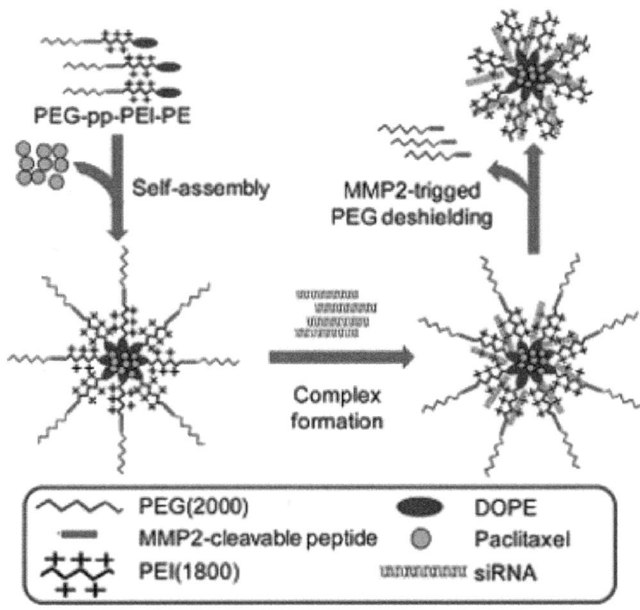

FIGURE 23.3   PEG-pp-PEI-PE micelles delivery approach [**69**]. (copy-right©2014 Elsevier).

and intra-cellular accumulation, respectively [66–68]. In the report of Zhu et al. was prepared polymeric micellar of PEG-pp-PEI-PE copolymer which are matrix metalloproteinase (MMP-2) sensitive through self-assembly for co-delivery of tumor-targeted siRNA and drugs. These synergistic functions ensure improved tumor targeting of the co-loaded siRNA and drugs, improved cancer cell internalization, and coordinated anti-tumor movement [69] as shown in Figure 23.3.

These effects together lead to strong anti-cancer immune response, and tumor inhibition with sustained the survival time. In another report, Targeting polymer micelles of tumor-associated macrophages (TAMs), which are galactose-functionalized zinc protoporphyrin IX (ZnPP) grafted with poly(L-lysine)-b-poly(ethylene glycol)) Polypeptide micelles (ZnPP PM), and these micelles can re-polarize TAM into M1 macrophages by generating reactive oxygen species (ROS) [70, 71].

23.4   APPLICATION PROSPECTS OF NANOMEDICINES IN CANCER IMMUNOTHERAPY

Immunotherapy has important innovation to improve anticancer treatment. This method will effectively increase the possibility of antigen targeted by immune-therapy, thereby overcoming the compensatory nature of cancer cells. However, conventional cancer immune-therapy delays the growth of cancer immunotherapy. With the development of nanomedicine technology, due to its inherent immunomodulatory activity, the use of nanomaterials has become an important tool for the treatment of tumors. We have proposed various applications to enhance the performance of nanomedicine and the effectiveness and safety of intelligent immunomodulatory therapy (Figure 23.4).

Nanomedicine practices the advantages of cancer immunotherapy in different as follows. 1) Nanomaterial-mediated photodynamic and photothermal therapy directly kill cancer cells by heating, which can prompt immunogenic cell death, thereby activating the systemic anti-cancer immunogenic response. 2) Immunomodulators that decrease off-targeting effects such as mRNA-based, scaffold-based vaccines, are new strategies to persist the result and decrease systemic adverse effects [72]. 3) Functionalized nanomaterials can stimulate cytotoxic T cells

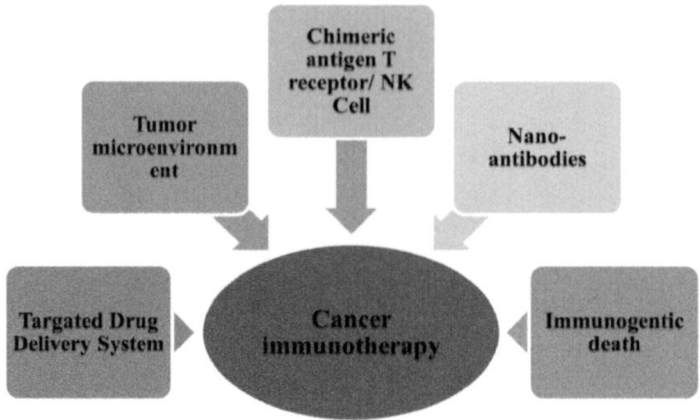

FIGURE 23.4 Different mechanism of nanomedicines on cancer immunotherapy.

and antigen-offering cells specific to TME, and inhibit macrophages by repolarizing them from M2- (tumor-promoting) macrophages to M1 (tumor-killing) macrophages cells, thereby effectively improving the killing effect of cancer [73]. The modified TME by hypoxia helps reduce the sensitivity of immune cells, thereby raising the metastatic activity of cancer cells, and may enhance the therapeutic efficacy of radiotherapy and cancer immunotherapy [74]. For all these reasons, Nanomedicine has extremely high variability in material with surface modification to improve the cancer immunology.

23.5 CONCLUSION

In last few decades, nano drug delivery and targeting the system has been at the leading edge within the chemotherapy. In spite of promising therapeutic approaches in tumor immunotherapy, there's static a scarcity of useful methods for cancers. In the near future, scientists will report specific tumor antigens for every sort of tumor to state targeted immune-therapies which will shows an essential character in producing a less toxic action and minimized cost effective [14]. Most significantly, with the medical appearance of various therapeutic factors, suitable biomarkers could be utilized to work out which, tumor will answer which treatments to calculate the probability of medicine resistance [75]. Moreover, T-cell immune checkpoint alleyways have been emphasized in several reports as a noticeable resistance device to immune response, especially beside tumor-specific T-cells [76]. Therefore, recognizing further immune checkpoints and explaining the original molecular actions which elaborated in immune check-point regulation may yield insight into effective anti-tumor immunity although preventive tumor immune evasion [77]. Moreover, it's possible that targeting various cytotoxic effectors as a mixture treatment might be simpler than using hybrid therapies against an equivalent effector population, delivering an efficacious stage in anti-cancer immunity [78]. To conclude, the innovative application of nano-medicines in cancer immunotherapy has shown potential results, which can diminish cancer growth and provide broad prospects for future cancer patients.

REFERENCES

1. Tian, T., et al., The origins of cancer robustness and evolvability. *Integr Biol (Camb)*, 2011. **3**(1): p. 17–30.
2. Pardoll, D.M., The blockade of immune checkpoints in cancer immunotherapy. *Nat Rev. Cancer*, 2012. **12**(4): p. 252–264.
3. Chen, D.S. and I. Mellman, Oncology meets immunology: the cancer-immunity cycle. *Immunity*, 2013. **39**(1): p. 1–10.

4. Motz, G.T. and G. Coukos, Deciphering and reversing tumor immune suppression. *Immunity*, 2013. **39**(1): p. 61–73.

5. Sheridan, C., Exosome cancer diagnostic reaches market. *Nat Biotechnol*, 2016. **34**(4): p. 359–360.

6. O'Neil, N.J., M.L. Bailey, and P. Hieter, Synthetic lethality and cancer. *Nat Rev Genet*, 2017. **18**(10): p. 613–623.

7. Soheilyfar, S., et al., In vivo and in vitro impact of miR-31 and miR-143 on the suppression of metastasis and invasion in breast cancer. *J Buon*, 2018. **23**(5): p. 1290–1296.

8. Harris, T.J. and C.G. Drake, Primer on tumor immunology and cancer immunotherapy. *J Immunother Cancer*, 2013. **1**(1): p. 12.

9. Seledtsov, V.I., A.G. Goncharov, and G.V. Seledtsova, Multiple-purpose immunotherapy for cancer. *Biomed Pharmacother*, 2015. **76**: p. 24–29.

10. Speiser, D.E., P.C. Ho, and G. Verdeil, Regulatory circuits of T cell function in cancer. *Nat Rev Immunol*, 2016. **16**(10): p. 599–611.

11. Martin, J.D., et al., Improving cancer immunotherapy using nanomedicines: progress, opportunities and challenges. *Nat Rev Clin Oncol*, 2020. **17**(4): p. 251–266.

12. Anselmo, A.C. and S. Mitragotri, Nanoparticles in the clinic: an update. *Bioeng Transl Med*, 2019. **4**(3): p. e10143.

13. Cabral, H., et al., Block copolymer micelles in nanomedicine applications. *Chem Rev*, 2018. **118**(14): p. 6844–6892.

14. Taefehshokr, N., et al., Promising approaches in cancer immunotherapy. *Immunobiol*, 2020. **225**(2): p. 151875.

15. Sengupta, S., Cancer nanomedicine: lessons for immuno-oncology. *Trends Cancer*, 2017. **3**(8): p. 551–560.

16. Krishnamachari, Y., et al., Nanoparticle delivery systems in cancer vaccines. *Pharm Res*, 2011. **28**(2): p. 215–236.

17. Hargadon, K.M., C.E. Johnson, and C.J. Williams, Immune checkpoint blockade therapy for cancer: an overview of FDA-approved immune checkpoint inhibitors. *Int Immunopharmacol*, 2018. **62**: p. 29–39.

18. Hinrichs, C.S. and S.A. Rosenberg, Exploiting the curative potential of adoptive T-cell therapy for cancer. *Immunol Rev*, 2014. **257**(1): p. 56–71.

19. Shirasu, N. and M. Kuroki, Functional design of chimeric T-cell antigen receptors for adoptive immunotherapy of cancer: architecture and outcomes. *Anticancer Res*, 2012. **32**(6): p. 2377–2383.

20. Weaver Jr., D.J., et al., C5a receptor-deficient dendritic cells promote induction of Treg and Th17 cells. *Eur J Immunol*, 2010. **40**(3): p. 710–721.

21. Aghebati-Maleki, L., et al., Phage display as a promising approach for vaccine development. *J Biomed Sci*, 2016. **23**(1): p. 66.

22. DeMaria, P.J. and M. Bilusic, Cancer vaccines. *Hematol Oncol Clin North Am*, 2019. **33**(2): p. 199–214.

23. Ohta, M., et al., Anomalies in transgenic mice carrying the human interleukin-2 gene. *Tokai J Exp Clin Med*, 1990. **15**(4): p. 307–15.

24. Carter, L., et al., PD-1: PD-L inhibitory pathway affects both CD4(+) and CD8(+) T cells and is overcome by IL-2. *Eur J Immunol*, 2002. **32**(3): p. 634–43.

25. Schmidt-Wolf, I.G., et al., Use of a SCID mouse/human lymphoma model to evaluate cytokine-induced killer cells with potent antitumor cell activity. *J Exp Med*, 1991. **174**(1): p. 139–149.

26. Kim, H.M., et al., Antitumor activity of cytokine-induced killer cells in nude mouse xenograft model. *Arch Pharm Res*, 2009. **32**(5): p. 781–787.

27. Rosenberg, S.A., et al., Durability of complete responses in patients with metastatic cancer treated with high-dose interleukin-2: identification of the antigens mediating response. *Ann Surg*, 1998. **228**(3): p. 307–319.

28. McDermott, D.F., The application of high-dose interleukin-2 for metastatic renal cell carcinoma. *Med Oncol*, 2009. **26**(Suppl 1): p. 13–17.

29. Beyer, M., Interleukin-2 treatment of tumor patients can expand regulatory T cells. *Oncoimmunology*, 2012. **1**(7): p. 1181–1182.

30. Schwartz, R.N., L. Stover, and J.P. Dutcher, Managing toxicities of high-dose interleukin-2. *Oncology (Williston Park)*, 2002. **16**(11 Suppl 13): p. 11–20.

31. Smyth, M.J., et al., IL-21 enhances tumor-specific CTL induction by anti-DR5 antibody therapy. *J Immunol*, 2006. **176**(10): p. 6347–6355.

32. Thompson, J.A., et al., Phase I study of recombinant interleukin-21 in patients with metastatic melanoma and renal cell carcinoma. *J Clin Oncol*, 2008. **26**(12): p. 2034–2039.

33. Sheng, W.Y. and L. Huang, Cancer immunotherapy and nanomedicine. *Pharm Res*, 2011. **28**(2): p. 200–214.

34. Micallef, M.J., et al., Interleukin 18 induces the sequential activation of natural killer cells and cytotoxic T lymphocytes to protect syngeneic mice from transplantation with Meth A sarcoma. *Cancer Res*, 1997. **57**(20): p. 4557–4563.

35. Robertson, M.J., et al., Clinical and biological effects of recombinant human interleukin-18 administered by intravenous infusion to patients with advanced cancer. *Clin Cancer Res*, 2006. **12**(14 Pt 1): p. 4265–4273.

36. Robertson, M.J., et al., A dose-escalation study of recombinant human interleukin-18 using two different schedules of administration in patients with cancer. *Clin Cancer Res*, 2008. **14**(11): p. 3462–3469.

37. Souza-Fonseca-Guimaraes, F., J. Cursons, and N.D. Huntington, The emergence of natural killer cells as a major target in cancer immunotherapy. *Trends Immunol*, 2019. **40**(2): p. 142–158.

38. Bottcher, J.P., et al., NK cells stimulate recruitment of cDC1 into the tumor microenvironment promoting cancer immune control. *Cell*, 2018. **172**(5): p. 1022–1037, e14.

39. Krasnova, Y., et al., Bench to bedside: NK cells and control of metastasis. *Clin Immunol*, 2017. **177**: p. 50–59.

40. Liu, E., et al., Cord blood NK cells engineered to express IL-15 and a CD19-targeted CAR show long-term persistence and potent antitumor activity. *Leukemia*, 2018. **32**(2): p. 520–531.

41. Muller, S., et al., High cytotoxic efficiency of lentivirally and alpharetrovirally engineered CD19-specific chimeric antigen receptor natural killer cells against acute lymphoblastic leukemia. *Front Immunol*, 2019. **10**: p. 3123.

42. Akbarzadeh, A., et al., Liposome: classification, preparation, and applications. *Nanoscale Res Lett*, 2013. **8**(1): p. 102.

43. Bulbake, U., et al., Liposomal formulations in clinical use: an updated review. *Pharmaceutics*, 2017. **9**(2): p. 12.

44. Lai, C., et al., The enhanced antitumor-specific immune response with mannose- and CpG-ODN-coated liposomes delivering TRP2 peptide. *Theranostics*, 2018. **8**(6): p. 1723–1739.

45. Hagan, C.T., Y.B. Medik, and A.Z. Wang, Chapter two—nanotechnology approaches to improving cancer immunotherapy. In *Advances in Cancer Research*, A.-M. Broome, Editor. 2018, Academic Press. p. 35–56.

46. Alhallak, K., et al., 18—biomaterials for cancer immunotherapy. In *Biomaterials for Cancer Therapeutics* (Second Edition), K. Park, Editor. 2020, Woodhead Publishing. p. 499–526.

47. Eatemadi, A., et al., Carbon nanotubes: properties, synthesis, purification, and medical applications. *Nanoscale Res Lett*, 2014. **9**(1): p. 393.

48. Daftarian, P., et al., Peptide-conjugated PAMAM dendrimer as a universal DNA vaccine platform to target antigen-presenting cells. *Cancer Res*, 2011. **71**(24): p. 7452–7462.

49. Zhang, W., Z. Zhang, and Y. Zhang, The application of carbon nanotubes in target drug delivery systems for cancer therapies. *Nanoscale Res Lett*, 2011. **6**(1): p. 555.

50. Qiu, H., et al., Nanomedicine approaches to improve cancer immunotherapy. *Wiley Interdiscip Rev Nanomed Nanobiotechnol*, 2017. **9**(5).

51. Anzaghe, M., S. Schülke, and S. Scheurer, Virus-like particles as carrier systems to enhance immunomodulation in allergen immunotherapy. *Curr Allergy Asthma Rep*, 2018. **18**(12): p. 71.

52. Bolli, E., et al., A virus-like-particle immunotherapy targeting epitope-specific anti-xCT expressed on cancer stem cell inhibits the progression of metastatic cancer in vivo. *Oncoimmunology*, 2018. **7**(3): p. e1408746.

53. Lizotte, P.H., et al., In situ vaccination with cowpea mosaic virus nanoparticles suppresses metastatic cancer. *Nat Nanotechnol*, 2016. **11**(3): p. 295–303.

54. Jain, S., D.G. Hirst, and J.M. O'Sullivan, Gold nanoparticles as novel agents for cancer therapy. *Brit J Radiol*, 2012. **85**(1010): p. 101–113.

55. Vines, J.B., et al., Gold nanoparticles for photothermal cancer therapy. *Front Chem*, 2019. **7**: p. 167–167.

56. Huang, X., et al., Cancer cell imaging and photothermal therapy in the near-infrared region by using gold nanorods. *J Am Chem Soc*, 2006. **128**(6): p. 2115–2120.

57. Lin, A.Y., et al., Gold nanoparticle delivery of modified CpG stimulates macrophages and inhibits tumor growth for enhanced immunotherapy. *PLOS One*, 2013. **8**(5): p. e63550.

58. Almeida, J.P.M., et al., In vivo gold nanoparticle delivery of peptide vaccine induces anti-tumor immune response in prophylactic and therapeutic tumor models. *Small (Weinheim an der Bergstrasse, Germany)*, 2015. **11**(12): p. 1453–1459.

59. Dreaden, E.C., et al., Small molecule-gold nanorod conjugates selectively target and induce macrophage cytotoxicity towards breast cancer cells. *Small (Weinheim an der Bergstrasse, Germany)*, 2012. **8**(18): p. 2819–2822.

60. Mueller, R., et al., Increased carcinoembryonic antigen expression on the surface of lung cancer cells using gold nanoparticles during radiotherapy. *Physica Medica*, 2020. **76**: p. 236–242.

61. Gholami, A., et al., Lipoamino acid coated superparamagnetic iron oxide nanoparticles concentration and time dependently enhanced growth of human hepatocarcinoma cell line (Hep-G2). *J Nanomater*, 2015. **2015**: p. 451405.

62. Inbaraj, B.S., et al., The synthesis and characterization of poly(γ-glutamic acid)-coated magnetite nanoparticles and their effects on antibacterial activity and cytotoxicity. *Nanotechnology*, 2011. **22**(7): p. 075101.

63. Motta, J.M. and V.M. Rumjanek, Sensitivity of dendritic cells to microenvironment signals. *J Immunol Res*, 2016. **2016**: p. 4753607.

64. Fogli, S., et al., Inorganic nanoparticles as potential regulators of immune response in dendritic cells. *Nanomedicine*, 2017. **12**(14): p. 1647–1660.

65. He, X.-Y., et al., Functional polymer/inorganic hybrid nanoparticles for macrophage targeting delivery of oligodeoxynucleotides in cancer immunotherapy. *Mater Today Chem*, 2017. **4**: p. 106–116.

66. Khatik, R., et al., Integrin $\alpha v\beta 3$ receptor overexpressing on tumor-targeted positive MRI-guided chemotherapy. *ACS Appl Mater Interfaces*, 2020. **12**(1): p. 163–176.

67. Letchford, K. and H. Burt, A review of the formation and classification of amphiphilic block copolymer nanoparticulate structures: micelles, nanospheres, nanocapsules and polymersomes. *Eur J Pharm Biopharm*, 2007. **65**(3): p. 259–269.

68. Croy, S.R. and G.S. Kwon, Polymeric micelles for drug delivery. *Curr Pharm Des*, 2006. **12**(36): p. 4669–4684.

69. Zhu, L., et al., Matrix metalloproteinase 2-sensitive multifunctional polymeric micelles for tumor-specific co-delivery of siRNA and hydrophobic drugs. *Biomaterials*, 2014. **35**(13): p. 4213–4222.

70. Yang, F., et al., Advanced biomaterials for cancer immunotherapy. *Acta Pharmacologica Sinica*, 2020. **41**(7): p. 911–927.

71. Kumar, A., et al., Enhanced apoptosis, survivin down-regulation and assisted immunochemotherapy by curcumin loaded amphiphilic mixed micelles for subjugating endometrial cancer. *Nanomed: Nanotechnol Biol Med*, 2017. **13**(6): p. 1953–1963.

72. Zhao, Z., et al., Delivery strategies of cancer immunotherapy: recent advances and future perspectives. *J Hematol Oncol*, 2019. **12**(1): p. 126.

73. Li, X., et al., Nanomedicine-based cancer immunotherapies developed by reprogramming tumor-associated macrophages. *Nanoscale*, 2021. **13**(9): p. 4705–4727.

74. Stylianopoulos, T., L.L. Munn, and R.K. Jain, Reengineering the physical microenvironment of tumors to improve drug delivery and efficacy: from mathematical modeling to bench to bedside. *Trends Cancer*, 2018. **4**(4): p. 292–319.

75. Moehler, M., et al., Immunotherapy in gastrointestinal cancer: Recent results, current studies and future perspectives. *Eur J Cancer*, 2016. **59**: p. 160–170.

76. Gubin, M.M., et al., Checkpoint blockade cancer immunotherapy targets tumour-specific mutant antigens. *Nature*, 2014. **515**(7528): p. 577–581.

77. Alard, E., et al., Advances in anti-cancer immunotherapy: car-T cell, checkpoint inhibitors, dendritic cell vaccines, and oncolytic viruses, and emerging cellular and molecular targets. *Cancers (Basel)*, 2020. **12**(7).

78. Marin-Acevedo, J.A., et al., Cancer immunotherapy beyond immune checkpoint inhibitors. *J Hematol Oncol*, 2018. **11**(1): p. 8.

24 Carbon Nanotubes and Fullerenes in Nanotheranostics

Naveen Rajana, Padakanti Sandeep Chary,
Valamla Bhavana, and Neelesh Kumar Mehra

24.1 INTRODUCTION

There is enormous development in the field of nanotherapeutics for the diagnosis and treatment of the numerous diseases. The United States Food and Drug Administration (USFDA) and European Medicines Agency (EMA) have approved several drug delivery–based medicines for therapeutic delivery such as liposomal formulations (Caelyx: Schering-Plough, North Ryde, New South Wales, Australia; Doxil: Centocor Ortho Biotech, Horsham, Pennsylvania; Myocet: Enxon Pharmaceuticals, Piscataway, New Jersey; DaunoXome, Diatos, Paris, France) and paclitaxel-loaded human albumin nanoparticles (ABraxane, Celgene, Summit, New Jersey). Both fullerenes and carbon nanotubes have received enormous attention in the development of nanotherapeutic medicine as "safe and more effective" because of their inimitable outstanding physicochemical properties [1–6].

24.1.1 CARBON NANOTUBES AS NANOTHERAPEUTIC CARRIERS

Currently, functionalized carbon nanotubes (CNTs) have drawn tremendous attention in the field of nanotheranostics. It is reported that Bacon first discovered CNTs in 1960 [7]. Further, Sumio Iijima defined and explored CNTs as tiny needle tubular structures during in his transmission electron microscopy (TEM) observation [8].

Carbon nanotubes are unique, three-dimensional *sp2* hybridized, composed of hollow nanoneedle tubular structure graphite sheets. CNTs belong to the fullerenes family, and have several unique and outstanding physicochemical properties, including ultra-light weight, aspect ratio (length/diameter) and greater surface area, nanoneedles, good surface chemistry, and non-immunogenicity. Further, biliary excretion, biocompatibility, quick internalization by cells because of anisotropic 'needle-like' morphology and greater entrapment efficiency, are some anticipated features that make them attractive nanocarriers in drug delivery [9–14].

24.1.1.1 Classification of Carbon Nanotubes

CNTs are broadly categorized into two classes based on the of number of walls, outlined in Figure 24.1. Single-walled carbon nanotubes (SWCNTs) are made up of a single graphite sheet and have diameter and length ranging from 0.4 to 3.0 and 20 to 1000 nm, respectively. Multi-walled carbon nanotubes (MWCNTs) are made up of many concentric layers of graphene (2–10 layers) with a diameter range from 1.4 to 100 nm and length range from 1 to 50 μm [10,15].

24.1.1.2 Advantages of Carbon Nanotubes

The advantages of functionalized CNTs are [10,16,17]:

1. High loading efficiency with endohedral filling
2. Photoluminescence and highly elastic nature

DOI: 10.1201/9781003130055-24

3. Biocompatible and non-immunogenic with minimal toxicity
4. Internalization in cells via endocytosis and nano-needle mechanisms
5. Biodegradability
6. Uniform ordered structure with high aspect ratio
7. More than 90% excreted out through biliary excretion (4% by feces and 96% by urine)
8. Ease of penetration into cell membrane because of small nanoneedle tubular structure
9. Endohedral filling of bioactive(s) into the interior cavity and both open ends
10. The pharmacokinetic properties and biodistribution can be altered easily through controlling size, degree of functionalization, cutting, and rich surface chemistry
11. Greater internal space for endohedral filling with respect to diameter results in greater drug encapsulation capacity with the ability to control the release of the drug

24.1.1.3 Disadvantages of Carbon Nanotubes

CNTs have several advantages; however, some disadvantages of CNTs [15,17] are as follows:

1. The hydrophobic nature of pristine CNTs means poor dispersibility
2. CNTs made up of Pristine are highly toxic and are not suitable for pharmaceutical applications
3. Aggregation/bundling phenomena
4. Amorphous and metallic impurities
5. Minimum possibilities of accumulation based on *in-vivo* studies

24.2 FUNCTIONALIZATION OF CNTS

Functionalization is the attachment of the several chemical functional moieties to the surface of CNTs. In the first generation, CNTs are poor in aqueous dispersibility and contain metallic and amorphous impurities. Functionalization enhances the aqueous dispersibility, eliminates impurities, and makes them more suitable for the development of novel and innovative diagnostic and imaging tools for biomedical purposes [15,18].

The functionalization of CNTs could be possible using covalent or non-covalent approaches between the surfaces of nanotubes and the free-chemical functional groups of bioactive moieties [19]. Covalent functionalization is a more effective method for conjugation of functional moieties on CNTs. In covalent functionalization, ends-defects and side-wall covalent functionalization are widely used approaches for functionalization; the former is more reactive than the latter. Another side-wall functionalization approach for covalent functionalization has been used to generate functional moieties on the sidewall of CNTs without the loss of Van Hove singularities. Under

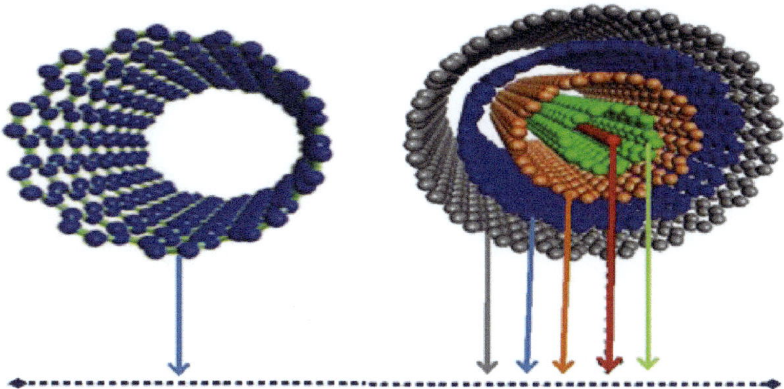

FIGURE 24.1 Available types of carbon nanotubes: (A) single-, and (B) multi-walled carbon nanotubes.

non-covalent functionalization, chemical functional groups can easily be conjugated on the surfaces of CNTs using hydrophobic, electrostatic, π–π stacking, and hydrogen bonding interactions and Van der Waals force [18–20].

24.3 CARBON NANOTUBES IN NANOTHERANOSTICS

Many biosensors with unique bio-sensing mechanisms have been available for the detection of different biological molecules for biomedical purposes. In this area, CNTs have been reported as a bioimaging and diagnostics tool utilizing biomedical imaging techniques like near infrared (NIR), photo acoustic imaging (PCA), contrast magnetic resonance, and nuclear imaging. In this section, we discuss biomedical imaging and diagnostics tools using CNTs in nanotheranostics applications [21,22].

Fluorescence imaging using CNTs is widely explored as a tool for *in vitro* and *in vivo* assay. They are capable of enhanced tissue penetration for imaging purpose in nanotheranostics. Functionalized or multifunctional CNTs exhibit higher fluorescence in the NIR region, and single-molecule fluorescence spectroscopy could be utilized to identify and measure electron band gaps on CNTs and DNA molecules [23,24].

In research investigations, CNTs are considered as NIR-II fluorescence materials that are required for tissue targetability in an angiographic probe. Since SWCNTs emit NIR fluorescence in the high wavelength region, that is, 1100–1400 nm, they show a deeper penetration and low scattering in the living body [25]. Particularly, SWCNTs show non-photo bleaching and non-blinking fluorescent emission properties and these characteristics play a crucial role in making them label-free, enabling in-situ real-time detection with both spatial and temporal resolution [26–28].

24.4 FULLERENES

Fullerenes are carbon allotropes similar with graphene structure and are rolled up to form a closed-carbon cage, hollow spheres, pentagonal and hexagonal rings with SP^2 hybridized molecules comprising 60 carbon atoms. They were discovered in 1985 [29] with nanosized dimensions and are defined as a soccer-ball-shaped truncated icosahedron with 12 pentagons (due to C5 single bonds) and 20 hexagons (C5 C6 double bonds). Polyhydroxy fullerenes (PHFs) are hydrophilic, biocompatible, anionic, functionalized fullerene molecules [3].

In fullerenes, the number of pentagons is limited to 13 to achieve the curvature required for formation of the optimized football shape. The cage or ring-like structure entirely depends on the arrangement of the pentagonal rings. These rings are distributed per the isolated pentagon rule, resulting in formation of a sphere, as mostly observed in C_{60} isomers [30].

$$\text{No of Hexagons} = \frac{(\text{Carbon atoms} - 20)}{2} \tag{1}$$

The two well-known isomers of fullerenes are C_{60} and C_{70}. C_{60} fullerenes are also known as Buckminster fullerenes. These two molecules can achieve the isolated pentagon rule only in their single configuration. These configurations are known to be highly stable and have been obtained for usage [29].

24.4.1 ADVANTAGES OF FULLERENES

1. Aqueous solubility and negative charge
2. Biocompatible

3. High encapsulation
4. Covalent and non-covalent functionalization for modification of fullerenes
5. Highly stable and lipophilic in nature

24.4.2 DISADVANTAGES OF FULLERENES

1. Do not overcome the complete solubility of the hydrophobic moiety even after the functionalization process.
2. Penetration of C60 loaded with additional moieties is not allowed into cell wall of bacteria due to their high molecular nature.
3. These are highly sensitive to light and oxygen [29].

24.4.3 FULLERENES IN NANOTHERANOSTICS

Fullerenes have been proved to be an attractive approach for diagnosis and therapy as they can detect, image, and control the delivery of the drug to the specific target site. In real time, the progression can be observed to evaluate the usefulness of treatment utilizing direct monitoring of the areas of interest through endohedral fullerenes' high-contrast capacity [31,32]. This type of multifunctional nanocarrier-based systems has been shown to be successful in mice, including in treatment and diagnosis of cancer, arthritis, and atherosclerosis [33,34].

Endohedral fullerenes contain a hollow carbon core shell that entraps inorganic metal ions during the synthesis. The cage of common C60 is smaller than that of endohedral fullerene. This may be because of size restrictions forced by the small size of the C60; therefore, C80 molecules can encapsulate the required quantity of desired metal ions, which includes gadolinium, yttrium, lanthanum, and scandium. The diagnostic property is strongly enhanced by the strong electronic properties of endohedral fullerenes. This type of compound is being explored as a platform to detect atherosclerosis, arthritis, and cancer [35–37]. Specificity and sensitivity are the main limitations for accurate and improved patient imaging.

Trimetaspheres, a C80 base, encloses the gadolinium in the cage, which is an example of endohedral fullerene. MRI is mostly used for the investigation of trimetaspheres, which uses the gadolinium-based contrast agents. There are several drawbacks, such as toxicity, inability to target the biomarkers of specific disease, and rapid clearance of the gadolinium chelate contrast agent, that limit the utilization of image guide interventions with MRI [38–40]. Trimetaspheres are able to overcome the drawbacks of contrast agents based on gadolinium. Since the gadolinium is entrapped inside the cage, it is isolated from the active targeting moieties present at outside the cage by a stable carbon shell. First, a carbon shell improves the safety by behaving like a barrier between the gadolinium (inside the cage) and active targeting ligands (outside the cage). Second, endohedral fullerenes that are encapsulated with gadolinium are more sensitive. Trimetaspheres enhance relaxivity by 20- to 50-fold when compared with gadolinium contrast agents. Third, as the targeting moieties are attached to cage, so the fullerene are able to target the precise disease biomarkers. The crux of the trimetaspheres serves as platform for diagnostic purpose where particular biomarkers are grafted to the gadolinium-encapsulated endohedral fullerene which is a MRI agent. This might be utilized to target any disease state for which certain expression of specific receptors are present. Based on previous works, trimetaspheres were formulated to study their internalization by glioblastoma cells and macrophage cells *in-vitro*. In glioblastoma, IL-3 receptors are overexpressed, and for diagnosing glioblastoma, MRI using gadolinium-based contrast agents was utilized [41]. The theranostic agents for glioblastoma can target the glioblastoma and decrease brain cancers that have been transplanted in mice. Endohedral fullerene MRI contrasts agents are used as diagnostics for atherosclerotic plaques [42].

Recently, a technique known as acoustic explosion was recommended for a few functionalized fullerenes, such as carboxy fullerenes ($C_{60}(C(COOH)_2)_3$) and polyhydroxy fullerenes

(C60(OH)$_x$O$_y$Na$_z$). Along with exposure to low-intensity (<102 W cm-2) continuous-wave laser irradiation in the absence or presence of O$_2$, glowing of functionalized fullerenes was sustained. A faint pop was heared upon irradiation when this process was carried out in tumor cells indicating the use of functionalized fullerene's photo acoustic properties in cancer targeting. In tumor-bearing nude mice, photoacoustic imaging gave positive results. Greater contrast was shown between non-tumor and tumor tissues after PHF intratumoral injection. The laser energy used was 1/3 of the maximum allowable exposure level of 29.5 mJ cm^{-2} for a 785-nm pulsed laser as established by the American National Standards Institute (ANSI). The results of this study indicate the possible utilization of functionalized fullerenes for acquiring photoacoustic images [43].

Photodynamic therapy is a non-invasive method utilized in the therapy of various cancers. The amalgamation of a focused irradiation and photosensitizing agent is utilized to induce free radical controlled production at a specific site, causing death of cells through various pathways, with low chances of collateral destruction to non-cancerous cells. When exposed to visible radiation, fullerenes produce reactive oxygen species [44].

Fullerenes are potential photosensitizers, and they are capable of absorbing photons in the electromagnetic spectrum of UV and visible range. Here, fullerene species are photo-excited in the triplet state and lead to the formation of O$_2$ free radical based on the medium's polarity. These can be attached to light-harvesting antennae, which enhances the production of free radicals. This indicates that fullerenes can be utilized in PDT of tumors and microorganism eradication. Ligands such as pullulan and polyethylene glycol conjugated with C60 showed strong suppression of tumors when intravenously injected into tumor-bearing mice associated with light irradiation [45]. To promote the PDT Gd3+-chelated C60-PEG was prepared by mixing C60-PEG-DTPA with gadolinium acetate solution that was obtained by addition of diethylentriaminepenta acetic acid to the end group of C60-PEG. The incorporation of Gd3+ ions in the photosensitizer provided MRI activity to the C60-PEG which was utilized as a non-invasive method to monitor the internalization in C60-PEG in cancer tissue. There was correlation between the time profile of photodynamic therapy and the detection of a positive signal of MRI [46].

N-methylpyrrolidinium-fullerene (BB4) is a good photosensitizer with the ability to destroy tumor cells in a mouse model containing peritoneal cancers and in-vitro after illumination with white light. N-methyl pyrrolidinium-fullerenes induce cell death by producing Type 1 ROS [47].

24.4.4 PHYSICOCHEMICAL PROPERTIES OF FULLERENES

24.4.4.1 Size Distribution

Dynamic light scattering technique is useful to determine the size distribution of the fullerene's derivatives usually measured at 25°C. The linear dimension (*do*) of the component is estimated to be approximately 1.8 nm; N distributions of the ith type of compound associated with the system are estimated by the following equation [48].

$$Ni - i + 1 = \left(di + \frac{1}{di}\right)3 \ .Kpack$$

where K_{pack} denotes the packing coefficient of the small spheres in the structure, and the value is equivalent to 0.52.

24.4.4.2 Iso-Thermal Solution Densities

Manyakina et al. calculated the partial molar volumes and average molar volumes of fullerene derivatives containing C60 and C70 structures. The following formula was used for calculation of the molar volume:

$$V = \frac{V}{nH2O + n\,derivative\,of\,fullerene}$$

The partial volume of water and fullerene derivates is given as follows:

$$VH2O = \left(\frac{\partial V}{\partial nH2O}\right) T, PV \text{ } derivative \text{ } offullerene = \left(\frac{\partial V}{\partial n \text{ } derivative \text{ } of \text{ } fullerene}\right)_{T,\,P}$$

For the calculation of partial volume, the dependence between the average and partial molar functions was used [49].

$$VH2O = V - x \text{ } derivatives \text{ } of \text{ } fullerene \left(\frac{\partial V}{\partial n \text{ } derivative \text{ } of \text{ } fullerene}\right), Vcarboxyfullerene$$

$$= V - XH2O\left(\frac{\partial V}{\partial xH2O}\right) T, P$$

24.4.4.3 Conductivity

The specific electric conductivities of the derivatives of fullerene are measured at 25°C. Here, conductivity is measured by locating the sample between two parallel electrodes that are maintained at 1 cm distance equal to 1 cm². Molar electric conductivity (λ – S·cm²·mol⁻¹) is calculated by the following equation [50].

$$k = \frac{1}{\rho}$$

$$\lambda = 1000k \,/\, Cm$$

$$\lambda = \lambda 0 - A.Cm$$

$$à = \lambda \,/\, \lambda 0$$

$$KD = \frac{CM\alpha 2}{1-\alpha}$$

24.4.4.4 Refractive Index

The refraction index of fullerene derivatives in aqueous solutions is denoted as *nD*. The specific refraction values of common derivatives of fullerenes associated with water solution were calculated by using the following equations.

$$r = \left(\frac{nD2-1}{nD2+2}\right)\cdot\left(\frac{1}{\rho}\right)$$

$$r = r(derivative).\omega(derivative) + rHOH\big(1 - \omega(derivative)\big)$$

$$R = \left(\frac{nD2-1}{nD2+2}\right)\cdot\left(\frac{M}{\rho}\right)$$

$$M = M(derivative).x(derivative) + M(HOH)\big(1 - x(derivative)\big)$$

where $M_{(derivative)}$ and M_{HOH} are the molecular masses of the derivatives of the fullerenes and water, respectively.

The following equation determines the specific refractive index [48].

$$Ri = ri.Mi$$

24.4.4.5 Viscosity

The dynamic viscosity of Newtonian liquid is determined by using the following equation

$$F1 - f = \eta \Delta VS$$

where $F_1 f$ is the force of the internal friction, η is dynamic viscosity, ΔV is gradient velocity, and S is surface area.

The kinematic viscosity is given as

$$v = \frac{\eta}{\rho}$$

where η is dynamic viscosity, v is kinematic viscosity, and ρ is the density of liquid.

Derivatives of fullerene viscosity depend on two types: (1) upon increasing the concentration of solution in a diluted sample, the $\eta(C)$ values simultaneously decrease, and (2) at a constant temperature, the viscosity of the derivatives present in solution form is clearly explained using the Bachinskii equation.

$$\eta = cB / (Vm - bB)$$

where cB and bB are Bachinskii constants, and Vm is the average molar volume of the derivatives.

By using these equations, the viscosities of the derivatives of the fullerenes can be derived.

24.4.4.6 Diffusion

Semenov et al. discussed Fick's first law of diffusion for fullerene derivatives by using the following formula.

$$\frac{dm}{dt} = C(derivatives).D.S.\partial C / \partial x$$

Where dm/dt is the amount of the mass passes across the surface per unit time rate. While analyzing this method for the derivatives of fullerenes, it depends on two factors (1) D (coefficient of diffusion) value and (2) radius of the particle.

By using the Smoluchowski–Stokes–Einstein law, the diffusion of the coefficient and radius of particles was correlated using the following equation.

$$D = \frac{KT}{6\pi\eta rD}$$

where D is the diffusion coefficient, K is the Boltzmann constant, rD is the radius of the particle, η is the viscosity, and T is temperature [48].

24.5 *IN VIVO* BIOFATE OF CARBON NANOTUBES AND FULLERENES

24.5.1 CARBON NANOTUBES

After cellular uptake, CNTs are internalized in any of various subcellular organelles such as nuclei, mitochondria, cytoplasm, lysosomes, cytoskeleton, and endoplasmic reticulum and can be relocated between these compartments via carrier-mediated transport [51]. Intracellular targeting can be controlled by conjugating a specific functional group to CNTs. The vacuoles are readily taken up by the Fluorescein isothiocyanate (FITC)-SWCNTs via carrier mediated transport mechanism, however, when these nanocarriers were functionalized with a carrier-mediated transport inhibitor, they are mainly internalized in the cytoplasm of the cell [52]. The internalization of SW-F in the cell and a summary of intracellular pathways are shown in Figure 24.2.

To determine the subcellular distribution of localized CNTs, various techniques such as confocal and fluorescent microscopy, transmission electron microscopy (TEM), Raman spectroscopy, and scanning electron microscopy (SEM) are used. Porter et al. used TEM and showed that SWCNTs were internalized in lysosomes after 2 days, and packs of SWCNTs were internalized in endosomes after 4 days, which were internalized in the nucleus by translocation through nuclear membrane [53].

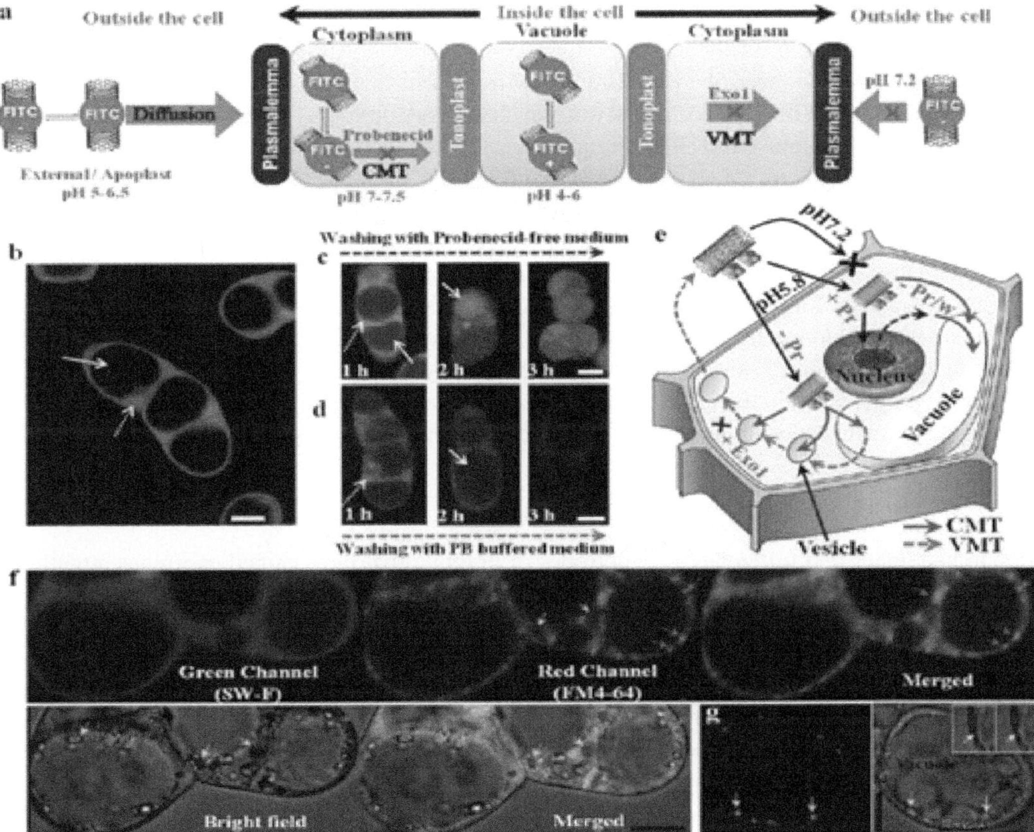

FIGURE 24.2 Controlled subcellular distribution of SW-F in *C. roseus* cells. (A) SW-F intracellular transport pathways. (B) Internalization of SW-F in the vacuole was inhibited by probenecid, represented by a solid arrow, and simultaneously promoted their accumulation in cytoplasm, represented by a dotted arrow. (C) The solid arrow represents the redistribution of SW-F into the vacuole after washing the cells treated with a probenecid in pH 5.8 medium free from probenecid. (D) After washing with a pH 7.2 phosphate buffer, increased cytoplasm clearance of SW-F was observed, represented with dotted lines. (E) Plant cell demonstrating SW-F controlled subcellular distribution. (F) Confocal microscopy images of *C. roseus* cell incubated in nutrient medium supplemented with 5 µg/mL SW-F and 5 mM probenecid. (G) Confocal microscopy images of *C. roseus* cell incubated in pH 7.2 phosphate buffer (adapted from Serag et al., 2011 with copyright permission).

Nunes et al. prepared an aqueous suspension of amine-functionalized MWCNTSs. They injected these MWCNTs stereotactically into the cortex of the mouse. They reported that these MWCNTs were mainly internalized in microglia at early time points. After 2 days of injection, degradation of MWCNTs started and exhibited structural deformations, loss of cylindrical structure, and reduced length. With time, the degree of structural defects in the MWCNTs was augmented, which was confirmed by Raman spectroscopy [54].

Zhang et al. prepared Gd_2O_3 nanoparticles and encapsulated these nanoparticles within carbon nanohorns (CNHs). After intravenous injection, they measured the biodistribution and clearance of CNHs in mice by determining the gadolinium concentration by inductively coupled plasma atomic emission spectroscopy. After 4 months of injection, in the liver, around 70% of CNHs were accumulated and 40% of injected CNHs were eliminated. About 25% of CNHs were degraded in the liver, and around 15% were eliminated in the feces [55].

24.5.2 FULLERENES

Various factors such as particle size, administration pathways, and various modifications affect the distribution of fullerenes in the body. The target tissue and toxicity at the specific target tissue can be recognized by the help of these factors. Intravenously injected C60 was cleared rapidly from the systemic circulation, however, if internalized, they remain in the liver for many days approximately 13 days, and cleared off from the liver slowly. Through the oral route, 14C-labeled C60 was not absorbed completely and was eliminated mainly through feces. These outcomes show that the liver is the major targeting organ for the accumulation and metabolism of fullerenes [56]. When compared to C60, water-soluble C60 had a larger distribution in tissue because of its hydrophilic nature. Li et al. fabricated (99m) Tc-labeled C(60)(OH)(x), injected it into mice and rabbits, and assessed the biodistribution. After injection through the tail vein into mice, the (99m) Tc-labeled compound was rapidly distributed throughout all organs except for low-perfusion tissues. The activity was retained for approximately 48 hrs in all organs, like bones, kidney, liver, and spleen. Bone showed enhanced localization within 24 hrs and all remaining tissues exhibited slow clearance for 48 hrs [57]. After inhalation, C60 and derivatives of C60 were partly accumulated in the lung and internalized by macrophages. At high concentrations (10 mg/kg), fullerenols exhibited an inflammatory response in the pulmonary system [58].

24.6 CONCLUSION

Carbon nanotubes and fullerenes are allotropes of graphite that have gained enormous attention in the development of safe and more effective nanotherapeutic medicine. CNTs are long and cylindrical in structure and used for diagnosing and targeting purposes, and they are classified into SWCNTs and MWCNTs. The addition of functional group moieties to CNTs results in increases of aqueous solubility by means of covalent and non-covalent approaches. Fullerenes based on structural carbon atoms exist as C60 and C70 (Buckminster fullerenes). Several physico-chemical properties of fullerene derivatives like isothermal densities, conductivity, size distribution, viscosities, refractive index, diffusion, etc. could be altered to make them suitable to detect, imaging and delivery of the drug to site of action. Acoustic explosion and photodynamic therapy are some of the mainly reported methods in the treatment of tumors. Endohedral fullerenes and polyhydroxy fullerenes are widely used theranostic fullerenes. Various factors such as particle size, administration pathways, and various modifications that affect the distribution of fullerenes in the body were discussed in the chapter.

24.7 ACKNOWLEDGMENTS

The authors would like to acknowledge the National Institute of Pharmaceutical Education, Hyderabad Department of Pharmaceuticals, Ministry of Chemical and Family Welfares, India, during writing this book chapter (manuscript communication number NIPER-H/2021/BC-015).

REFERENCES

1. Jain, N. K., Mishra, V., & Mehra, N. K. 2013. Targeted drug delivery to macrophages. *Expert Opinion in Drug Delivery*, 10(3), 353–367.
2. Jain, K., Mehra, N. K., & Jain, N. K. 2014. Potentials and emerging trends in nanopharmacology. *Current Opinion in Pharmacology*, 15, 97–106.
3. Mehra, N. K., & Palakurthi, S. 2016. Interactions between carbon nanotubes and bioactives: A drug delivery perspective. *Drug Discovery Today*, 21(4), 585–597.
4. Mehra, N. K., Jain, A. K., & Nahar, M. 2018. Carbon nanomaterials in oncology: An expanding horizon. *Drug Discovery Today*, 23(5), 1016–1025.
5. Jain, H., Bairagi, A., Srivastava, S., Singh, S. B., & Mehra, N. K. 2020. Recent advances in the development of microparticles for pulmonary administration. *Drug Discovery Today*, 25(10), 1865–1872.
6. Koppa Raghu, P., Bansal, K. K., Thakor, P., Bhavana, V., Madan, J., Rosenholm, J. M., & Mehra, N. K. 2020. Evolution of nanotechnology in delivering drugs to eyes, skin and wounds via topical route. *Pharmaceuticals*, 13(8), 167.
7. Bacon, R. 1960. Growth, structure, and properties of graphite whiskers. *Journal of Applied Physics*, 31(2), 283–290.
8. Iijima, S. 1991. Helical microtubules of graphitic carbon. *Nature*, 354(6348), 56–58.
9. Pastorin, G., Wu, W., Wieckowski, S., Briand, J. P., Kostarelos, K., Prato, M., & Bianco, A. 2006. Double functionalisation of carbon nanotubes for multimodal drug delivery. *Chemical Communications*, 11, 1182–1184.
10. Chen, C., Zhang, H., Hou, L., Shi, J., Wang, L., Zhang, C., Zhang, M., Zhang, H., Shi, X., Li, H., & Zhang, Z. 2013. Single-walled carbon nanotubes mediated neovascularity targeted antitumor drug delivery system. *Journal of Pharmacy and Pharmaceutical Sciences*, 16(1), 40–51.
11. Niu, L., Meng, L., & Lu, Q. 2013. Folate-conjugated PEG on single walled carbon nanotubes for targeting delivery of doxorubicin to cancer cells. *Macromolecular Bioscience*, 13(6), 735–744.
12. Mehra, N. K., & Jain, N. K. 2013. Development, characterization and cancer targeting potential of surface engineered carbon nanotubes. *Journal of Drug Targeting*, 21(8), 745–758.
13. Mehra, N. K., Mishra, V., & Jain, N. K. 2013. Receptor-based targeting of therapeutics. *Therapeutic Delivery*, 4(3), 369–394.
14. Mehra, N. K., Mishra, V., & Jain, N. K. 2014. A review of ligand tethered surface engineered carbon nanotubes. *Biomaterials*, 35(4), 1267–1283.
15. Wong, B. S., Yoong, S. L., Jagusiak, A., Panczyk, T., Ho, H. K., Ang, W. H., &Pastorin, G. 2013. Carbon nanotubes for delivery of small molecule drugs. *Advanced Drug Delivery Reviews*, 65(15), 1964–2015.
16. Lacerda, L., Russier, J., Pastorin, G., Herrero, M. A., Venturelli, E., Dumortier, H., Al-Jamal, K. T., Prato, M., Kostarelos, K., & Bianco, A. 2012. Translocation mechanisms of chemically functionalised carbon nanotubes across plasma membranes. *Biomaterials*, 33(11), 3334–3343.
17. Kotchey, G. P., Zhao, Y., Kagan, V. E., & Star, A. 2013. Peroxidase-mediated biodegradation of carbon nanotubes in vitro and in vivo. *Advanced Drug Delivery Reviews*, 65(15), 1921–1932.
18. Zhou, Y., Fang, Y., & Ramasamy, R. P. 2019. Non-covalent functionalization of carbon nanotubes for electrochemical biosensor development. *Sensors*, 19(2), 392.
19. Saka, C. 2018. Overview on the surface functionalization mechanism and determination of surface functional groups of plasma treated carbon nanotubes. *Critical Reviews in Analytical Chemistry*, 48(1), 1–14.
20. Caoduro, C., Hervouet, E., Girard-Thernier, C., Gharbi, T., Boulahdour, H., Delage-Mourroux, R., & Pudlo, M. 2017. Carbon nanotubes as gene carriers: Focus on internalization pathways related to functionalization and properties. *Acta Biomaterialia*, 49, 36–44.
21. Roy, S., Korzeniowska, B., Dixit, C. K., Manickam, G., Daniels, S., & McDonagh, C. 2015. Biocompatibility and bioimaging application of carbon nanoparticles synthesized by phosphorus pentoxide combustion method. *Journal of Nanomaterials*, 2015, 1–10.
22. Ceppi, L., Bardhan, N. M., Na, Y., Siegel, A., Rajan, N., Fruscio, R., Del Carmen, M. G., Belcher, A. M., & Birrer, M. J. 2019. Real-time single-walled carbon nanotube-based fluorescence imaging improves survival after debulking surgery in an ovarian cancer model. *ACS Nano*, 13(5), 5356–5365.
23. Bhunia, S. K., Saha, A., Maity, A. R., Ray, S. C., & Jana, N. R. 2013. Carbon nanoparticle-based fluorescent bioimaging probes. *Scientific Reports*, 3(1), 1–7.
24. Rani, R., Kumar, V., & Rizzolio, F. 2018. Fluorescent carbon nanoparticles in medicine for cancer therapy: An update. *ACS Medicinal Chemistry Letters*, 9(1), 4–5.

25. Yudasaka, M., Yomogida, Y., Zhang, M., Tanaka, T., Nakahara, M., Kobayashi, N., . . . & Kataura, H. 2017. Near-infrared photoluminescent carbon nanotubes for imaging of brown fat. *Scientific Reports*, 7(1), 1–12.
26. Bisker, G., Dong, J., Park, H. D., Iverson, N. M., Ahn, J., Nelson, J. T., Landry, M. P., Kruss, S., & Strano, M. S. 2016. Protein-targeted corona phase molecular recognition. *Nature Communications*, 7(1), 1–14.
27. Beyene, A. G., Delevich, K., Yang, S. J., & Landry, M. P. 2018. New optical probes bring dopamine to light. *Biochemistry*, 57(45), 6379–6381.
28. Dinarvand, M., Neubert, E., Meyer, D., Selvaggio, G., Mann, F. A., Erpenbeck, L., & Kruss, S. 2019. Near-infrared imaging of serotonin release from cells with fluorescent nanosensors. *Nano Letters*, 19(9), 6604–6611.
29. Kroto, H. W., Heath, J. R., O'Brien, S. C., Curl, R. F., & Smalley, R. E. 1985. C60: Buckminsterfullerene. *Nature*, 318(6042), 162–163.
30. Tan, Y. Z., Xie, S. Y., Huang, R. B., & Zheng, L. S. 2009. The stabilization of fused-pentagon fullerene molecules. *Nature Chemistry*, 1(6), 450–460.
31. Patra, C. R., Jing, Y., Xu, Y. H., Bhattacharya, R., Mukhopadhyay, D., Glockner, J. F., Wang, J. P., & Mukherjee, P. 2010. A core-shell nanomaterial with endogenous therapeutic and diagnostic functions. *Cancer Nanotechnology*, 1(1–6), 13–18.
32. Yigit, M. V., Zhu, L., Ifediba, M. A., Zhang, Y., Carr, K., Moore, A., & Medarova, Z. 2011. Noninvasive MRI-SERS imaging in living mice using an innately bimodal nanomaterial. *ACS Nano*, 5(2), 1056–1066.
33. Jaffer, F. A., Nahrendorf, M., Sosnovik, D., Kelly, K. A., Aikawa, E., & Weissleder, R. 2006. Cellular imaging of inflammation in atherosclerosis using magneto-fluorescent nanomaterials. *Society of Nuclear Medicine and Molecular Imaging*, 5(2), 85–92.
34. Von Maltzahn, G., Ren, Y., Park, J. H., Min, D. H., Kotamraju, V. R., Jayakumar, J., Fogal, V., Sailor, M. J., Ruoslahti, E., & Bhatia, S. N. 2008. In vivo tumor cell targeting with "click" nanoparticles. *Bioconjugate Chemistry*, 19(8), 1570–1578.
35. Nitta, N., Seko, A., Sonoda, A., Ohta, S., Tanaka, T., Takahashi, M., Murata, K., Takemura, S., Sakamoto, T., & Tabata, Y. 2008. Is the use of fullerene in photodynamic therapy effective for atherosclerosis? *Cardiovascular and Interventional Radiology*, 31(2), 359–366.
36. Bolskar, R. D. 2008. Gadofullerene MRI contrast agents. In *Nanomedicine*. Future Medicine Ltd, London, UK, 3(2), 201–213.
37. Mody, V. V., Nounou, M. I., & Bikram, M. 2009. Novel nanomedicine-based MRI contrast agents for gynecological malignancies. *Advanced Drug Delivery Reviews*, 61(10), 795–807.
38. Chewning, R. H., & Murphy, K. J. 2007. Gadolinium-based contrast media and the development of nephrogenic systemic fibrosis in patients with renal insufficiency. *Journal of Vascular and Interventional Radiology*, 18(3), 331–333.
39. Ledneva, E., Karie, S., Launay-Vacher, V., Janus, N., & Deray, G. 2009. Renal safety of gadolinium-based contrast media in patients with chronic renal insufficiency 1. *Pubs.Rsna.Org*, 250(3), 618–628.
40. Runge, V. M. 2009. Gadolinium and nephrogenic systemic fibrosis. *American Journal of Roentgenology*, 192(4), 195–196.
41. Madhankumar, A. B., Slagle-Webb, B., Mintz, A., Sheehan, J. M., & Connor, J. R. 2006. Interleukin-13 receptor–targeted nanovesicles are a potential therapy for glioblastoma multiforme. *Molecular Cancer Therapeutics*, 5(12), 3162–3169.
42. MacFarland, D. K., Walker, K. L., Lenk, R. P., Wilson, S. R., Kumar, K., Kepley, C. L., & Garbow, J. R. 2008. Hydrochalarones: A novel endohedral metallofullerene platform for enhancing magnetic resonance imaging contrast. *Journal of Medicinal Chemistry*, 51(13), 3681–3683.
43. Satoh, M., & Takayanagi, I. 2006. Pharmacological studies on fullerene (C60), a novel carbon allotrope, and its derivatives. *Journal of Pharmacological Sciences*, 100(5), 513–518.
44. Liu, J., & Tabata, Y. 2010. Photodynamic therapy of fullerene modified with pullulan on hepatoma cells. *Journal of Drug Targeting*, 18(8), 602–610.
45. Liu, J., & Tabata, Y. 2011. Photodynamic antitumor activity of fullerene modified with poly(ethylene glycol) with different molecular weights and terminal structures. *Journal of Biomaterials Science, Polymer Edition*, 22(1–3), 297–312.
46. Liu, J., Ohta, S. I., Sonoda, A., Yamada, M., Yamamoto, M., Nitta, N., & Tabata, Y. 2007. Preparation of PEG-conjugated fullerene containing Gd3+ ions for photodynamic therapy. *Journal of Controlled Release*, 117(1), 104–110.
47. Mroz, P., Xia, Y., Asanuma, D., Konopko, A., Zhiyentayev, T., Huang, Y.-Y., Sharma, S. K., Dai, T., Khan, U. J., Wharton, T., & Hamblin, M. R. 2011. Intraperitoneal photodynamic therapy mediated by a fullerene in a mouse model of abdominal dissemination of colon adenocarcinoma. *Nanomedicine: Nanotechnology, Biology and Medicine*, 7(6), 965–974.

48. Semenov, K. N., Charykov, N. A., Murin, I. V., & Pukharenko, Y. V. 2015. Physico-chemical properties of the C60-tris-malonic derivative water solutions. *Journal of Molecular Liquids*, 201, 50–58.
49. Manyakina, O. S., Semenov, K. N., Charykov, N. A., Ivanova, N. M., Keskinov, V. A., Sharoyko, V. V., Letenko, D. G., Nikitin, V. A., Klepikov, V. V., & Murin, I. V. 2015. Physico-chemical properties of the water-soluble C70-tris-malonic solutions. *Journal of Molecular Liquids*, 211, 487–493.
50. Damaskin, B. B., & Petrii, O. A. 1983. *Introduction to electrochemical kinetics*. Russian Edition, Vysshaya shkola, Moscow, 278–289.
51. Zhao, F., Zhao, Y., Liu, Y., Chang, X., Chen, C., & Zhao, Y. 2011. Cellular uptake, intracellular trafficking, and cytotoxicity of nanomaterials. *Small*, 7(10), 1322–1337.
52. Serag, M. F., Kaji, N., Venturelli, E., Okamoto, Y., Terasaka, K., Tokeshi, M., Mizukami, H., Braeckmans, K., Bianco, A., & Baba, Y. 2011. Functional platform for controlled subcellular distribution of carbon nanotubes. *ACS Nano*, 5(11), 9264–9270.
53. Porter, A. E., Gass, M., Muller, K., Skepper, J. N., Midgley, P. A., & Welland, M. 2007. Direct imaging of single-walled carbon nanotubes in cells. *Nature Nanotechnology*, 2(11), 713–717.
54. Nunes, A., Bussy, C., Gherardini, L., Meneghetti, M., Herrero, M. A., Bianco, A., Prato, M., Pizzorusso, T., Al-Jamal, K. T., & Kostarelos, K. 2012. In vivo degradation of functionalized carbon nanotubes after stereotactic administration in the brain cortex. *Nanomedicine*, 7(10), 1485–1494.
55. Zhang, M., Tahara, Y., Yang, M., Zhou, X., Iijima, S., & Yudasaka, M. 2014. Quantification of whole body and excreted carbon nanohorns intravenously injected into mice. *Advanced Healthcare Materials*, 3(2), 239–244.
56. Gharbi, N., Pressac, M., Hadchouel, M., Szwarc, H., Wilson, S. R., & Moussa, F. 2005. Fullerene is a powerful antioxidant in vivo with no acute or subacute toxicity. *Nano Letters*, 5(12), 2578–2585.
57. Qingnuan, L., Yan, X., Xiaodong, Z., Ruili, L., Qieqie, D., Xiaoguang, S., Shaoliang, C., & Wenxin, L. 2002. Preparation of 99mTc-C60(OH)x and its biodistribution studies. *Nuclear Medicine and Biology*, 29(6), 707–710.
58. Fujita, K., Morimoto, Y., Ogami, A., Myojyo, T., Tanaka, I., Shimada, M., Wang, W.-N., Endoh, S., Uchida, K., Nakazato, T., Yamamoto, K., Fukui, H., Horie, M., Yoshida, Y., Iwahashi, H., & Nakanishi, J. 2009. Gene expression profiles in rat lung after inhalation exposure to C60 fullerene particles. *Toxicology*, 258(1), 47–55.

Pramod Kumar

25.1 INTRODUCTION

Traditional disease management approaches have previously been widely developed and are primarily based on using small molecules and proteins for therapeutic benefit. These drugs are effective in treating a variety of diseases; however, they have several drawbacks. For example, most small molecules become active when they bind to a target protein, but very few proteins have these effective binding sites [1]. Furthermore, the limiting factor is the stability or complication in the production and tissue penetration of protein-based drug molecules [2]. Overall, the likelihood of developing effective drug candidate is low.

For therapeutic benefit, gene therapy is a promising approach to disease management that requires the delivery and insertion of desired genes into the patient's cells. Deoxyribonucleic acid (DNA) and ribonucleic acid (RNA)–based biological macromolecules are used as medicines in this technique to treat or prevent diseases. One of the most recent emerging fields studied and accepted by academia and industry research is RNA-based therapeutic approaches. More than 15 RNA candidates have already entered clinical trials, and a number of molecules are in advanced clinical trials and will hit the market soon [3].

RNA-based therapeutic agents, such as siRNA, microRNA (miRNA), and mRNA, work through a variety of mechanisms, such as target gene knockdown, target gene upregulation, or specific gene expression [4]. The primary benefit of using an RNA-based approach is that it can generate multiple folds of protein molecules upon successful delivery. Aside from that, RNA-based therapeutics are simple to design using an in vitro transcription system or even chemical synthesis. These properties of RNA therapeutics have the potential to lead to the development of effective medicines to manage mutation-based cancer disease or even epidemics. Short interfering RNA (siRNA), which typically has 20–27 base pairs, is an effective therapeutic macromolecule that works at the RNA interference level. Because of a variety of biological barriers, only a few RNA-based molecules have entered clinical trials and been successfully translated. The reason for the limited success of RNA-based medicine is that these molecules are too large and anionic, resulting in limited intracellular delivery. The naked RNA is extremely susceptible to elimination from the body through renal and hepatic clearance, as well as degradation by intrinsic factors such as RNase, exonuclease, or endonuclease. They can activate the innate immune response via a TLR-dependent or TLR-independent signaling pathway. To ensure effective delivery to target cells, RNA molecules must be protected from clearance or intrinsic mechanisms. Physical methods such as microinjection and electroporation could be used to easily introduce siRNA into cells. Such methods, however, are not optimized for most in vivo applications. To this end, a potential approach for intracellular delivery of RNA therapeutics using nanocarrier systems could significantly improve such molecular medicine's therapeutic potential.

25.2 NUCLEIC ACID-BASED APPROACH FOR DISEASE MANAGEMENT

The detailed study of the human genome has suggested a wide range of possibilities for identifying the genes involved in disease pathology and paving the way for the advancement of nucleic

DOI: 10.1201/9781003130055-25

acid-based medicine to combat genetic conditions [5]. Despite the fact that most nucleic acid-based medicines are still in the early stages of development, they are highly effective in the treatment of a wide range of disease classes, including cystic fibrosis; cardiovascular, inflammatory, neurodegenerative, and infectious diseases; cancer; diabetes; hemophilia; pulmonary diseases; and other genetic diseases. The traditional approach to nucleic acid-based therapy is based on either DNA or RNA genetic materials, as shown in the following [6].

25.2.1 DNA-BASED THERAPEUTICS

DNA therapeutics include gene transfer technologies such as plasmids, oligonucleotides for antisense and antigene applications (antisense oligonucleotides), DNA aptamers, and DNA acidzymes. Plasmids are small circular DNA-based constructs with a high molecular weight that encode proteins. The plasmid guides the DNA transcription and translation apparatus within the nucleus to synthesize the specific protein upon cellular uptake [7]. Antisense single DNA strand oligonucleotides that are complementary to the mRNA target bind to the target RNA. This DNA–RNA heterocomplex is typically cleaved by RNase H endonuclease activity, resulting in a decrease in target gene translation. Aptamers based on DNA are also double-stranded DNA moieties that directly interact with target proteins to inhibit their activity. Aptamers are sometimes more effective than antibodies in inhibiting protein functions due to their specificity, non-immunogenicity, and better stability in pharmaceutical formulations [8]. Similarly, ribozyme analogs such as DNAzymes are used as therapeutics in which RNA backbone chemistry is modified using DNA motifs to improve biological stability and obtained through in vitro selection. They are programmed to cleave a specific mRNA in order to suppress gene activity [9].

25.2.2 RNA-BASED THERAPEUTICS

RNA aptamers, RNA decoys, antisense RNA, ribozymes, micro-ribonucleic acid, and siRNA are examples of RNA-based medicines. RNA aptamers, for example, recognize the target on the base of a complementary shape and bind to target proteins. RNA aptamers are single-stranded RNA fragments with high specificity and affinity for target proteins [10]. Ribozymes and antisense RNA techniques inhibit transcription in the same way that ASO and DNAzymes do. MiRNAs are endogenous, small noncoding RNA molecules of 21–25 nucleotides in length. They are partially complementary to mRNA and are responsible for downregulating gene expression through a variety of mechanisms, such as translational suppression, mRNA cleavage, or mRNA deadenylation. MiRNAs function by base-pairing with complementary mRNA sequences [11]. The most extensively researched nucleic acid-based medicine is siRNA, which acts at the post-transcriptional level through chromatin remodeling, protein translation inhibition, and ubiquitous mRNA breakdown. siRNA are short, double-stranded RNA segments that complement target mRNA sequences [12].

25.2.3 KEY FEATURES OF siRNA-BASED THERAPEUTICS (siRNA AS THERAPEUTIC AGENTS)

The transfer of existing molecules to the target site is an important success factor in molecular medicine. siRNA has already been established as a potential molecular medicine with major clinical implications against a number of lethal pathologies. It has a significant capacity to counter specific gene signaling via the delivery of double-stranded RNA (dsRNA, primarily), which induces downregulation in target gene via RNA interference. siRNA primarily targets the complementary mRNA, depriving it of its function. Figure 25.1 depicts the mechanism of siRNA activity in blocking target mRNA translation [13].

One potential advantage of RNA therapeutics over DNA-based approaches is the ability to test the RNA mechanism both in vitro and in vivo. Despite the high therapeutic potential of siRNA in molecular medicine, clinical translation is still limited due to the fact that unmodified RNAs are

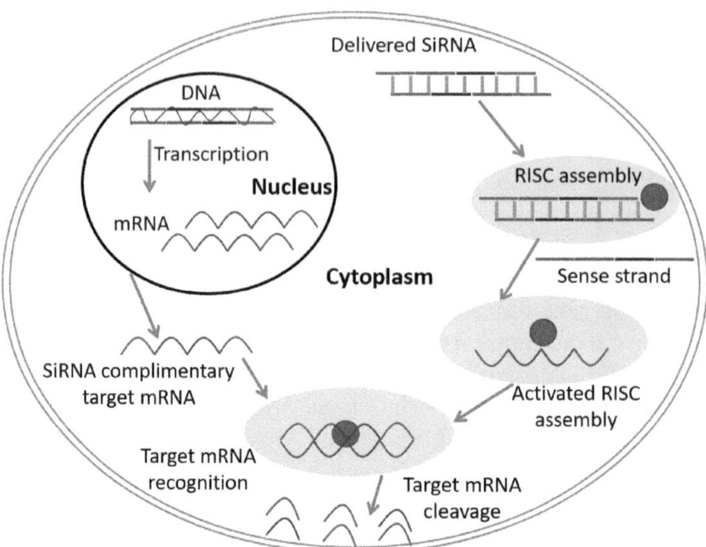

FIGURE 25.1   The mechanism of siRNA in the lysis of target mRNA.

easily degraded by endogenous enzymes (e.g. RNAse) and the lack of effective delivery systems to improve stability [13, 14].

Furthermore, their low half-life in circulation and poor chemical stability result in low turnover, which is only useful in easily transfectable cells with transient inhibition. The development of resilient delivery vectors could be extremely beneficial in avoiding such constraints [14, 15] Furthermore, the potential of siRNA-based nanomedicines could lead the technology in subsequent clinical trials and clinics (table 25.1).

25.3   CHALLENGES IN THE DELIVERY OF SIRNAS AND THEIR ADAPTATION

The investigation of siRNA therapy's broad application is hampered by its suboptimal delivery to diseased tissues. There are several barriers to intracellular siRNA delivery, including rapid degradation in physiological fluids, rapid renal filtration, phagocyte degradation, and transport from blood to diseased tissues. For effective cellular uptake, siRNA molecules must cross the vascular barrier once they reach the target tissue. Their migration from the endosome to the cytoplasm, as well as their release to form the RNA-induced silencing complex (RISC) in order to activate the machinery, are also challenges [16]. The following are potential barriers to siRNA delivery to the target tissue.

25.3.1   DELIVERY BARRIERS

Because of the susceptibility of intestinal degradation and lower intestinal barrier permeability, intravenous or infusion injections are the most commonly used route of administration for siRNA-based medicines [17]. To protect siRNA from hydrolytic enzymes, a delivery platform is required. To that end, the particulate delivery vehicle can enhance siRNA therapeutic value by modifying biodistribution and localization at the target site. The optimal platform for siRNA delivery could be nanoparticles.

25.3.2   VASCULAR BARRIERS

A delivery platform is required to protect siRNA from hydrolytic enzymes. To that end, the particulate delivery vehicle can improve the therapeutic value of siRNA by altering biodistribution

TABLE 25.1

Key Advancements in Nanoparticle Development and Clinical Translation

S. No.	Description	Diseases/Target Gene	Clinical Stage	Company/Name of Product	Remarks
1	Lipid nanoparticles made of DSPC, DLin-MC3-DM, APEG$_{2000}$-C-DMG	Hereditary transthyretin amyloidosis/hATTR	In market	Alnylam Pharma./ONPATTRO (patisiran, ALN-TTR02)	First nanocarrier-based siRNA drug; many under development process on same platform
2	SNALP MC3 lipid	Hypercholesteremia/ApoB	Phase I	Tekmira Pharma. Corporation/PRO-040201/TKM-ApoB	Trial terminated due to immune system stimulation
3	LNP (liposomes)	Melanoma, liver cancer, mir-34 mimic	Phase I/II	Mirna Therapeutics Inc./MRX34	A liposomal miR-34a mimic
4	Anionic liposomes	Chronic myeloid leukemia/BCR-ABL	Phase I	University of Duisburg-Essen/BCR-ABL siRNA	Three consecutive doses given
5	SNALP MC3 lipid	Hypercholesterolemia/ApoB	Phase I	Tekmira Pharma. Corporation/PRO-040201/TKM-ApoB	Direct tumor cell death and sensitization of tumor cells to help in chemotherapy
6	Mesenchymal stromal cell–derived exosomes (KRAS G12D siRNA)	Stage IV pancreatic cancer, pancreatic adenocarcinoma, ductal adenocarcinoma/AJCC v8/KRAS	Phase I	M.D. Anderson Cancer Center/iExosomes-KrasG12D siRNA	Endogenous derived gene delivery system
7	Cationic lipid AtuFECT01, 1,2-diphytanoyl-sn-glycero-3-phospho-ethanolamine (DPhyPE), DSPE-PEG	Advanced solid tumor/sprotein kinase N3	Phase I/II	Silence therapeutics/Atuplex (Atu027)	Discontinued after phase I
8	Cationic [O,Oȼ-ditetradecanoyl-N-(a-trimethylammonioacetyl) diethanol amine chloride (DC-6–14), cholesterol, dioleoylphosphatidylethanolamine; molar ratio of 4:3:3]	Liver fibrosis and idiopathic pulmonary fibrosis/HSP47	Phase I/II	Bristol-Myers Squibb/BMS 986263 ND-L02-s0201	Developed by Nitto Denko Corporation
9	18:1 PC (cis) 1,2-dioleoyl-*sn*-glycero-3-phosphocholine (DOPC)	Advanced cancer/EphA2	Phase I	MD Anderson Cancer Center/siRNA-EphA2-DOPC	Neutral liposomes

(Continued)

TABLE 25.1 (Continued)

Key Advancements in Nanoparticle Development and Clinical Translation

S. No.	Description	Diseases/Target Gene	Clinical Stage	Company/Name of Product	Remarks
10	Spherical nucleic acid (SNA)–coated gold nanoparticles	Gliosarcoma/BCL2L12	Phase I	Northwestern University/ NU-0129	Actively crosses the blood–brain barrier
11	SNALP MC3 lipid	Liver or adrenocarcinoma/PKL1	Phase I/II	National Cancer Institute/ Tekmira Pharm./TKM 080301	Well tolerated and good antitumor efficacy
12	LNP EnCore	Solid cancer/MYC	Phase I/II	Dicerna Pharma., Inc./ DCR-MYC	Dicerna involved different GalXC technology against lactate dehydrogenase useful in primary hyperoxaluria type I
13	LNP EnCore	Primary hyperoxaluria type I/ glycolate oxidase	Phase I	Dicerna Pharma., Inc./ DCR-PH1	Discontinued, as preliminary results do not meet expectations
14	Cyclodextrin nanoparticles, transferrin, PEG	Solid tumor/M2 subunit of ribonucleotide reductase/RRM2	Phase I	Calando Pharma./CALAA-01	Systemically deliver siRNA nanoparticles using receptor-mediated approach; 21% of patients suffered adverse event; trial ended
15	SNALP, MC3 lipid	Solid tumors with liver involvement/ VEGF, KSP	Phase I	Alnylam Pharma./ALN-VSP02	Multiple genes
16	SNALP, cationic PEGylated liposomes, DSPC, DLin-MC3-DMA, DMG-PEG, and cholesterol	Solid tumors IV I, or recruiting solid tumors with liver involvement/ polo-kinase-1	Phase I/II	Tekmira Pharma/TKM-080301	Similar drugs under testing for Apo B in hypercholesterolemia, VP24, VP35, l-polymerase Ebola virus infection
17	SNALP MC3 lipid	Hepatitis B, chronic/HBV proteins	Phase II	Arbutus Biopharma/ ARB-001467	3-siRNAs delivered simultaneously using LNP technology

and localization at the target site. Nanoparticles may be the best platform for siRNA delivery [18]. The beneficial feature of disease tissue (e.g., cancer tissue) is that it allows nanocarrier accumulation, and the defective lymphatic system prevents filtration, so enhanced permeability and retention (EPR) of particulate siRNA nanocarrier is very helpful in avoiding vascular obstacles.

25.3.3 Cellular Barriers

The eukaryotic cell membrane is made up of net negatively charged lipid bilayers. The use of cationic lipids to induce endocytosis is very promising for improving cellular uptake. The use of targeting ligands such as folate, transferring or aptamers (protein based), N-acetylgalactosamine (sugar based), or estrogen (steroid based) could be very beneficial in improving targeted endocytosis [19].

25.3.4 Intracellular Barriers

The endosomal escape of the delivered engineered drug delivery vehicle is the final barrier to effective siRNA delivery. Otherwise, the endosome will fuse with the lysosomes, potentially leading to the lysosomal degradation of active siRNA. To that end, the use of cationic polymers that induce endosomolysis or neutrally charged ionizable lipids that become positive inside endosomes improves siRNA release by disrupting lysosomes [20].

25.3.5 Immunological Barriers

Any therapeutic approach must be concerned about the induction of immune modulation when using external materials. To avoid this effect, 21–23 base pair siRNA selection and/or siRNA methylation at the 2' position are effective approaches. The delivery vehicle should be chosen so that it is not recognized as foreign material and does not cause unwanted side effects or off-target silencing [21].

25.4 PREREQUISITES OF SIRNA DELIVERY FOR DISEASE MANAGEMENT

Specificity, efficiency, and safety once delivered in the cell are critical measurement criteria for selecting siRNA. Because siRNA is highly sensitive to degradation in body fluid, integral siRNA delivery at the target location is critical for the success of siRNA therapeutics. Importantly, effective and well-controlled siRNA in vivo delivery remains difficult due to the larger size (13,000 Mw) and anionic nature of most eukaryotic cells. As a result, unmodified siRNA molecules are difficult to uptake efficiently, resulting in suboptimal gene silencing in vivo [22].

As a result, developing safe and efficient gene delivery methods is critical for siRNA therapeutics.

However, no single strategy can guarantee their success. Several vectors have been evaluated and found to be highly effective in providing specificity in siRNA delivery [23]. Many of the previously mentioned barriers to siRNA delivery can be overcome by engineering the delivery vehicle. Significant progress has been made in optimizing siRNA delivery to target sites by modulating effective delivery systems. RNA delivery systems are broadly classified into viral and non-viral delivery methods, as shown in the following [24].

25.4.1 siRNA Delivery Based on Viral Vectors

The use of viral gene delivery carriers has the distinct advantage of strong interaction with cellular receptors, resulting in rapid intracellular delivery. The viral vectors are effective in siRNA delivery because they can carry a large amount of siRNA [25]. Retrovirus, adenovirus, adeno-associated virus (AAV), and lentivirus are the most common viral-based gene delivery carriers. Adenoviruses have a high transduction efficiency and high levels of transgene expression, allowing them to be used to transduce a variety of complex organs [26, 27]. However, the use of a viral vector raised concerns about biosafety and immunogenicity. As a result, the use of a viral-based delivery system necessitates a high level of technical expertise. Recently, the engineering of viral vectors by producing replication incompetent delivery systems has revealed limited safety issues.

25.4.2 siRNA Delivery Based on Non-Viral Vectors

The biosafety of viral-based vectors motivates scientists to look into non-viral-based RNA delivery systems. These systems rely on either physical methods (e.g., electroporation, microinjection, or the use of ballistic particles) or chemical methods (e.g., calcium phosphate, lipid, protein complexes). There has been significant progress in the development of non-viral vectors, particularly scaffold-based approaches. Because of higher physicochemical stability and increased efficiency of diseased protein correction by using cells as bioreactors, localized siRNA delivery using hydrogel-based systems represents a potential substitute. However, systemic administration of siRNA is still associated with a number of limitations, including insufficient blood half-life, ineffective targeting, and associated cytotoxicity.

25.5 NANOPARTICLES FOR SIRNA DELIVERY

In comparison to their viral counterparts, the primary advantage of using non-viral vectors is their lower immunogenicity. They could include a mix of genetic cargos useful in a variety of applications. Simultaneously, the non-viral system suffers from poor clinical translation due to insufficient therapeutic efficacy prediction. Several advances in RNA carrier systems have been made, and it is expected that these advances will lead to siRNA therapeutics as a foundation for many unmet clinical needs in the near future. Multivalent electrostatic interactions in positively charged delivery vector and negatively charged siRNA molecules produce lipid and polymer-based non-viral vectors.

Recent significant advancements in non-viral delivery systems include increased loading capacity [28], faster scale-up for mass production [29], ability of functionalization for better permeability [30], and better targeting [31], as well as higher intracellular uptake [32]. Nanoparticles, in particular, have the potential to meet a number of challenges in siRNA therapeutics due to their unique ability to be modified for physical, chemical, mechanical, and targeting properties for specific clinical applications. Furthermore, they are an excellent platform for assisting in the retention and promotion of sustained siRNA within the structure. Figure 25.2 suggests that after cellular uptake of nanocarriers, conformational changes in their ingredients can induce siRNA release from endosomes to protect them from lysosomal degradation [33]. Nanoparticles can be made of lipids, proteins, synthetic polymers, carbon materials, or even metals, depending on their chemical composition. They are divided into three types: lipid-based organic systems, non-lipid organic systems (polymers and peptides), and non-lipid inorganic systems. These carriers assemble the siRNA into supramolecular complexes, allowing the beneficial functional properties to be integrated during gene delivery. Table 25.2 describes the important and common properties of the nanoparticles used in siRNA delivery.

25.5.1 Organic Lipid-Based Nanoparticles

Liposomal nanocarriers based on lipids are the most widely investigated delivery vehicle tested for siRNA delivery. Liposomes are composed of concentric outer lipid bilayers surrounding an inner hydrophilic core. As a result, they can transport both hydrophobic and hydrophilic therapeutic molecules. Liposomes can also be customized to achieve the best results in terms of siRNA load, vesicle size, and transfection yield. Lipoplex, lipopolyplexes, stable nucleic-acid-lipid particles (SNALPs), and membrane/core nanoparticles (MCNPs) are liposome-based lipid carriers that are useful in siRNA delivery (Figure 25.3) [24, 34]. Liposome-polycation DNA complexes, lipidoids, lipid nanoparticles (LNPs), solid lipid nanoparticles (SLNs), nanostructured lipid carriers (NLCs), and exosomes are examples of lipid-based systems.

TABLE 25.2

Common Features of Various Nanocarriers

S. No.	Characteristics	Organic Lipid-Based Nanocarriers	Organic Polymer-Based Nanocarriers	Inorganic Nanocarriers
1	Composition	Cholesterol, cationic lipid and lipid derivatives are primary ingredients	Cationic polymer is primary ingredient	Inorganic elements, surfactants
2	Development approach	Electrostatic interactions between positively charged carrier and siRNA. The external core is stabilized by surfactants and emulsifiers	Electrostatic attraction of siRNA with cationic polymers. Loading via conjugation on the surface, in the core, or physical encapsulation	The crystallization of inorganic salts creates a 3D arrangement of linked atoms via covalent or metallic binding. Loading via direct conjugation, non-covalent, encapsulation, surface adsorption
3	Preparation method	Difficult	Easy	Easy
4	Loading capacity	High	Good	High loading capacity
5	Functionalization	Easy	Easy	Good
6	Targeting approach	Active and passive	Active and passive	Active and passive
7	Batch to batch deviation	High	High	Low
8	Examples	Liposomes, LNP, lipoplex, solid lipid nanoparticles	Synthetic: PEI, PLL, PAMAM; natural: chitosan	MSNs, carbon nanotubes, QDS, CaP, gold nanoparticles
9	Stability	Relatively short shelf life/ relative low stability, good serum stability	Better shelf life, protection against enzymatic degradation, high thermodynamic stability and dynamic stability	Long shelf life, stabile over wide a range of temperature, pH, and enzymatic degradation
10	Vital mechanism of action	Cationic lipid induces the cellular integration, clathrin- and caveolae-mediated endocytosis, drug release via conformation change of lipid ingredients	Cationic polymer induces cellular uptake. Endosomal escape via conformation change, pH sensitivity, proton sponge effect, cationic polymer configuration, etc.	Easy and rapid internalization, endosomal escape takes place because of "proton sponge" effect
11	Transferring effect	Low	Low	Low
12	Primary application	In vitro/in vivo	In vitro	In vitro
13	Cellular toxicity	Toxic at high dose	Low, relatively toxic at high dose	Moderate, toxicity issues (long-term safety)
14	Biocompatibility	High	Intermediate	Low
15	Biodegradability	High	Intermediate	Low
16	Immunogenicity	Low/no immunogenicity	Intermediate	Immunogenic issues
17	Other features/remarks	Safe development Sterilization possible Freeze drying possible Controlled drug release Rapid clearance (uptake by RES) Successful in clinical trails Already in market High cost of development	Small size Narrow distribution High cationic potential Controlled drug release Low transfection efficiency Moderate siRNA protection Biocompatibility issues	Large surface and pore volume Adequate surface plasmon resonance absorption Antibacterial and antiviral Tunable size and shape Remote controlled (e.g., magnetic NPs) Wide availability Optical properties for imaging Lack of clinical trails Low cost/scalable

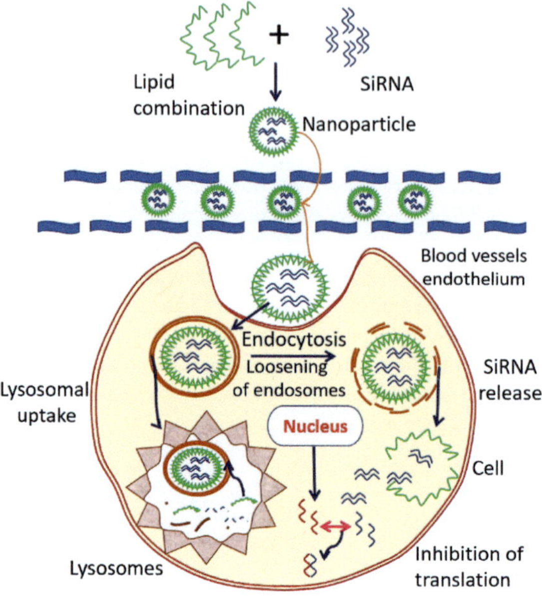

FIGURE 25.2 Application of nanotechnology in the delivery of siRNA to the target site.

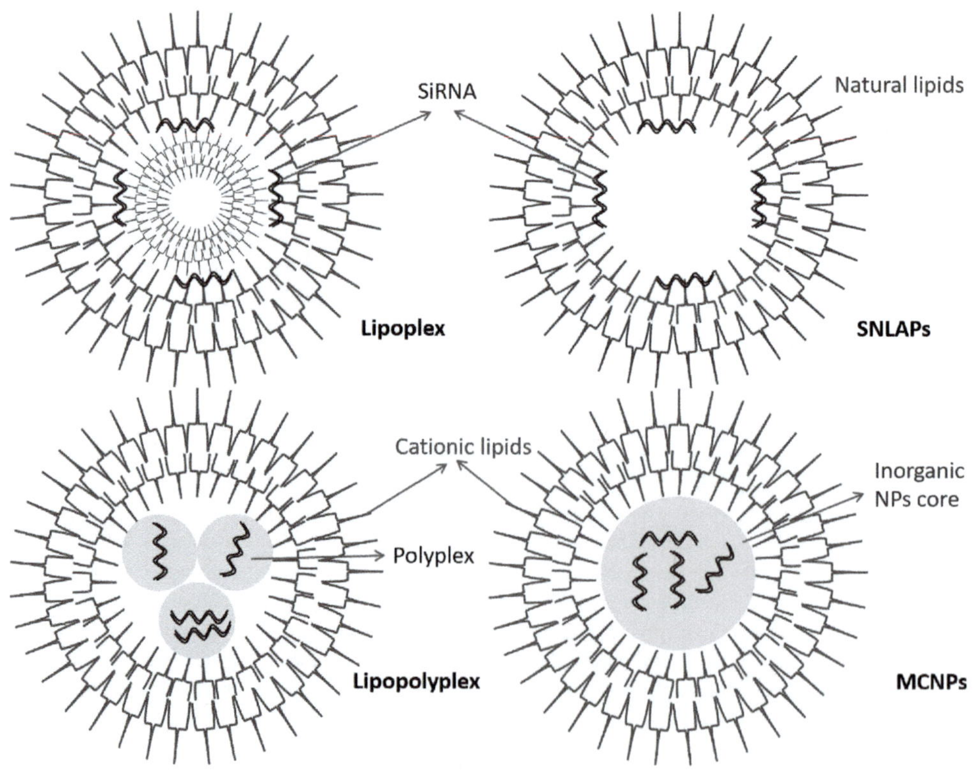

FIGURE 25.3 Some potential examples of lipid-based siRNA nanoparticle delivery systems.

25.5.1.1 Lipoplex

The most common liposome-based gene delivery carrier system is lipoplex, in which cationic lipids play a critical role in inducing liposome aggregation and lipid membrane breaking. Finally, ruptured lipid membranes cover the siRNA-coated liposomes [19]. The use of neutral lipids rather than cationic counterparts has resulted in better biocompatibility and pharmacokinetics. Furthermore, modifications in neutral lipoplexes similar to cationic lipoplexes could improve siRNA entrapment efficiency [35]. The most extensively researched cationic lipids used to create lipoplexes with negatively charged siRNA are dioleoyl phosphatidylethanolamine (DOPE) and 1,2-dioleoyl-3-trimethylammonium-propane (DOTAP).

25.5.1.2 Lipopolyplex

Polyplex development typically necessitates the electrostatic compaction of polyanionic nucleic acids and polycationic polymers (PEI, dendrimer peptide or lipoplex). However, due to its large positive surface, it suffers from limited loading, low gene transfection efficacy, and cytotoxicity. Lipopolyplex combines the characteristics of polyplex and lipoplex, with the core-shell assembly consisting of siRNA, polycation, and lipid. Lipopolyplex (liposomes containing polymers) are a potential alternative to lipoplex because the polymer component has natural binding ability with siRNA. In the case of lipopolyplex, it is possible to reduce cationic polymer-induced cell cytotoxicity by replacing cationic lipid with anionic lipid and peptide components [36]. Overall, lipopolyplex are second-generation non-viral nanocarrier systems with improved biocompatibility, low immunogenicity, low toxicity, and high delivery efficiency as a result of the synergistic effect of polycation and lipid constituents [37, 38].

25.5.1.3 Stable Nucleic-Acid-Lipid Particles

Similar to liposomes, nucleic acid–lipid particles (SNALPs) are used to mask the negative charges of the siRNA phosphodiester backbone and facilitate efficient cellular uptake. SNALPs are lipid bilayer systems with an outer layer of neutral lipids and an inner layer of cationic lipids. Because of the attraction with cationic lipids, siRNA within SNALPs is typically bound to the inner layer. Polyethylene glycol (PEG)-conjugated lipids are added to improve the pharmacokinetics of SNALPs and provide better stability to the nanocarriers [39].

25.5.1.4 Membrane/Core Nanoparticles

Membrane/core nanoparticles (MCNPs) are dual-controlled nanocarrier systems in which the core of one or more inorganic nanoparticles is surrounded by lipid bilayers, allowing for dual control over siRNA release. Calcium phosphate (CaP)-based RNA nanoparticles exhibit excellent biocompatibility due to the lipid ingredients, as well as sensitivity to the acidic environment of the cytoplasm to efficiently release the loaded siRNA. Furthermore, lipid-coated CaP nanoparticles exhibit negligible immunogenicity, with 70–80% in vitro silencing of target RNA in a tumor xenograft model. When anisamide-coated CaP nanoparticles enter the cytoplasm, they cause endosome swelling, resulting in siRNA release [40]. Zinc-based porous metal-organic framework nanoparticles coated with platelet-derived complex exhibit pH-dependent siRNA release in the cytoplasm with high efficacy in vitro against multiple targets and antitumor activity in a murine xenograft model [41].

These nanoparticles, when coated with cell membrane, adapt the natural physiochemical properties of the cell membrane, such as proteins, antigens, and immunological moieties. Overall, the developed system has biological properties as well as biological functions, such as immunosuppressive activity, increased circulation time, and targeted identification. These membranes can be derived from or made up of red cells, platelet membranes, endoplasmic reticulum, immune cells, bacterial cells, and cancer cells [42]. Endoplasmic reticulum–coated siRNA nanoparticle hybrid complex (DATAP and DOPE lipid ingredient nanoparticles) exhibits significantly higher gene silencing (EGFR) in cell culture system as well as in an in vivo MCF7 breast tumor model [43].

However, due to complex development methods, sensitivity to deactivation, inability for large-scale synthesis, and preservation methods, cell membrane-covered nanoparticles are still of limited value in clinical translation.

25.5.1.5 Liposome-Polycation-DNA Complexes

Liposome-polycation-DNA (LPD) complexes are another liposome-based siRNA delivery system modification that allows for a dual-controlled mechanism for SiRNA, similar to MCNPs. siRNA is condensed with protamine (arginine-rich cationic polypeptide) in this study, and the synthesized core material containing siRNA is surrounded by lipid bilayers [39, 44]. LPDs were created by complexing a synthetic cationic pyridium derived lipid, 1-methyl-4-(cis-9-dioleyl) methyl-pyridinium-chloride) (SAINT-C18) with a SiRNA carrier (S-LPD). Even in the presence of blood serum, these carriers maintain their size integrity and RNA activity, which is critical for in vivo activity. When compared to DOTAP-LPD, these carriers demonstrated higher siRNA loading, lower toxicity, and superior gene downregulation effectiveness [45]. This carrier also exhibits excellent selective siRNA delivery by incorporating a small amount of PEG or, in the case of endothelial cells, targeting ligand anti E selectin [45] or RGD peptide, which selectively targets integrins useful in cancer targeting [46].

25.5.1.6 Lipidoids

Lipidoid nanoparticles are delivery systems for lipid-like molecules (rather than truly lipid-based moieties) composed of cholesterol and PEG-modified synthetic degradable lipids. Lipidoids are effective at delivering functional siRNA to reverse target gene expression while causing minimal toxicity due to the lower siRNA dose [47]. High-throughput screening of compound libraries can generate a large amount of structure–activity data with a higher likelihood of identifying the target mRNA. The screening of such synthetic chemicals is inexpensive, and the in vitro screening steps can be avoided using the predictive structure activity functions relationship [48, 49]. The ability of the lipidoids system to deliver multiple payloads to multiple in vitro and in vivo cell lines demonstrated its importance in future siRNA-based delivery systems.

25.5.1.7 Lipid Nanoparticles

Lipid nanoparticles are distinguished by their ease of production, limited immune induction, multi-dosing capabilities, high payloads, improved penetration into tissues to deliver therapeutics, design flexibility, and ability to induce high transfection. They are the most advanced siRNA therapeutic delivery systems, as the LNP-siRNA formulation has already been approved by the Food and Drug Administration (FDA) as the world's first RNAi-based medicine, Onpatro, against hereditary transthyretin amyloidosis [50]. Because of the multifactorial benefits of LNPs, many other life sciences companies, including BioNtech and Curevac (Germany), eTheRNA (Netherlands), ModeRNA, and Precision Nanosystem (USA), are working on their development. It has been discovered that ionizable cationic lipid DLin-MC3-DMA–based LNP-siRNA formulations can target human chronic myeloid leukemia (CML) at both the in vitro and in vivo levels, resulting in a reduction in CD34+ CML residual colonies [51]. The balance of cationic lipids and PEG lipids has proved an excellent strategy for high encapsulation and favorable LNP pharmacokinetic parameters with triggered endosomal escape before lysosomal uptake [52].

25.5.1.8 Solid Lipid Nanoparticles and Nanostructured Lipid Carriers

Solid lipid nanoparticles (SLNs) are lipid, surfactant, and therapeutic molecules in appropriate ratios that remain solid at body temperature. The key ingredients in SLNs are solid lipids (e.g., tristearin, trimyristin, trilaurin, palmitic, or stearic acids) and stabilizers (e.g., phospholipids, Pluronic F68, or Tween 80). The lipid core of SLNs provides the fluidity that distinguishes them from other existing drug carriers. However, SLNs are underutilized for siRNA delivery due to suboptimal loading of hydrophilic medicine in the hydrophobic core. The reason for this phenomenon is that charged siRNA interacts less with solid hydrophobic core materials. According to some studies, the siRNA cationic polymer complex (dispersed in oil phase) incorporated in the solid lipid core may provide effective sustained release [53]. The hydrophobic ion pairing (HIP) of siRNA and the formation of drug-surfactant complexes (e.g., siRNA with DOTAP lipid) approach is another suitable method for incorporating hydrophilic siRNA in a hydrophobic core to improve the sustained release property [54].

One advancement in lipid-based carriers is the development of NLCs by lipid matrix formulation via mixing solid lipid with liquid lipid to provide better modulation in terms of high payload with less leakage and sustained drug release. Overall, it results in a less ordered structure that can hold more therapeutic compounds [55, 56]. When tested in siRNA delivery in lung cancer therapy, NLC exhibits promising properties in terms of localization and superior activity in delivering anticancer agents [55, 57]. Once administered via freeze-dried collagen extracellular matrix (ECM) hydrogel, the DOPE (1,2-dioleoyl-sn-glycero-3-phosphoethanolamine) shell (cNLC)–based NLC carrier outperformed chitosan and DOTAP (1,2-dioleoyl-3-trimethylammonium-propan)–based nanocarriers in the targeted downregulation of ERK-1 (protein involved in proliferation and wound healing).

25.5.1.9 Exosome Nanoparticles

The use of the body's own extracellular shuttle service exosomes is a recent advancement in nanoparticles for siRNA delivery (30–120 nm). Exosomes are nanosized endocytic vehicles that are produced by many cells, including T-cells, B-cells, mast cells, epithelium, and tumor cells, and are primarily involved in cell–cell communication for mRNA and microRNA. As a result, exosomes act as a natural carrier for siRNA delivery. Exosomes are endogenous lipid-based nanocarriers that have recently been studied for a variety of applications. They are released into the extracellular environment upon fusion of the plasma membrane during endosome inward budding. Because they are endogenous, they can successfully deliver molecular medicine to target cells while avoiding immunogenic induction. As a result of their superior biodegradability and immunocompetence, they are a potential candidate for effective siRNA delivery [58, 59].

25.5.2 ORGANIC POLYMER-BASED NANOPARTICLES

Polymer-based nanoparticles are solid, biodegradable colloids with high clinical value, and they have found widespread use in drug and gene delivery. The majority of polymeric biodegradable formulations include siRNA within a polymeric core. Polymeric nanoparticles can be either natural or synthetic in nature. Natural polymers include cyclodextrin, chitosan, and atelocollagen, whereas synthetic polymers include polyethyleneimine (PEI), poly(dl-lactide-co-glycolide) (PLGA), and dendrimers [47].

25.5.2.1 Cyclodextrin Nanoparticles

Cyclodextrins are cyclic oligosaccharides derived from starch by an enzymatic reaction in which glucose macrocyclic rings are joined by -1,4 glycosidic bonds. They are primarily used to improve the solubility of hydrophobic drug compounds. Recently, cyclodextrin has been demonstrated to be useful in the preparation of nanoparticles with high drug loading and solubility, improved stability, drug absorption in nanosystems, and the ability to modify for site-specific delivery. Overall, it can demonstrate a significant improvement in bioavailability, with controlled release properties exhibiting improved safety and efficacy profiles. PEG was used as a steric stabilization agent and coupled with transferrin to target the transferrin receptor in the first cyclodextrin-siRNA nanocarrier platform (using electrostatic attraction) reported in 2009. The components self-assembled into nanoparticles, and when administered intravenously (iv) to patients, this platform has the potential to inhibit specific genes in human volunteers [60, 61]. The modified cyclodextrin reacts with polycationic lipids to form inclusion complexes adamantyl-PEG-dianisidine, which has demonstrated the ability to act as a potential delivery platform for siRNA to cancer cells and cause significant downregulation of reference gene [62].

25.5.2.2 Chitosan Nanoparticles

Chitosan (derived from chitin; linear polysaccharides containing N-acetylglucosamine and glucosamine) is being tested for drug delivery due to its excellent biocompatibility, low immunogenicity, and mucosal adhesion properties. Overall, its ability to promote cell permeation and endosomal escape makes it an excellent vector for siRNA delivery. In contrast, the clinical success of chitosan-based gene delivery platforms remains unsatisfactory due to critical challenges such as poor aqueous solubility, charge inference at body pH, and poor targeting capability. Nonetheless, several studies have suggested that chitosan modification may have the potential to improve the therapeutic potential of siRNA-based therapeutics, such as chemical modification (PEGylation) to increase solubility, chemical modifications of siRNA to improve stability, or the addition of negatively charged ingredients to stabilize nanoparticles [63, 64].

25.5.2.3 Polyethyl Imine Complexes

Linear cationic polymer polyethylenimine (PEI)–based nanocomplexes are suitable for therapeutic siRNA delivery, as they can protect it from nucleolytic degradation, deliver it into target tissues (promote cellular uptake), provide intracellular release, and increase overall therapeutic efficacy in preclinical in vivo models. Because of the buffering capacity of secondary or tertiary amines, these polymers sequester protons after entering the acidic lysosome compartment. The chloride ions are pumped into the endosome by the protonation of polyamine carriers. Water influx in the endosomes causes swelling and degradation, allowing the siRNA to be released into the cytoplasm [65, 66].

Non-covalent binding with lipopolyplexes to form the ternary complex gives the PEI-based delivery platform a synergistic advantage. This step reduces cytotoxicity and increases siRNA delivery to downregulate the oncogenic receptor tyrosine kinase HER2 and the survival factor surviving [67]. By introducing cationic charges at the particle surface as well as the PLGA matrix, PEI can facilitate the use of PLGA nanoparticles in siRNA therapeutics by improving the retention of anionic siRNA molecules [68, 69]. When polycationic 25kDa PEI polymer was covalently coupled to the SiO_2 surface, it favored silica-based (SiO_2) nanoparticles for efficient siRNA delivery. The study clearly shows that the level of dual-reporter luciferase transfected osteosarcoma U2OS cells is downregulated, resulting in significantly lower cytotoxicity [70].

25.5.2.4 Poly(d,l-lactide-co-glycolide) Nanoparticles

PLGA is a clinically approved synthetic polymer with excellent biocompatibility and biodegradability in a variety of applications. PLGA-based nanoparticles are a good carrier for gene silencing in vivo. After internalization via endocytosis, PLGA has the ability to bypass endo-lysosomal degradation. As a result, the gene load is efficiently delivered in the cytoplasm [71, 72]. To improve electrostatic interaction and encapsulation of nucleotide-based therapeutics, the PLGA matrix can be easily modified by adding cationic polymer. This stable formulation results in increased cellular uptake and gene silencing capacity without cytotoxicity [68]. For such purposes, a small amount of cationic polymer is enough for high payload of siRNA [73]. When PLGA nanoparticles are encapsulated with dual siRNAs MDR1 and BCL2, they help to improve the anticancer activity of potential drug molecules such as paclitaxel and cisplatin by inhibiting drug efflux or cell death defense pathways (the genes responsible for drug efflux and cellular defense, respectively). As a result, PLGA may serve as a potential siRNA delivery vehicle carrier to combat cancer cell drug resistance [74].

25.5.2.5 Dendrimer Nanocarriers

Dendrimers are special polymeric structure–based nanocarrier platforms that are synthesized by adding monomeric units one at a time to form a well-defined dendron-shaped structure. Dendrimers have three key elements: a central core (which guides branching), repetitive branches (which regulate dendrimer generations), and terminal groups (which allow the charge, targeting ligand binding, or interaction with siRNA other therapeutics). They can be synthesized using either a divergent method (first the central core, then the outer part) or a convergent method (first peripheral core, followed by central core). Dendrimers are expected to be an ideal nanocarrier delivery platform due to their precise structure, low polydispersity index, selective geometry, and multivalent property [75]. Dendrimers can be conjugated with a wide range of drugs, targeting ligands, and solubilizing agents, giving them an advantage over other linear polymers [76].

The cationic charge of dendrimers allows for effective siRNA loading via dendrimer for active dendrimer–siRNA complexation. The positive charge on the surface of the dendrimer allows siRNA complex hydration under physiological conditions and high intracellular uptake of encapsulated siRNA. To release siRNA molecules into the cytosol, siRNA/dendrimer complexes bind to the cell surface. Dendrimer tertiary amines in their interior promote siRNA release via the "proton sponge" process. As a result, the siRNA that is released combines the RNAi mechanism for gene down-regulation [75]. Because of their ease of synthesis and modification, as well as their commercial availability, poly(amidoamine) (PAMAM) dendrimers are the most widely studied for siRNA. Poly (propylene imine), poly(I-lysine), carbosilane, triazine, polyglycerol, and many other molecules have been tested for siRNA delivery in dendrimers [77].

There is a minor fact about the cellular cytotoxicity of dendritic carriers caused by the positive peripheral charge, which can be mitigated by identifying a new core unit, functionalizing the dendrimer surface, and using biocompatible/bioactive species [75, 78]. The use of neutral or anionic biocompatible dendrimers or the use of chemical modifications to mask the peripheral positive charge [79] is also a potential strategy to reduce dendrimer-associated cytotoxicity. Dendrimers' active peripheral structure allows for functionalization with a variety of biocompatible molecules such as PEGylation, acetylation, glycosylation, and amino acids. Dendrimer amino acid functionalization is a highly effective method in dendrimer-based cancer therapy [80].

25.5.3 Inorganic Nanocarriers

Inorganic nanoparticles have been introduced as a replacement for viral, polymeric, and liposome systems. Because of their flexibility in preparation and surface-functionalization efficacy, they are particularly useful for siRNA delivery. These properties enable inorganic nanoparticles to overcome the numerous challenges presented by organic materials. Other advantages of inorganic nanoparticles include their high surface area (which allows for high entrapment via encapsulation or chemical coupling) and their unique physical and optical properties, which may allow for tracking siRNA delivery in cells and tissues. The primary goal of developing inorganic nanoparticles should be to achieve effective intracellular delivery using a biocompatible vehicle with low immunogenicity, allowing for clinical applications of siRNA delivery. A variety of inorganic nanoparticles have been investigated, including potential candidates such as gold nanoparticles, magnetic nanoparticles, mesoporous silica nanoparticles (MSNs), calcium phosphate nanoparticles (CaP), and others, as listed in the following.

25.5.3.1 Gold Nanoparticles

Among the inorganic nanoparticles used to deliver siRNA because of their positive properties such as inertness, non-toxicity, and biocompatibility, gold nanoparticles are a stable and safe siRNA delivery carrier. The ability of gold nanoparticles to modify their surfaces enhances their ability to tune therapeutic agent delivery and release. Furthermore, well-studied surface features of gold nanoparticles enable siRNA coupling via covalent and non-covalent encapsulation techniques.

After the addition of PEI or other positively charged PEI derivatives, gold nanoparticles can be modified for endosomal escape via the proton sponge effect [81]. External force NIR irradiation of hollow gold nanoparticles resulted in significant endosomal siRNA release in the cytoplasm [82]. Recently, nanoparticle-stabilized nanocapsules were tested for siRNA delivery, in which siRNA was complexed first via electrostatic interactions with positively charged arginine-functionalized gold nanoparticles, and then these nanoparticles were allowed to self-assemble on the surface of fatty acid droplets. It enables rapid siRNA delivery into the cytosol via a cholesterol-dependent membrane fusion [83]. As a result, several strategies for improving siRNA loading and triggered cytosolic delivery could be easily incorporated into gold nanoparticles.

25.5.3.2 Magnetic Nanoparticles

The principle of MNPs (which contain iron oxide as a key component) is that external magnetic fields are used to deploy their distribution for precise siRNA delivery, and thus it can be coupled with magnetic resonance imaging (MRI) to assess siRNA delivery [84]. Furthermore, MNPs were used for targeted drug delivery by introducing a targeting legend at the surface. RGD peptide attached to magnetic nanoparticles against the v3 integrin receptor overexpressing tumor target, for example, was highly effective in guiding localized drug delivery at target sites. This formulation was administered intravenously and was tracked using MRI. Near-infrared optical imaging indicates the importance of MNP formulation in any human cancer studies, including basic tumor biology and tumor therapy development [85]. The formulation of magnetic nanoparticles also allows for surface modification with cationic polymers such as PEI and cationic lipid to facilitate electrostatic encapsulation of siRNA [86].

25.5.3.3 Mesoporous Silica Nanoparticles

MSNs are a promising delivery reagent because of their advantageous chemical properties, thermal stability, surface properties, and biocompatibility. Their mesoporous nature allows for high load and subsequent delivery to target locations. The properties of silica-based nanoparticles can be altered by manipulating the additives. The active silica surface allows for surface manipulation in order to link the drug molecules [87]. Mesoporous silica's large surface area provides enough space and binding sites for siRNA-like large molecules via non-covalent loading or direct covalent coupling. In one potential study, thiolated siRNA was efficiently conjugated to the surfaces of mesoporous nanoparticles. Furthermore, using cationic polymers (e.g., polyethyleneimine, polyamidoamine, or polylysine) to coat the polymeric surface can improve siRNA encapsulation via electrostatic interaction [88, 89].

25.5.3.4 Calcium Phosphate Nanoparticles

The osteoinductivity, osteoconductivity, and high affinity of the biocompatible and biodegradable natural element CaP for nucleic acids is especially useful in gene delivery in bone tissue engineering [90]. The primary binding of CaP to gene cargos occurs through the chelation of calcium ions and phosphates in siRNA nucleic acid. However, CaP-based siRNA delivery is currently plagued by low endosome escape efficiency and unfavorable CaP/siRNA nanoparticle growth in physiological environments. To improve endosomal escape, pH-responsive block polymers such as poly(ethylene glycol)-block-poly(methacrylic acid) could be used to create CaP-siRNA nanoparticles (PMA). Thus, in an acidic environment, the nanoparticles become hydrophobic, disrupting the endosomal surface and allowing siRNA to be released [91]. The incorporation of an asymmetric lipid bilayer into the CaP/siRNA/DOPA-HA nanoparticles improves tumor-targeted siRNA delivery by preserving the encapsulated siRNA integrity and stability for a longer period of time [92].

25.5.3.5 Miscellaneous Inorganic Nanoparticle Systems

Other inorganic or combination of organic-inorganic material based nanoparticles have been investigated, such as carbon nanotubes (CNTs), graphene oxide (GO), fullerenes, and hollow manganese oxide (MgO). Because of their nano-needle structure, CNTs permeate the plasma membrane and deliver siRNA into the cytoplasm via an endocytosis-independent pathway without causing cell death. The payload's protection in physiological fluids (blood), cell membrane penetration, and low toxicity make them an excellent carrier for siRNA delivery with successful biological activity in vivo [92, 93]. Hollow inorganic nanoparticles such as MgO, fullerene, and GO can also be used to create biocompatible nanoparticles with simple synthesis routes, functionalization capability, and high therapeutic loading. These materials may improve the efficacy of siRNA delivery [94]. CNT- and graphene-based nanosheet-based allotropic nanostructures are being developed as shuttle nano-vehicles for siRNA delivery applications. The high surface area, which exposes every carbon atom on the surface, allows for flexible functionalization and adequate loading efficiency of CNTs [94]. However, these carbon-based materials are not biodegradable in vivo, which can lead to a number of negative health consequences. Combining inorganic nanocarriers with organic cationic polymer or cationic lipid (hybrid nanocarriers) may improve the stability of organic nanoparticles and the low compatibility of inorganic materials for siRNA delivery [95].

25.6 SUMMARY AND FUTURE OUTLOOK

One of the most significant innovations in current medical sciences is the use of nanoparticle-based medicinal approaches. siRNA is a nucleic acid-based medicine that can be used to treat a variety of diseases. However, siRNA technology must be improved to deliver therapeutics intracellularly without degradation in body fluids, enzymes, the immune system, or lysosomal degradation. The unique properties of nanoparticles, such as their high surface area, ability to attach the targeting ligand at the surface, use of disease tissue's EPR effect, and ability of intracellular uptake, distinguish them as a unique vehicle for siRNA-based applications. Furthermore, because of their high siRNA encapsulation, nanoparticles can protect cargos from physiological fluid, intracellular uptake, and controlled release in the cytoplasm before reaching the lysosomal degradation machinery. Because of these advancements in nanoparticle development, more and more research is being conducted for the delivery of siRNA for the correction of protein defects for the treatment of molecular diseases. Furthermore, nanoparticle-based siRNA formulations have already been introduced to the market, and some other siRNA nanoparticle formulations are being considered by drug regulatory bodies in the United States and the European Union. As a result, nanoparticles are expected to play a significant role in siRNA delivery to combat various lethal diseases associated with gene mutation, gene deletion, or protein defects.

REFERENCES

1. Hopkins, A.L. and C.R. Groom, The druggable genome. *Nature Reviews Drug Discovery*, 2002. **1**(9): p. 727–730.
2. Chames, P., et al., Therapeutic antibodies: successes, limitations and hopes for the future. *British Journal of Pharmacology*, 2009. **157**(2): p. 220–233.
3. Wang, F., T. Zuroske, and J.K. Watts, RNA therapeutics on the rise. *Nature Reviews Drug Discovery*, 2020. **19**: p. 441–442.
4. Sahin, U., K. Karikó, and Ö. Türeci, mRNA-based therapeutics—developing a new class of drugs. *Nature Reviews Drug Discovery*, 2014. **13**(10): p. 759–780.
5. Baker, B.F., The role of antisense oligonucleotides in the wave of genomic information. *Nucleosides, Nucleotides & Nucleic Acids*, 2001. **20**(4–7): p. 397–399.
6. Saraswat, P., A. Pareek, and A. Bhandari, Nucleic acids as therapeutics. In *From Nucleic Acids Sequences to Molecular Medicine*, V.A. Erdmann and J. Barciszewski, Editors. 2012, Springer, Berlin, Heidelberg. p. 19–45.
7. Uherek, C. and W. Wels, DNA-carrier proteins for targeted gene delivery. *Advanced Drug Delivery Reviews*, 2000. **44**(2–3): p. 153–166.
8. Jayasena, S.D., Aptamers: an emerging class of molecules that rival antibodies in diagnostics. *Clinical Chemistry*, 1999. **45**(9): p. 1628–1650.
9. Akhtar, S., et al., The delivery of antisense therapeutics. *Advanced Drug Delivery Reviews*, 2000. **44**(1): p. 3–21.
10. Kaur, G. and I. Roy, Therapeutic applications of aptamers. *Expert Opinion on Investigational Drugs*, 2008. **17**(1): p. 43–60.

11. Bartel, D.P., MicroRNAs: target recognition and regulatory functions. *Cell*, 2009. **136**(2): p. 215–233.

12. Dorsett, Y. and T. Tuschl, SiRNAs: applications in functional genomics and potential as therapeutics. *Nature Reviews Drug Discovery*, 2004. **3**(4): p. 318–329.

13. Bumcrot, D., et al., RNAi therapeutics: a potential new class of pharmaceutical drugs. *Nature Chemical Biology*, 2006. **2**(12): p. 711–719.

14. Jeong, J.H., S.W. Kim, and T.G. Park, Molecular design of functional polymers for gene therapy. *Progress in Polymer Science*, 2007. **32**(11): p. 1239–1274.

15. Watts, J.K., G.F. Deleavey, and M.J. Damha, Chemically modified siRNA: tools and applications. *Drug Discovery Today*, 2008. **13**(19): p. 842–855.

16. Kim, H.J., et al., Recent progress in development of siRNA delivery vehicles for cancer therapy. *Advanced Drug Delivery Reviews*, 2016. **104**: p. 61–77.

17. Haussecker, D., Current issues of RNAi therapeutics delivery and development. *Journal of Controlled Release*, 2014. **195**: p. 49–54.

18. Cho, K., et al., Therapeutic nanoparticles for drug delivery in cancer. *Clinical Cancer Research*, 2008. **14**(5): p. 1310–1316.

19. Xia, Y., J. Tian, and X. Chen, Effect of surface properties on liposomal siRNA delivery. *Biomaterials*, 2016. **79**: p. 56–68.

20. Semple, S.C., et al., Rational design of cationic lipids for siRNA delivery. *Nature Biotechnology*, 2010. **28**(2): p. 172–176.

21. Tatiparti, K., et al., SiRNA delivery strategies: a comprehensive review of recent developments. *Nanomaterials (Basel)*, 2017. **7**(4).

22. Dykxhoorn, D.M. and J. Lieberman, Knocking down disease with siRNAs. *Cell*, 2006. **126**(2): p. 231–235.

23. Sondhi, D., et al., Genetic modification of the lung directed toward treatment of human disease. *Human Gene Therapy*, 2016. **28**(1): p. 3–84.

24. Marquez, A.R., C.O. Madu, and Y. Lu, An overview of various carriers for siRNA delivery. *Oncomedicine*, 2018. **3**: p. 48–58.

25. Putnam, D., Polymers for gene delivery across length scales. *Nature Materials*, 2006. **5**(6): p. 439–451.

26. Zhang, W.-W., Development and application of adenoviral vectors for gene therapy of cancer. *Cancer Gene Therapy*, 1999. **6**(2): p. 113–138.

27. Yeh, P. and M. Perricaudet, Advances in adenoviral vectors: from genetic engineering to their biology. *The FASEB Journal*, 1997. **11**(8): p. 615–623.

28. Yin, H., et al., Non-viral vectors for gene-based therapy. *Nature Reviews Genetics*, 2014. **15**(8): p. 541–555.

29. Zhang, L., et al., Nanoparticles in medicine: therapeutic applications and developments. *Clinical Pharmacology & Therapeutics*, 2008. **83**(5): p. 761–769.

30. Wang, Y.Y., et al., Addressing the PEG mucoadhesivity paradox to engineer nanoparticles that "slip" through the human mucus barrier. *Angewandte Chemie International Edition*, 2008. **47**(50): p. 9726–9729.

31. Zhou, J. and J.J. Rossi, Cell-type-specific, aptamer-functionalized agents for targeted disease therapy. *Molecular Therapy—Nucleic Acids*, 2014. **3**: p. e169.

32. Son, S., et al., Bioreducible polymers for gene silencing and delivery. *Accounts of Chemical Research*, 2012. **45**(7): p. 1100–1112.

33. Hu, B., et al., Therapeutic siRNA: state of the art. *Signal Transduction & Targeted Therapy*, 2020. **5**(1): p. 101.

34. Zhen, S. and X. Li, Liposomal delivery of CRISPR/Cas9. *Cancer Gene Therapy*, 2020. **27**(7): p. 515–527.

35. Wu, S.Y. and N.A.J. McMillan, Lipidic systems for in vivo siRNA delivery. *The AAPS Journal*, 2009. **11**(4): p. 639–652.

36. Chen, W., et al., Lipopolyplex for therapeutic gene delivery and Its application for the treatment of Parkinson's disease. *Frontiers in Aging Neuroscience*, 2016. **8**: p. 68.

37. Xue, H.Y., et al., Lipid-based nanocarriers for RNA delivery. *Current Pharmaceutical Design*, 2015. **21**(22): p. 3140–3147.

38. Mishra, P., et al., Steroid receptors as molecular targets for cancer diagnosis and therapy. *Critical Reviews™ in Therapeutic Drug Carrier Systems*, 2009. **26**(3): p. 207–273.

39. Zhang, J., X. Li, and L. Huang, Non-viral nanocarriers for siRNA delivery in breast cancer. *Journal of Controlled Release*, 2014. **190**: p. 440–450.

40. Li, J., et al., Biodegradable calcium phosphate nanoparticle with lipid coating for systemic siRNA delivery. *Journal of Controlled Release*, 2010. **142**(3): p. 416–421.

41. Zhuang, J., et al., Targeted gene silencing in vivo by platelet membrane–coated metal-organic framework nanoparticles. *Science Advances*, 2020. **6**(13): p. eaaz6108.
42. Xuan, M., J. Shao, and J. Li, Cell membrane-covered nanoparticles as biomaterials. *National Science Review*, 2019. **6**(3): p. 551–561.
43. Qiu, C., et al., Regulating intracellular fate of siRNA by endoplasmic reticulum membrane-decorated hybrid nanoplexes. *Nature Communications*, 2019. **10**(1): p. 2702.
44. Zhang, Y., A. Satterlee, and L. Huang, In vivo gene delivery by nonviral vectors: overcoming hurdles? *Molecular Therapy*, 2012. **20**(7): p. 1298–304.
45. Kowalski, P.S., et al., SAINT-liposome-polycation particles, a new carrier for improved delivery of siRNAs to inflamed endothelial cells. *European Journal of Pharmaceutics & Biopharmaceutics*, 2015. **89**: p. 40–47.
46. Vader, P., et al., Targeted delivery of small interfering RNA to angiogenic endothelial cells with liposome-polycation-DNA particles. *Journal of Controlled Release*, 2012. **160**(2): p. 211–216.
47. Lee, J.-M., T.-J. Yoon, and Y.-S. Cho, Recent developments in nanoparticle-based siRNA delivery for cancer therapy. *BioMed Research International*, 2013. **2013**: p. 782041.
48. Whitehead, K.A., et al., Degradable lipid nanoparticles with predictable in vivo siRNA delivery activity. *Nature Communications*, 2014. **5**(1): p. 4277.
49. Zhang, Y.-M., et al., Small combinatorial library of lipidoids as nanovectors for gene delivery. *ACS Applied Nano Materials*, 2018. **1**(8): p. 3925–3934.
50. Anselmo, A.C. and S. Mitragotri, Nanoparticles in the clinic: an update. *Bioengineering & Translational Medicine*, 2019. **4**(3): p. e10143.
51. Jyotsana, N., et al., Lipid nanoparticle-mediated siRNA delivery for safe targeting of human CML in vivo. *Annals of Hematology*, 2019. **98**(8): p. 1905–1918.
52. Kulkarni, J.A., et al., Lipid nanoparticle technology for clinical translation of siRNA therapeutics. *Accounts of Chemical Research*, 2019. **52**(9): p. 2435–2444.
53. Xue, H.Y. and H.L. Wong, Tailoring nanostructured solid-lipid carriers for time-controlled intracellular siRNA kinetics to sustain RNAi-mediated chemosensitization. *Biomaterials*, 2011. **32**(10): p. 2662–2672.
54. Lobovkina, T., et al., In vivo sustained release of siRNA from solid lipid nanoparticles. *ACS Nano*, 2011. **5**(12): p. 9977–9983.
55. Garbuzenko, O.B., et al., Strategy to enhance lung cancer treatment by five essential elements: inhalation delivery, nanotechnology, tumor-receptor targeting, chemo- and gene therapy. *Theranostics*, 2019. **9**(26): p. 8362–8376.
56. Müller, R.H., M. Radtke, and S.A. Wissing, Solid lipid nanoparticles (SLN) and nanostructured lipid carriers (NLC) in cosmetic and dermatological preparations. *Advanced Drug Delivery Reviews*, 2002. **54**(Suppl 1): p. S131–S155.
57. Taratula, O., et al., Nanostructured lipid carriers as multifunctional nanomedicine platform for pulmonary co-delivery of anticancer drugs and siRNA. *Journal of Controlled Release*, 2013. **171**(3): p. 349–357.
58. van den Boorn, J.G., et al., SiRNA delivery with exosome nanoparticles. *Nature Biotechnology*, 2011. **29**(4): p. 325–326.
59. Shtam, T.A., et al., Exosomes are natural carriers of exogenous siRNA to human cells in vitro. *Cell Communication & Signaling*, 2013. **11**(1): p. 88.
60. Davis, M.E., The first targeted delivery of siRNA in humans via a self assembling, cyclodextrin polymer-based nanoparticle: from concept to clinic. *Molecular Pharmaceutics*, 2009. **6**(3): p. 659–668.
61. Davis, M.E., et al., Evidence of RNAi in humans from systemically administered siRNA via targeted nanoparticles. *Nature*, 2010. **464**(7291): p. 1067–1070.
62. Malhotra, M., et al., Cyclodextrin-siRNA conjugates as versatile gene silencing agents. *European Journal of Pharmaceutical Sciences*, 2018. **114**: p. 30–37.
63. Hu-Lin, J., et al., Chemical modification of chitosan as a gene transporter. *Current Organic Chemistry*, 2018. **22**(7): p. 668–689.
64. Malhotra, M., et al., Development and characterization of chitosan-PEG-TAT nanoparticles for the intracellular delivery of siRNA. *International Journal of Nanomedicine*, 2013. **8**: p. 2041–2052.
65. Dominska, M. and D.M. Dykxhoorn, Breaking down the barriers: siRNA delivery and endosome escape. *Journal of Cell Science*, 2010. **123**(8): p. 1183.
66. Ma, D., Enhancing endosomal escape for nanoparticle mediated siRNA delivery. *Nanoscale*, 2014. **6**(12): p. 6415–6425.
67. Ewe, A., et al., Optimized polyethylenimine (PEI)-based nanoparticles for siRNA delivery, analyzed in vitro and in an ex vivo tumor tissue slice culture model. *Drug Delivery & Translational Research*, 2017. **7**(2): p. 206–216.

68. Patil, Y. and J. Panyam, Polymeric nanoparticles for siRNA delivery and gene silencing. *International Journal of Pharmaceutics*, 2009. **367**(1–2): p. 195–203.

69. Takashima, Y., et al., Spray-drying preparation of microparticles containing cationic PLGA nanospheres as gene carriers for avoiding aggregation of nanospheres. *International Journal of Pharmaceutics*, 2007. **343**(1–2): p. 262–269.

70. Buchman, Y.K., et al., Silica nanoparticles and polyethyleneimine (PEI)-mediated functionalization: a new method of PEI covalent attachment for siRNA delivery applications. *Bioconjugate Chemistry*, 2013. **24**(12): p. 2076–2087.

71. Panyam, J., et al., Rapid endo-lysosomal escape of poly(DL-lactide-co-glycolide) nanoparticles: implications for drug and gene delivery. *The FASEB Journal*, 2002. **16**(10): p. 1217–1226.

72. Perlstein, I., et al., DNA delivery from an intravascular stent with a denatured collagen-polylactic-polyglycolic acid-controlled release coating: mechanisms of enhanced transfection. *Gene Therapy*, 2003. **10**(17): p. 1420–1428.

73. Pantazis, P., et al., Preparation of siRNA-encapsulated PLGA nanoparticles for sustained release of siRNA and evaluation of encapsulation efficiency. *Methods in Molecular Biology*, 2012. **906**: p. 311–319.

74. Risnayanti, C., et al., PLGA nanoparticles co-delivering MDR1 and BCL2 siRNA for overcoming resistance of paclitaxel and cisplatin in recurrent or advanced ovarian cancer. *Scientific Reports*, 2018. **8**(1): p. 7498.

75. Liu, X., P. Rocchi, and L. Peng, Dendrimers as non-viral vectors for siRNA delivery. *New Journal of Chemistry*, 2012. **36**(2): p. 256–263.

76. Jain, V. and P.V. Bharatam, Pharmacoinformatic approaches to understand complexation of dendrimeric nanoparticles with drugs. *Nanoscale*, 2014. **6**(5): p. 2476–2501.

77. Biswas, S. and V.P. Torchilin, Dendrimers for siRNA delivery. *Pharmaceuticals (Basel, Switzerland)*, 2013. **6**(2): p. 161–183.

78. Wu, J., W. Huang, and Z. He, Dendrimers as carriers for siRNA delivery and gene silencing: a review. *The Scientific World Journal*, 2013. **2013**: p. 630654.

79. Tsai, H.-C. and T. Imae, Fabrication of dendrimers toward biological application. In *Progress in Molecular Biology and Translational Science*, A. Villaverde, Editor. 2011, Academic Press, Cambridge. p. 101–140.

80. Cheng, Y., et al., Design of biocompatible dendrimers for cancer diagnosis and therapy: current status and future perspectives. *Chemical Society Reviews*, 2011. **40**(5): p. 2673–2703.

81. Ding, Y., et al., Gold nanoparticles for nucleic acid delivery. *Molecular Therapy*, 2014. **22**(6): p. 1075–1083.

82. Lu, W., et al., Tumor site-specific silencing of NF-kappaB p65 by targeted hollow gold nanosphere-mediated photothermal transfection. *Cancer Research*, 2010. **70**(8): p. 3177–3188.

83. Jiang, Y., et al., Direct cytosolic delivery of siRNA using nanoparticle-stabilized nanocapsules. *Angewandte Chemie International Edition*, 2015. **54**(2): p. 506–510.

84. Lee, J.-H., et al., All-in-one target-cell-specific magnetic nanoparticles for simultaneous molecular imaging and siRNA delivery. *Angewandte Chemie International Edition*, 2009. **48**(23): p. 4174–4179.

85. Kumar, M., et al., Image-guided breast tumor therapy using a small interfering RNA nanodrug. *Cancer Research*, 2010. **70**(19): p. 7553–7561.

86. Liu, G., et al., N-Alkyl-PEI-functionalized iron oxide nanoclusters for efficient siRNA delivery. *Small*, 2011. **7**(19): p. 2742–2749.

87. Bharti, C., et al., Mesoporous silica nanoparticles in target drug delivery system: a review. *International Journal of Pharmaceutical Investigation*, 2015. **5**(3): p. 124–133.

88. Bhattarai, S.R., et al., Enhanced gene and siRNA delivery by polycation-modified mesoporous silica nanoparticles loaded with chloroquine. *Pharmaceutical Research*, 2010. **27**(12): p. 2556–2568.

89. Xia, T., et al., Polyethyleneimine coating enhances the cellular uptake of mesoporous silica nanoparticles and allows safe delivery of siRNA and DNA constructs. *ACS Nano*, 2009. **3**(10): p. 3273–3286.

90. Levingstone, T.J., et al., Calcium phosphate nanoparticles-based systems for RNAi delivery: applications in bone tissue regeneration. *Nanomaterials (Basel)*, 2020. **10**(1).

91. Pittella, F., et al., Enhanced endosomal escape of siRNA-incorporating hybrid nanoparticles from calcium phosphate and PEG-block charge-conversional polymer for efficient gene knockdown with negligible cytotoxicity. *Biomaterials*, 2011. **32**(11): p. 3106–3114.

92. Kirkpatrick, D.L., et al., Carbon nanotubes: solution for the therapeutic delivery of siRNA? *Materials (Basel, Switzerland)*, 2012. **5**(2): p. 278–301.

93. Varkouhi, A.K., et al., SiRNA delivery with functionalized carbon nanotubes. *International Journal of Pharmaceutics*, 2011. **416**(2): p. 419–425.
94. Varshosaz, J. and S. Taymouri, Hollow inorganic nanoparticles as efficient carriers for siRNA delivery: a comprehensive review. *Current Pharmaceutical Design*, 2015. **21**(29): p. 4310–4328.
95. Dizaj, S.M., S. Jafari, and A.Y. Khosroushahi, A sight on the current nanoparticle-based gene delivery vectors. *Nanoscale Research Letters*, 2014. **9**(1): p. 252.

26 Green Synthesis of Nanoparticles
From Protocols to Applications

Aanjaneya Mamgain, Nilosha Parveen, Rameshroo Kenwat, Ravindra Shukla, Shivani Rai Paliwal, and Rishi Paliwal

26.1 INTRODUCTION

Green synthesis of nanoparticles may be defined as the non-toxic, nature-friendly, safe reagent [1], and less expensive or cost of preparation is minimal and process for synthesis nanoparticles without use of chemicals, high pressure, temperature, and emission of hazardous waste materials [2]. This area has gained pace in the recent times due to its employment of green methods like plants (leaves, fruits, roots, and flowers) and microorganisms (Bacteria, Yeast, Virus, Algae, and Fungi) to produce nanomaterials. Several plants materials i.e., leaves, flowers, seeds, and stems are used to produce plant extract and extract contain biomolecules i.e., sugars, polyphenols, terpenoids, phenolic acid, enzymes, vitamins, and protein, etc) which are used as a reducing agent for this bio-reduction process which produce nanoparticles having various size and shape. Nanoparticles are having chemical, mechanical, optical, and magnetic properties due to their shape, size, surface area, and surface charge. The techniques like UV/vis spectroscopy, FTIR, SEM, AFM, TEM, DLS and zeta potential analysis are used for detection and characterization of such biosynthesized nanoparticles. Biogenic nanoparticles are full of several properties such as antimicrobial, antitumor, and antioxidant agents for the control of the phytopathogens and bioremediative factors. They are also widely used for textile industry, food, smart agriculture, and sewage treatment [3].

26.2 COMMON APPROACHES OF SYNTHESIS OF GREEN NANOPARTICLES

Nanoparticles are commonly synthesized by the two methods i.e., top-down, and bottom-up approach. For generating required nanostructure, top-down method disintegrates the bulk materials whereas bottom-up method formulates the larger nanostructure from the single atoms and molecules. The common synthetic approaches are classified into physical, chemical, and biological green synthesis [4].

26.2.1 PHYSICAL METHOD

Several researchers have developed various physical methods for achieving nanoparticles like geometries which can be used for diverse applications. Physical methods such as ball milling, ion beam lithography, thermal evaporate, microcontact printing, layer by layer growth, diffusion flame, molecular beam epitasis, laser desorption, sputter deposition, dip pen lithography, and photolithography are employed for this purpose [1, 3]. Physical methods produce nanoparticles which are free from any organic solvents; however, employment of high energies may be barrier for some nanoparticles and their subsequent applications.

DOI: 10.1201/9781003130055-26

26.2.2 CHEMICAL METHOD

Some commonly employed chemical methods of nanoparticle synthesis include sol-gel process, chemical solution deposition, electrochemical method, microemulsion method, pyrolysis, photochemical method, Langmuir Blodgett method, hydrolysis co-precipitation, catalytic route, wet chemical method, and solvothermal synthesis. In chemical method, organic solvent or aqueous colloidal dispersion solution are used to reduce the metal salts (gold, iron, zinc oxide, copper, silver, platinum and palladium etc) for producing nanoparticles [1, 5].

26.2.3 BIOLOGICAL (BIOGENIC) METHOD

Both physical and chemical methods need high concentration of reducing agent, stabilizing agent and high radiation, which can be harmful for both the environment and human health. Relatively, green synthesis requires low energy for synthesizing nanoparticles, and it is also single step or one pot environment friendly bio reduction method. Biological synthesis or green synthesis nanoparticles have been used exploring biological resources involving plants, virus, micro-organism (bacteria, yeast, algae, and fungi), and there by product (proteins and lipids). Green synthesis ignores highly toxic, highly expensive, and high energy and adopted an easy and simple process for producing nanoparticles [1, 5]. Natural biogenic synthesis is divided into bio-reduction and biosorption. Biological methods are successfully utilized to synthesis various metals salts nanoparticles such as silver, gold, copper, platinum, cadmium sulfide, zinc oxide, titanium dioxide, palladium, and copper etc [6, 7] and are shown in Figure 26.1.

26.2.3.1 Green Synthesis of Nanoparticles: A simple protocol

In order to develop nanoparticles using green synthesis, firstly, fresh biological resource for example here plant leaves are collected and then subsequently it is cut into fine pieces and then treated with water. Afterwards, the mixture solution is heated either in hot plate or heating mantle or sometime

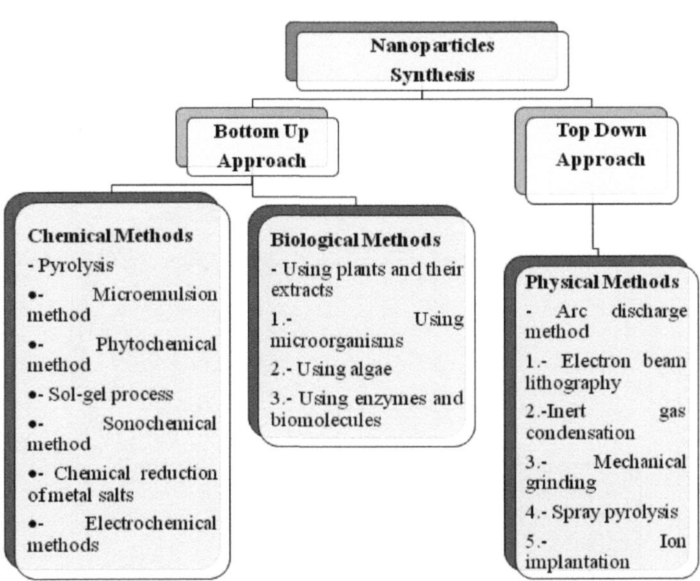

FIGURE 26.1 Methods of preparation of nanoparticles (NPs).

directly heated from sun or macerated only. After heating, the solution is filtered, and an aqueous leaf extract is collected. Finally, a precursor solution is added in to the leaf extract and stirred it in magnetic stirrer. The so formed nanoparticles are collected and the same is characterized by various techniques like particle size analyzer, TEM, and XRD etc (Figure 26.2). Figure 26.3 shows a simple protocol for the green synthesis of nanoparticles using plants.

26.2.3.1.1 Silver Nanoparticles

As discussed above synthesis of silver nanoparticles is also reported using different method i.e., physical, chemical, biological method. Since silver nanoparticles synthesized from chemical methods represents a process which may be harmful for environment and causes toxicity and adverse effects during biomedical applications. Due to this, researchers tried to synthesis silver nanoparticles using biological method which is eco-friendly process and do not use toxic chemical substances [8]. In a recent study, Tailor et al. (2020) reported green synthesis of silver nanoparticles using *Ocimum canum* and their anti-bacterial activity. In this study, authors characterized silver nanoparticles using SEM, and XRD and found a crystallographic spherical structure of nanoparticle which

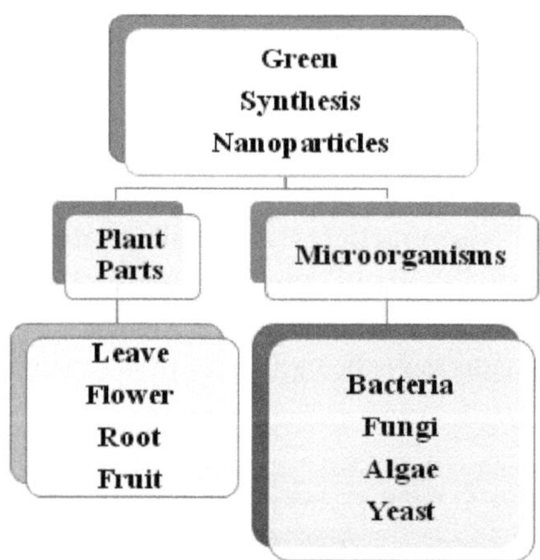

FIGURE 26.2   Flow chart showing various methods of green synthesis of nanoparticles.

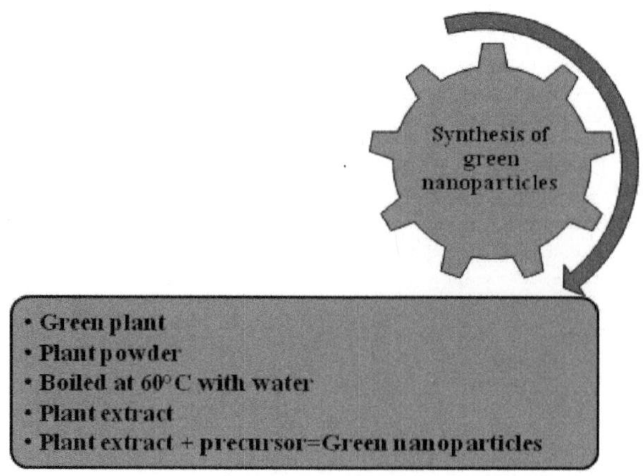

FIGURE 26.3   Procedure showing development of plant based green nanoparticles.

was in the size range of 15.72 nm. Nanoparticles were tested against *Escherichia coli* bacterium for antibacterial activity and at 30 ppm concentration a maximum of 2.45 cm zone of inhibition was observed. Some other biological sources reported for synthesizing silver nanoparticles include *Morinda citrifolia* L. [8], *Ctenolepis garcini* L. [9], *Scutellaria barbata* [10], flower extract of *Abelmoschus esculentus* [11], safflower waste extract of *Carthamus tinctorius* L. [12], *Kalanchoe pinnata* leaves [13] and flower extract of *Aerva lanata* [14]. Some of these studies are summarized in Table 26.1.

26.2.3.1.2 Gold Nanoparticles

Due to their unique electrical, mechanical, thermal, chemical, and optical characteristics, gold nanoparticles are a type of nanomaterial that has attracted significant interest in the field of biomedicine. With these huge potentials, gold nanoparticles synthesized using organic reductions come with the threat of some harmful events as a result of their interactions with biological tissues and molecules. Therefore, green synthesis is being advocated for developing them. For example, in a study, Wang et al. (2020) reported green synthesis and characterization of gold nanoparticles using lignin nanoparticles. Authors used LNPs as reducing agent, stabilizing agent for synthesizing LNPs@AuNPs where no chemical were used [34]. Several other research reports for synthesizing gold nanoparticles using biological entities uses flower of *Jatropha integerrima* Jacq [35], seed extract of *Ricinus communis* L [36] and leaf extract of *Alhagi graecorum* [37].

26.2.3.1.3 Copper Nanoparticles

Copper nanoparticles with various structural characteristics and useful biological effects have been engineered utilizing simple, new and useful green manufacturing techniques. The methods have ability to alter particle size and hence subsequently the size-dependent characteristics of copper nanoparticles. Copper nanoparticles can be synthesized using a variety of techniques, including chemical, physical, biological, and green synthesis techniques. Biological techniques make use of fungus, bacteria, and plant extracts [38]. Amaliyah and co-workers reported green synthesis and characterization of copper nanoparticle using *Piper retrofractum* vahl extract as bioreductor and capping agent. Authors used sonication and stirring process during synthesis and found that for preparation of copper nanoparticles stirring process is more uniform distribution of size comparison to sonication process [39]. Several research reports utilized diverse biological agents such as *Artemisia* plant extract [40], leaves of *Cordia myxa* L. [41], Cotton [42] and peels of *Citrus paradisi* fruit [43] for synthesis of copper nanoparticles.

26.2.3.1.4 Palladium Nanoparticles

Palladium NPs showed admirable physicochemical properties such as chemical stability, great thermal stability, highly photocatalytic activity, optical and electronic properties. Pd-NPs having various applications such as pollutant dyes degradation, antifungal activity, bactericidal, and antifungal activity [44]. In a recent study, Bathula and colleagues reported ultrasonically driven green synthesis of palladium nanoparticles by *Coleus amboinicus* for catalytic reduction and Suzuki-Miyaura reaction. In this study, authors characterized nanoparticles using XRD analysis which show cubic formation with range of 52 nm crystalline sizes and HRTEM image showed a sphere-shape with 20 nm ranges of particles. It was noted that green synthesis is less expensive process that evade severe condition and toxic reagents use [45].

26.2.3.1.5 Titanium Dioxide Nanoparticles

A recent increase in scientific interest about titanium dioxide (also known as titania, TiO_2) is due to its photoactivity. TiO_2 generates a variety of reactive oxygen species (ROS) after being exposed to UV radiation in aqueous solutions. Photodynamic therapy (PDT) uses the capacity to generate ROS and subsequently cause cell death to treat a variety of diseases, from psoriasis to cancer. In cancerous tumors therapy and in the photodynamic inactivation of antibiotic-resistant bacteria,

TABLE 26.1

List of Some Recent Reports Showing Synthesis of Silver Nanoparticles

S. No.	Plant Name	Part used	Size	Shape	Application	References
1	*Crataegus oxyacantha*	Twigs	35–85 nm, 40–70 nm, 45–85 nm 25–65 nm	Spherical Oval	Urease inhibitory	[15]
2	*Moringa oleifera*	Flower	8 nm	Spherical	Anti-microbial and sensing properties	[16]
3	*Phyla dulcis*	Leaves	63–76 nm	-	Anti-microbial	[17]
4	*Populus ciliata*	Leaves	4 nm	Spherical	Anti-bacterial	[18]
5	*Scoparia dulcis*	Leaves	8.2 nm	Spherical	Anti-microbial	[19]
6	*Dryopteris Cochleata*	Rhizomes	-	-	Venom neutralization	[20]
7	*Atropa acuminata*	Leaves	5–20 nm	Spherical	antioxidant, anti-inflammatory, anticancer and larvicidal activities	[21]
8	*Solibacillusisronensis*	-	80–120 nm	Quasi-spherical	Biofilm inhibition	[22]
9	*Parthenium Hysterophorus*	Leaves	187.87± 4.89	Spherical	antibacterial, antifungal, anti-inflammatory, and antioxidant properties	[23]
10	*Dietziamaris*	-	40–50 nm	Spherical	human keratinocyte cell line	[24]
11	*Astragalus tribuloides*	Roots	16.2 to 51.5 nm.	Spherical	Antioxidant, Antibacterial, and Anti-Inflammatory Activities	[25]
12	*Jasminum officinal*	Leaves	87.6 ± 2.11 nm	Spherical	Evaluation of Cytotoxic Activity Towards Bladder (5637) and Breast Cancer (MCF-7) Cell Lines	[26]
13	*Brillantaisiapatula, Crossopteryx febrifuga and Senna siamea*	Leaves	45 nm 115 nm and 47 nm respectively	Spherical	antimicrobial	[27]
14	*Ocimum canum*	Leaves	15.76 nm	Spherical and rod	Anti-bacterial	[28]
15	*Nigella sativa*	Seeds	25.2 nm	Spherical	anti-inflammatory and antioxidant effects	[29]
16	*Lysiloma acapulcensis*	Stem and roots	1.2–62 nm	Spherical and quasi spherical	Anti-microbial	[30]
17	*Artocarpus hirsutus*	Seed	25–40 nm	Spherical	Anti-bacterial	[31]
18	**17 Eriobotrya japonica** **18**	Peels	17–35 nm	Spherical	**19 Cancer cells proliferation, inflammation, allergic disorders and phagocytosis induction**	[32]
19	**20 Jasmine flowers**	Flowers	10–40 nm	Nanofibers	**21 Anti-microbial**	[33]
20	**22 Morinda citrifolia L.**	Fresh leaves, Fruit pulp and Dried seeds	11 nm (Leaves), 7 nm (Fruit pulp) and 3 nm (Dried seeds)	Spherical	**23 Antibacterial activity**	[8]

titanium dioxide nanoparticles (TiO_2) have been investigated as photosensitizing agents. TiO_2 NPs can be utilized as photosensitizers in PDT both by themselves and in composites and mixtures with other chemicals or biomolecules. Furthermore, different organic compounds can also be grafted on TiO_2 nanoparticles, resulting in hybrid materials; these nanostructures can reveal increased light absorption, allowing their further use in targeted therapy in medicine [46]. Green synthesis of these nanoparticles has been advocated recently. In a study, Ahmad and co-workers reported green synthesis of TiO_2-NPs by using *Mentha arvensis* leaves extract and its antimicrobial properties [47]. Similarly, titanium dioxide nanoparticle synthesis using bio-reductant such as leaf of *Phyllanthus niruri* [48], leaf of *Laurus nobilis* [49], and leaf of *Moringa oleifera* [50] has been tremendously explored.

26.2.1.3.6 Iron Nanoparticles

Nowadays, there is a lot of interest in the synthesis of iron nanoparticles (INPs) utilizing plant extract to provide a new and sustainable strategy for green chemistry. This approach substitutes phytochemicals and aqueous matrixes for chemical compounds and organic solvents. Like any chemical or biological reaction, the reaction yield is greatly influenced by variables such as reaction temperature, iron precursor concentration, leaf extract concentration, and reaction period. Due to their numerous uses, iron oxide nanoparticles of various morphologies and sizes have been thoroughly researched. For example, the treatment of organic or inorganic water contaminants as well as site cleanup have sparked interest in iron nanoparticles (Fe-NPs) [51, 52]. In another study, Chen and colleagues reported green synthesis of iron nanoparticles using leaf aqueous extract of *Ziziphora clinopodioides*. After several studies, authors found that Fe-NPs could be given as an anti-hemolytic anemia drug, and hematoprotective in clinical trial [53].

26.2.1.3.7 Bismuth Oxide Nanoparticles

Due to their distinctive physicochemical characteristics, bismuth-based nanoparticles (BBNs) display enormous promise and are consequently widely used in a variety of technologies. On this account, green synthesis of BBNs has attracted a lot of interest since it is a technique that is safe for the environment, non-toxic, stable, and offers a variety of nanoscale manufacturing possibilities [54]. It is now known that in comparison to traditional radiosensitizers, bismuth oxide nanoparticles have more cell penetration and fewer side effects [55]. In another report, Motakef-Kazemi and colleagues utilized a green method of bismuth oxide nanoparticles synthesis using aqueous extract of *Mentha pulegium*. The biological studies showed excellent potential of anti-bacterial activity and UV blocking of such bismuth oxide nanoparticles [56].

26.2.3.1.8 Chromium Oxide NPs

A wide bandgap, a high melting temperature, and improved stability are just a few of the distinctive physicochemical characteristics of the chromium oxide nanoparticles. Numerous applications, such as catalysis, photonics, coating materials and improved colourants have been included in the use of chromium oxide nanoparticles [57]. In a study, Khan and co-workers reported green synthesis of Cr_2O_3 NPs using *Abutilon indicum* L. leaf extract. These chromium oxide nanoparticles showed antioxidant and anticancer activity against Linoleic acid system and MCF-7 cancer cell line compared to standard antioxidant and standard anti-cancer drug. Authors claimed that such nanoparticles are economical, biocompatible for application of several use i.e., antioxidant, anticancer, and antibacterial [58].

26.2.3.1.9 Zinc oxide NPs

Zinc oxide nanoparticles (ZnO-NPs), a key ceramic substance, are now used in a variety of industrial fields, including the pharmaceutical, cosmetic, and concrete industries, as opposed to the microbiological, textile, and automobile industries. For the preparation of ZnO-NPs, a variety of chemical and physical techniques were used, but biological methods as "green" routes in various substrates (such as microorganisms, enzymes, bacteria, and plant extracts) are potentially steered as environmentally friendly alternatives to chemical and/or physical techniques. In both microscale and nanoscale formulations, ZnO-NPs are being studied as potential of antibacterial activity. Further, ZnO-NPs have anticancer capabilities and are frequently used to treat a variety of various skin problems. Additionally, ZnO-NPs have become an effective tool for administering drugs and sensing [59]. In a study, Annapoorani and co-workers reported an eco-friendly synthesis of zinc oxide nanoparticles using leaf extract of *Rivina humilis*. Such nanoparticles have shown antioxidant effect against R. humilis and antibacterial effect against agar diffusion method. Further authors also found these nanoparticles active apoptosis cell death in Neuro2a cells, and hence are very helpful in biomedical applications [60].

26.2.3.2　Bacteria Based Green Synthesis of Nanoparticles

The unique capacity of bacteria to decrease heavy metal ions makes them one of the greatest options for nanoparticle production among the wide variety of bioresources. In fact, the mechanism of metal bioreduction in bacteria, particularly dissimulator metal-reducing bacteria, is now well characterized and has greatly aided in the understanding of the microbial processes involved in the production of nanoparticles. Looking in to these potential, in a recent study, Rajesekar and colleagues reported synthesis of gold nanoparticles using marine bacteria (*Rastrelliger kanagurta*, *Selachimorpha* esp., and *Panna microdon*). Authors found a relatively less toxicity of these gold nanoparticles at 50 μg/ml as showed in Zebrafish larvae. Overall, it was claimed that gold nanoparticles prepared from bacteria were having antibacterial and anti-mycobacterial activity. Further, the nanoparticles were less toxic and more biocompatible and could be used for pharmaceutical application [49].

26.2.3.3　Fungi Based Green Synthesis of Nanoparticles

Fungi and yeast products that are biologically active serve as better scaffolds for the stabilization and reduction of nanoparticles. Since fungus and yeast are excellent extracellular enzyme secretors and there are many species, cultivating and maintaining them in the lab is quite easy. Using reducing enzymes intracellular or extracellular, they may create metal nanoparticles and nanostructures. For example, in a study, Molnar and co-workers reported that fungi (intracellular or extracellular extract) are best for synthesizing metal nanoparticles because of scalability and economical effective for growth of fungal for industrial application [61]. In another study, green synthesis of gold nanoparticles using endophytic strain Fusarium solani ATLOY-8 which is isolated from chonemorpha fragrans plant is reported [62]. Authors found that such nanoparticles are pink-ruby red in color and with the size range of 40 and 45 nm which were tested against MCF-7 cell line and He La cancer cell line and showed cytotoxicity effect.

26.2.3.4　Yeast Based Green Synthesis of Nanoparticles

As a bioreductant, the yeast strains have additional advantages than bacteria as they offer capacity of bulk production of nanoparticles, ease of managing yeasts in the laboratory conditions, the development of various enzymes and their rapid growth using basic nutrients. Several researches utilized yeast in the manufacture of metallic nanoparticles. For example, in a study, Niknejad and colleagues reported green synthesis of nanoparticles using yeast for sustainable properties for nanotechnology. In this study, researcher synthesized silver nanoparticles using yeast *Saccharomyces cerevisiae* and observed their antifungal activity against *Candida albicans* [63]. In another study, Sivaraj and co-workers reported green synthesis of silver nanoparticles using commercial yeast extract which showed anti-mycobacterial activity against *Mycobacterium tuberculosis* [64].

26.2.3.5　Algae Based Green Synthesis of Nanoparticles

Algae are a desirable substrate for the manufacture of a variety of nanomaterials, largely because their cell extracts include bioactive substances that function as biocompatible reductants, such as pigments and antioxidants. Gold (Au), silver (Ag), and other metallic nanoparticles have been synthesized using both intracellular and extracellular bioactives presents in Cyanophyceae, Chlorophyceae, Phaeophyceae, and Rhodophyceae algae. In-depth research has been done on Chlorella species and Sargassum species for the manufacture of nanoparticles with antibacterial capabilities that may potentially replace traditional antibiotics. In a recent report, Devi and colleagues reported green synthesis of gold nanoparticles and silver nanoparticles using *Sargassum ilicifolium* [65]. In another study, Elgamouz and colleagues reported green synthesis of AgNPs using Algae based natural source. For capping shell of nanoparticles, authors used *Noctiluca scintillans* green algae bioactive compounds. Such silver nanoparticles showed antimicrobial and anticancer activity [66].

26.2.4 FACTORS AFFECTING OF GREEN NANOPARTICLE SYNTHESIS

The key properties of synthesized nanoparticles using green methods are highly affected by several factors of process. Several reaction parameters like temperature, concentration of capping agents, reaction time, solvents, pH condition (acidic, alkaline, or neutral), time and preparation cost heavily affect features like particle size, size distribution, surface charge and shape, pore size and many more [5, 6, 67–69]. Some of these features are summarized in Table 26.2 for readers' benefits.

26.3 APPLICATIONS OF GREEN NANOPARTICLES

As discussed above in several section, application of nanotechnology contains various fields i.e., medicine, environment, pharmaceutical, and agriculture. Mostly green synthesized metallic nanoparticles are utilized for their biomedical applications such as antifungal, anticancer, antimicrobial and antioxidant potential. In addition, they have been explored in waste water treatment and environment protection. Figure 26.4 summarizes the key application of green synthesized nanoparticles. Table 26.3 enlists some reports related to applications of green nanoparticles.

26.4 CONCLUSION AND FUTURE PERSPECTIVES

Altogether, green synthesis of metallic nanoparticles is a relatively safer, eco-friendly, less expensive process as compare to physical and chemical methods. In this chapter, we discussed different approaches that have been commonly used for the development of the nanoparticles using, physical,

TABLE 26.2

Factor Affecting Green Synthesis of Nanoparticles

S. No.	Parameters	Effect on Green Synthesis NPs	References
1	pH	Variability in size and shape	[70, 71]
2	Reactants concentration	Variability in size and shape	[70, 72]
3	Reaction temperature	Size, shape, yield, and stability	[70, 71]
4	Reaction time	Size	[72]
5	Capping Agent	Size, shape, chemical and physical properties	[73]
6	Choice of the Organism	Growth rate, biochemical pathways and enzyme activities;	[74]
7	Solvent	Toxic/non-toxic Formulation	[75]

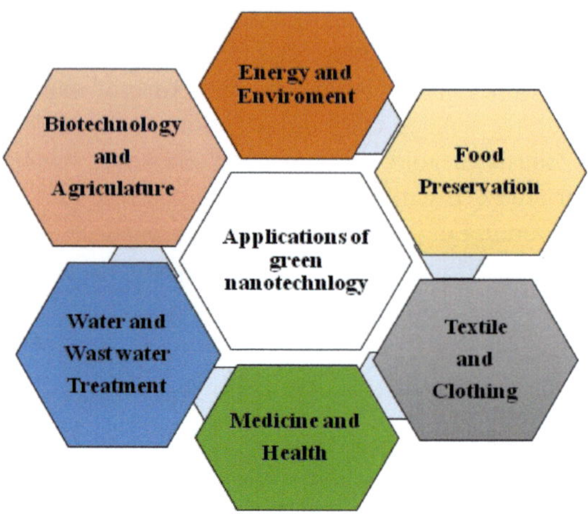

FIGURE 26.4   Application of green nanotechnology in different domains.

TABLE 26.3
Different Green Synthesized Metal/Metal Oxide Nanoparticles and Their Applications

S. No.	Nanosystems	Plant Name	Applications	References
1	Copper nanoparticles	*Citrus limon*	Anti-bacterial activity	[76]
2	Silver nanoparticles	*Melia azedarach*	Anti-fungal activity	[77]
3	Zinc Oxide nanoparticles	*Phoenix dactylifera*	Antibacterial	[78]
4	Zinc nanoparticles	*Atrocarpusgomezians*	Antioxidant	[79]
5	Silver	*Azadirachta indica*	Biolarvicidal	[80]
6	Palladium	*Catharanthus roseus*	Catalytic activity in dye degradation	[81]
7	Silver	*Red ginseng*	Antibacterial	[82]
8	Silver	*Pistacia atlantica*	Antibacterial	[83]
9	Silver	*Pinus densifolia*	Antibacterial	[84]
10	Silver	*Nigella sativa*	Cytotoxicity	[85]
11	Titanium dioxide and Silver	*Euphorbia prostrata*	Leishmanicidal	[86]
12	Gold	*Cymbopogon citratus*	Mosqutitocidal	[87]
13	Lead	*Cocos nucifera*	Antibacterial	[88]
14	Gold	*Ferula persica*	Anticancer	[89]
15	Iron oxide	*Carica papaya*	Antibacterial activity	[90]
16	Iron oxide	*Ramalina sinensis*	Removing Heavy Metals	[91]
17	Palladium	*Salvia hispanica*	Antibacterial	[92]
18	MgO nanoparticles (MgONPs)	*Saussureacostus*	Anticancer	[93]
19	Titanium dioxide	*Trianthemaportulacastrum and Chenopodium quinoa*	Antifungal	[94]
20	**24 Selenium Nanoparticles**	**25 Withaniasomnifera**	Antibacterial	[95]

TABLE 26.3 (*Continued*)

Different Green Synthesized Metal/Metal Oxide Nanoparticles and Their Applications

S. No.	Nanosystems	Plant Name	Applications	References
21	26 Copper Nanoparticles	27 Artemisia	Infectious illness	[40]
22	28 Copper Nanoparticles	29 Cordia myxa L.	Antibacterial activity	[41]
23	30 Copper Nanoparticles	31 Vitis vinifera L.	Anti-diabetic efficacy	[96]
24	32 Palladium Nanoparticles	33 Punica granatum	Catalytic activity	[97]
25	34 Titanium Dioxide Nanoparticles	35 Laurus nobilis	Antioxidant and antimicrobial activities	[49]
26	36 Iron Nanoparticles	37 Peltophorumpterocarpum	Photocatalytic	[98]
27	38 Iron Nanoparticles	39 Coriandrum sativum	Anti-liver cancer	[99]
28	40 Zinc oxide Nanoparticles	41 Cucumis melo	Anti-bacterial activity	[100]

chemical and green synthesis method and found that a large number of reports are advocating for green methods of nanoparticle synthesis. Bioreductants obtained from plant sources and form microorganism (bacteria, algae, fungi and yeast) could successfully derived gold, silver and iron oxide nanoparticles etc. In future, more controlled process utilizing green nanotechnology will be explored for scaled nanoparticle synthesis process.

REFERENCES

1. Parveen, K., V. Banse, and L. Ledwani. Green synthesis of nanoparticles: their advantages and disadvantages. In *AIP Conference Proceedings*. 2016. AIP Publishing.
2. Goutam, S.P., et al., Green synthesis of nanoparticles and their applications in water and wastewater treatment. *Bioremediation of Industrial Waste for Environmental Safety: Volume I: Industrial Waste and Its Management*, 2020: p. 349–379.
3. Salem, S.S. and A. Fouda, Green synthesis of metallic nanoparticles and their prospective biotechnological applications: an overview. *Biological Trace Element Research*, 2021. **199**: p. 344–370.
4. Lee, S.H. and B.-H. Jun, Silver nanoparticles: synthesis and application for nanomedicine. *International Journal of Molecular Sciences*, 2019. **20**(4): p. 865.
5. Singh, J., et al., 'Green' synthesis of metals and their oxide nanoparticles: applications for environmental remediation. *Journal of Nanobiotechnology*, 2018. **16**(1): p. 1–24.
6. Zhang, D., et al., Green synthesis of metallic nanoparticles and their potential applications to treat cancer. *Frontiers in Chemistry*, 2020. **8**.
7. Ijaz, I., et al., Detail review on chemical, physical and green synthesis, classification, characterizations and applications of nanoparticles. *Green Chemistry Letters and Reviews*, 2020. **13**(3): p. 223–245.
8. Morales-Lozoya, V., et al., Study of the effect of the different parts of Morinda citrifolia L. (noni) on the green synthesis of silver nanoparticles and their antibacterial activity. *Applied Surface Science*, 2021. **537**: p. 147855.
9. Narayanan, M., et al., Green synthesis of silver nanoparticles from aqueous extract of Ctenolepis garcini L. and assess their possible biological applications. *Process Biochemistry*, 2021. **107**: p. 91–99.
10. Veeraraghavan, V.P., et al., Green synthesis of silver nanoparticles from aqueous extract of Scutellaria barbata and coating on the cotton fabric for antimicrobial applications and wound healing activity in fibroblast cells (L929). *Saudi Journal of Biological Sciences*, 2021. **28**(7): p. 3633–3640.
11. Devanesan, S. and M.S. AlSalhi, Green synthesis of silver nanoparticles using the flower extract of Abelmoschus esculentus for cytotoxicity and antimicrobial studies. *International Journal of Nanomedicine*, 2021: p. 3343–3356.

12. Rodríguez-Félix, F., et al., Sustainable-green synthesis of silver nanoparticles using safflower (Carthamus tinctorius L.) waste extract and its antibacterial activity. *Heliyon*, 2021. **7**(4).

13. Mehata, M.S., Green synthesis of silver nanoparticles using Kalanchoe pinnata leaves (life plant) and their antibacterial and photocatalytic activities. *Chemical Physics Letters*, 2021. **778**: p. 138760.

14. Palithya, S., et al., Green synthesis of silver nanoparticles using flower extracts of Aerva lanata and their biomedical applications. *Particulate Science and Technology*, 2022. **40**(1): p. 84–96.

15. Ali, S., et al., Green synthesis of silver and gold nanoparticles using Crataegus oxyacantha extract and their urease inhibitory activities. *Biotechnology and Applied Biochemistry*, 2021. **68**(5): p. 992–1002.

16. Bindhu, M., et al., Green synthesis and characterization of silver nanoparticles from Moringa oleifera flower and assessment of antimicrobial and sensing properties. *Journal of Photochemistry and Photobiology B: Biology*, 2020. **205**: p. 111836.

17. Carson, L., et al., Green synthesis of silver nanoparticles with antimicrobial properties using Phyla dulcis plant extract. *Foodborne Pathogens and Disease*, 2020. **17**(8): p. 504–511.

18. Hafeez, M., et al., Populus ciliata mediated synthesis of silver nanoparticles and their antibacterial activity. *Microscopy Research and Technique*, 2021. **84**(3): p. 480–488.

19. Parvataneni, R., Biogenic synthesis and characterization of silver nanoparticles using aqueous leaf extract of Scoparia dulcis L. and assessment of their antimicrobial property. *Drug and Chemical Toxicology*, 2020. **43**(3): p. 307–321.

20. Singh, P., et al., Green synthesis of silver nanoparticles using Indian male fern (Dryopteris Cochleata), operational parameters, characterization and bioactivity on Naja naja venom neutralization. *Toxicology Research*, 2020. **9**(5): p. 706–713.

21. Rajput, S., D. Kumar, and V. Agrawal, Green synthesis of silver nanoparticles using Indian Belladonna extract and their potential antioxidant, anti-inflammatory, anticancer and larvicidal activities. *Plant Cell Reports*, 2020. **39**: p. 921–939.

22. Singh, P., et al., A sustainable approach for the green synthesis of silver nanoparticles from Solibacillus isronensis sp. and their application in biofilm inhibition. *Molecules*, 2020. **25**(12): p. 2783.

23. Ahsan, A., et al., Green synthesis of silver nanoparticles using Parthenium hysterophorus: optimization, characterization and in vitro therapeutic evaluation. *Molecules*, 2020. **25**(15): p. 3324.

24. Venil, C., et al., Green synthesis of silver nanoparticles using canthaxanthin from Dietzia maris AURCCBT01 and their cytotoxic properties against human keratinocyte cell line. *Journal of Applied Microbiology*, 2021. **130**(5): p. 1730–1744.

25. Sharifi-Rad, M., et al., Green synthesis of silver nanoparticles using Astragalus tribuloides delile. root extract: characterization, antioxidant, antibacterial, and anti-inflammatory activities. *Nanomaterials*, 2020. **10**(12): p. 2383.

26. Elhawary, S., et al., Green synthesis of silver nanoparticles using extract of jasminum officinal L. leaves and evaluation of cytotoxic activity towards bladder (5637) and breast cancer (MCF-7) cell lines [retraction]. *International Journal of Nanomedicine*, 2022. **17**: p. 2805–2806.

27. Kambale, E.K., et al., Green synthesis of antimicrobial silver nanoparticles using aqueous leaf extracts from three Congolese plant species (Brillantaisia patula, Crossopteryx febrifuga and Senna siamea). *Heliyon*, 2020. **6**(8).

28. Tailor, G., et al., Green synthesis of silver nanoparticles using Ocimum canum and their anti-bacterial activity. *Biochemistry and Biophysics Reports*, 2020. **24**: p. 100848.

29. Alkhalaf, M.I., R.H. Hussein, and A. Hamza, Green synthesis of silver nanoparticles by Nigella sativa extract alleviates diabetic neuropathy through anti-inflammatory and antioxidant effects. *Saudi Journal of Biological Sciences*, 2020. **27**(9): p. 2410–2419.

30. Garibo, D., et al., Green synthesis of silver nanoparticles using Lysiloma acapulcensis exhibit high-antimicrobial activity. *Scientific Reports*, 2020. **10**(1): p. 12805.

31. Shobana, S., et al., Green synthesis of silver nanoparticles using Artocarpus hirsutus seed extract and its antibacterial activity. *Current Pharmaceutical Biotechnology*, 2020. **21**(10): p. 980–989.

32. Jabir, M.S., et al., Green synthesis of silver nanoparticles from Eriobotrya japonica extract: a promising approach against cancer cells proliferation, inflammation, allergic disorders and phagocytosis induction. *Artificial Cells, Nanomedicine, and Biotechnology*, 2021. **49**(1): p. 48–60.

33. Aravind, M., et al., Critical green routing synthesis of silver NPs using jasmine flower extract for biological activities and photocatalytical degradation of methylene blue. *Journal of Environmental Chemical Engineering*, 2021. **9**(1): p. 104877.

34. Wang, B., et al., Green synthesis and characterization of gold nanoparticles using lignin nanoparticles. *Nanomaterials*, 2020. **10**(9): p. 1869.

35. Cai, F., et al., Green synthesis of gold nanoparticles for immune response regulation: Mechanisms, applications, and perspectives. *Journal of Biomedical Materials Research Part A*, 2022. **110**(2): p. 424–442.

36. Rahman, T.U., et al., Phytochemical screening, green synthesis of gold nanoparticles, and antibacterial activity using seeds extract of Ricinus communis L. *Microscopy Research and Technique*, 2022. **85**(1): p. 202–208.

37. Hawar, S.N., et al., Green synthesis of silver nanoparticles from Alhagi graecorum leaf extract and evaluation of their cytotoxicity and antifungal activity. *Journal of Nanomaterials*, 2022. **2022**: p. 1–8.

38. Din, M.I. and R. Rehan, Synthesis, characterization, and applications of copper nanoparticles. *Analytical Letters*, 2017. **50**(1): p. 50–62.

39. Amaliyah, S., et al., Green synthesis and characterization of copper nanoparticles using Piper retrofractum Vahl extract as bioreductor and capping agent. *Heliyon*, 2020. **6**(8).

40. Al-Khafaji, M.A.A., R.A. Al-Refai'a, and O.M.Y. Al-Zamely, Green synthesis of copper nanoparticles using Artemisia plant extract. *Materials Today: Proceedings*, 2022. **49**: p. 2831–2835.

41. Abbas, S.F., et al. Green synthesis of copper nanoparticles from Cordia myxa L. leaves ethanol extract and their antibacterial activity. In *AIP Conference Proceedings*. 2022. AIP Publishing.

42. Pérez-Alvarez, M., et al., Green synthesis of copper nanoparticles using cotton. *Polymers*, 2021. **13**(12): p. 1906.

43. Ghaffar, A., et al., Citrus paradisi fruit peel extract mediated green synthesis of copper nanoparticles for remediation of disperse yellow 125 dye. *Desalination and Water Treatment*, 2021. **212**(7): p. 368–375.

44. Sonbol, H., et al., Padina boryana mediated green synthesis of crystalline palladium nanoparticles as potential nanodrug against multidrug resistant bacteria and cancer cells. *Scientific Reports*, 2021. **11**(1): p. 5444.

45. Bathula, C., et al., Ultrasonically driven green synthesis of palladium nanoparticles by Coleus amboinicus for catalytic reduction and Suzuki-Miyaura reaction. *Colloids and Surfaces B: Biointerfaces*, 2020. **192**: p. 111026.

46. Ziental, D., et al., Titanium dioxide nanoparticles: prospects and applications in medicine. *Nanomaterials*, 2020. **10**(2): p. 387.

47. Ahmad, W., K.K. Jaiswal, and S. Soni, Green synthesis of titanium dioxide (TiO2) nanoparticles by using Mentha arvensis leaves extract and its antimicrobial properties. *Inorganic and Nano-Metal Chemistry*, 2020. **50**(10): p. 1032–1038.

48. Shanavas, S., et al., Green synthesis of titanium dioxide nanoparticles using Phyllanthus niruri leaf extract and study on its structural, optical and morphological properties. *Materials Today: Proceedings*, 2020. **26**: p. 3531–3534.

49. Rajeswari, V.D., et al., Green synthesis of titanium dioxide nanoparticles using Laurus nobilis (bay leaf): antioxidant and antimicrobial activities. *Applied Nanoscience*, 2021: p. 1–8.

50. Patidar, V. and P. Jain, Green synthesis of TiO2 nanoparticle using Moringa oleifera leaf extract. *International Research Journal of Engineering and Technology*, 2017. **4**(3): p. 1–4.

51. Ebrahiminezhad, A., et al., Plant-mediated synthesis and applications of iron nanoparticles. *Molecular Biotechnology*, 2018. **60**: p. 154–168.

52. Fahmy, H.M., et al., Review of green methods of iron nanoparticles synthesis and applications. *BioNanoScience*, 2018. **8**: p. 491–503.

53. Chen, S., et al., Ziziphora clinopodioides Lam leaf aqueous extract mediated novel green synthesis of iron nanoparticles and its anti-hemolytic anemia potential: a chemobiological study. *Arabian Journal of Chemistry*, 2022. **15**(3): p. 103561.

54. Prakash, M., et al., Green synthesis of bismuth based nanoparticles and its applications-a review. *Sustainable Chemistry and Pharmacy*, 2022. **25**: p. 100547.

55. Zulkifli, Z., et al., Synthesis and characterisation of bismuth oxide nanoparticles using hydrothermal method: the effect of reactant concentrations and application in radiotherapy. In *Journal of Physics: Conference Series*. 2018. IOP Publishing.

56. Motakef-Kazemi, N. and M. Yaqoubi, Green synthesis and characterization of bismuth oxide nanoparticle using mentha pulegium extract. *Iranian Journal of Pharmaceutical Research: IJPR*, 2020. **19**(2): p. 70.

57. Iqbal, J., et al., Facile green synthesis approach for the production of chromium oxide nanoparticles and their different in vitro biological activities. *Microscopy Research and Technique*, 2020. **83**(6): p. 706–719.

58. Khan, S.A., et al., Green synthesis of chromium oxide nanoparticles for antibacterial, antioxidant anticancer, and biocompatibility activities. *International Journal of Molecular Sciences*, 2021. **22**(2): p. 502.

59. Mirzaei, H. and M. Darroudi, Zinc oxide nanoparticles: biological synthesis and biomedical applications. *Ceramics International*, 2017. **43**(1): p. 907–914.

60. Annapoorani, A., et al., Eco-friendly synthesis of zinc oxide nanoparticles using Rivina humilis leaf extract and their biomedical applications. *Process Biochemistry*, 2022. **112**: p. 192–202.

61. Molnár, Z., et al., Green synthesis of gold nanoparticles by thermophilic filamentous fungi. *Scientific Reports*, 2018. **8**(1): p. 3943.

62. Clarance, P., et al., Green synthesis and characterization of gold nanoparticles using endophytic fungi Fusarium solani and its in-vitro anticancer and biomedical applications. *Saudi Journal of Biological Sciences*, 2020. **27**(2): p. 706–712.

63. Niknejad, F., et al., Green synthesis of silver nanoparticles: advantages of the yeast Saccharomyces cerevisiae model. *Current Medical Mycology*, 2015. **1**(3): p. 17.

64. Sivaraj, A., et al., Commercial yeast extracts mediated green synthesis of silver chloride nanoparticles and their anti-mycobacterial activity. *Journal of Cluster Science*, 2020. **31**: p. 287–291.

65. Devi, T.A., et al., Green synthesis of plasmonic nanoparticles using Sargassum ilicifolium and application in photocatalytic degradation of cationic dyes. *Environmental Research*, 2022. **208**: p. 112642.

66. Elgamouz, A., et al., Green synthesis, characterization, antimicrobial, anti-cancer, and optimization of colorimetric sensing of hydrogen peroxide of algae extract capped silver nanoparticles. *Nanomaterials*, 2020. **10**(9): p. 1861.

67. Patra, J.K. and K.-H. Baek, Green nanobiotechnology: factors affecting synthesis and characterization techniques. *Journal of Nanomaterials*, 2015. **2014**: p. 219.

68. Patil, S. and R. Chandrasekaran, Biogenic nanoparticles: a comprehensive perspective in synthesis, characterization, application and its challenges. *Journal of Genetic Engineering and Biotechnology*, 2020. **18**: p. 1–23.

69. Uzair, B., et al., Green and cost-effective synthesis of metallic nanoparticles by algae: safe methods for translational medicine. *Bioengineering*, 2020. **7**(4): p. 129.

70. Shah, M., et al., Green synthesis of metallic nanoparticles via biological entities. *Materials*, 2015. **8**(11): p. 7278–7308.

71. Ghaemi, M. and S. Gholamipoor, Controllable synthesis and characterization of silver nanoparticles using Sargassum angostifolium. *Iranian Journal of Chemistry and Chemical Engineering*, 2017. **36**(1): p. 1–10.

72. Aboelfetoh, E.F., R.A. El-Shenody, and M.M. Ghobara, Eco-friendly synthesis of silver nanoparticles using green algae (Caulerpa serrulata): reaction optimization, catalytic and antibacterial activities. *Environmental Monitoring and Assessment*, 2017. **189**: p. 1–15.

73. San, K.A. and Y.-S. Shon, Synthesis of alkanethiolate-capped metal nanoparticles using alkyl thiosulfate ligand precursors: a method to generate promising reagents for selective catalysis. *Nanomaterials*, 2018. **8**(5): p. 346.

74. Rai, M. and C. Posten, *Green Biosynthesis of Nanoparticles: Mechanisms and Applications*. 2013. CABI.

75. Er, H., et al., Formation of silver nanoparticles from ionic liquids comprising N-alkylethylenediamine: effects of dissolution modes of the silver (I) ions in the ionic liquids. *Colloids and Surfaces A: Physicochemical and Engineering Aspects*, 2017. **522**: p. 503–513.

76. Amer, M. and A. Awwad, Green synthesis of copper nanoparticles by Citrus limon fruits extract, characterization and antibacterial activity. *Chemistry International*, 2021. **7**(1): p. 1–8.

77. Jebril, S., R.K.B. Jenana, and C. Dridi, Green synthesis of silver nanoparticles using Melia azedarach leaf extract and their antifungal activities: in vitro and in vivo. *Materials Chemistry and Physics*, 2020. **248**: p. 122898.

78. Rambabu, K., et al., Green synthesis of zinc oxide nanoparticles using Phoenix dactylifera waste as bioreductant for effective dye degradation and antibacterial performance in wastewater treatment. *Journal of Hazardous Materials*, 2021. **402**: p. 123560.

79. Suresh, D., et al., Artocarpus gomezianus aided green synthesis of ZnO nanoparticles: Luminescence, photocatalytic and antioxidant properties. *Spectrochimica Acta Part A: Molecular and Biomolecular Spectroscopy*, 2015. **141**: p. 128–134.

80. Poopathi, S., et al., Synthesis of silver nanoparticles from Azadirachta indica—a most effective method for mosquito control. *Environmental Science and Pollution Research*, 2015. **22**: p. 2956–2963.

81. Kalaiselvi, A., et al., Synthesis and characterization of palladium nanoparticles using Catharanthus roseus leaf extract and its application in the photo-catalytic degradation. *Spectrochimica Acta Part A: Molecular and Biomolecular Spectroscopy*, 2015. **135**: p. 116–119.

82. Singh, P., et al., Biogenic silver and gold nanoparticles synthesized using red ginseng root extract, and their applications. *Artificial Cells, Nanomedicine, and Biotechnology*, 2016. **44**(3): p. 811–816.

83. Sadeghi, B., A. Rostami, and S. Momeni, Facile green synthesis of silver nanoparticles using seed aqueous extract of Pistacia Atlantica and its antibacterial activity. *Spectrochimica Acta Part A: Molecular and Biomolecular Spectroscopy*, 2015. **134**: p. 326–332.

84. Velmurugan, P., et al., Synthesis and characterization of nanosilver with antibacterial properties using Pinus densiflora young cone extract. *Journal of Photochemistry and Photobiology B: Biology*, 2015. **147**: p. 63–68.

85. Amooaghaie, R., M.R. Saeri, and M. Azizi, Synthesis, characterization and biocompatibility of silver nanoparticles synthesized from Nigella sativa leaf extract in comparison with chemical silver nanoparticles. *Ecotoxicology and Environmental Safety*, 2015. **120**: p. 400–408.

86. Zahir, A.A., et al., Green synthesis of silver and titanium dioxide nanoparticles using Euphorbia prostrata extract shows shift from apoptosis to G0/G1 arrest followed by necrotic cell death in Leishmania donovani. *Antimicrobial Agents and Chemotherapy*, 2015. **59**(8): p. 4782–4799.

87. Murugan, K., et al., Cymbopogon citratus-synthesized gold nanoparticles boost the predation efficiency of copepod Mesocyclops aspericornis against malaria and dengue mosquitoes. *Experimental Parasitology*, 2015. **153**: p. 129–138.

88. Elango, G. and S.M. Roopan, Green synthesis, spectroscopic investigation and photocatalytic activity of lead nanoparticles. *Spectrochimica Acta Part A: Molecular and Biomolecular Spectroscopy*, 2015. **139**: p. 367–373.

89. Hosseinzadeh, N., et al., Green synthesis of gold nanoparticles by using Ferula persica Willd. gum essential oil: production, characterization and in vitro anti-cancer effects. *Journal of Pharmacy and Pharmacology*, 2020. **72**(8): p. 1013–1025.

90. Bhuiyan, M.S.H., et al., Green synthesis of iron oxide nanoparticle using Carica papaya leaf extract: application for photocatalytic degradation of remazol yellow RR dye and antibacterial activity. *Heliyon*, 2020. **6**(8).

91. Arjaghi, S.K., et al., Retracted article: green synthesis of iron oxide nanoparticles by RS lichen extract and its application in removing heavy metals of lead and cadmium. *Biological Trace Element Research*, 2021. **199**: p. 763–768.

92. Kiani, M., et al., High-gravity-assisted green synthesis of palladium nanoparticles: the flowering of nanomedicine. *Nanomedicine: Nanotechnology, Biology and Medicine*, 2020. **30**: p. 102297.

93. Amina, M., et al., Biogenic green synthesis of MgO nanoparticles using Saussurea costus biomasses for a comprehensive detection of their antimicrobial, cytotoxicity against MCF-7 breast cancer cells and photocatalysis potentials. *PLOS One*, 2020. **15**(8): p. e0237567.

94. Irshad, M.A., et al., Synthesis and characterization of titanium dioxide nanoparticles by chemical and green methods and their antifungal activities against wheat rust. *Chemosphere*, 2020. **258**: p. 127352.

95. Alagesan, V. and S. Venugopal, Green synthesis of selenium nanoparticle using leaves extract of withania somnifera and its biological applications and photocatalytic activities. *Bionanoscience*, 2019. **9**: p. 105–116.

96. Vardhana, J., et al., Biogenic synthesis of copper nanoparticles using Vitis vinifera L. seed extract, and its in-vitro biological applications. *Journal of Plant Biochemistry and Biotechnology*, 2022. **31**(3): p. 684–687.

97. Şahin Ün, Ş., et al., Green synthesis, characterization and catalytic activity evaluation of palladium nanoparticles facilitated by Punica granatum peel extract. *Inorganic and Nano-Metal Chemistry*, 2021. **51**(9): p. 1232–1240.

98. Shah, Y., M. Maharana, and S. Sen, Peltophorum pterocarpum leaf extract mediated green synthesis of novel iron oxide particles for application in photocatalytic and catalytic removal of organic pollutants. *Biomass Conversion and Biorefinery*, 2022: p. 1–14.

99. Zhan, Q., J. Han, and L. Sheng, Iron nanoparticles green-formulated by Coriandrum sativum leaf aqueous extract: investigation of its anti-liver-cancer effects. *Archives of Medical Science*, 2021. https://doi.org/10.5114/aoms/144627.

100. Archana, P., et al., Concert of zinc oxide nanoparticles synthesized using Cucumis melo by green synthesis and the antibacterial activity on pathogenic bacteria. *Inorganic Chemistry Communications*, 2022. **137**: p. 109255.

Index